PRE-COURSE/POST-COURSE ASSESSM

D0077415

Name: _____ Date: _____

As you complete the key fitness/wellness lab assessments in this course, record your results in the "Pre-Course [...] the end of the course, re-do the labs, record your results in the "Post-Course Assessment" column, and see the progress you have made!

Lab	Pre-Course Assessment	Post-Course Assessment
Lab 3.2: Assessing Your Cardiorespiratory Fitness Level	**3-minute step test** 1 minute recovery HR:_____ (bpm) Fitness rating: _____ **1-mile walk test** VO₂ max: _____ Fitness rating: _____ **1.5-mile run test** VO₂ max: _____ Fitness rating: _____	**3-minute step test** 1 minute recovery HR:_____ (bpm) Fitness rating: _____ **1-mile walk test** VO₂ max: _____ Fitness rating: _____ **1.5-mile run test** VO₂ max: _____ Fitness rating: _____
Lab 4.1: Assessing Your Muscular Strength	**Chest press** S/BW ratio: _____ Rating: _____ **Leg press** S/BW ratio: _____ Rating: _____	**Chest press** S/BW ratio: _____ Rating: _____ **Leg press** S/BW ratio: _____ Rating: _____
Lab 4.2: Assessing Your Muscular Endurance	**20RM assessment** Chest press 20RM weight lifted: _____ Leg press 20RM weight lifted: _____ **Push-up assessment** Repetitions: _____ Rating: _____ **Curl-up assessment** Repetitions: _____ Rating: _____	**20RM assessment** Chest press 20RM weight lifted: _____ Leg press 20RM weight lifted: _____ **Push-up assessment** Repetitions: _____ Rating: _____ **Curl-up assessment** Repetitions: _____ Rating: _____
Lab 5.1: Assessing Your Flexibility	**Sit-and-reach test** Reach distance (in or cm): _____ Rating: _____	**Sit-and-reach test** Reach distance (in or cm): _____ Rating: _____
Lab 6.1: How to Calculate Your BMI	BMI: _____ kg/m² Weight classification: _____	BMI: _____ kg/m² Weight classification: _____
Lab 6.2: Measure and Evaluate Your Body Circumferences	Waist: _____ Hip: _____ WHR Ratio: _____ Upper arm: _____ (right) _____ (left) Forearm: _____ (right) _____ (left) Thigh: _____ (right) _____ (left) Calf: _____ (right) _____ (left) Neck: _____ Disease risk rating for WHR: _____ Disease risk rating for WC: _____	Waist: _____ Hip: _____ WHR Ratio: _____ Upper arm: _____ (right) _____ (left) Forearm: _____ (right) _____ (left) Thigh: _____ (right) _____ (left) Calf: _____ (right) _____ (left) Neck: _____ Disease risk rating for WHR: _____ Disease risk rating for WC: _____
Lab 6.3: Estimate Your Percent Body Fat (Skinfold Test)	Sum of 3 skinfolds: _____ % body fat estimate: _____ Rating: _____	Sum of 3 skinfolds: _____ % body fat estimate: _____ Rating: _____
Lab 7.2: Keeping a Food Diary and Analyzing Your Daily Nutrition **Lab 7.3:** Improving Your Nutrition	Milk intake: _____ cups Meat and beans intake: _____ oz. Vegetables intake: _____ cups Fruits intake: _____ cups Grains intake: _____ oz.	Milk intake: _____ cups Meat and beans intake: _____ oz. Vegetables intake: _____ cups Fruits intake: _____ cups Grains intake: _____ oz.
Lab 8.1: Calculating Energy Balance and Setting Energy Balance Goals	Estimated calorie intake: _____ Estimated calorie expenditure: _____ Calorie balance (intake minus expenditure): _____	Estimated calorie intake: _____ Estimated calorie expenditure: _____ Calorie balance (intake minus expenditure): _____
Lab 8.3: Your Weight Management Plan	% body fat: _____ Weight: _____ lb. BMI: _____ kg/m²	% body fat: _____ Weight: _____ lb. BMI: _____ kg/m²
Lab 9.1: How Stressed Are You?	Score: _____ Stress level: _____	Score: _____ Stress level: _____
Lab 10.1: Understanding Your CVD Risk	Family risk for CVD, total points: _____ Lifestyle risk for CVD, total points: _____ Additional risks for CVD, total points: _____	Family risk for CVD, total points: _____ Lifestyle risk for CVD, total points: _____ Additional risks for CVD, total points: _____
Lab 12.1: Assessing Your Personal Risk of Cancer	Breast cancer risk, total points: _____ Skin cancer risk, total points: _____ Reproductive cancer risk, total points: _____ General cancer risk, total points: _____	Breast cancer risk, total points: _____ Skin cancer risk, total points: _____ Reproductive cancer risk, total points: _____ General cancer risk, total points: _____
Lab 13.1: Assessing Your Alcohol Use and Risk of Abuse	Drinking patterns and abuse risk score: _____ How risky is your alcohol use?_____	Drinking patterns and abuse risk score: _____ How risky is your alcohol use?_____

BEHAVIOR CHANGE CONTRACT

Choose a health behavior that you would like to change, starting this quarter or semester. Sign the contract at the bottom to affirm your commitment to making a healthy change and ask a friend to witness it.

My behavior change will be:

_____

My long-term goal for this behavior change is:

_____

Barriers I must overcome to make this behavior change are (things I am currently doing or situations that contribute to this behavior or make it harder to change):

1. _____

2. _____

3. _____

The strategies I will use to overcome these barriers are:

1. _____

2. _____

3. _____

Resources I will use to help me change this behavior include:

A friend/partner/relative _____

A school-based resource _____

A community-based resource _____

A book or reputable website _____

In order to make my goal more attainable, I have devised these short-term goals:

Short-Term Goal _____ **Target Date**_____ **Reward** _____

Short-Term Goal _____ **Target Date**_____ **Reward** _____

Short-Term Goal _____ **Target Date**_____ **Reward** _____

When I make the long-term behavior change described above, my reward will be:

Short-Term Goal _____ **Target Date**_____ **Reward** _____

I intend to make the behavior change described above, I will use the strategies and rewards to achieve the goals that will contribute to a healthy behavior change.

Signed _____ **Date**_____

Witness _____ **Date**_____

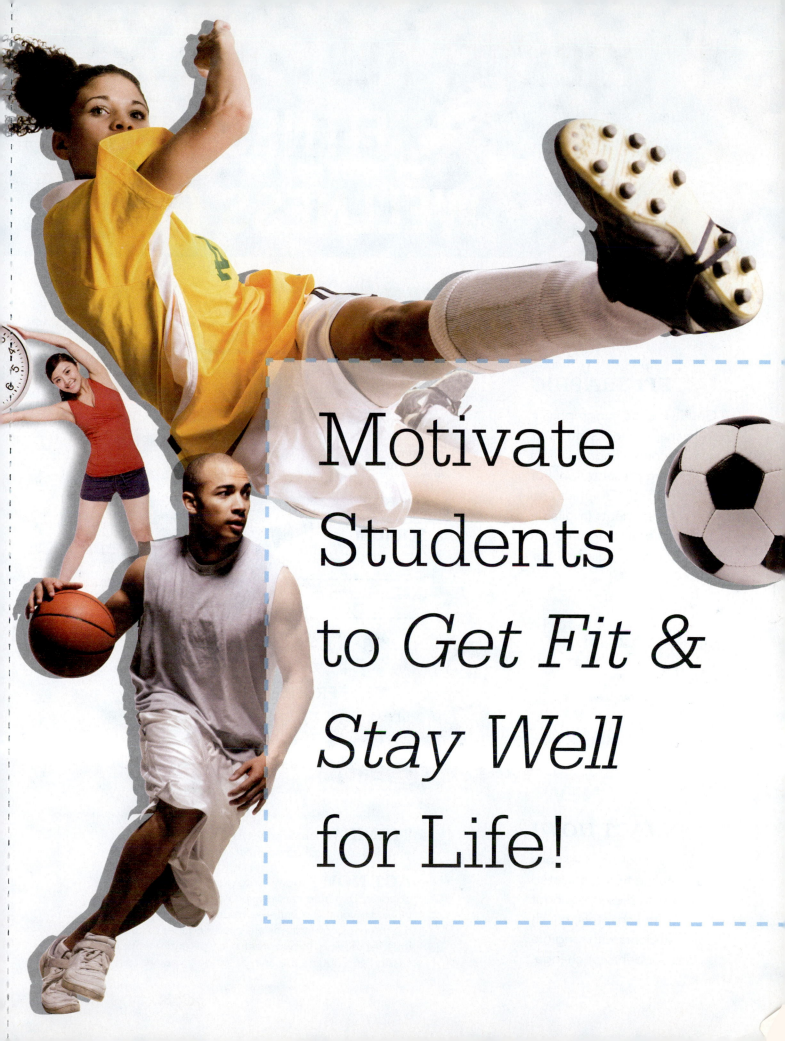

Motivate Students to *Get Fit & Stay Well* for Life!

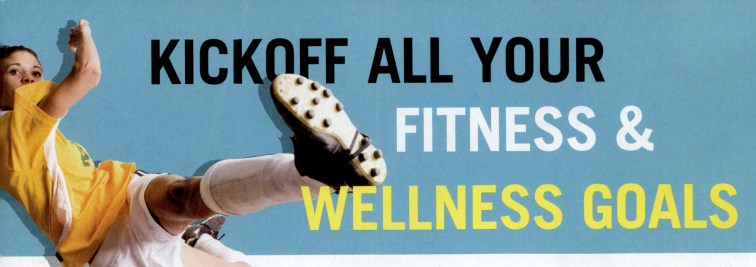

KICKOFF ALL YOUR FITNESS & WELLNESS GOALS

NEW!

GETFITGRAPHIC

A GetFitGraphic infographic in every chapter hooks students with a compelling topic in a visually stunning presentation. For instructors, GetFitGraphics and related assessments (available online) provide a jumping off point for classroom discussions.

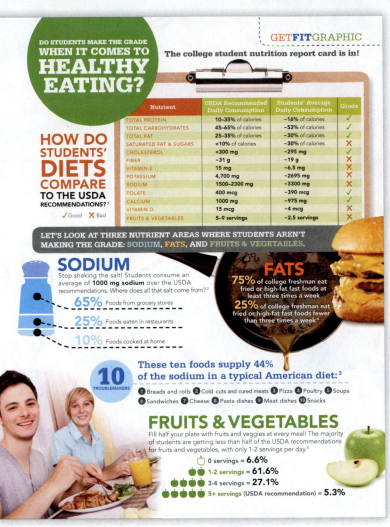

DO STUDENTS MAKE THE GRADE WHEN IT COMES TO HEALTHY EATING?

GET**FIT**GRAPHIC

The college student nutrition report card is in!

HOW DO STUDENTS' DIETS COMPARE TO THE USDA RECOMMENDATIONS?[1]

✓ Good ✗ Bad

Nutrient	USDA Recommended Daily Consumption	Students' Average Daily Consumption	Grade
TOTAL PROTEIN	10–35% of calories	~16% of calories	✓
TOTAL CARBOHYDRATES	45–65% of calories	~53% of calories	✓
TOTAL FAT	25–35% of calories	~30% of calories	✓
SATURATED FAT & SUGARS	<10% of calories	~30% of calories	✗
CHOLESTEROL	<300 mg	~295 mg	✓
FIBER	~31 g	~19 g	✗
VITAMIN E	15 mg	~6.5 mg	✗
POTASSIUM	4,700 mg	~2695 mg	✗
SODIUM	1500–2300 mg	~3300 mg	✗
FOLATE	400 mcg	~390 mcg	✓
CALCIUM	1000 mg	~975 mg	✓
VITAMIN D	15 mcg	~4 mcg	✗
FRUITS & VEGETABLES	5–9 servings	~2.5 servings	✗

LET'S LOOK AT THREE NUTRIENT AREAS WHERE STUDENTS AREN'T MAKING THE GRADE: SODIUM, FATS, AND FRUITS & VEGETABLES.

SODIUM
Stop shaking the salt! Students consume an average of **1000 mg sodium** over the USDA recommendations. Where does all that salt come from?[2]

- **65%** Foods from grocery stores
- **25%** Foods eaten in restaurants
- **10%** Foods cooked at home

FATS
75% of college freshman eat fried or high-fat fast foods at least three times a week
25% of college freshman eat fried or high-fat fast foods fewer than three times a week[4]

10 TROUBLEMAKERS These ten foods supply 44% of the sodium in a typical American diet:[3]
❶ Breads and rolls ❷ Cold cuts and cured meats ❸ Pizza ❹ Poultry ❺ Soups ❻ Sandwiches ❼ Cheese ❽ Pasta dishes ❾ Meat dishes ❿ Snacks

FRUITS & VEGETABLES
Fill half your plate with fruits and veggies at every meal! The majority of students are getting less than half of the USDA recommendations for fruits and vegetables, with only 1-2 servings per day.[5]

- 0 servings = **6.6%**
- 1-2 servings = **61.6%**
- 3-4 servings = **27.1%**
- 5+ servings (USDA recommendation) = **5.3%**

NEW!

THINK!/ACT NOW!

Critical thinking questions with timeline tips, associated with case studies throughout the chapters, coach students with tangible goals for behavior change.

THINK! Which energy system do you think Angela's friend relied on most while hitting her serves?

ACT NOW! Today, write out activities you would do for a 10-minute cardiorespiratory warm-up. This week, try your 10-minute warm-up and think about how the three energy systems are providing fuel to keep your muscles moving. In two weeks, log an entire workout session and outline the energy systems you are using.

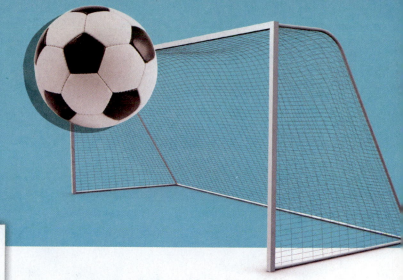

Activate, Motivate,
& ADVANCE YOUR WELL-BEING

A YOGA PROGRAM

ACTIVATE!

Yoga is a fun physical and psychological practice that incorporates stretching, relaxation, and breathing movements to bring greater balance to our body and mind. Yoga's benefits range from enhancing flexibility and muscular strength to reducing tension and stress. The postures can renew, invigorate, and heal the body through stretching and strengthening. Breathing techniques can release tension and stress and bring an overall calmness of mind and spirit. These programs will help you learn how to get started with basic yoga.

What Do I Need?

MATERIALS: Choose a mat at least 1/8 of an inch thick—the thicker the mat the more cushion it will provide for your body. You may also want to use blocks and straps. They aid in supporting the body for postures that might be challenging, especially in the beginning.

LOCATION: You can practice yoga anywhere big enough to lay down a mat. Choose a space that is calm, quiet, and comfortable in light and temperature.

CLOTHING: Wear comfortable clothing that allows you to freely move your body.

How Do I Start?

BREATH: Your breath (referred to as *pranayama* in yoga exercises) is the most important part of yoga. Aim for deep breaths, inhaling and exhaling from the belly. Never force or strain your breathing.

The most common breath used during yoga is called *ujjayi* (pronounced *ooo-ja-i-aa*). Practice this breath while in a seated position. Once you can sustain your ability to breathe in this manner, begin using it during yoga practice.

To perform ujjayi breathing, inhale and exhale slowly and deeply through the nose. You will begin to slightly constrict the passage of air. Your breathing will sound like Darth Vader or like you are fogging up a pair of glasses.

During your yoga practice, every time you lift your chest, inhale, and when you drop your chest, exhale. If you are holding a pose, breathe deeply and slowly so you can hear yourself breathe.

SCAN TO SEE IT ONLINE!

NEW!

Activate, Motivate,
& ADVANCE YOUR WELL-BEING

Activate, Motivate, & Advance programs now target key wellness goals in addition to fitness. Programs for nutrition and yoga encourage students to eat healthfully and reduce stress. The new programs complement the existing Activate, Motivate, & Advance programs for cardiorespiratory endurance, strength training, flexibility, meditation, and more.

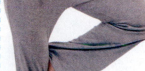

25 Oblique Curl

Lie on your back with one foot on the mat and knee bent to 90 degrees. Rest the opposite ankle on the bent knee. With one arm providing support on the ground and the other hand behind the head, contract your oblique abdominals and lift your opposite shoulder toward the lifted knee (elbow stays out). Keep the supporting arm and elbow on the floor and refrain from pulling on the head and neck with your hand. Return to the starting position slowly and repeat on the other side.

SCAN TO SEE IT ONLINE!

Muscles targeted:

4 External obliques

NEW!

QR Codes for Training on the Go

QR codes in the text link to Mobile Activate, Motivate, & Advance programs and exercise videos, so students can serve up fitness and wellness content anytime, anywhere with their mobile phone. Just scan the code and the content loads instantly.

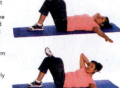

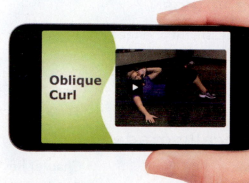

Oblique Curl

MAKE THE CONNECTION
BETWEEN LECTURE
AND BEHAVIOR CHANGE

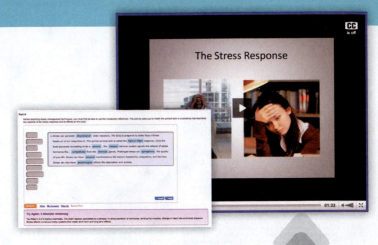

MasteringHealth™

Mastering is the most effective and widely used online homework, tutorial, and assessment system for the sciences. It delivers self-paced tutorials that focus on your course objectives, provide individualized coaching, and responds to each student's progress.

FOR STUDENTS

Proven, assignable, and automatically graded health activities reinforce course learning objectives.

Health and Fitness Coaching Activities

Coaching activities guide students through key health and fitness concepts with interactive mini-lessons that provide hints and feedback.

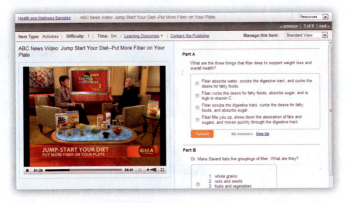

51 *ABC News* Videos

Timely videos, with assessment and feedback, help health come to life and show how it's related to the real world.

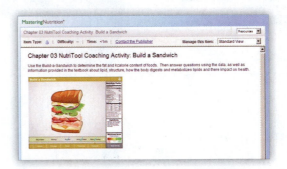

NutriTools Build-A-Meal Activities

These unique activities allow students to combine and experiment with different food options and learn firsthand how to build healthier meals.

Other automatically graded health and fitness activities include:

- Behavior Change Video Activities
- Chapter Reading Quizzes
- Chapter Review MP3s
- Exercise Videos
- GetFitGraphic Activities

DO YOUR STUDENTS WANT TO PRACTICE ON THEIR OWN?

MasteringHealth also provides students with the tools to study effectively and practice on their own time at their own pace.

eText

The Pearson eText gives students access to the text whenever and wherever they can access the Internet. The eText can be viewed on PCs, Macs, and tablets, including iPad and Android.

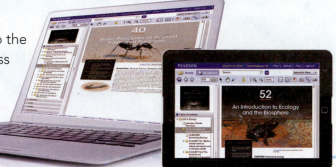

Study Area

Students can access the Study Area for use on their own or in a study group.

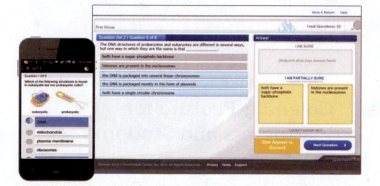

NEW! Dynamic Study Modules

Dynamic Study Modules enable students to study effectively on their own in an adaptive format. Students receive an initial set of questions with a unique answer format asking them to indicate their confidence level. Once completed, reviews include explanations using materials taken directly from the text. These modules can be accessed on smartphones, tablets, and computers.

Labs and Self Assessments

All labs and self assessments are available under the Study Area in an interactive PDF format.

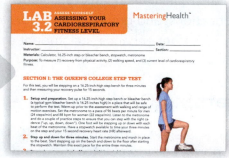

Chapter Review MP3s Sessions

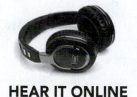

HEAR IT ONLINE

Downloadable MP3 tutor sessions with rapid review explain the big picture concepts for each chapter and can be downloaded to student smartphones, tablets, and computers.

The Study Area also includes:

Cumulative Test, RSS Feeds, Audio Case Studies, ABC Videos, and book specific activities.

EASY TO GET STARTED, USE, AND MAKE YOUR OWN

FOR INSTRUCTORS

MasteringHealth™ helps instructors maximize class time with easy-to-assign, customizable, and automatically graded assessments that motivate students to learn outside of the class and arrive prepared for lecture.

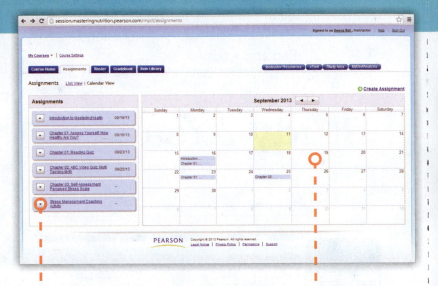

Customize Publisher-provided Problems or Quickly Add Your Own

MasteringNutrition™ makes it easy to edit any questions or answers, import your own questions, and quickly add images or links to further enhance the student experience.

Calendar Feature for Instructors and Students

The Course Home default page now features a Calendar View displaying upcoming assignments and due dates.

- Instructors can schedule assignments by dragging and dropping the assignment onto a date in the calendar.
- The calendar view lets students see at-a-glance when an assignment is due, and resembles a syllabus.

Learning Outcomes

Tagged to book content and tied to Bloom's Taxonomy, Learning Outcomes are designed to let Mastering do the work in tracking student performance against your learning outcomes. Mastering offers a data supported measure to quantify students' learning gains and to share those results quickly and easily:

- Add your own or use the publisher-provided learning outcomes.
- View class performance against the specified learning outcomes.
- Export results to a spreadsheet.

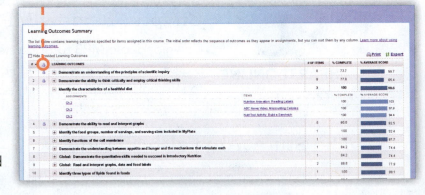

Now that students come more prepared to class with MasteringHealth

Flip Your Classroom

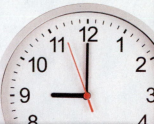

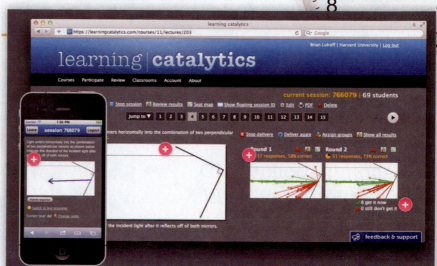

LEARNING CATALYTICS™

Learning Catalytics allows students to use their smartphones, tablets, or laptops to respond to questions in class.

With Learning Catalytics you can:

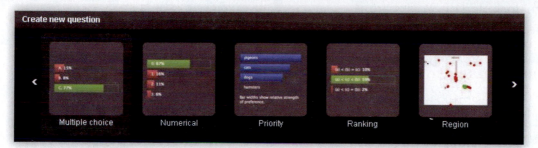

Use a wide variety of question types to engage students: multiple choice, word clouds, sketch a graph, annotate art, highlight a passage, compute a numeric answer, and more.

Use multiple question types to get into the minds of students to understand what they do or don't know and adjust lectures accordingly.

- Access rich analytics to understand student performance.
- Add your own questions to make Learning Catalytics fit your course exactly.
- Assess and improve students' critical-thinking skills, and so much more.

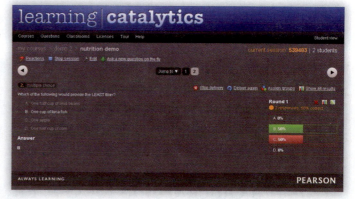

Learning Catalytics is included with the purchase of MasteringHealth.

EVERYTHING YOU
NEED TO TEACH
IN ONE PLACE!

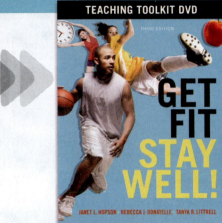

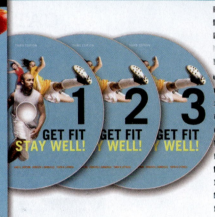

Teaching Toolkit DVD for *Get Fit, Stay Well!*

The Teaching Toolkit DVD replaces the former printed Teaching Toolbox by providing everything you need to prep for your course and deliver a dynamic lecture in one convenient place. Included on 3 disks are these valuable resources:

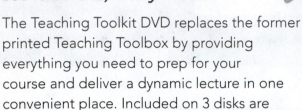

DISK 1 — Robust media assets for each chapter

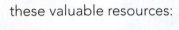

- 51 ABC News Lecture Launcher videos
- Exercise and assessment videos
- PowerPoint® Lecture Outlines
- PowerPoint clicker questions and Jeopardy-style quiz show questions
- Files for all illustrations and tables and selected photos from the text
- Transparency Masters

DISK 2 — Comprehensive Test Bank

- Test Bank in Word and RTF formats
- Computerized Test Bank, which includes all the questions from the test bank in a format that allows you to easily and intuitively build exams and quizzes

DISK 3 — Additional innovative supplements for instructors and students

FOR INSTRUCTORS:
- Instructor's Resource Support Manual
- Introduction to MasteringHealth
- Introductory video for Learning Catalytics
- Great Ideas: Active Ways to Teach Health & Wellness
- Teaching with Student Learning Outcomes
- Teaching with Web 2.0

FOR STUDENTS:
- Take Charge of Your Health Worksheets
- Behavior Change Log Book and Wellness Journal
- Eat Right! Healthy Eating in College and Beyond
- Live Right! Beating Stress in College and Beyond
- Food Composition Table

User's Quick Guide for Get Fit, Stay Well!

This easy-to-use printed supplement accompanies the Teaching Toolkit and offers easy instructions for both experienced and new faculty members to get started with the rich Toolkit content, how to access assignments within MasteringNutrition, and how to flip the classroom with Learning Catalytics.

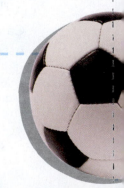

GET
FIT
STAY
WELL!

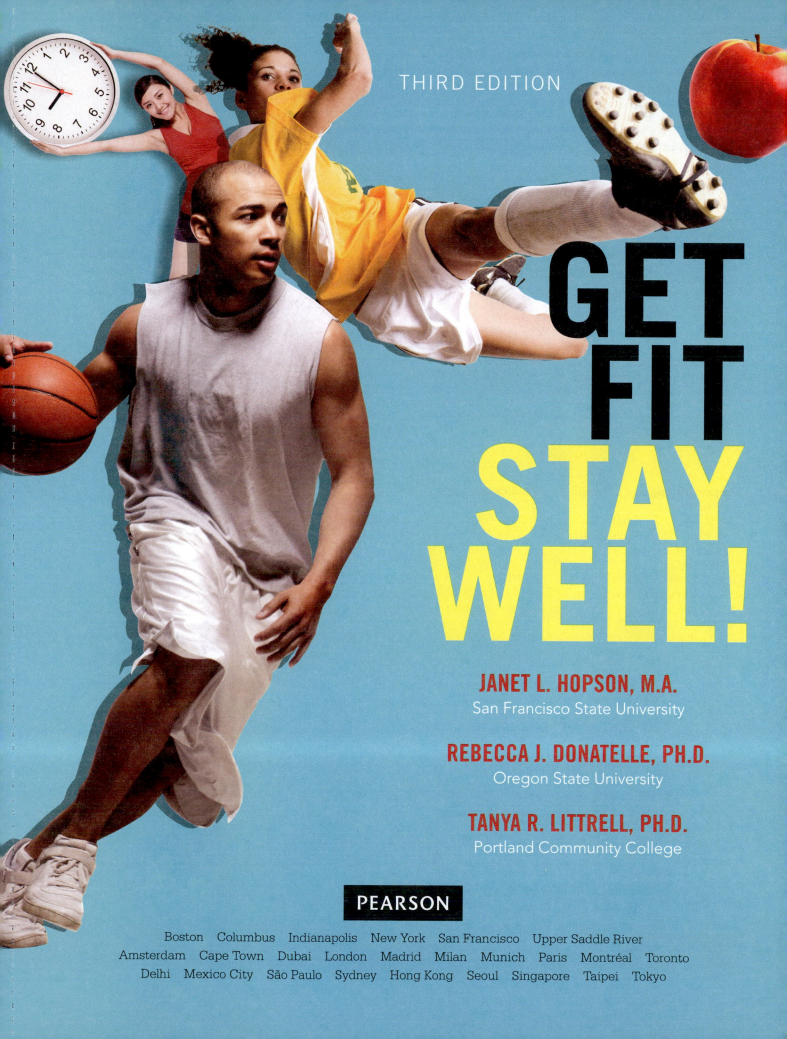

THIRD EDITION

GET
FIT
STAY
WELL!

JANET L. HOPSON, M.A.
San Francisco State University

REBECCA J. DONATELLE, PH.D.
Oregon State University

TANYA R. LITTRELL, PH.D.
Portland Community College

PEARSON

Boston   Columbus   Indianapolis   New York   San Francisco   Upper Saddle River
Amsterdam   Cape Town   Dubai   London   Madrid   Milan   Munich   Paris   Montréal   Toronto
Delhi   Mexico City   São Paulo   Sydney   Hong Kong   Seoul   Singapore   Taipei   Tokyo

Executive Editor: Sandra Lindelof
Associate Editor: Erin Schnair
Editorial Manager: Susan Malloy
Editorial Assistant: Tu-Anh Dang-Tran
Assistant Editor: Briana Verdugo
Production Project Manager: Dorothy Cox
Managing Editor: Mike Early
Assistant Managing Editor: Nancy Tabor
Content Producer: Julia Akpan
Production Management and Compositor: PreMediaGlobal
Cover and Interior Designer: Tandem Creative, Inc.
Senior Manufacturing Buyer: Stacey Weinberger
Executive Marketing Manager: Neena Bali

Cover Photos: Mike Kemp/Getty Images; Rubberball/Mark Andersen/Getty Images; Lane Oatey/Blue Jean Images/Getty Images; Andrey_Kuzmin/Shutterstock; domnitsky/Shutterstock

Credits and acknowledgments for materials borrowed from other sources and reproduced, with permission, in this textbook appear on the appropriate page within the text [or on p. C-1–C-2].

Library of Congress Cataloging-in-Publication Data
Hopson, Janet L.
  Get fit stay well! / Janet L. Hopson, M.A., San Francisco State University, Rebecca J. Donatelle,
Ph.D., Oregon State University, Tanya R. Littrell, Ph.D., Portland Community College.
—Third edition.
  pages cm
ISBN-13: 978-0-321-91184-1
ISBN-10: 0-321-91184-9
1. Physical fitness—Textbooks.   2. Health—Textbooks.   I. Title.
RA781.H65H67 2013
613.7—dc23   2013036486

4 5 6 7 8 9 10—V003—17 16 15

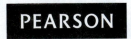

www.pearsonhighered.com

ISBN 10: 0-321-93395-8; ISBN 13: 978-0-321-93395-9 (Student Edition)
ISBN 10: 0-321-95746-6; ISBN 13: 978-0-321-95746-7 (Instructor's Review Copy)
ISBN 10: 0-321-95763-6; ISBN 13: 978-0-321-95763-4 (a la Carte Edition)

To the memory of Ruth and David Hopson, who taught me, by example and encouragement, to love fitness activity.—JLH

To the strong, intelligent, loving, and hard-working women who have motivated me and taught me to care about the important things—especially my mom, Agnes E. Donatelle.—RJD

To the memory of my loving grandmother Doretta Littrell Lawrence, a dance, fitness, and physical education professional who influenced many lives and inspired us all.—TRL

About the Authors

Janet L. Hopson, M.A.

A full-time author and lecturer, Janet L. Hopson has written or co-authored nine books, including two popular nonfiction books on human pheromones and human brain development, and eight textbooks on general biology and wellness for college and high school students. Ms. Hopson currently teaches science writing at San Francisco State University. She holds B.A. and M.A. degrees from Southern Illinois University and the University of Missouri. She has won awards for magazine writing, and her articles have appeared in *Smithsonian*, *Psychology Today*, *Science Digest*, *Science News*, *Outside*, *Scientific American Mind*, and others. She is married and enjoys golfing, swimming, reading, traveling, competitive tennis, and equestrian sports.

Rebecca J. Donatelle, Ph.D.

Dr. Rebecca J. Donatelle is a professor emeritus in public health at Oregon State University, having served as the department chair, Coordinator of the Public Health Promotion and Education Programs, and faculty member and researcher in the College of Health and Human Sciences. She has a Ph.D. in community health/health education, an M.S. in health education, and a B.S. with majors in both health/physical education and English. Her main research and teaching focus has been on the factors that increase risk for chronic diseases and the use of incentives and social supports in developing effective interventions for high-risk women and families. Her research has been published in numerous journals, and she has been a consultant, guest speaker, and presenter at professional conferences throughout the country. Dr. Donatelle is also the author of the highly successful introductory health textbooks *Access to Health* and *Health: The Basics*, as well as the new *My Health: An Outcomes Approach*.

Tanya R. Littrell, Ph.D.

Dr. Tanya R. Littrell is a full-time faculty member in fitness technology and physical education at Portland Community College in Portland, Oregon. Dr. Littrell worked as a fitness director for many years before attending graduate school at Oregon State University, where she earned both a master's degree in human performance/exercise physiology and a doctoral degree in exercise science/exercise physiology. Dr. Littrell has been teaching lifetime fitness classes for undergraduates since 1998. When she is not teaching, preparing to teach, or writing, you can find Dr. Littrell on the trails running or mountain biking, hiking, traveling, or spending quality time with family and friends.

Brief Contents

Available as an additional electronic chapter in the eText of MasteringHealth™

Contents

1 Changing Personal Behaviors for Optimal Wellness 1

2 Understanding Fitness Principles 29

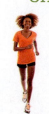

3 Conditioning Your Cardiorespiratory System 64

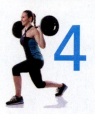

4 Building Muscular Strength & Endurance 112

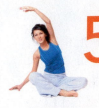

5 Maintaining Flexibility & Back Health 168

6 Understanding Body Composition 212

7 Improving Your Nutrition 234

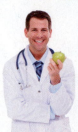
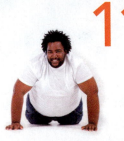

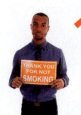

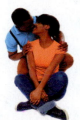

14 Reducing Your Risk of Sexually Transmitted Infections 446

Available as an additional electronic chapter in the eText of MasteringHealth™

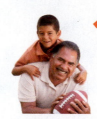

15 Maintaining Lifelong Fitness and Wellness 467

Feature Boxes

Note: Page numbers followed by an asterisk refer to Chapter 15, available as an additional electronic chapter in the eText of MasteringHealth.

Labs and Programs

LABS

Activate, Motivate, & ADVANCE YOUR FITNESS

Note: Page numbers followed by an asterisk refer to Chapter 15, available as an additional electronic chapter in the eText of MasteringHealth.

Preface

You may have noticed that health, fitness, and wellness are highly popular topics! Open a newspaper, turn on the TV, or surf the Internet and you will undoubtedly find articles about the benefits of exercise, the health risks associated with obesity, or the results of a recent nutritional study. At the same time, if you are a college student taking a fitness and wellness course, you may feel a sense of disconnect between those stories and your own life. You might wonder: What has any of this got to do with me?

Our primary goal in writing this textbook was simple: to get students to realize that the lifestyle choices you make now—regardless of your current age—have real and lasting effects on your lifelong wellness. We also wanted to write a textbook that takes into account the many challenges facing today's students and offers maximum flexibility for creating a personalized fitness and wellness program that you can tailor to your own goals and time demands. Finally, we wanted this textbook to address a common fact of life: the gap between knowing what we *ought* to do (e.g., exercise more, eat healthier foods, quit smoking, etc.) and actually *doing it*. Throughout this textbook, we emphasize that effective behavior change is a gradual process, based on having realistic expectations and setting achievable short-term and long-term goals.

With these aims in mind, the following are some of the unique features you'll find in *Get Fit, Stay Well!*

New to This Edition

- *New GetFitGraphic infographics* in every chapter presents a thought-provoking topic in a visually stunning presentation. GetFitGraphics help students understand information effectively and provide a jumping off point for instructors to stimulate classroom discussions.

- *New Activate, Motivate, & Advance Nutrition and Yoga programs* at the ends of Chapters 7 and 9 expand the Activate, Motivate, & Advance programs in Chapters 2–5, 8, and 9. Together, these function like having your own built-in personal trainer. Each program contains guidance on three parts of a fitness or wellness program: getting started, motivating to continue, and taking it to the next level. The

customizable "pre-fab" programs and the related tracking features and technique videos on the mobile website make it easy to jump into a behavior change project.

- *New Think!/Act Now!* questions and timeline tips throughout the text encourage critical thinking and help students apply the foregoing material to their own lives, with step-by-step coaching suggestions and goals for behavior change.

- *New QR codes* make fitness mobile, with links to exercise videos and the Activate, Motivate, Advance mobile website. Just scan the QR code with a reader on a smartphone or a tablet, and the device loads up the relevant content.

- *New Reflection questions* appear at the end of the labs, asking students to reflect on the choices they made or their results from the assessments.

- *Chapter 15, Maintaining Lifelong Fitness & Wellness* is available as an additional chapter in the eText of MasteringHealth, so students can easily access the chapter and plan for their lifelong fitness and wellness.

Chapter-by-Chapter Changes

The authors have updated the Third Edition line by line to provide students with the most current information plus references for further exploration. This includes all data and statistics throughout the text. We have reorganized portions of chapters to improve the flow of topics, and added, updated, and improved upon figures, tables, photos, and feature boxes. The following is a chapter-by-chapter listing of noteworthy changes, updates, and additions.

Chapter 1: Changing Personal Behaviors for Optimal Wellness

- New GetFitGraphic on financial wellness
- New Diversity box on the disparities in life expectancy by age, race, and other factors
- Revised Tools for Change box on sticking with an exercise program
- New coverage on provisions of the Affordable Care Act that are relevant to students

Chapter 2: Understanding Fitness Principles

- New GetFitGraphic on exercise's effects on the brain
- Updated Tools for Change box to include motivational tips for adding physical activity
- Updated coverage on the latest American College of Sports Medicine (ACSM) recommendations
- Updated pre-exercise screening questionnaire in Lab 2.1

Chapter 3: Conditioning Your Cardiorespiratory System

- New GetFitGraphic on short workouts
- Updated figure containing a sample cardiorespiratory workout
- Updated figure to illustrate perceived exertion
- New figure on shopping for exercise shoes

Chapter 4: Building Muscular Strength & Endurance

- New GetFitGraphic on women and strength training
- Updated muscular anatomy figure to show a more detailed presentation
- Updated curl-up test in Lab 4.1

Chapter 5: Maintaining Flexibility & Back Health

- New GetFitGraphic on back pain and college students
- New section and table on commonly used flexibility tools

Chapter 6: Understanding Body Composition

- New GetFitGraphic on spot reduction
- New Q&A box on muscle tone and body composition
- New table on body fat norms for men and women
- Addition of bioelectrical impedance analysis (BIA) assessment to Lab 6.3

Chapter 7: Improving Your Nutrition

- New GetFitGraphic on college students and healthy eating
- New figure with healthy eating recommendations for vegetarian diets
- Reorganized section clarifying recommended nutrient intakes
- Updated tips for using SuperTracker.gov in Lab 7.2
- New Activate, Motivate, Advance Nutrition program on increasing fruit and vegetable intake and variety

Chapter 8: Managing Your Weight

- New GetFitGraphic on weight loss myths
- Updated coverage and figure on obesity and overweight in America
- New Lab 8.2 on determining readiness for weight change
- New Lab 8.4 on identifying and cutting back junk food

Chapter 9: Managing Stress

- New GetFitGraphic on exercising to improve mental health
- Updated Q&A box on sleep and mood
- Revised section on changing behavioral responses to stress
- Enhanced text coverage on yoga
- New Lab 9.1 with a stress assessment specifically designed for students
- New Activate, Motivate, Advance program for managing stress through yoga

Chapter 10: Reducing Your Risk of Cardiovascular Disease

- New GetFitGraphic on the societal impacts of CVD
- Updated figure on plaque buildup in arteries
- Updated sections on the risks for CVD

Chapter 11: Reducing Your Risk of Diabetes and Other Chronic Diseases

- New GetFitGraphic on lifestyle choices and chronic disease
- Updated coverage on reducing risks for chronic diseases

Chapter 12: Reducing Your Risk of Cancer

- New GetFitGraphic on college students and melanoma
- Updated figures and Tools for Change boxes on breast and testicular self-exams

Chapter 13: Avoiding Substance Use, Abuse, and Addiction

- New GetFitGraphic on college students and substance abuse
- New figure on the Centers of Disease Control and Prevention (CDC) nonsmoking campaign
- Enhanced text coverage on pre-gaming and binge drinking by college students
- Additional coverage on blackouts, including a new key term
- Revised coverage on long-term effects of alcohol abuse
- Additional coverage on hookahs
- New Lab 13.3 on drug abuse

Chapter 14: Reducing Your Risk of Sexually Transmitted Infections

- New GetFitGraphic on preventing STIs in college students
- Updated discussion of current treatments for various STIs and AIDS
- Updated coverage of positive communication between sexual partners in Lab 14.2

Chapter 15: Maintaining Lifelong Fitness and Wellness

- Chapter is available as an additional chapter in the eText of MasteringHealth
- New GetFitGraphic on physiological age versus actual age
- New Diversity box on pregnancy and exercise
- New figure on aging in the United States
- New figure on America's effort to recycle solid waste
- New coverage on fitness, wellness, and aging
- Additional coverage on self-care and health care
- Updated sections on environmental wellness

- Updated coverage of effective communication between relationship partners in Lab 15.1

Updates to the Media Program

- *New! MasteringHealth for Get Fit, Stay Well!* is an online homework, tutorial, and assessment product designed to improve results by helping students quickly master concepts. Students benefit from self-paced tutorials that feature immediate wrong-answer feedback and hints that emulate the office-hour experience to help keep students on track. With a wide range of interactive, engaging, and assignable activities, students are encouraged to actively learn and retain course concepts.
- *51 New ABC News videos* with accompanying quizzes and discussion questions are available on the Teaching Toolkit DVD and in MasteringHealth.

Other Key Features

- *Unique Case Studies presented in each chapter* introduce a "character" who reflects the concerns, questions, and thought processes that students are likely to have themselves. Think!/Act! and Think!/Act Now! questions at the end of the case studies encourage critical thinking and help students consider how the material applies to their own lives.
- *Labs employ a unique three-pronged approach:* (1) skill-acquisition labs, (2) self-assessment labs, and (3) action-plan labs. The labs not only measure a student's current level of fitness/wellness, but also teach practical lifelong skills and encourage real behavior change. Many additional labs are offered online on the book's website. All labs are also available online in interactive PDF format and are assignable through MasteringHealth.
- *The most modern strength-training presentation available* includes photos of more than 100 strength-training and flexibility exercises featuring actual college students, modern gym equipment, and options for students with limited access to equipment. Videos of the exercises in the book, as well as many alternate exercises, are available online in MasteringHealth and on the Teaching Toolkit DVD.
- *A separate chapter on diabetes and other chronic diseases* makes this text a valuable reference for fitness and wellness courses, as it emphasizes one of today's national health epidemics.

- *A strong emphasis is placed on behavior change throughout the text.* Think!/Act Now! features suggest immediate action while Tools for Change boxes provide tools for longer-term change. The "Plan for Change" labs ask students to write out an action plan for behavior change.

- *Q&A boxes* investigate common questions and concerns students may have in relation to chapter topics.

- *Diversity boxes* address topics relevant to diverse student populations, acknowledging that age, race, gender, disability, and individual life circumstances can result in specific fitness and wellness needs.

- *A running glossary* helps students easily review and master key terms.

- *End-of-chapter review questions and critical thinking questions* encourage students to evaluate material they have just learned.

- *Research citations* demonstrate the accuracy, currency, and scientific grounding for information presented in the text.

- *A pre- and post-course progress worksheet* included at the beginning of the book and available online allows students to assess their progress on key fitness/ wellness assessments.

- *A mobile fitness programs website* associated with the Activate, Motivate, Advance features throughout the book contains tracking tools for customizing and logging a behavior change project.

Instructor Supplements

This textbook comes with unparalleled supplemental resources to assist instructors with classroom preparation and presentation.

Teaching Toolkit DVD

Instructors can save hours of valuable planning time with a single comprehensive DVD containing numerous supplements and resources that reinforce key learning from the text and suit virtually any teaching style. The Teaching Toolkit DVD includes:

- All art, photos, and tables from the text; PowerPoint® lecture slides; a computerized test bank; 51 new *ABC News* videos; exercise demonstration videos, Active Lecture (clicker) Questions; Quiz Show Game PowerPoint slides; interactive PDF lab worksheets; PDF transparency masters, Instructor Resource and Support Manual PDFs, and Test Bank Word files

- *Instructor Resource and Support Manual* with detailed chapter outlines incorporating Toolkit assets, in-class discussion questions, and activities, additional resources, first-time teaching tips, sample syllabi, and tips for using MasteringHealth

- *Test Bank* with over 1,000 questions in multiple-choice, true/false, and short-essay formats, tagged to Bloom's taxonomy and global and book-specific student learning outcomes

- *User's Quick Start Guide* with instructions for getting up and running using the materials in the Teaching Toolkit DVD, accessing assignments within MasteringHealth, and flipping the classroom with Learning Catalytics

- *Great Ideas: Active Ways to Teach Health and Wellness,* a manual of ideas for classroom activities related to fitness and wellness topics, including activities that can be adapted to various topics and class sizes

- *Teaching with Student Learning Outcomes* publication containing useful suggestions and examples for successfully incorporating outcomes into a fitness and wellness course

- *Teaching with Web 2.0* handbook introducing popular new online tools and offering ideas for incorporating them into a fitness and wellness course

- *Behavior Change Log Book with Wellness Journal,* which includes updated worksheets, nutrition information, journals, and fitness logs

- *Food Composition Table* containing detailed nutrition information about thousands of foods

- *Live Right! Beating Stress in College and Beyond* booklet on handling life's challenges including sleep, finances, time management, academic pressure, and relationships

- *Eat Right! Healthy Eating in College and Beyond* booklet of guidelines, tips, and recipes for healthy eating

- *Take Charge of Your Health!* self-assessment worksheets

MasteringHealth

www.masteringhealthandnutrition.com
(or www.pearsonmastering.com)

This new online course management program is loaded with valuable teaching resources that make it easy to give assignments and track student progress. The preloaded content in MasteringHealth includes unsurpassed resources for teaching online or hybrid courses:

- *Fitness & Wellness Coaching Activities* guide students through key health concepts with interactive mini-lessons.

- *Reading Quizzes* (20 questions per chapter) ensure that students have completed the assigned reading before class.

- *51 ABC News Videos* bring health to life and spark discussion with up-to-date hot topics and include multiple-choice questions that provide wrong-answer feedback to redirect students to the correct answer.

- *NutriTools Coaching Activities* in the nutrition chapter allow students to combine and experiment with different food options and learn firsthand how to build healthier meals.

- *MP3s* relate to chapter content and come with multiple-choice questions that provide wrong-answer feedback.

- *Learning Catalytics* provides open-ended questions students can answer in real time. Through targeted assessments, Learning Catalytics helps students develop the critical thinking skills they need for lasting behavior change.

- *The Study Area* is broken down into learning areas and includes videos, MP3s, practice quizzing, labs, and much more.

- *Pearson eText* gives students access to the text whenever and wherever they have access to the Internet.

- *More than 100 exercise videos* demonstrate strength-training and flexibility exercises with resistance bands, stability balls, free weights, and gym machines, as well as lab assessment techniques. The videos are also available for download onto iPods® or other media players, and some have related quizzing.

- *Audio cases studies* from the text pertain to each chapter's content. All are available for download as MP3 files and have related assignable and gradable quizzing.

- *Interactive labs* automatically perform calculations on students' input. Completed labs can be submitted to instructors by digital drop box, e-mail, or print. Additional labs available only online are designed to accommodate varying skill levels, differing access to equipment, and the specific needs of students with disabilities.

- *A mobile website for the Activate, Motivate, & Advance programs* from the text help students commit to and track a new fitness or wellness routine. Links to exercise demonstration and technique videos provide further guidance for students just getting started on a new fitness program.

Student Supplements

A wealth of materials is available to help students review and explore course content and enact behavior change in their own lives.

- *The Study Area of MasteringHealth* is organized by learning areas. *Read It* houses the Pearson eText, with which users can create notes, highlight text in different colors, create bookmarks, zoom, click hyperlinked words for definitions or associated media, and change page view. *See It* includes 51 ABC News videos on important health topics and more than 100 exercise videos. *Hear It* contains MP3 Chapter Review files and audio case studies. *Do It* contains critical-thinking questions and weblinks. *Review It* contains study quizzes for each chapter. *Live It* will help jump-start students' behavior-change projects with assessments and resources to plan change.

- *Behavior Change Log Book and Wellness Journal* This booklet helps students track their daily exercise and nutritional intake and create a personalized long-term nutrition and fitness program.

- *Eat Right! Healthy Eating in College and Beyond* This handy, full-color booklet provides practical guidelines, tips, shopper's guides and recipes for putting healthy eating principles into action.

- *Live Right! Beating Stress in College and Beyond* This booklet gives students useful tips for coping with stressful life challenges both during college and for the rest of their lives.

- *Take Charge of Your Health! Worksheets* This pad of 50 self-assessment activities allows students to explore their health behaviors.

- *New Lifestyles Pedometer* Take strides to better health with this pedometer, a first step toward overall health and wellness.

- *MyDietAnalysis* Powered by ESHA Research, Inc., MyDietAnalysis features a database of nearly 20,000 foods. This easy-to-use program allows students to track their diet and activity for up to three profiles and to assess the nutritional value of their food consumption.

- *Food Composition Table* This comprehensive booklet provides detailed nutritional information on thousands of foods and is correlated with MyDietAnalysis.

Acknowledgments

From Janet Hopson

Preparing a new edition of a college program such as *Get Fit, Stay Well!*—including the book and all of its accompanying study and instructional materials—is an enormous undertaking. The authors' efforts are just part of a complex, well-integrated, and coordinated effort. We would like to thank the following members of the Pearson staff: Erin Schnair, who handled with skill and grace the daily demands of upgrading, updating, and shepherding our author team through this new edition and all its innovations. Kari Hopperstead, who so ably managed the second edition text and ancillary revision to create the foundation upon which we built this third version; Barbara Yien, Frank Ruggirello, Sandra Lindelof, and Deirdre Espinoza, who all championed and greatly improved this book in its early stages; Claire Alexander, who so nimbly functioned as development editor in earlier editions; our superb marketing manager Neena Bali; Dorothy Cox and Jared Sterzer, our production coordinators; the talented composition and production team at PreMediaGlobal; Yvo Riezebos and Tandem Creative Inc. Design Group, who are responsible for this book's dynamic design; and former students Christine Blackman, who so skillfully helped us research the scientific literature, and Briana Verdugo, who cheerfully and creatively smoothed our pathway as an editorial assistant. Finally, and in many ways primarily, I would like to personally thank my co-authors Becky and Tanya for their years of effort and their superb knowledge and experience.

From Rebecca Donatelle

After working on several college textbooks over the years, one thing has become very clear to me: the publishing house you choose to work with is the single most important factor in producing a quality textbook that is going to be successful in the marketplace. Pearson has assembled a truly remarkable group of top-notch acquisition, editorial, production, marketing, sales, and ancillary staff to help nurture a text through its development and growth. I am fortunate to have had the opportunity to work with individuals who worry the details and possess an incredible degree of creativity and professionalism. You are truly THE BEST . . . thank you so much to each and every one of you. A special thank you to Erin Schnair for her painstaking attention to detail, creative approach to revisions, and wonderful oversight on this project. She did a simply wonderful job as project editor, building on the outstanding work of her predecessor, Kari Hopperstead. Additionally, I would like to thank my amazing co-authors, Jan and Tanya. From conceptualization to final product, this text would not have happened without your efforts.

From Tanya Littrell

I would like to first and foremost thank my family and friends for all of their support through the long hours of creating and revising this textbook. Thank you to my co-authors, Jan and Becky, whose expertise and experience have really guided this textbook. Working with the staff at Pearson has been wonderful. Thank you to Sandra Lindelof for bringing me into this project, Barbara Yien for her unending patience on the first edition, Kari Hopperstead for keeping me on track with the many second edition updates,

Acknowledgments (continued)

and Erin Schnair for her support and dedication to this third edition. I would also like to thank fellow faculty members at Portland Community College who have been supportive throughout this project; in particular, Janeen Hull, a faculty peer and friend. Ms. Hull was the knowledgeable and creative mind behind most of the Activate, Motivate, & Advance programs. My graduate work and teaching at Oregon State University really set the stage for my work on this project, and so I would like to thank Anthony Wilcox, department chair of Nutrition and Exercise Sciences, for having faith in me as an instructor and giving me teaching and supervisory experience that led to this opportunity.

From The Publisher

Many thanks go to Lauren Tobey of Oregon State University and Launda Wheatley of Albion College for their contributions to the new Activate, Motivate, & Advance programs; Karen Vail-Smith of East Carolina University for her creative contributions to the new GetFitGraphics; and Leah Robinson of Auburn University for her research efforts on several chapters. We're also grateful for the contribution of Stephen Ball of the University of Missouri for his expertise in helping revise Chapter 6, Understanding Body Composition. For work on the ancillary materials, we thank Southern Editorial and Molly Ward.

Reviewers for the Third Edition

Many thanks to the hundreds of instructors and students who reviewed and class-tested the previous editions of this text, and to the following reviewers who contributed feedback for this revision: Kym Atwood (University of West Florida), Don Bard (University of California, Santa Cruz), Tara Brown (Georgia Highlands College), Tony Caterisano (Furman University), Karen K. Dennis (Illinois State University), Bart Desender (Tarrant County College), Erin Driver (Oregon State University), Gail Freedman (Northern Virginia Community College), Kathy Hanlon O'Connell (Dutchess Community College), Ellis Jensen (Utah Valley University), Stasi Kasianchuk (Oregon State University), Holly Molella (Dutchess Community College), Allison H. Nye (Cape Fear Community College), Kristina Shelton (Northern Virginia Community College), Ingrid Skoog (Oregon State University), Jen Spry-Knutson (Des Moines Area Community College), Sheila Stepp (Orange County Community College), Virginia Trummer (University of Texas at San Antonio), Doc Wilson (Cape Fear Community College).

Reviewers for MasteringHealth

We thank the following members of the Faculty Advisory Board, who offered us valuable insights that helped develop MasteringHealth: Steve Hartman (Citrus College), William Huber (County College of Morris), Kris Jankovitz (Cal Poly), Stasi Kasaianchuk (Oregon State University), Lynn Long (University of North Carolina Wilmington), Ayanna Lyles (California University of Pennsylvania), Steven Namanny (Utah Valley University), Karla Rues (Ozarks Technical Community College), Debra Smith (Ohio University), Sheila Stepp (SUNY Orange), and Mary Winfrey-Kovell (Ball State University).

1 Changing Personal Behaviors for Optimal Wellness

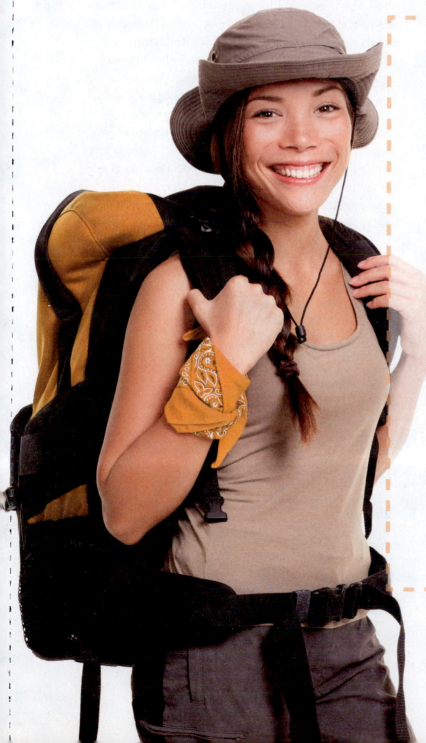

LEARNINGoutcomes

1. Identify your current place on the wellness continuum.

2. Describe the dimensions of wellness and how they are interconnected.

3. Explain the benefits of wellness for individuals and for society as a whole.

4. Determine your stage in the behavior change process for one or more behaviors.

5. Write out a wellness goal using the SMART goal-setting guidelines.

6. Commit to fitness and wellness by filling in a behavior change contract.

7. Learn and use strategies for keeping your behavior change on track.

MasteringHealth™

www.masteringhealthandnutrition.com
(or www.pearsonmastering.com)
Go online for chapter quizzes, interactive assessments, videos, and more!

casestudy

CARLOS

"Hi, I'm Carlos. I just started my freshman year in college. It's my first time living away from home, and I'm getting used to lots of new things. I know my family had to sacrifice for me to be here, so I feel pressure to do well. I also miss my girlfriend, Liz—she's a senior in high school and it's been really hard being away from her. I like my classes so far, but I am never caught up with my reading, and I haven't had a good night's sleep in about a month. To top it all off, I caught a cold that's been going around, and I feel miserable! What can I do to better manage my life?"

HEAR IT! ONLINE

C an you relate to any of Carlos's problems? If so, you are not alone. Many college students report that stress, depression, inadequate sleep, frequent colds, and relationship problems negatively affect their academic performance (**Figure 1.1**).[1] When asked to rate their overall **wellness**, at least one-third of college students described it as only "good"

---

wellness Achieving the highest level of health possible in each of several dimensions

physical fitness The ability to perform moderate to vigorous levels of physical activity without undue fatigue

---

FIGURE **1.1** The top 10 wellness impacts on college performance.

Data from: American College Health Association, *American College Health Association—National College Health Assessment II (ACHA-NCHA II): Reference Group Executive Summary Fall 2012* (Hanover, MD: American College Health Association, 2013).

compared to "very good" or "excellent." About 10 percent rated it as just "fair" or "poor."

Wellness is an optimal soundness of body and mind. To understand wellness, it helps to first consider the concept of health. While historically the term *health* meant merely the absence of disease, experts today view it as an inclusive term that encompasses everything from environmental health to the health of populations. The term *wellness* conveys a more personalized definition of *health*. It is the achievement of the highest level of health possible in physical, social, intellectual, emotional, spiritual, and environmental dimensions. It describes a vibrant state in which a person enjoys life to the fullest, adapts relatively easily to life's many challenges, feels that life is meaningful, and functions effectively in society. In this book, we will sometimes use the terms *health* and *wellness* interchangeably, but *wellness* always refers to a more individualized, dynamic concept, requiring significant personal effort, but with the potential to bring great rewards.

Central to wellness is **physical fitness**, or simply *fitness*, the ability to perform moderate to vigorous levels of physical activity without undue fatigue. Fitness is just one dimension of wellness, but we give it special attention in this book because it influences so many of the other dimensions and because the tools for improving fitness are readily available while you are a college student—a period

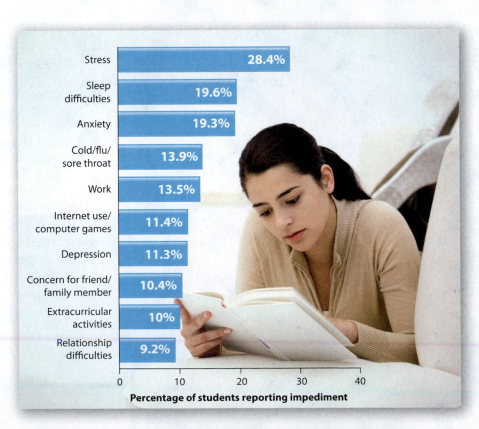

	Percentage of students reporting impediment
Stress	28.4%
Sleep difficulties	19.6%
Anxiety	19.3%
Cold/flu/sore throat	13.9%
Work	13.5%
Internet use/computer games	11.4%
Depression	11.3%
Concern for friend/family member	10.4%
Extracurricular activities	10%
Relationship difficulties	9.2%

Percentage of students reporting impediment
0   10   20   30   40

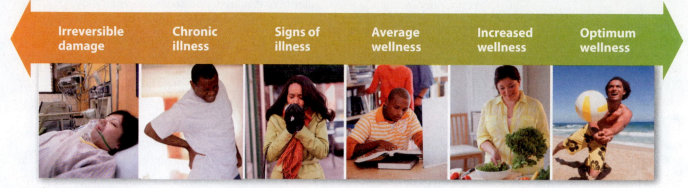

| Irreversible damage | Chronic illness | Signs of illness | Average wellness | Increased wellness | Optimum wellness |

FIGURE **1.2** The double-headed arrow depicts the continuum of wellness states.

in your life when you can establish personal habits that will increase your current happiness as well as benefit you for a lifetime.[2]

Where Am I on the Wellness Continuum?

Improving your wellness—moving toward that vibrant multidimensional state—is an ambitious but achievable goal. The wellness patterns you establish during this course can change how you live each day, how fit, happy, and relaxed you feel, and can positively affect your quality of life for years to come. However, no single college course can address every health concern or guarantee a lifetime of wellness. Your age, personal history, genetic susceptibility to medical conditions, and your physical environment all affect your wellness. Additionally, having access to high-quality medical care, nutritious food, good exercise facilities, and social support networks enhance positive behaviors.

The first step in achieving optimal wellness is assessing how close you are at present to that long-term goal. We can picture wellness as a continuum of greater or lesser total soundness of body and mind (**Figure 1.2**). Understanding your current place on the **wellness continuum** is important for setting goals and changing wellness behaviors.

What Are the Dimensions of Wellness?

We can think of wellness as consisting of six primary dimensions (physical, social, intellectual, emotional, spiritual, and environmental) (**Figure 1.3**). Wellness is a process, and at times you may experience faster growth in one dimension than in others. The dimensions are interconnected, however, so positive effort in one area can help you make progress in others and move you toward greater overall health and well-being.

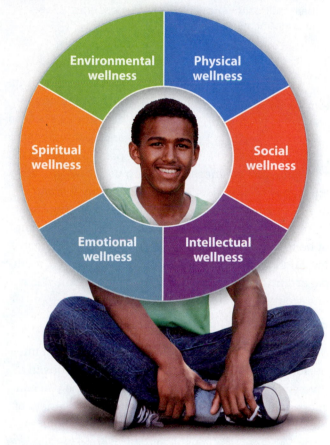

FIGURE **1.3** Wellness is an optimal level of health in six interconnected dimensions of human experience.

Physical Wellness

Physical wellness encompasses all aspects of a sound body, including body size, shape, and composition; sensory sharpness and

wellness continuum A spectrum of wellness states from irreversible damage to optimum wellness

physical wellness A state of physical health and well-being that includes body size and shape, body functioning, measures of strength and endurance, and resistance to disease

responsiveness; body functioning; physical strength, flexibility, and endurance; resistance to diseases and disorders; and recuperative abilities. The physical state we call fitness includes measures of physical wellness and allows a person to exert physical effort without undue stress, strain, or injury. Many of your day-to-day choices and habits can support or undermine your physical wellness, including your diet; amount and types of exercise; sleep patterns; level of stress; use of tobacco, drugs, or alcohol; participation in unsafe sex; observance of traffic laws and the wearing of helmets and seat belts; daily hygiene (e.g., flossing and brushing teeth); and access to quality medical attention (e.g., regular checkups, vaccinations, and treatment).

Social Wellness

Social wellness is the ability to have satisfying interpersonal relationships and maintain connections in a diverse range of social networks. This means you can successfully interact with others, adapt to a variety of social situations, and act appropriately in various settings. Whether you are shy and introverted or outgoing and extroverted, social wellness includes the ability to communicate clearly and effectively; the capacity to establish intimacy through trust and acceptance; a willingness to ask for and give support; the ability to maintain friendships over time; and skills for interacting within groups, such as on the job or in the community.

Intellectual Wellness

Intellectual wellness is the ability to use your brain power effectively to solve problems and meet life's

challenges. It allows you to think clearly, quickly, creatively, and critically; use good reasoning and make careful decisions; continually learn from your successes and mistakes; organize and streamline your tasks; and maintain a sense of humor.[3]

Emotional Wellness

Emotional wellness refers to the ability to control your emotions and express them appropriately at the right times. Social and emotional concerns—such as stress, anxiety, depression, and relationship problems—are increasingly common on college campuses and can impede academic success. In fact, students list depression as the number one reason for withdrawal from college.[4] Improving emotional wellness requires developing good self-esteem; gaining self-confidence; being able to cope with sadness, anger, resentment, and negativity; and developing an appropriate balance of emotional dependence and independence.

Spiritual Wellness

For some people, **spiritual wellness** may involve a belief in a supreme being or a way of life prescribed by a particular religion. For others, spiritual wellness is a feeling of unity or oneness with others and with nature, and a sense of meaning or value in life. Developing spiritual wellness may deepen one's understanding of life's purpose; allow a person to feel a part of a greater spectrum of existence; and promote feelings of love, joy, peace, contentment, and wonder over life's experiences.

Environmental Wellness

Our home, work, community, and school environments can be relaxing, safe havens or toxic, threatening, and

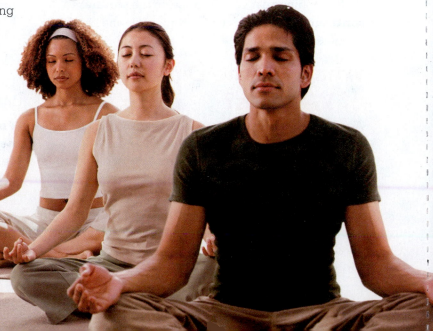

casestudy

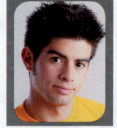

CARLOS

"I know that my life is pretty good. I'm in college, studying what interests me, and I'm excited about the future. I just constantly feel behind. I fall asleep in class sometimes, eat a lot of junk food, and I'm not exercising—who has time? Then I got this cold, partly because I have been stressed out and not sleeping much. I've made some friends in my dorm, and it helps to know that a lot of them are going through the same things. Talking to Liz every night on the phone helps, too."

THINK! In which dimensions of wellness could Carlos be stronger? Where would you place him on the wellness continuum? Where would you place yourself?

ACT NOW! Today, identify your strongest wellness dimensions, your weakest ones, and the first one you would like to improve. This week, create a wellness balance chart and plan the balance you would like to achieve (see Lab 1.2). In two weeks, chart any improvements and readjust your plan, if necessary.

DO IT! ONLINE   HEAR IT! ONLINE

---

stressful places to be. **Environmental wellness** entails understanding how the environment can positively or negatively affect you; the role you play in preserving, protecting, and improving the world around you; and what you can do to conserve dwindling resources for future generations.

Related Dimensions of Wellness

Occupational and financial wellness overlap with other wellness areas, and are sometimes considered their own dimensions. Your wellness in these areas can dramatically affect your overall wellness and add to your life's balance (or lack thereof). If you ask family members and friends about their current problems, many will identify their jobs or finances as the top stressors in their lives.

Occupational Wellness
Occupational wellness is the level of happiness and fulfillment you experience in your work. An important component of occupational wellness is finding a non-toxic, hazard-free work environment that provides contact with managers and co-workers who value your skills and opinions. Contrary to what people often think, job satisfaction is not closely tied to high

wages.[5] You can reach optimal occupational wellness when your personal goals align closely with those of your employer, and when you feel that you are making significant contributions to both sets of goals.

Financial Wellness
Financial wellness is the ability to successfully balance and manage your financial needs and wants with your income, debts, savings, and investments. If you cannot pay your bills, it can be hard to think of much else and this dimension can overshadow and unbalance the others. Even people who are managing their finances still need to make wise consumer choices, carefully control debt, and continually prioritize expenses. A positive benefit is that students who successfully navigate financial challenges have a greater chance of completing their education.[6] (See the GetFitGraphics: Dealing with Debt in College on page 7.)

Balancing Your Wellness Dimensions

You may have healthy relationships, but no fondness for exercise. Perhaps your spiritual life is rich, but you have trouble juggling academic demands. Virtually everyone is stronger in some dimensions of wellness than others. Striving for improvement in all six wellness dimensions is a lifelong process. One good approach is to concentrate on those dimensions that present the most pressing need, while working on the others in a steady but relaxed and motivated way. Over time, a balance of work on all the dimensions—one or two now, others later—will eventually promote overall wellness. Your brain and body, your thoughts and emotions, your actions and reactions, your relationship to yourself and others—all are interconnected and integrated. Likewise, the dimensions of wellness are interrelated. For example, increasing your exercise and general activity will help you manage stress, mood, sleep, body composition, and so on.[7]

Lab 1.1 and **Lab 1.2** at the end of the chapter will help you assess your wellness in each of the primary dimensions, analyze the areas that need improvement, and begin to plan changes.

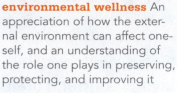

environmental wellness An appreciation of how the external environment can affect oneself, and an understanding of the role one plays in preserving, protecting, and improving it

occupational wellness A level of happiness and fulfilment in work, including harmony with personal goals, appreciation from bosses and co-workers, and a safe workplace

financial wellness The ability to balance and manage financial needs and wants with income, debts, savings, and investments

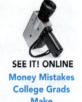

SEE IT! ONLINE
Money Mistakes
College Grads
Make

DO IT! ONLINE

Why Does Wellness Matter?

Wellness has many benefits for individuals, as well as for society as a whole.

Good Wellness Habits Can Help You Live a Longer, Healthier Life

In the United States, federal health experts consider the average life expectancy at birth for males to be 75.6 years and for females to be 80.6 years.[8] Equally important is our average *healthy* life expectancy—the years a person can expect to live without disability or major illness: about 65 for males and 67 for females (**Figure 1.4**).[9] Another way to analyze our national health is to identify disparities in health information, access, and care that might be associated with race, education, and economic levels. The impact can be widespread. Certain groups of people may experience obstacles to wellness due to inaccessible health care. See the box Diversity: The Life Expectancy Gap on page 8 to learn more about how health disparities affect racial and socioeconomic groups.

As a college student, you can make an enormous change in your own healthy life expectancy by learning more about wellness, making decisions to improve your own wellness dimensions, and by establishing and maintaining good wellness habits. For example, if you look closely at the causes of death for people ages 15 to 24, you find that more died from accidents than from most other causes combined (**Figure 1.5**).[10] By making better wellness choices—such as wearing seat belts and bike helmets, and avoiding risky behaviors such as driving under the influence of drugs or

SEE IT! ONLINE
Women's Life Expectancy in Decline

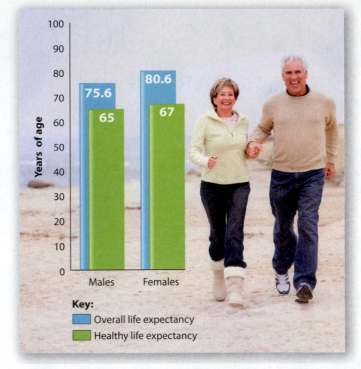

FIGURE **1.4** Healthy life expectancy is a subset of overall life expectancy. Lengthening the span of your healthy years is an important wellness goal.

Data from: J. A. Salomon et al., "Healthy Life Expectancy for 187 Countries, 1990–2010: A Systematic Analysis for the Global Burden Disease Study 2010," *The Lancet* 380, no. 9859 (2012): 2144–62, doi:10.1016/S0140-6736(12)61690-0.

alcohol—you can reduce your risk of premature death in an accident.

Most Americans die of heart disease or cancer due to their national tendencies to eat too much, exercise too little, and ignore wellness advice (**Figure 1.6**).[11] However, *many* risk factors for America's biggest killers are *modifiable*—within your control: They include high blood pressure, tobacco use, alcohol use, high

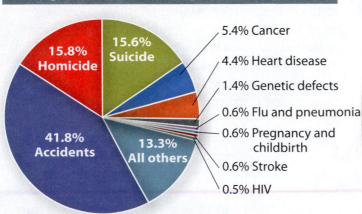

FIGURE **1.5** The leading causes of death among Americans of ages 20–24.

Data from: S. L. Murphy, J. Xu, and K. D. Kochanek, "Deaths: Final Data for 2010," *National Vital Statistics Reports* 61, no. 4 (2013).

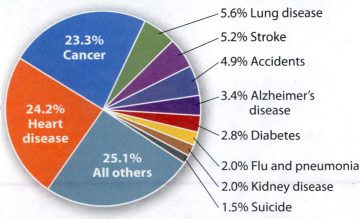

FIGURE **1.6** The leading causes of death among Americans overall.

Data from: S. L. Murphy, J. Xu, and K. D. Kochanek, "Deaths: Final Data for 2010," *National Vital Statistics Reports* 61, no. 4 (2013).

DEALING WITH **DEBT** IN COLLEGE

Figuring out how to manage one's money can be tough for college students—and owing money on credit cards and loans can be a major strain in college and beyond. A recent survey of 15,000 college students found that 60 percent worried often or very often about meeting regular expenses, and over half also worry frequently about paying for school.[1]

WHY SHOULD COLLEGE STUDENTS WORRY?

(Educated Americans are in debt.)

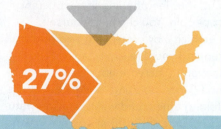

27%

27% of Americans spent more than 40% of their income on mortgage and credit card debt in 2008.[2]

Those with college educations were more likely to
SPEND OVER 40% OF THEIR INCOME ON DEBT
than those with high school diplomas or less.[3]

Of a **$50,360** salary (median income for those holding a bachelor's degree), that means

TYPICAL DEBT = $20,144[4]

CREDIT CARD CHARGES CAN ALSO STACK UP, DIGGING STUDENTS DEEPER INTO THE DEBT HOLE.[5]

80% students with debit cards

35% students with credit cards

$755 is the average outstanding balance students owe on credit cards

41% of students graduate with some student loan debt[6]

$22K Average debt[7]

10YRS or more to repay that size loan at an average payment of about **$250** per month[8]

DEBT STARTS BUILDING IN COLLEGE WITH STUDENT LOANS.

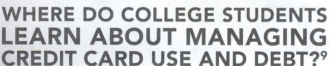

WHERE DO COLLEGE STUDENTS LEARN ABOUT MANAGING CREDIT CARD USE AND DEBT?[9]

Most learn from personal experience only

Some learn from discussions with friends and family

A few learn from financial classes or seminars

Avoid mounting debt now.

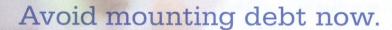

▶ **BUY ONLY** items you truly need—and pay cash when you can.

▶ **PAY BILLS** on time to protect your financial reputation for future borrowing.

▶ **CONSIDER DEBT** as a last resort, not a first choice.

▶ **KEEP A MINIMUM** of credit cards and try to pay the total balance each month.

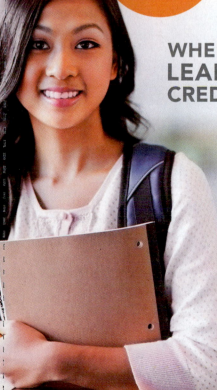

DIVeRSiTY
The Life Expectancy Gap

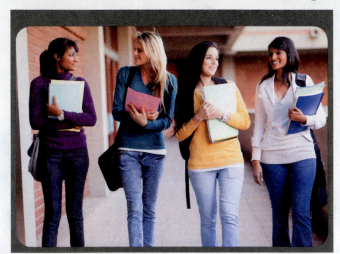

According to the head of a large research team studying social impacts on life expectancy, "there are essentially two Americas." They identify one subgroup that is increasing life expectancy and another that is experiencing decreasing life expectancy. To uncover the reasons behind these "two Americas," public health researcher S. Jay Olshansky of the University of Chicago led American and European researchers in an investigation of the disparities in U.S. life expectancy based on race and education.[1]

Your maximum age in America is strongly affected by your race and education levels. Based on race alone, white males live an average of seven years longer than black males; white women five years longer than black women.[2] Adding education to the equation doubles the disparity: There is a 14-year gap between college-educated white males and black males without a high school diploma, and a 10-year gap between well-educated white women and poorly educated black women.[3]

Researchers also analyze mortality statistics by the impact of specific social factors. In another large study,

researchers calculated that fully half of the deaths in the United States can be attributed to social factors such as low education, racial segregation, poverty, lack of health insurance, or living in an economically depressed area.[4]

Nationally, the Affordable Care Act and various anti-discrimination laws are aimed at narrowing the nation's health disparities and thus lengthening life expectancy for many groups of people. You can help yourself, regardless of your ethnicity, by employing two powerful approaches to extending your life expectancy: (1) getting a college education to increase your lifelong socio-economic level; and (2) incorporating healthy behaviors to improve your lifelong fitness and wellness. Congratulations, as taking this course means that you are making strides toward both!

THINK! Why do you think having a college education leads to a longer life? Think about your family and friends. Do the more educated ones seem to live longer and/or have longer healthy lives without major disability?

ACT NOW! Today, list the direct and indirect benefits of having a college education on your lifelong fitness and wellness. This week, pull out your college graduation plan (or create one) and make sure that you have a clear path to your goal. Write out any questions you have. In two weeks, meet with a college advisor or financial aid advisor to get your questions answered and ensure that you are on track with your education.

Sources:
1. S. J. Olshansky et al., "Differences in Life Expectancy Due to Race and Educational Differences are Widening, and Many May Not Catch Up," *Health Affairs* 31, no. 8 (2012): 1803, doi: 10.1377/hlthaff.2011.0746
2. N. Bharmal et al., "State-Level Variations in Racial Disparities in Life Expectancy," *Health Services Research* 47, no. 1 p. 2 (2012): 544, doi: 10.1111/j.1475 -6773.2011.01345.x
3. Olshansky, "Differences in Life Expectancy Due to Race and Educational Differences are Widening, and Many May Not Catch Up," 2012.
4. G. Sandro et al., "Estimated Deaths Attributed to Social Factors in the United States," *American Journal of Public Health* 101, no. 8 (2011): 1456–65.

cholesterol, obesity, low fruit and vegetable intake, and physical inactivity.

Researchers have made a compelling case for the role of physical inactivity in chronic disease. Medical researchers have shown in hundreds of studies that the vast majority of all illnesses of middle age and later years

sedentary Physically inactive; exerting physical effort only for required daily tasks and not for leisure-time exercise

(including heart disease, cancer, and type 2 diabetes) are related to, and exacerbated by, a lack of physical activity.[12] Living a **sedentary** life also increases the danger of *hypokinetic diseases*—conditions that can be triggered or worsened by too little movement or activity, such as obesity, back pain, arthritis, and high blood pressure. In fact, watching television or sitting at a desk for six hours per day could shorten your life by five years, while engaging in sufficient leisure-time activity could lengthen it by nearly that much.[13] **Figure 1.7**

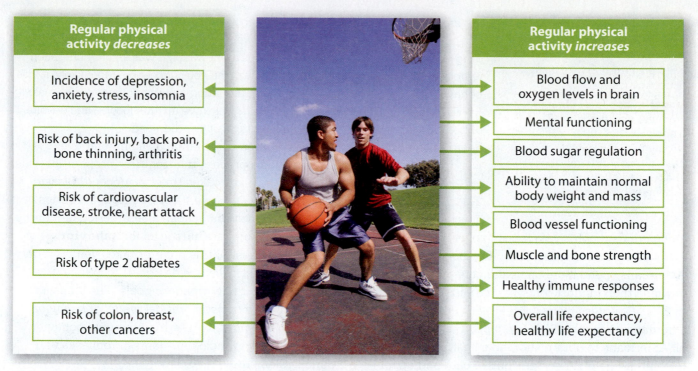

Regular physical activity *decreases*		Regular physical activity *increases*
Incidence of depression, anxiety, stress, insomnia		Blood flow and oxygen levels in brain
Risk of back injury, back pain, bone thinning, arthritis		Mental functioning
Risk of cardiovascular disease, stroke, heart attack		Blood sugar regulation
Risk of type 2 diabetes		Ability to maintain normal body weight and mass
Risk of colon, breast, other cancers		Blood vessel functioning
		Muscle and bone strength
		Healthy immune responses
		Overall life expectancy, healthy life expectancy

FIGURE **1.7** Regular physical activity results in many health benefits.

illustrates some of the health benefits of regular physical activity.

The American College of Sports Medicine recommends that all healthy adults between the ages of 18 and 65 strive for at least 150 minutes of moderate exercise per week (or 75 minutes of vigorous exercise or a combination of the two).[14] However, in 2011, 26.2 percent of all adults reported no physical activity in the last month.[15] The high percentages of overweight and obese adults provide more evidence that most Americans are too inactive (**Figure 1.8**).[16] Indeed, we are one of the most sedentary and overweight nations on earth.[17]

Good Wellness Habits Benefit Society as a Whole

If Americans could raise their levels of wellness, they would be happier, more productive, and spend less money on health care. Achieving better wellness and combating today's chronic diseases have therefore become important national priorities.

The Office of the Surgeon General of the United States has summarized its health priorities in *Healthy People 2020*, a report that outlines four broad goals: (1) attain high-quality, longer lives free of preventable disease, disability, injury, and premature death; (2) achieve health equity, eliminate disparities, and improve the health of all groups; (3) create social and physical environments that promote good health for all; and (4) promote quality of life, healthy

development, and healthy behaviors across all life stages.[18] Accordingly, the Surgeon General advises Americans to eat healthier, be more physically active,

SEE IT! ONLINE
Hunger at Home

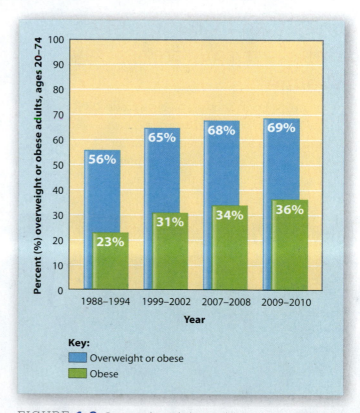

FIGURE **1.8** Overweight and obese adults are now clearly the majority, with percentages rising steadily in the past 30 years.

Data from: C. L. Ogden et al., "Prevalence of Obesity in the United States, 2009–2010," *NCHS Data Brief* 82 (2012), www.cdc.gov; Centers for Disease Control and Prevention, FastStats, "Obesity and Overweight," October 2012, www.cdc.gov

behavior change An organized, deliberate effort to alter or replace an existing habit or pattern of activity

stages of behavior change From the transtheoretical model, a set of states most people pass through in their awareness of, determination to alter, and efforts to replace existing habits or actions

not smoke, limit alcohol, and avoid drugs—all of which are wellness behaviors.

The high cost of health care and health insurance is a major concern for Americans. In 2011, Americans spent $2.7 trillion on health care, which averages to over $8,600 for every man, woman, and child.[19] Further, although Americans spend more on health care, their health is worse than in most other industrialized nations.[20] In 2010, Congress passed the Patient Protection and Affordable Care Act (PPACA) to provide a means for all Americans to obtain affordable health care and to encourage more to seek preventive care and adopt wellness behaviors.[21] One of the key ACA provisions allows parents to keep young adults on their existing insurance policies through age 26. Because of this, more than 3 million additional 19- to 25-year-olds now have health insurance.[22]

How Can I Change My Behavior to Increase My Wellness?

If you are like most people, you have made a New Year's resolution on January 1, have worked hard to adopt some new behavior until about the 10th, have started slipping back to your old habits by the 15th, and

SEE IT! ONLINE
Life-Changing Resolutions

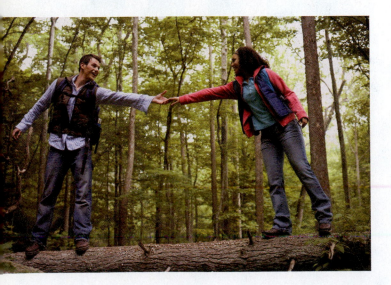

have forgotten about the whole thing by the 31st. Your resolution may well have been a new wellness behavior—lots of resolutions are. Perhaps it was an easy one, such as "eat more fruit," and you succeeded. More likely, it was a harder one—"start lifting weights three times a week," or "lose 20 pounds," or "give up junk food"—and despite your good intentions, it just didn't stick.

People often see change as a singular event instead of as a process that requires preparation, has several stages, and takes time to succeed. Classic research shows that we must go through a series of mental and emotional stages over a period of months to adequately prepare ourselves for **behavior change**. The rest of this chapter takes you through a series of practical steps designed to help you succeed at your new wellness goals. The steps are inspired by the *transtheoretical model of behavior change,* a blueprint for altering your own behavior developed by psychologists James Prochaska and Carlo DiClemente.[23]

Step One: Understand the Stages of Behavior Change

The transtheoretical model of behavior change delineates six **stages of behavior change**: pre-contemplation, contemplation, preparation, action, maintenance, and termination. The model shows that changing behaviors usually involves a gradual process of awareness, preparation, and then action. Understanding this process can help you proceed more deliberately to identify and successfully change a problem behavior. Keep in mind that the steps of this model are general and people often backtrack as they work on them.

Precontemplation People in the precontemplation stage have no current intention of changing. They may have tried to change an old habit and given up, or they may be in denial and unaware of the problem.

Contemplation In this stage, people recognize that they have a problem and begin to contemplate the need to change within six months or so. People can languish in this stage for months or years, however, realizing that they have a negative wellness pattern, yet lacking the time, energy, or commitment to make the change.

Preparation Most people at this stage are within a month or so of taking action. They have thought about what they might do and may even have come up with a plan. Rather than thinking about why they can't begin, they have started to focus on what they can do.

Action In this stage, people begin to execute their action plans. Unfortunately, many people try to take shortcuts; they start behavior change here rather than going through the earlier stages. However, without making a plan, publicly stating the desire to change, enlisting other people's help, and setting realistic goals, they are likely to fail.

Maintenance In the maintenance stage, people work to prevent a relapse into old habits through a conscious application of wellness tools and techniques. Maintenance requires vigilance, attention to detail, and long-term commitment. You are in the maintenance stage after you have incorporated the new action and have continued it for six months or longer without relapse into old habits.

Relapse While not an original stage of behavior change, relapse is something that happens periodically for most people trying to change behaviors. Common causes of relapse include overconfidence, daily temptations, stress or emotional distractions, and putting yourself down.

Termination At the termination stage, the new behavior is ingrained; you are maintaining it and are no longer at risk for relapse. The new behavior has become a part of the way you live and thus the temptation to return to former behaviors is greatly reduced.

Step Two: Increase Your Awareness

Wellness behaviors that are important to college students can be simple to think about but are often challenging to achieve. An important starting point is to become aware of what is required to achieve wellness in each of the following areas.

LIVE IT! ONLINE
Worksheet 1
Health Behavior
Self Assessment

Staying Physically Fit Nowhere does the phrase "Use it or lose it" apply more fully than to your physical fitness. Over 16 percent of people of ages 16–24 reported no physical activity in the last month.[24] The same is true for many of the non-traditional students (over age 25, often married and working full- or part-time) who make up 40 percent of today's college enrollees. They report being so busy juggling responsibilities and deadlines that there is often little time for physical activity.[25] Much of the decline people expect with advancing age is, in fact, a reflection of inactivity and its toll on the body rather than the effects of aging themselves. Staying active every day is probably the single most important wellness behavior you can adopt.

Eating Healthy Foods The American diet tends to be light on nutrition and heavy on calories. Most Americans consume more calories than they burn off each day.

casestudy

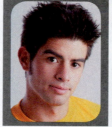

CARLOS

"In an ideal world I'd reduce my stress by sleeping eight hours a night, eating healthier food, and exercising more. Maybe then I would ace my exams and still have time for a social life. But I know I can't just snap my fingers and make all of that happen. Right now, I really have to get more sleep—it doesn't do me any good to stay up all night studying and then fall asleep in class. Some of my friends take 'power naps' in the afternoon. I might try that! I'm also thinking of signing up for a gym class next quarter. That way I can be sure to work some exercise into my schedule. Beyond that—well, I think I should probably take things one at a time."

THINK! What are Carlos's main wellness goals? What is his current stage of behavior change for each goal?

ACT NOW! Today, name a wellness behavior that you have identified for change and write down your stage of behavior change for that item. This week, tape this up where you can see it each morning, and do one thing each day to advance your stage, such as finding more information, or looking for a counselor or group on campus that can help you. In two weeks, reevaluate where you are in changing your behavior and make plans to move into the next stage.

HEAR IT! ONLINE

They also tend to eat more protein, salt, sugar, animal fat, and solidified vegetable oils (*trans* fats) than are recommended.[26] They consume too little fiber and too few helpings of fruits and vegetables.[27] Important factors in their consumption are the ubiquity of unhealthy foods in their everyday environments (including college campuses); aggressive marketing campaigns that promote unhealthy foods; the short-term pleasure they get from eating rich, salty, soft, and sweet foods; and the habits and automatic responses they develop around unhealthy foods.[28] Conversely, establishing good nutrition habits has many wellness benefits, including increased energy, greater stamina, better weight management, stronger disease resistance, and reduced risk of chronic illness.

Managing Your Weight As we saw in Figure 1.8 (page 9), 68 percent of American adults have a body weight and mass (fat-to-lean ratio) above recommended ranges.

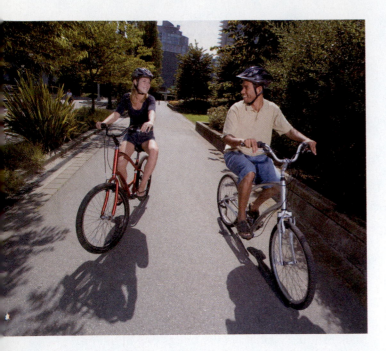

Overweight and obesity rates are better among college students (39 percent), but the proportion is higher (43 percent) among non-traditional students.[29] Overweight and obesity are correlated with arthritis, bone and joint problems, back pain, decreased physical performance, more chronic illness, and a shorter life expectancy. Modifying your activity level, exercise habits, eating habits, and stress levels can all contribute to maintaining a healthy weight.

Managing Your Stress
Most students find college stressful. Whether you went straight to college after high school or have returned as a non-traditional student after military service, working, or starting a family, the lifestyle changes and the competing demands of academics, work, and social commitments can take an emotional and physical toll. Stressful stimuli can trigger automatic coping behaviors such as drinking or drug use, poor sleep habits, loss of concentration, and over-eating. These, in turn, can disrupt thinking and memory, disturb sleep, increase depression, impair immunity to infections, and contribute to weight gain.[30] Over many years, unrelieved stress may also contribute to higher blood pressure, premature aging, and increased risk for chronic illnesses.

Avoiding Drugs, Smoking, and Alcohol Abuse
Using drugs, smoking, and abusing alcohol are all ways of manipulating the brain chemically. Unfortunately, the use and abuse of these substances carry high risks for illness and injury and can undermine multiple dimensions of wellness.

Practicing Accident, Injury, and Disease Prevention
Prevention has several practical meanings for wellness behavior. It can mean preventing injuries and the accidents that account for most deaths among young adults. It can mean self-care such as daily dental hygiene and regular body checks for skin and tissue changes (i.e., tracking moles and performing breast self-exams). And it can mean preventing disease through medical checkups and vaccinations.

Step Three: Contemplate Change

Habits are usually deeply ingrained, and even minor habits can be surprisingly hard to change. As we have discussed, research has confirmed that people are more successful when they prepare for change emotionally and mentally rather than starting right in on the change itself. For example, people who believe they can change their physical activity levels and make specific plans to do so are significantly more successful at launching new exercise patterns.[31] Contemplating change can include examining your current patterns, identifying your beliefs and attitudes, solidifying your motivation, and choosing a realistic target for your efforts to change.

Examine Current Habits and Patterns
What current behavior should you work on changing? The assessment in **Lab 1.1** will help you identify habits that lower your wellness. When considering a habit, ask yourself the following:

DO IT! ONLINE

- How long has it been going on?
- How often does it happen?
- How serious are the consequences of the habit or problem?
- What are some of my reasons for continuing this problematic behavior?
- What kinds of situations trigger the behavior?
- Are other people involved in this habit? If so, in what way?

Habits involve elements of deliberate choice but are also influenced by automatic, subconscious processes as well as demographics, personal attitudes and beliefs, and many other factors. Age, sex, race, income, family background, education, and access to health care all increase or decrease the likelihood of developing certain health habits. For example, people are more likely to eat snacks after seeing junk food advertisements on TV, or to drink alcohol after seeing TV or movie characters drinking.[32] Likewise, if your peers smoke, you yourself are much more likely to smoke based on simple imitation, not on direct pressure from them.[33] Identifying factors that may encourage negative behaviors or block positive ones can help you prepare for behavior change. Analyzing the factors that reinforce your current habit patterns can also help you understand why you developed and maintained unwanted habits and where you need to make changes in order to succeed.

Assess Current Beliefs and Attitudes Your attitudes about health and wellness affect your daily choices. When reaching for another cigarette, smokers, for example, sometimes tell themselves, "I'll stop tomorrow" or "They'll have a cure for lung cancer by the time I get it." These beliefs allow them to continue smoking. One model suggests that several factors must be in place before you successfully change a habit that diminishes wellness.[34] Among these factors are the following:

- You must believe that your current pattern could lead you to a serious problem. The more severe the consequences, the more likely you are to change the behavior. For example, smoking can cause cancer and emphysema and promote heart disease. The fear of developing those diseases can help a person stop smoking.

- You must believe that you personally are quite susceptible to developing the health problem. For example, losing a parent to lung cancer could make a person work harder to stop smoking.

What beliefs underlie your current pattern of wellness habits, both positive and negative?

Assess Your Motivation What is your **motivation**, or inducement, to change a wellness behavior? For some, a rewarding result, such as looking better, can motivate change. For others, a sense of accomplishment or just feeling better every day may do it. See the box What Gets You Moving? on page 14 to explore exercise motivation in students.

Motivations can be external (come from someone or something outside yourself) or internal (come from inside yourself), but in either case are part of your sense of self. The degree to which you believe in your own abilities is your **self-efficacy**. Your conviction that you can control events and factors in your life is your **locus of control**. An *internal* locus of control usually gives you a strong belief in your ability to effect change. An *external* locus of control usually leads you to see other people and things as controlling what you do and whether you can change.

A person with a strong sense of self-efficacy and a largely internal locus of control has a better chance of following through with a decision to change wellness behavior. For example, suppose you wish to bring your weight down to a healthy range. If your parents are both overweight, you may think "My weight is controlled by my genes" and thus be resigned to being overweight. However, by gathering information about weight

management, by identifying behaviors that are within your power to change (such as food choices, eating habits, and exercise), and by acknowledging their importance, you can shift to a more internalized locus of control and increase your chances of successful weight management. Likewise, you can help boost your own self-efficacy through this shift to more internalized control.

- -

THINK! Where is your locus of control? Are you motivated by external factors (e.g., your genes) or internal factors (e.g., your own power)?

ACT NOW! Today, write down three things you can control about the behavior you want to change. For example, if you want to lose weight, one thing you can control is rerouting your walk to class so that you don't pass tempting vending machines. This week, try controlling one of those behaviors, such as taking that new route. In two weeks, think specifically about what factors trigger automatic behaviors, such as increased stress leading to increased snacking, and make a plan to work on the root cause of the automatic behavior.

- -

Choose a Target Behavior The last preparatory step is to choose one well-defined habit, or **target behavior**, as your initial focus for change. It is a much better strategy to start small and build on success than to try for too much and end up failing. To choose potential target behaviors, ask yourself these questions:

- *What do I want?* What is your ultimate goal? To lose weight? Exercise more? Reduce stress? Sleep better? Have a lasting relationship? Whatever it is, you need a clear picture of your target outcome.

- *Which change is my greatest priority at this time?* People often decide to change several things at once. Suppose you are gaining unwanted weight. Rather than saying, "I need to eat less and start exercising," identify one specific behavior that contributes significantly to this problem and tackle that first.

motivation One's inducement to do something such as change a current behavior

self-efficacy The degree to which one believes in his or her ability to achieve something

locus of control Belief that control over life events and changes comes primarily from outside of oneself (external locus of control) or from within (internal locus of control)

target behavior One well-defined habit chosen as a primary focus for change

LIVE IT! ONLINE
Worksheet 3 Health Locus of Control

TOOLS FOR CHANGE

What Gets You Moving?

Like many students, you may need powerful motivation to start a fitness program and follow it through. Researchers have discovered several interesting facts about student motivation to be active and fit. If you have trouble sticking with exercise programs, apply these tips to your own fitness and wellness plan and increase your chances of following through!

1. **Make it FUN!** What types of things make you happy? Can those be turned into active pursuits? Read or watch a movie while on the exercise bike or while stretching. Recruit friends for a hike to catch up on your social time while being active too. Researchers have also confirmed that the social aspect of sports and activities—a sense of belonging to a team, a gym, or simply a group of friends who like to take bike rides or play frisbee in the park—helps people enjoy fitness activities and stick with them.[1]

2. **Have a plan, start small, and build.** Just five minutes every other day doing push-ups and abdominal curl-ups can really help increase your muscle strength and endurance. Over time and with your increasing fitness, you will naturally want to increase your time. Before you know it, you have developed a habit of working on your upper body and core muscles for 20 minutes 3–4 times per week!

3. **Do it for yourself!** Researchers have shown that exercisers who list intrinsic (internally focused) motivations and self-regulation are much more apt to stick with a regular fitness program.[2] In fact, having physical activity regulated by someone else (external regulation) was negatively associated with activity levels.[3] So, spend some time figuring out what your internal motivations are and use those to get yourself moving.

4. **Use technology.** Researchers have found that college students who used exercise video games, such as Wii Fit™, had more intention to continue over traditional exercise programs.[4] In addition to video games, there are a number of ways to get active via technology. Search for health and fitness apps on your smart phone that will help you design and track your fitness activities.

5. **Start where you are.** Think about things you already do that can be expanded or changed to count as exercise and physical activity. Do you have a dog? Try walking your dog faster or work up to jogging. Do you walk from the bus stop to campus? Walk faster or take a route that is longer or incorporates a hill.

6. **Don't be too hard on yourself.** Allow yourself a few setbacks along the way. Don't let those setbacks stop you from reaching your goals, but take them *in stride.*

THINK! What are your main motivations for fitness and physical activity? Are they primarily external or internal? Do you participate in sports? Are you active with friends? Why or why not? Which of your activities are the most fun, and what makes them so?

ACT NOW! Today, make a list of activities that you could add for (a) more social contact; (b) more fun and enjoyment, and (c) for five minutes each day. This week, try adding one new activity or change a current activity in your life to make it more active. In two weeks, assess your motivation level: Do you look forward to your new or changed activity and is it becoming part of your regular routine?

Sources:
1. B. Kwan and A. Bryan, "Affective Response to Exercise as a Component of Exercise Motivation: Attitudes, Norms, Self-Efficacy, and Temporal Stability of Intentions," *Psychology of Sport and Exercise* 11, no. 1 (2010): 71–9.
2. J. Brunet and C. Sabiston, "Exploring Motivation for Physical Activity across the Adult Lifespan," *Psychology of Sport and Exercise* 12, no. 2 (2011): 99–105.
3. Ibid.
4. A. Garn, B. Baker, E. Beasley, and M. Solomon, "What Are the Benefits of a Commercial Exergaming Platform for College Students? Examining Physical Activity, Enjoyment, and Future Intentions," *Journal of Physical Activity and Health* 9, no. 2 (2012): 311–8.

- *Why is this important to me?* Think through why you want to change. Are you doing it because of your health? To improve your academic performance? To look better? To win someone else's approval? It's best to target a behavior because it's right for you rather than because you think it will help you win others' approval.

- *Fill in the details.* Rather than using a generality ("I need to eat better"), consider specific behaviors that relate to the general problem. What are your unhealthy eating habits? Do you eat too few fruits and vegetables? Do you have fast food for lunch every day? Identifying the specific behavior you would like to change will help you set clear goals.

Step Four: Prepare for Change

Once you have assessed your current status and chosen a target behavior, you are ready to make specific preparations, including observing role models, setting realistic goals, anticipating barriers, and making a commitment to change.

Observe Role Models Watching others successfully change their behavior can give you ideas and encouragement for your own changes. This process of modeling, or learning from role models, can be very helpful. Suppose you have trouble talking to strangers or new acquaintances and want to improve your communication skills. Try observing friends whose social skills you admire and note how they make conversation. What techniques help make them successful communicators? If you see behaviors that work well, separate their components so you can model your behavior change on a proven approach.

Set Realistic Goals and Objectives Your wellness goals and objectives should be both achievable for you and in line with what you truly want.[35] Achievable, truly desired goals increase motivation, and this, in turn, leads to a better chance of success at behavior change.

To set successful goals, try using the SMART system. SMART goals are *specific, measurable, action-oriented, realistic,* and *time-oriented.* A vague goal would be "Get into better shape by exercising more." A SMART goal would be

- *specific*—"Start weight training";

- *measurable*—"Increase the amount of weight I can safely lift";

- *action-oriented*—"Go to the gym three times per week";

- *realistic*—"Increase the weight I can lift by 20 percent [not 200 percent]";

- *time-oriented*—"Try my new weight program for eight weeks, then reassess."

Anticipate and Overcome Barriers to Change

Anticipating **barriers to change**, or possible stumbling blocks, will help you prepare for behavior change. A majority of students, for example, want to lose or gain weight but have failed to do so permanently.[36] Diet-control failure is based on several barriers to change, including internal drives to eat high-calorie foods and external temptations such as snacks and fast foods on sale in most campus buildings. An awareness of these facts might encourage you, for example, to bring a bag full of carrot sticks, apple slices, or sunflower seeds to eat as snacks rather than getting hungry between classes, letting your unhealthy food habits take over, and heading straight for the campus hamburger, pizza, or taco stand. The following are a few general barriers to wellness change:

- *Overambitious goals* can derail behavior change. Most people cannot lose weight, stop smoking, and begin running three miles a day all at the same time. It tends to be equally unsuccessful to try for dramatic change within an unrealistically short time frame—such as losing 20 pounds in one month. Habits are best changed one at a time, taking small, progressive steps; rewarding successes; and being patient with yourself.

- *Self-defeating beliefs and attitudes* can impede successful change. Believing that you are too young to worry about fitness and wellness can bar you from making a solid commitment to change. Likewise, thinking you are helpless to change your weight, smoking, or fitness habits could undermine your efforts. Greater self-efficacy and more positive expectations may help.

- *Failing to accurately assess your current state of wellness* could block progress. You might assume that you are strong and flexible, for example, when you are actually below average for your age. Failing to gather enough data on wellness risks and benefits can also be a barrier that leaves you with weakened motivation and commitment.

- *Lack of support and guidance* can act as a barrier. Supportive friends are a good start. You should also seek guidance from your fitness and wellness instructor; from counselors and other campus resources; from up-to-date, trusted health sources on the Internet (see the box How Can I Find Reliable Wellness Information? on page 17); and from health professionals.

barriers to change Stumbling blocks faced in the efforts to alter a current behavior

behavior change contract
A formal document that clarifies the goals and steps needed to change a current habit or habit pattern

countering Substituting a desired behavior for an undesirable one

A formal written document called the **behavior change contract** functions

- as a promise to yourself,
- as a public declaration of intent,
- as an organized plan that lays out start and end dates and daily actions,
- as a listing of barriers or obstacles you may encounter,
- as a place to brainstorm strategies for overcoming those impediments,
- as a collected set of sources of support, and
- as a reminder of the rewards you plan to give yourself for sticking with the program.

Writing a behavior change contract will help you clarify your goals, make a commitment to change, and, if you wish, announce your intentions to supportive friends and family. In **Lab 1.3** you will create a behavior change contract as part of your fitness and wellness plan.

DO IT! ONLINE

Step Five: Take Action to Change

Now that you've put some thought into it, and made a plan for change, it's time to take action! The following are some strategies to keep your behavior change process on track.

Visualize New Behavior Athletes often use a form of mental practice called *imagined rehearsal* or simply *visualization* to reach their performance goals. Picturing themselves accomplishing an action in their minds ahead of time helps prepare them for real competition. Visualization can help you imagine the way a current negative behavior unfolds, and then allows you to practice in advance what you will say and do to counter it.

Make a Commitment The more strongly you state an intention to change a wellness habit, either verbally or on paper, the more likely it is you will succeed.

Control Your Environment If you are trying to quit drinking, going to a bar could lead you to resume an undesired behavior. Going to dinner and a movie with a sympathetic friend, on the other hand, could help reinforce your abstinence. If you are trying to lose weight but need to eat out, plan ahead by only visiting restaurants that have healthy options you enjoy. Think about which people and settings tend to trigger your unwanted behavior, and then stay away from them as much as possible and set up supportive situations instead.

Change Your Self-Talk Your *self-talk*—that is, the way you think and talk to yourself—matters. Think about what you say to yourself when something goes badly or when something succeeds. Purposely blocking or stopping negative thoughts and replacing them with positive ones can help you change a habit.

Learn to "Counter" **Countering** is another term for substituting a desired behavior for an undesirable one. You may want to stop eating junk food, for example, but quitting "cold turkey" just isn't realistic. Instead, compile a list of substitute foods and places to get them. Then, have your healthy options ready before your mouth starts watering at the smell of french fries, tacos, or pizza.

Practice "Shaping" *Shaping* is a stepwise process of making a series of small changes, starting slowly and mastering one step before moving on to the next. Suppose you want to start jogging three miles every other day, but right now you get tired and winded after half a mile. Shaping would dictate a process of slow, progressive steps such as walking one hour every other day at a slow, relaxed pace for the first week; walking for an hour every other day but at a faster pace the second week; and speeding up to a slow run the third week. Regardless of the change you plan, remember that current habits did not develop overnight, and they will not change overnight, either.

Reward Yourself Setting up a system of rewards can help you keep new behavior on track. Rewards can be consumable, like a cookie or a gourmet meal. They can be active, like going to a concert or playing Frisbee. They can be

Q&A How Can I Find Reliable Wellness Information?

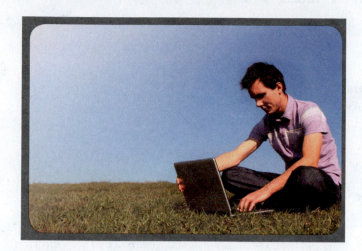

Fitness and wellness are important American preoccupations—and major industries as well. It can be hard to distinguish legitimate information from thinly disguised advertising for products and services. Here are some general tips and specific sources of reliable information.

Look for organizations without a direct interest in your wallet.

Examples are health-related agencies of the state and federal government (e.g., CDC or FDA); major colleges and universities; big-name hospitals and medical centers (e.g., Mayo Clinic or Cooper Institute); and well-known nonprofit organizations (e.g., American College of Sports Medicine or American Medical Association). Cross-check any information you gather from other sources against these kinds of known and reliable sources to see whether facts and figures are consistent.

If a newspaper or magazine quotes a research report, look up the research itself.

Consider details of the study, noting whether the researcher works for a large, recognizable university, government agency, or research institute; whether the study had human subjects or inferred conclusions from

lab animals; and whether the conclusions were based on dozens or hundreds of research subjects or just a few.

Take fitness advice only from experts who represent reliable sources.

Well-meaning friends often have misinformation, and promoters of products and services are usually strongly biased.

Read consumer health newsletters published by distinguished universities, research institutes, and nonprofit organizations.

Examples include the *Harvard Health Letter; Mayo Clinic Health Letter*, and *Nutrition Action Health Letter*.

Finally, use established, widely respected websites such as the following to learn more about fitness and wellness topics:

CDC Wonder (wonder.cdc.gov)

Mayo Clinic (www.mayoclinic.com)

National Center for Health Statistics (www.cdc.gov/nchs)

National Health Information Center (www.health.gov/nhic)

Harvard School of Public Health, *World Health News* (www.worldhealthnews.harvard.edu)

American Cancer Association (www.cancer.org)

American Heart Association (www.americanheart.org)

American Lung Association (www.lung.org)

American Medical Association (www.ama-assn.org)

Healthy People 2020 (www.healthypeople.gov)

U.S. Department of Health and Human Services (www.healthfinder.gov)

World Health Organization (www.who.int)

American College of Sports Medicine (www.acsm.org)

President's Council on Physical Fitness and Sports (www.fitness.gov)

FDA Information for Consumers (www.fda.gov/ForConsumers/default.htm)

Note: Web links are always subject to change. Visit the Study Area in MasteringHealth to view updated Web links for each chapter.

---

possessions, like getting a new MP3 player or downloading music or a movie. A reward can be an incentive, like being taken to a special event by a friend. It can be social, like receiving praise or a hug. And it can be intrinsic, meaning a new behavior feels so enjoyable it becomes its own reward. Whatever your motivating rewards may be, build a few (but not too many) into your program.

Use Writing as a Wellness Tool Throughout the labs in this textbook, you will examine your current wellness habits and analyze them through writing. **Journaling**,

or writing personal experiences, interpretations, and results in a journal or notebook, is an important skill for behavior change. Journaling can help you monitor your daily efforts, measure how much you have learned, record how you feel about your progress, and note ideas for improving your program.

> **journaling** Keeping a written record of personal experiences, interpretations, and results

LIVE IT! ONLINE
Worksheet 2
Weekly Behavior
Change Evaluation

CHAPTER IN REVIEW

MasteringHealth™

www.masteringhealthandnutrition.com (or www.pearsonmastering.com)
Build your knowledge—and wellness!—in the Study Area of MasteringHealth with a variety of study tools.

SEE IT! ONLINE

videos

Money Mistakes College Grads Make

Women's Life Expectancy in Decline

Hunger at Home

Life-Changing Resolutions

HEAR IT! ONLINE

audio tools

Audio case study

MP3 chapter review

REVIEW IT! ONLINE

chapter review

Chapter reading quizzes

Glossary flashcards

LIVE IT! ONLINE

programs & behavior change

Take Charge of Your Health! Worksheets:

Worksheet 1 Health Behavior Self-Assessment

Worksheet 2 Weekly Behavior Change Evaluation

Worksheet 3 Multidimensional Health Locus of Control

Behavior Change Log Book and Wellness Journal

DO IT! ONLINE

labs

Lab 1.1 How Well Are You?

Lab 1.2 Chart Your Personal Wellness Balance

Lab 1.3 Create a Behavior Change Contract

reviewquestions

1. How does *wellness* differ from *health*?
   a. Wellness is the absence of disease.
   b. Wellness is the achievement of the highest level of health possible in physical, social, intellectual, emotional, environmental, and spiritual dimensions.
   c. Wellness and health are equivalent.
   d. Health is a more individualized, dynamic concept than wellness.

2. Which dimension of wellness includes good organizational skills?
   a. Social
   b. Intellectual
   c. Emotional
   d. Environmental

3. Which of the following is a modifiable risk factor for disease?
   a. Age
   b. Race
   c. Genetics
   d. Tobacco use

4. The American College of Sports Medicine recommends that all healthy adults between the ages of 18 and 65 strive for
   a. at least 50 minutes of moderate exercise per week.
   b. at least 100 minutes of moderate exercise once a week.
   c. at least 150 minutes of moderate exercise per week.
   d. at least 200 minutes of moderate exercise per week.

5. Which of the following is a top cause of death among Americans of ages 20–24?
   a. Accidents
   b. Heart disease
   c. Stroke
   d. Lung disease

6. Which of the following is a stage of the transtheoretical model of behavior change?
   a. Increased wellness
   b. Preparation
   c. Social wellness
   d. Motivation

7. What is meant by the term *healthy life expectancy*?
   a. How many years a person can expect to live
   b. How many years a person can expect to live without disability or major illness
   c. A realistic attitude toward how long a person can expect to live
   d. How many years a person believes he or she has to live
8. Imagined rehearsal is a form of
   a. countering.
   b. modeling.
   c. rewarding.
   d. visualization.
9. What is "shaping"?
   a. A stepwise process of change, designed to change one small piece of a target behavior at a time
   b. A model of behavior change that uses mental imaging to reshape the brain's signals
   c. A journaling strategy
   d. A way of learning behaviors by watching others perform them
10. Which action strategy for behavior change can help you monitor your daily efforts, measure how much you have learned, and record how you feel about your progress?
   a. Journaling
   b. Shaping
   c. Visualization
   d. Countering

---

critical thinkingquestions

1. What does it mean to be well? What are the benefits of wellness?
2. Why is it important to find your current place on the wellness continuum? Identify your place on the wellness continuum in Figure 1.2.
3. Describe the SMART goal-setting guidelines.
4. Name the dimensions of wellness and assign yourself a score (1 to 5) for your degree of wellness in each dimension. Which of your dimensions of wellness needs the most attention? Name one thing you could do today to increase your commitment and effort toward that dimension.
5. Which risk-lowering choices do you incorporate into your lifestyle? Choose two or three of them and discuss the personal attitudes and beliefs that underlie your present behavior.
6. Using the stages of change (transtheoretical) model, discuss what you might do (in stages) to help a friend stop smoking. Why is it important that a person be ready to change before trying to change?
7. Which habits (wellness-related or not) have you tried to change in the past? Why do you think your efforts succeeded or failed? Using the skills for behavior change from this chapter, write a plan that will help you approach each habit more successfully.

---

references

1. American College Health Association, *American College Health Association—National College Health Assessment II (ACHA-NCHA II): Reference Group Executive Summary Fall 2012* (Hanover, MD: American College Health Association, 2013).
2. S. Harper, D. Rushani, and S. J. Kaufman, "Trends in Black-White Life Expectancy Gap, 2003 to 2008," *Journal of the American Medical Association Research Letters* 307, no. 21 (2012).
3. G. Greengross and G. Miller, "Humor Ability Reveals Intelligence, Predicts Mating Success, and Is Higher in Males," *Intelligence* 39 (2011): 188–92.
4. T. J. Pleskac et al., "A Detection Model of College Withdrawal," *Organizational Behavior and Human Decision Processes* 115 no. 1 (2011): 85–98.
5. T. A. Judge et al., "The Relationship Between Pay and Job Satisfaction: A Meta-Analysis of the Literature," *Journal of Vocational Behavior* 77 (2010): 157–67.
6. Pleskac et al., "A Detection Model of College Withdrawal," 2011.
7. P. D. Loprinzi and B. J. Cardinal, "Association Between Objectively-Measured Physical Activity and Sleep, NHANES 2005–2006," *Mental Health and Physical Activity* 3, no. 2 (2011): 65–9.
8. E. Arias, "United States Life Tables, 2008." *National Vital Statistics Report* 61, no. 3 (Hyattsville, MD: National Center for Health Statistics, 2012); D. Hoyert and J. Xu, "Deaths, Preliminary Data for 2011," *National Vital Statistics Report* 61, no. 6 (Hyattsville, MD: National Center for Health Statistics, 2012); World Health Organization, "World Health Statistics 2012," 2013, www.who.int
9. J. A. Salomon et al., "Healthy Life Expectancy for 187 Countries, 1990–2010: A Systematic Analysis for the Global Burden Disease Study 2010," *The Lancet* 380, no. 9859 (2012): 2144–62, doi: 10.1016/S0140-6736(12)61690-0.
10. S. L. Murphy et al., "Deaths, Preliminary Data for 2012," *National Vital Statistics Report* 61, no. 4 (2012).
11. Hoyert and Xu, "Deaths, Preliminary Data for 2011" (2012); G. Danaei et al., "The Preventable Causes of Death in the United States: Comparative Risk Assessment of Dietary, Lifestyle, and Metabolic Risk Factors," *PLoS Medicine* 6, no. 4 (2009): e1000058, www.plosmedicine.org; Centers for Disease Control and Prevention, *Chronic Disease Overview*, 2009.
12. World Health Organization, "Diet and Physical Activity: A Public Health Priority," Global Strategy on Diet, Physical Activity and Health, 2013, www.who.int
13. J. H. O'Keefe et al., "Exercise and Life Expectancy," *The Lancet* 379, no. 9818 (2012): 799; P. T. Katzmarzyk and M. Lee, "Sedentary Behavior and Life Expectancy in the USA: A Cause-Deleted Life Table Analysis," *British Medical Journal Open* 2, no. 4 (2012), 2:e000828, doi: 10.1136/bmjopen-2012-000828; J. Lennert Veerman

et al., "Television Viewing Time and Reduced Life Expectancy: A Life Table Analysis," *Diabetologia* 55, no. 11 (2012): 2895–905; I. Janssen et al., "Years of Life Gained Due to Leisure-Time Physical Activity in the U.S.," *American Journal of Preventative Medicine* 44, no. 1 (2013): 23–9.

14. C. E. Garner et al., "American College of Sports Medicine Position Stand: Quantity and Quality of Exercise for Developing and Maintaining Cardiorespiratory, Musculoskeletal, and Neuromotor Fitness in Apparently Healthy Adults: Guidance for Prescribing Exercise," *Medicine and Science in Sports and Exercise* 43, no. 7 (2011): 1334–59.

15. Centers for Disease Control Office of Surveillance, Epidemiology, and Laboratory Services, Behavioral Risk Factor Surveillance System, Prevalence and Trends Data, Nationwide 2011, Exercise (January 2013), www.cdc.gov

16. C. L. Ogden et al., "Prevalence of Obesity in the United States, 2009–2010," *NCHS Data Brief* 82 (2012), www.cdc.gov; K. M. Flegal et al., "Prevalence of Obesity and Trends in the Distribution of Body Mass Index Among US Adults, 1999–2010," *Journal of the American Medical Association* 307, no. 5 (2012): 491–97.

17. National Research Council, *U.S. Health in International Perspective: Shorter Lives, Poorer Health,* ed. S. H. Woolf and L. Aron (Washington, DC: The National Academies Press, 2013), WHO Global Infobase, www.who.int

18. Healthy People 2020, Framework: The Vision, Mission, and Goals of Healthy People 2020, www.healthypeople.gov

19. Centers for Medicare and Medicaid Services (CMS), National Health Expenditure Projections 2011–2021 Forecast Summary, 2011, www.cms.gov; Centers for Medicare and Medicaid Services, NHE Fact Sheet, January 2013, www.cms.gov

20. National Research Council, *U.S. Health in International Perspective: Shorter Lives, Poorer Health,* 2013.

21. U.S. Department of Health and Human Services, "Understanding the Affordable Health Care Act: Introduction" (2011), www.healthcare.gov

22. HealthCare.gov, Fact Sheet, "State Level Estimates of Gains in Insurance Coverage Among Young Adults" (June 2012), www.healthcare.gov

23. J. Prochaska, C. DiClemente, and J. Norcross, "In Search of How People Change: Application to Addictive Behaviors," *American Psychologist* 47, no. 9 (1983): 1102–14.

24. Centers for Disease Control Office of Surveillance, Epidemiology, and Laboratory Services, Behavioral Risk Factor Surveillance System, "Prevalence and Trends Data, Nationwide 2011, Exercise" (January 2013), www.cdc.gov

25. D. A. Hermon and G. A. Davis, "College Student Wellness: A Comparison Between Traditional- and Nontraditional-Age Students," *Journal of College Counseling* 7, no. 1 (2004): 32–9, doi: 10.1002/j.2161-1882.2004.tb00257.x

26. U.S. Department of Agriculture and U.S. Department of Health and Human Services, *Dietary Guidelines for Americans, 2010,* 7th edition (Washington, DC: U.S. Government Printing Office, December 2010).

27. U. S. Department of Agriculture, Center for Nutrition Policy and Promotion, "Report of the Dietary Guidelines Advisory Committee on the Dietary Guidelines for Americans, 2010" (January 2011), www.cnpp.usda.gov

28. T. M. Marteau, G. J. Hollands, and P. C. Fletcher, "Changing Human Behavior to Prevent Disease: The Importance of Targeting Automatic Processes," *Science* 337, no. 6101 (2012): 1492–95.

29. American College Health Association, *ACHA-NCHA II,* 2013, K. M. Leung et al., "Predictors of Physical Activities in Non-Traditional College Students," Abstract of Presented Paper, American Alliance for Health, Physical Education, Recreation, and Dance Annual Convention, Charlotte, North Carolina (April 2013).

30. Marteau, "Changing Human Behavior to Prevent Disease: The Importance of Targeting Automatic Processes," 2012.

31. M. Koring et al., "Synergistic Effects of Planning and Self-Efficacy on Physical Activity," *Health Education and Behavior* 39, no. 2 (2012): 152–8.

32. Marteau, "Changing Human Behavior to Prevent Disease: The Importance of Targeting Automatic Processes," 2012.

33. Z. Harakeh and W. A. Vollebergh, "The Impact of Active and Passive Peer Influence on Young Adult Smoking: An Experimental Study," *Drug and Alcohol Dependence* 121, no. 3," (2012): 220–3.

34. E. P. Sarafino, *Health Psychology* (New York: Wiley, 1990) 189–91.

35. University of Iowa Advising Center, "Motivation, Goal Setting, and Success," www.uiowa.edu

36. American College Health Association, *ACHA-NCHA II,* 2013.

getfitgraphic references

1. National Survey of Student Engagement, "NSSE Annual Results 2012: Promoting Student Learning and Institutional Improvement: Lessons from NSSE at 13," November 2012, http://nsse.iub.edu

2. S. D. Hanna, Y. Yuh, and S. Chatterjee, "The Increasing Financial Obligations Burden of US Households: Who Is Affected?" *International Journal of Consumer Studies* 36, no. 5 (2012): 588–94; American College Health Association, *American College Health Association—National College Health Assessment II (ACHA-NCHA II): Reference Group Executive Summary Fall 2012,* 2013.

3. Ibid.

4. State Higher Education Executive Officers Association, "The Economic Value of Post-Secondary Degrees," December 2012, www.sheeo.org

5. Data are from Sallie Mae, "How America Pays for College 2012," 2012, www.salliemae.com

6. Adapted from American Sociological Association, "Study: Young Adults from Middle Income Families at Higher Risk for Student Loan Debt Than Their Poorer Peers," August 2012, Based on paper "Disparities in Debt: Parents' Socioeconomic Resources and Young Adult Student Loan Debt" presented by J. Houle at ASA 107th Annual Meeting (Denver, CO: August 2012).

7. Ibid.

8. The Project on Student Debt, "State by State Data," 2012, http://projectonstudentdebt.org

9. Data adapted from L. Peñaloza and M. Barnhart, "Living U.S. Capitalism: The Normalization of Credit/Debt," *Journal of Consumer Research* 38, no. 4 (2011): 743–62, doi: 10.1086/660116

Name: _____ **Date:** _____

Instructor: _____ **Section:** _____

Purpose: This lab will help you assess your current level of wellness in each of the six dimensions and identify which wellness areas to target for behavior change.

Directions: Complete sections I–VI. For each item, indicate how often you think the statements describe you by checking the box under the relevant score. After each section, total your scores for that section and write your score in the space provided. After completing all sections, you will summarize, analyze, and reflect on your results in section VII.

SECTION I: PHYSICAL WELLNESS

	Never 1	Rarely 2	Sometimes 3	Often 4	Always 5
1. I listen to my body and make adjustments or seek professional help when something is wrong.					
2. I do moderate activity every day, such as taking the stairs instead of riding the elevator.					
3. I engage in vigorous exercise three to four times per week.					
4. I do exercises for muscular strength and endurance at least two times per week.					
5. I do stretching and limbering exercises at least five times per week.					
6. I do yoga, Pilates, tai chi, or other exercises for balance and core strength two or three times per week.					
7. I feel good about the condition of my body. I have lots of energy and can get through the day without being overly tired.					
8. I get adequate rest at night and wake on most mornings feeling ready for the day ahead.					
9. My immune system is strong, and my body heals quickly when I get sick or injured.					
10. I eat nutritious foods daily and avoid junk food.					
Total for Section I: Physical Wellness = _____					

SECTION II: SOCIAL WELLNESS

	Never 1	Rarely 2	Sometimes 3	Often 4	Always 5
1. I am open, honest, and get along well with others.					
2. I participate in a variety of social activities and enjoy all kinds of people.					
3. I try to be a *better person* and work on behaviors that have caused friction in the past.					
4. I am open and accessible to a loving and responsible relationship.					
5. I have someone I can talk to about private feelings.					
6. When I meet people, I feel good about the impression they have of me.					
7. I get along well with members of my family.					
8. I consider the feelings of others and do not act in hurtful or selfish ways.					
9. I try to see the good in my friends and help them feel good about themselves.					
10. I am good at listening to friends and family who need to talk.					
Total for Section II: Social Wellness = _____					

SECTION III: INTELLECTUAL WELLNESS

	Never 1	Rarely 2	Sometimes 3	Often 4	Always 5
1. I carefully consider options and possible consequences as I make choices.					
2. I am alert and ready to respond to life's challenges in ways that reflect thought and sound judgment.					
3. I learn from my mistakes and try to act differently the next time.					
4. I actively learn all I can about products and services before buying them.					
5. I manage my time well rather than letting time manage me.					
6. I follow directions or recommended guidelines and act in ways likely to keep myself and others safe.					
7. I consider myself to be a wise health consumer and check for reliable sources of information before making decisions.					
8. I have at least one personal-growth hobby that I make time for every week.					
9. My credit card balances are low, and my finances are in good order.					
10. I examine my own perceptions and then check evidence to see whether I was correct.					
Total for Section III: Intellectual Wellness = _____					

SECTION IV: EMOTIONAL WELLNESS

	Never 1	Rarely 2	Sometimes 3	Often 4	Always 5
1. I find it easy to laugh, cry, and show emotions such as love, fear, and anger and I try to express them in positive ways.					
2. I avoid using alcohol or drugs as a means to forget my problems or relieve stress.					
3. My friends regard me as a stable, well-adjusted person whom they trust and rely on for support.					
4. When I am angry, I try to resolve issues in nonhurtful ways rather than stewing about them.					
5. I try not to worry unnecessarily, and I try to talk about my feelings, fears, and concerns rather than letting them build up.					
6. I recognize when I'm stressed and take steps to relax through exercise, quiet time, or calming activities.					
7. I view challenging situations and problems as opportunities for growth.					
8. I feel good about myself and believe others like me for who I am.					
9. I try not to be too critical or judgmental of others.					
10. I am flexible and adapt to change in a positive way.					
Total for Section IV: Emotional Wellness = _____					

SECTION V: SPIRITUAL WELLNESS

	Never 1	Rarely 2	Sometimes 3	Often 4	Always 5
1. I take time alone to think about life's meaning and where I fit in to the greater whole.					
2. I believe life is a gift we should cherish.					
3. I look forward to each day as an opportunity for further growth.					
4. I experience life to the fullest.					
5. I take time to enjoy nature and the beauty around me.					
6. I have faith in a greater power, nature, or the connectedness of all living things.					
7. I engage in acts of care and goodwill without expecting something in return.					
8. I look forward to each day as an opportunity to grow and be challenged in life.					
9. I work for peace in my interpersonal relationships, my community, and the world at large.					
10. I have a great love and respect for all living things and regard animals as important links in a vital living chain.					
Total for Section V: Spiritual Wellness = _____					

SECTION VI: ENVIRONMENTAL WELLNESS

	Never 1	Rarely 2	Sometimes 3	Often 4	Always 5
1. I am concerned about environmental pollution and actively try to preserve and protect natural resources.					
2. I buy recycled paper and purchase biodegradable products whenever possible.					
3. I recycle my garbage, reuse containers, and try to minimize the amount of paper and plastics that I use.					
4. I consider whether my clothes are truly dirty before washing them to save on water and reduce detergent in our water sources.					
5. I try to reduce my use of gasoline and oil by limiting my driving.					
6. I write my elected leaders about environmental concerns.					
7. I turn down the heat and wear warmer clothes at home in the winter and use the air conditioner only when really necessary.					
8. I am aware of potential hazards in my area and try to reduce my exposure whenever possible.					
9. I use both sides of the paper when taking notes and doing assignments.					
10. I try not to leave the water running too long when I shower, shave, or brush my teeth.					
Total for Section VI: Environmental Wellness = _____					

SECTION VII: REFLECTION—YOUR PERSONAL WELLNESS CONTINUUM

1. Enter your totals for sections I–VI below:

Physical Wellness _____   **Emotional Wellness** _____

Social Wellness _____   **Spiritual Wellness** _____

Intellectual Wellness _____   **Environmental Wellness** _____

2. Understanding your scores:

Scores of 35–50: Outstanding! Your answers show that you are aware of the importance of these behaviors in your overall wellness, and that you are putting your knowledge to work by practicing good habits that should reduce your overall risks.

Scores of 30–34: Your wellness practices in these areas are very good, but there is room for improvement. What changes could you make to improve your score?

Scores of 20–29: Your wellness risks are showing. Find information about the risks you face and why it is important to change these behaviors.

Scores below 20: You may be taking unnecessary risks to your wellness. Identify each dimension and, whenever possible, seek additional resources for changing your behavior, either on your campus or through your local community health resources.

3. Which dimension did you score highest on? Which dimension did you score lowest on? Were you surprised by these results?

_____

_____

4. Discuss the potential health implications of your scores on the individual dimensions and your overall score.

_____

_____

Name: _____ Date: _____

Instructor: _____ Section: _____

Purpose: To learn how to chart your current personal wellness balance and identify the wellness areas in which you would like to improve.

Materials: Results from Lab 1.1

Directions: Follow the instructions below.

SECTION I: YOUR PERSONAL WELLNESS BALANCE

1. Create a personal wellness balance chart with your scores from sections I–VI of Lab 1.1. Allocate a larger "piece of the pie" for dimensions of wellness where your scores are higher and a smaller slice for dimensions with lower scores. Another option—allocate a larger slice for areas where you spend most of your time during a week.

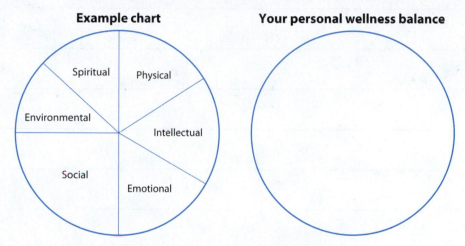

Example chart

Spiritual, Physical, Environmental, Intellectual, Social, Emotional

Your personal wellness balance

2. Now create your **goal wellness balance chart**. Change your current balance chart to reflect your desired scores in each wellness dimension, or to reflect the optimal percentage of time you would like to allocate to each dimension.

Goal wellness balance chart

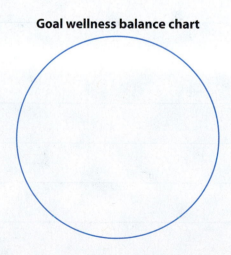

SECTION II: REFLECTION

Reflect on your answers, your wellness balance charts, and your wellness continuum (from the **Think! Act Now!** on page 5). What are your major areas of concern regarding your wellness? What two or three behaviors could you change easily to improve your wellness? Which one needs attention first?

_____

_____

_____

_____

_____

_____

_____

_____

_____

_____

_____

_____

_____

_____

_____

_____

_____

_____

_____

LAB 1.3

CREATE A BEHAVIOR CHANGE CONTRACT

MasteringHealth™

Name: _____ Date: _____

Instructor: _____ Section: _____

Purpose: To introduce students to the process of writing a behavior change contract and planning for new lifestyle behaviors. This introduction will serve as a model for other behavior change plans in subsequent chapters.

Directions: Complete the following sections.

SECTION I: PERSONAL WELLNESS REVIEW

1. Review your answers from Lab 1.1 and Lab 1.2.

2. Consider the stages of change (precontemplation, contemplation, preparation, action, maintenance) and evaluate your readiness to make a behavior change.

3. Choose a target behavior to change. For this behavior, you should be in the contemplation or preparation stages. Write the behavior below.

My behavior to change is _____

SECTION II: SHORT- AND LONG-TERM GOALS

1. **Long-Term Goal:** Long-term goals are those set for six months to a year or more. These goals should be achievable and may take many steps and an extended time to accomplish. Be sure to use SMART (specific, measurable, action-oriented, realistic, time-oriented) goal-setting guidelines when creating your long-term goal. After writing out your long-term goal, choose an appropriate target date and a reward for completing your goal.

   a. Long-Term Goal: _____

   b. Target Date: _____

   c. Reward: _____

2. **Short-Term Goals:** Short-term goals are those you want to achieve in less than six months. These goals will often help you reach your long-term goal. They may also be part of your long-term goal. Again, use SMART goal-setting guidelines when setting short-term goals. After writing out your short-term goals, choose appropriate target dates and rewards.

   a. Short-Term Goal #1: _____

   b. Target Date: _____

   c. Reward: _____

   a. Short-Term Goal #2: _____

   b. Target Date: _____

   c. Reward: _____

SECTION III: BEHAVIOR CHANGE OBSTACLES AND STRATEGIES

1. Below are **three obstacles** to changing this behavior (things I am currently doing or situations that contribute to this behavior or make it harder to change):

a. _____

b. _____

c. _____

2. Here are **three strategies** I will use to overcome the three obstacles:

a. _____

b. _____

c. _____

SECTION IV: GETTING SUPPORT

1. Resources I will use to help me change this behavior:

a. A friend/partner/relative: _____

b. A school-based resource: _____

c. A community-based resource: _____

d. A book or reputable website: _____

2. How will you use these supportive resources to help you with your goals?

_____

_____

SECTION V: CONTRACT, TRACKING, AND FOLLOW-UP

1. Contract: I intend to make the behavior change described above. I will use the strategies and rewards to achieve the goals that will contribute to a healthy behavior change.

Signed _____ Date _____

Witness _____ Date _____

2. Tracking: Tracking progress toward your goals is very important to ensure successful behavior change. As you move through this course, you will be asked to monitor your progress on several of your health, wellness, and fitness goals. Accurate and regular record-keeping is important.

3. Follow-up: When reaching your target date, it is important to follow up and reassess your program. During this course, you will be answering questions such as, Did you accomplish your goal? Do you need to set a new and more challenging goal? Do you need to alter your goals or program to make it more realistic? This section in your labs is important to modify your goals and your program and to set future goals.

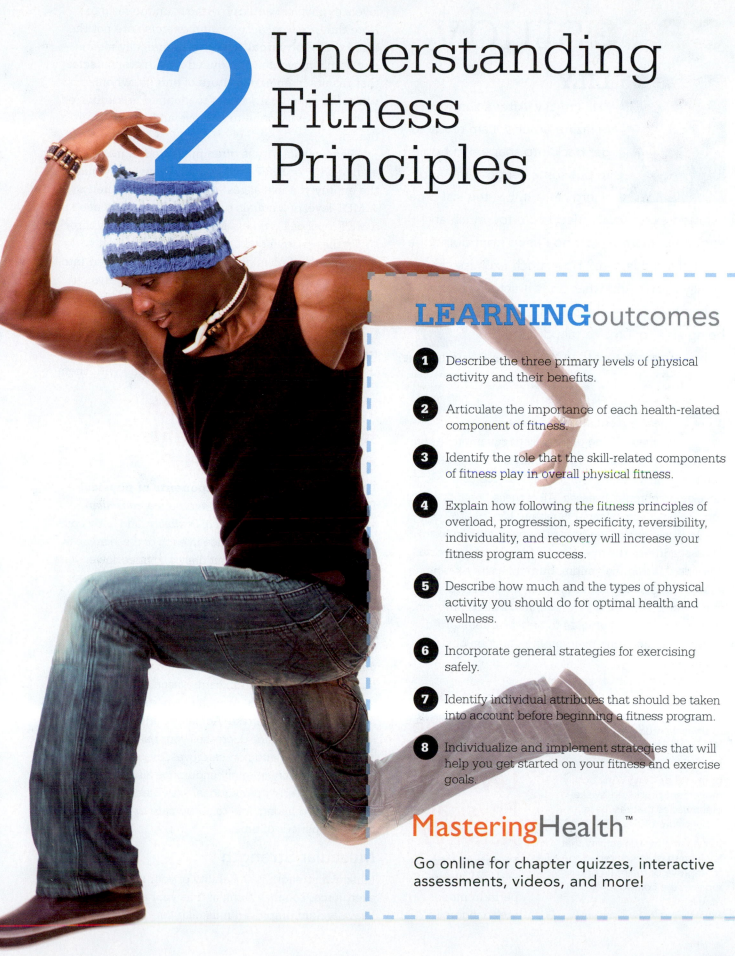

2 Understanding Fitness Principles

LEARNINGoutcomes

1 Describe the three primary levels of physical activity and their benefits.

2 Articulate the importance of each health-related component of fitness.

3 Identify the role that the skill-related components of fitness play in overall physical fitness.

4 Explain how following the fitness principles of overload, progression, specificity, reversibility, individuality, and recovery will increase your fitness program success.

5 Describe how much and the types of physical activity you should do for optimal health and wellness.

6 Incorporate general strategies for exercising safely.

7 Identify individual attributes that should be taken into account before beginning a fitness program.

8 Individualize and implement strategies that will help you get started on your fitness and exercise goals.

MasteringHealth™

Go online for chapter quizzes, interactive assessments, videos, and more!

casestudy

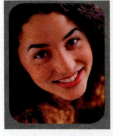

LILY

"Hi, I'm Lily. After a summer of lazing around, I am ready to get back into shape. I'm hoping to put some serious time and energy into it, but the last time I started exercising, I tried to do too much and ended up injured. How do I keep from doing the same thing this time? How much exercise do I really need? And what does it actually mean to be fit, anyway—does it just mean being able to run a certain distance, or is there more to it than that?"

HEAR IT! ONLINE

Fitness is a critical component of overall wellness. Being physically fit can improve your mood, give you more energy for daily activities, help you maintain a healthy weight, and reduce your risk of developing chronic diseases. All of these benefits can, in turn, help you live a longer, healthier life.

In this chapter, we cover the basic principles of fitness, address the question of how much exercise you need, introduce general guidelines for exercising safely, and discuss individual factors you should consider when designing your personal fitness program. Also, we go over strategies to help you get started exercising, including overcoming common obstacles to success.

physical fitness A set of attributes that relate to one's ability to perform moderate to vigorous levels of physical activity without undue fatigue

physical activity Any bodily movement produced by skeletal muscles that results in an expenditure of energy

exercise Physical activity that is planned or structured, done to improve or maintain one or more of the components of fitness

What Are the Three Primary Levels of Physical Activity?

Physical fitness is the ability to perform moderate to vigorous

levels of physical activity without undue fatigue. Note that *physical activity* and *exercise* are not the same thing: **physical activity** technically means any bodily movement produced by skeletal muscles that results in an expenditure of energy, whereas **exercise** specifically refers to planned or structured physical activity done to achieve and maintain fitness.

Physical activity is often measured in metabolic equivalents, or **MET** levels. A MET level of 1 equals the energy you use at rest or while sitting quietly. A MET level of 2 equals two times the energy used at a MET level of 1, while a MET level of 3 equals three times the energy used at a MET level of 1, and so forth. Levels of physical activity can be grouped into three primary categories: (1) *light/lifestyle/physical activities* (<3 METS), (2) *moderate physical activities* (3 to 6 METS), and (3) *vigorous physical activities* (>6 METS). **Figure 2.1** on the following page illustrates examples of each of these levels of physical activity, and the benefits that are associated with them.

What Are the Health-Related Components of Physical Fitness?

The five **health-related components of physical fitness** are *cardiorespiratory endurance, muscular strength, muscular endurance, flexibility,* and *body composition.* Minimal competence in each of these areas is necessary for you to carry out daily activities, lower your risk of developing chronic diseases, and optimize your health and well-being.

Cardiorespiratory Endurance

Cardiorespiratory endurance (also called *cardiovascular fitness/endurance, aerobic fitness,* and *cardiorespiratory fitness*) is the ability of the cardiovascular and respiratory systems to provide oxygen to working muscles during sustained exercise. Achieving adequate cardiorespiratory endurance decreases your risk of dying of cardiovascular and non-cardiovascular diseases.[1] Increased cardiorespiratory endurance also improves your ability to enjoy recreational activities, such as bicycling and hiking, and to participate in them for extended periods of time.

Muscular Strength

Muscular strength is the ability of your muscles to exert force. You may think of it as your ability to lift a heavy weight. Improved muscular strength decreases

Light/Lifestyle Physical Activities (<3 METS)	Examples:	Benefits:
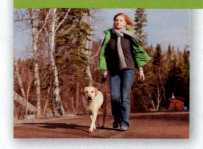	Light yard work and housework, leisurely walking, self-care and bathing, light stretching, light occupational activity	A moderate increase in health and wellness in those who are completely sedentary; reduced risk of some chronic diseases
Moderate Physical Activities (3–6 METS)	Examples:	Benefits:
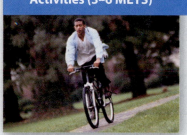	Walking 3–4.5 mph on a level surface, weight training, hiking, climbing stairs, bicycling 5–9 mph on a level surface, dancing, softball, recreational swimming, moderate yard work and housework	Increased cardiorespiratory endurance, lower body fat levels, improved blood cholesterol and pressure, better blood glucose management, decreased risk of disease, increased overall physical fitness
Vigorous Physical Activities (>6 METS)	Examples:	Benefits:
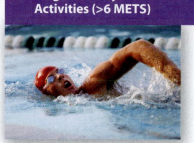	Jogging, running, circuit training, backpacking, aerobic classes, competitive sports, swimming laps, heavy yard work or housework, hard physical labor/construction, bicycling over 10 mph up steep terrain	Increased overall physical fitness, decreased risk of disease, further improvements in overall strength and endurance

FIGURE **2.1** Examples and benefits of light/lifestyle physical activity, moderate physical activity, and vigorous physical activity.

your risk of low bone density and musculoskeletal injuries.[2] In order to improve muscular strength, you need to tax your muscles in a controlled setting. This typically involves a weight room, as well as supervision to avoid injury.

Muscular Endurance

Muscular endurance is the ability of your muscles to contract repeatedly over time. Along with cardiorespiratory endurance, muscular endurance allows you to participate in recreational sports without undue fatigue. For example, in order to play a continuous game of basketball, you need to have good cardiorespiratory endurance to move up and down the court for the entire 90 minutes—and you need to have good muscular endurance to keep guarding, blocking, and shooting the ball effectively.

Flexibility

Flexibility is the ability to move your joints in a full range of motion. This component of fitness is often overlooked, but maintaining a minimal level of flexibility is important for overall wellness. Flexibility in your joints increases your ability to do the activities you enjoy and work toward specific fitness goals. Although we don't know whether stretching reduces overall injury rates, it may reduce specific muscle and tendon injuries.[3]

MET The standard metabolic equivalent used to estimate the amount of energy (oxygen) used by the body during physical activity; 1 MET = resting or sitting quietly

health-related components of physical fitness Components of physical fitness that have a relationship with good health

Having an adequate joint range of motion can be especially important to prevent neck and back pain when you are older and help prevent the decreased physical function associated with aging.[4]

Body Composition

Body composition refers to the relative amounts of fat and lean tissue in your body. Lean tissue consists of muscle, bone, organs, and fluids. A healthy body composition has adequate muscle tissue with moderate to low amounts of fat tissue. The recommendations for fat percentages will vary based upon your gender and age. Increased levels of fat will put you at risk for diabetes, heart disease, and certain cancers.

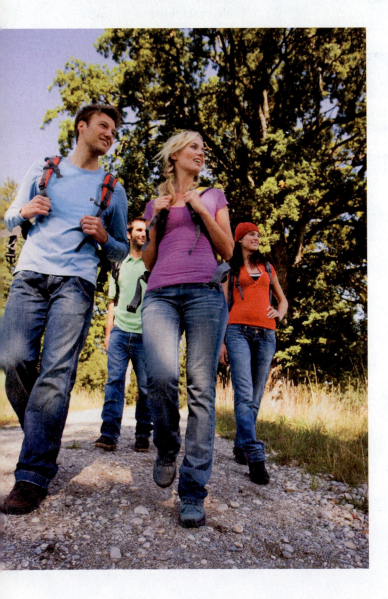

What Are the Skill-Related Components of Physical Fitness?

In addition to the five health-related components of fitness, physical fitness involves attributes that improve your ability to perform athletic, exercise, and daily functional tasks. These attributes are called the **skill-related components of fitness**. Often termed *sport skills,* these are qualities that athletes target to gain a competitive edge. Recreational athletes and general exercisers can also benefit from improving these sport skills. Maintaining a minimal level in each of these areas can help you in the long term, as well, by reducing the risk of falls as you age and by allowing you to maintain your independence. The six skill-related components of fitness are:

- *Agility:* The ability to rapidly change the position of your body with speed and accuracy

- *Balance:* The maintenance of equilibrium while you are stationary or moving

- *Coordination:* The ability to use both your senses and your body to perform motor tasks smoothly and accurately

- *Power:* The ability to perform work or contract muscles with high force quickly

- *Speed:* The ability to perform a movement in a short period of time

- *Reaction time:* The time between a stimulus and the initiation of your physical reaction to that stimulus

Although skill-related fitness is largely determined by heredity, regular training can result in significant improvements.[5] In order to improve skill-related components of fitness, athletes and exercisers first need to target the skills important to their specific sport or exercise. For instance, a runner can benefit from increasing power for hill running and speed for winning races, whereas a tennis player can benefit from increased agility and reaction time.

Improving your fitness skills can be as easy as participating regularly in any sport or activity. Playing football will increase reaction time and power, while dancing will increase balance, agility, and coordination. Another way to increase these skills is to perform drills that mimic a sport-specific skill, or work specifically on any of the skill-related components of fitness. You can practice drills in group exercise classes, or you can work with a personal trainer. Specialized equipment is often used in such drills: For example, exercises utilizing obstacles such as hurdles or cones can help you improve your speed, agility, and coordination, whereas using balance boards or exercise balls can help you improve your balance.

What Are the Principles of Fitness?

In order to design an effective fitness program, you need to consider the basic **principles of fitness** (also called *principles of exercise training*). These guiding principles explain how the body responds or adapts to exercise training.

Overload

The principle of **overload** states that in order to see improvements in your physical fitness, the amount or dose of training you undertake must be more than your body or specific body system is accustomed to. This applies to any of the components of physical fitness discussed earlier. For example, in order to increase your flexibility, you must stretch a little farther than you are used to.

Training Effects Consistent overloads or stresses on a body system will cause an *adaptation* to occur (**Figure 2.2**). An adaptation is a change in the body as a result of an overload. In exercise training this is called a *training effect*. For example, if you normally run two laps around a track each day but gradually increase this to four laps each day, the overload to your cardiorespiratory and muscular systems will cause adaptations in those systems. While you may feel tired and out of breath the first time you run four laps, after a few weeks of running those four laps the adaptations in your body will allow you to cover that distance with greater ease.

Dose-Response The amount of adaptation you can expect is directly related to the amount of overload or training dose that you complete. This is called the *dose-response relationship*. An increase in your "dose," or amount of training, will result in increased responses or adaptations to that training. How much response or adaptation you can expect is dependent upon the body system trained, the health or fitness outcome measured, and your individual physical and genetic characteristics.

Diminished Returns According to the concept of *diminished returns* (also called the *initial values principle*), the rate of fitness improvement diminishes over

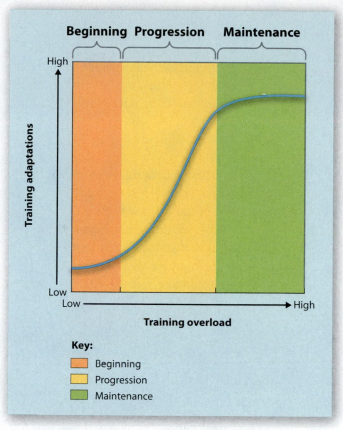

FIGURE **2.2** After adjusting to new training overloads at the beginning of your exercise program, you will see larger adaptations and improvements during the progression phase. As you approach your goal or genetic limits, your increases in overload will not result in further adaptations. This is a sign that you have reached a plateau and should maintain (if satisfied) or adjust your program for further improvement.

time as fitness levels approach genetic limits. Initial fitness levels determine the amount of improvement that you can achieve from exercise training overloads. If you are sedentary and far from your genetic limits, you might experience large increases in fitness levels from moderate amounts of training. If you are active and closer to your genetic limits already, you may gain only small increases in fitness from larger amounts of training.

Progression

The principle of **progression** states that in order to effectively and safely increase fitness, you need to apply an optimal level of overload to the body within a certain time period. Simply

principles of fitness General principles of exercise adaptation that guide fitness programming

overload Subjecting the body or body system to more physical activity than it is accustomed to

progression A gradual increase in a training program's intensity, frequency, and/or time

stated, you need to increase your workout levels enough to see results, but not so much that you increase your risk of injury. Your body will then progressively adapt to the overloads presented to it. To make sure that you are not progressing too quickly, follow the "10 percent rule": increase your program frequency, intensity, or duration by no more than 10 percent per week.

Specificity

The principle of **specificity** states that a body system will improve only if that specific body system is stressed or progressively overloaded by the physical activity. To follow this principle, make sure that you are training targeted muscle groups specific to your sport or that your program is specifically designed to meet your goals. For instance, if you are planning to walk a marathon, you should primarily *walk* during your training. If, instead, you decide to swim laps for the majority of your training, you may increase your cardiorespiratory fitness levels, but you will not be specifically training your lower body muscles to walk 26 miles.

Reversibility

All fitness gains are reversible, according to the principle of **reversibility**. This is the "use it or lose it" principle. If you do not maintain a minimal level of physical activity and exercise, your fitness levels will slip. Unfortunately, you cannot accumulate fitness or workout sessions in a "bank" for later. Doing a great deal of exercise in one week will not compensate for a subsequent month of doing no exercise. Whenever you stop exercising, it takes only one to two weeks to start losing fitness gains you may have made while training. Most of your improvements could be gone in a few months.[6] For example, if you spent four months running four miles three times a week, you could lose any fitness gains from those four months within two months of *no* training.

Individuality

The principle of **individuality** states that adaptations to a training overload may vary greatly from person to person. Genetics influence all individual differences in training adaptations. Two

specificity The principle that only the body systems worked during training will show adaptations

reversibility The principle that training adaptations will revert toward initial levels when training is stopped

individuality The variable nature of physical activity dose-response or adaptations in different persons

rest and recovery Taking a short time off from physical activities to allow the body to recuperate and improve

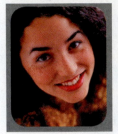
people may participate in the same training program but have very different responses. While you cannot control your genetic makeup, understanding how you respond to exercise is important in designing your personal fitness plan. A person who responds well to a training program is considered a *responder*. One who does not respond well is considered a *nonresponder*. Of those individuals who show improvements, some may respond better to increases in total amount of physical activity, while others may show more improvement with increases in exercise intensity. Figuring out your individual responses to certain exercise programs is a trial-and-error process. Complete regular fitness assessments and training logs to track your progress and then adjust your program accordingly to meet your goals.

Rest and Recovery

The principle of **rest and recovery** (also called the *principle of recuperation*) is critical to ensuring continued progress toward your fitness goals. As you will recall, the overload principle states that you must subject your body to more exercise than it is accustomed to doing. However, your body also needs time to recover from the increased physiological and structural training stresses that you place on it. In *resistance training* (also called *weight training*) in particular, most of the training adaptations actually take place during the rest periods between workouts.

Constant training day after day with insufficient rest periods can result in reduced health benefits and can eventually lead to **overtraining**. If you are exercising consistently and start feeling more fatigue and muscle soreness than usual during and after exercise, you could be doing too much. Reduce the duration or intensity of your exercise and rest for a day or two. To prevent overtraining and to gain optimal benefits from your training program, schedule regular rest days (one to three per week) in any cardio-respiratory endurance program and every other day for any strength training program. Another important tip to avoid overtraining and injury is to alternate hard workout days with easier workout days during your weekly plan.

How Much Exercise Is Enough?

How much exercise or physical activity do you really need? The answers will vary, depending on which sources you turn to and on your individual fitness goals. Most agree that the first step is to avoid inactivity, particularly sitting too much. A recent, large study found that the more you sit each day, the greater your risk of chronic health problems and diseases, like heart disease and diabetes.[7] Researchers found that even if you exercise some, the more you sit during the day, the higher your risk. Sitting more than four hours per day increased the risk for health problems, and sitting more than eight hours per day resulted in the highest risk levels. Whereas *any* amount of physical activity can confer basic health benefits, also aim to decrease your daily sitting time. Start by making sure that you are getting the minimal activity level recommendations given next. For additional health benefits and fitness improvements, follow the guidelines outlined in the Physical Activity Pyramid and the FITT Principle.

LIVE IT! ONLINE
Worksheet 26
How Much Do
I Move?

Minimal Physical Activity Level Guidelines

Guidelines for physical activity and exercise are issued by various organizations that rely on credible scientific research in developing their recommendations. These organizations can be *government agencies* (e.g., the President's Council on Physical Fitness and Sports), *professional organizations* (e.g., the American College of Sports Medicine), or *private organizations* (e.g., the American Heart Association). In 2008, the U.S. Department of Health and Human Services issued the first ever national physical activity guidelines designed to "provide achievable steps for youth, adults, and seniors, as well as people with special conditions to live healthier and longer lives."[8] The recommendations are echoed by other leading organizations, such as the World Health Organization and American College of Sports Medicine.[9]

As a nation, Americans are doing better meeting these guidelines, but there is still room to improve. When the guidelines were released in 2008, 18 percent of adults in the United States reported meeting both the aerobic and strength training guidelines.[10] In 2012, 20 percent of adults met the current guidelines for both aerobic and muscle strengthening activities. College-aged adults (18–24 years) fared a little better, with 28 percent meeting those same guidelines. However, the percentages drop as people age: Fewer than 13 percent of people 65 years and older reported enough aerobic and muscle strengthening activities in 2012 to meet the guidelines. The good news is that Americans have met the *Healthy People 2020* target for the number of adults getting both aerobic and muscle strengthening, the bad news is that still leaves 80 percent not getting enough of both types of activity.[11] How close are you to meeting these recommendations? Look at the guidelines in **Table 2.1** to find out.

The Physical Activity Pyramid Guides Weekly Choices

The Physical Activity Pyramid (**Figure 2.3** on the following page) visually summarizes minimal physical activity and exercise guidelines for optimal health and wellness. The Physical Activity Pyramid's bottom layer represents light or lifestyle activities that you should strive to incorporate into your everyday life. Light physical activity every day, such as walking and gardening,

is a great way to start and to ensure a strong "base" to your pyramid! The next layer of the pyramid represents moderate-to-vigorous aerobic and/or sports activities that you should try to do three to five times per week in order to build cardiorespiratory endurance and fitness. Aim to accumulate at least 150 minutes of moderate physical activity each week, such as quick walking or flat bicycling, or 75 minutes of vigorous activity each week, such as swimming or jogging. The third layer of the pyramid represents strength-training and flexibility-building exercises that you should try to incorporate at least two days per week. The top layer of the pyramid represents the activities that should ideally receive the least amount of your time—sedentary activities such as watching TV or surfing the Web—in favor of more active pursuits.

The box Tips for Getting Up and Moving on the following page provides suggestions for how to incorporate more physical activity into your daily life.

TABLE **2.1** Physical Activity Guidelines for Americans			
	Key Guidelines for Health*	For Additional Fitness or Weight Loss Benefits*	PLUS
Adults	150 min/week moderate-intensity OR 75 min/week of vigorous-intensity OR Equivalent combination of moderate- and vigorous-intensity (i.e., 100 min moderate-intensity + 25 min vigorous-intensity)	300 min/week moderate-intensity OR 150 min/week of vigorous-intensity OR Equivalent combination of moderate- and vigorous-intensity (i.e., 200 min moderate-intensity + 50 min vigorous-intensity) OR More than the previously described amounts	Muscle strengthening activities for all the major muscle groups at least 2 days/week
Older Adults	If unable to follow above guidelines, then as much physical activity as your condition allows	If unable to follow above guidelines, then as much physical activity as your condition allows	In addition to muscle strengthening activities, those with limited mobility should add exercises to improve balance and reduce risk of falling
Children and Adolescents	60 min or more of moderate- or vigorous-intensity physical activity daily	Add vigorous-intensity physical activities within the 60 daily minutes at least 3 days/week	Include muscle and bone strengthening activities within the 60 daily minutes at least 3 days/week Activities should be age-appropriate, enjoyable, and varied

*Notes: Avoid inactivity, some activity is better than none; accumulate physical activity in sessions of 10 minutes or more at one time; and spread activity throughout the week.

Source: "2008 Physical Activity Guidelines for Americans: Be Active, Healthy, and Happy!" from the Office of Disease Prevention and Health Promotion, U.S. Department of Health and Human Services website, 2008, www.hhs.gov

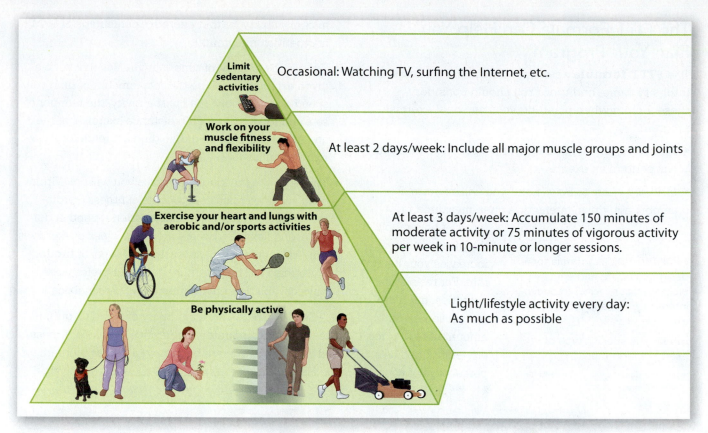

FIGURE **2.3** The Physical Activity Pyramid presents recommended levels of activity for optimal health and wellness.

 TOOLS FOR **CHANGE**

Tips for Getting Up and Moving

You can improve your fitness level simply by adding more physical activity to your daily life and reducing your sitting time. Below are a few ways you can incorporate more physical activity:

- Instead of driving your car or taking the bus to campus, ride your bike or walk.

- If you must drive or bus to campus, park your car farther from your destination or get off a bus stop earlier than usual.

- If you have a dog, walk it daily. If you already do that, add a second daily walk—your dog will love you for it!

- Carry a handbasket while grocery shopping instead of pushing a cart (assuming your grocery list is not very long).

- If you have children, play actively with them.

- If you have a desk job or study for long periods of time, get up and walk around often. Try doing push-ups or curl-ups while waiting for files to download.

- If you sit a lot during the day for work or school, can you create a standing work area instead? Try putting your computer or books on a counter at standing height, or ask if work stations that can transform from sitting to standing are available at your workplace.

- Stand or walk around inside while talking on the phone. On hold? Use that time to do a few stretches!

- Study while exercising! Complete class readings or study notes while on a stationary bike.

- Don't sit while watching TV or movies. Stretch or do exercises during commercial breaks, or watch TV from an exercise bike or treadmill.

THINK! Examine the Physical Activity Pyramid. How does your weekly physical activity match up to its recommendations? In which areas of the pyramid could you improve?

ACT! Draw your current physical activity pyramid. Now draw your physical activity pyramid incorporating the simple suggestions above. This week, list the activities you could add to your week to become more active.

The FITT Formula Can Help You Plan Your Program

The **FITT formula** acronym stands for frequency, intensity, time, and type. You should consider these factors when planning your personal exercise program.

- *Frequency* is the number of times per week that you will perform an exercise.

- *Intensity* refers to how "hard" you will exercise. For aerobic activities, intensity is often measured in terms of how much the given activity increases your heart rate. For resistance activities, intensity is represented in the amount of resistance or weight lifted as a percentage of your maximal ability for that exercise (percentage of 1RM or repetition maximum).

- *Time* is the amount of time that you will devote to a given exercise. It can be the total amount of time you spend on an aerobic or a sport activity, the number of sets and repetitions for a resistance exercise, or the amount of time you spend holding a stretch for a flexibility exercise.

- *Type* refers to the kind of exercise you will do. Within each of the exercise components of fitness (cardiorespiratory endurance, muscular strength and endurance, and flexibility), there are many types of exercises that will increase fitness levels. Your type, or **mode**, of exercise will be determined by your preferences, physical abilities, environment, and personal goals.

See **Figure 2.4** for a summary of the FITT guidelines for cardiorespiratory endurance, muscular fitness, and flexibility. If you are beginning a fitness program for the first time, you may want to start with the physical

FITT formula A formula for designing a safe and effective program that specifies frequency, intensity, time, and type of exercise

mode The specific type of exercise performed

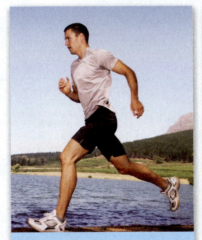 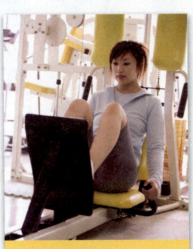 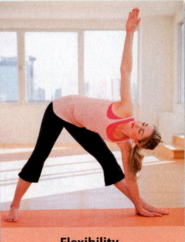

	Cardiorespiratory Endurance	**Muscular Fitness**	**Flexibility**
Frequency	3–5 days per week	2–3 days per week	Minimally 2–3 days per week
Intensity	Moderate and/or vigorous intensity	50–80% of 1RM	To the point of tightness
Time	20–60 minutes	8–10 exercises, 1–4 sets, 8–20 reps	10–30 seconds per stretch, 2–4 reps
Type	Any rhythmic, continuous, large muscle group activity	Resistance training (with body weight and/or external resistance) for all major muscle groups	Stretching, dance, or yoga exercises for all major muscle groups

FIGURE **2.4** The FITT principle applied to summary guidelines for cardiorespiratory endurance, muscular fitness, and flexibility.

Data from: American College of Sports Medicine, *ACSM's Guidelines for Exercise Testing and Prescription*, 9th edition (Baltimore: Lippincott Williams & Wilkins, 2014).

activity guidelines in Table 2.1. When you are ready, add appropriate levels of the Physical Activity Pyramid and then customize your program using the FITT formula to suit your personal goals.

What Does It Take to Exercise Safely?

Exercise-related injuries have risen in recent decades. More than 7 million Americans receive medical attention for sports-related injuries each year, with the greatest numbers of injuries affecting 5- to 24-year-olds.[12] To reduce your risk of exercise injury, follow the guidelines below.

Warm Up Properly Before Your Workout

A proper warm-up consists of two phases: a general warm-up and a specific warm-up. In a *general warm-up,* your goal is to warm up the body by doing 5–10 minutes of light physical activity similar to the activities you will be performing during exercise. During this period of time (called the *rest-to-exercise transition*), you are preparing your body to withstand the more vigorous exercise to come. Your core body temperature should rise a few degrees, and you should break a slight sweat. This movement and temperature rise will increase your overall blood flow, ready the joint fluid and structures, and improve muscle elasticity.

During a *specific warm-up,* your goal is to focus on the particular muscle groups and joints that you will be using during the activity set. This part of the warm-up should consist of three to five minutes of **range-of-motion** movements. You should move the joints involved in your exercise through the range of motion that they will experience

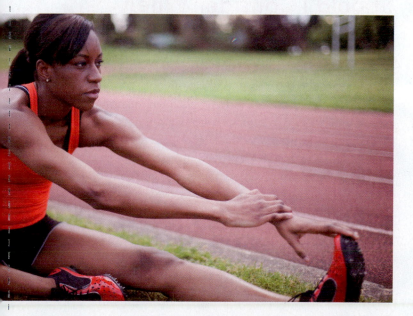

during the activity. Move joints through a full range of motion in a relaxed and controlled manner. If you want to add light stretching to your warm-up, do so at the end of your specific warm-up.

Cool Down Properly After Your Workout

After you finish your workout, cool down in a manner that is appropriate to the activity that you performed. This *exercise-to-rest transition* should last anywhere from 5 to 15 minutes. If your heart rate and temperature rose during your workout, you should perform a *general cool-down* in which your goal is to bring your heart rate, breathing rate, and temperature closer to resting levels. This cool-down is usually a less vigorous version of the activity you just performed. For example, if you jogged for 25 minutes, your general cool-down may consist of 10 minutes of walking.

If you have just finished a resistance-training program and your heart rate is not elevated, you should perform a *specific cool-down* for the joints and muscles you have exercised. A specific cool-down can be performed after a general cool-down for aerobic activities and right after exercise for resistance training activities. During a specific cool-down, you should stretch the muscle groups worked during the activity.

Take the Time to Properly Learn the Skills for Your Chosen Activity

There are hundreds of different activities that you can do to increase your health and fitness, each with a specific set of physical skills required for participation. You might choose simple activities, such as walking or jogging, which require little skill and have short learning curves, or you might choose difficult activities, such as fencing or hockey, which require more complex skills. Whatever you choose, properly learn the physical skills required for the activity to enhance your enjoyment and to avoid injury. If you are just beginning a sport for the first time—for example, skiing—do not immediately approach the sport the way a more experienced athlete would. Take lessons, start on the beginner slopes, and give yourself time to safely perform your chosen activity.

> **range-of-motion** The movement limits that limbs have around a specific joint

Consume Enough Energy and Water for Exercise

Deciding how much to eat and drink prior to exercise can be tricky. You need enough energy to work out, but you should not exercise on a full stomach. Eating a small meal 1½ to 2 hours before exercise is a good way to make sure that you have energy (but not an upset stomach) during the workout. A light snack 30–60 minutes before your workout is acceptable as well.

Dehydration is more likely than food intake to affect your exercise performance. During the hours before your workout, be sure to drink enough water so that you do not feel thirsty as you go into your exercise session. Guidelines for drinking before, during, and after exercising should be tailored to the individual and the exercise session.[13] General guidelines are 17–20 oz. of fluid two to three hours before exercise and 7–10 oz. of fluid 10–20 minutes prior to exercise.[14] During your workout, hydrate when you feel thirsty, and increase the amount of water you consume as you start to sweat more profusely.

Select Appropriate Footwear and Clothing

Consider this: Your feet will typically strike the ground 1,000 times during one mile of running. Over weeks of training, that translates to a great deal of wear and tear on your feet and lower body. Needless to say, proper footwear is critical to a safe and successful training program—regardless of the activity you choose.

While some sports require specialized footwear, most beginning exercisers just need one pair of good, all-around cross-trainers or running shoes. The most important aspect of footwear is proper fit and cushioning. Always try on shoes before purchasing them, and, if possible, spend a few minutes mimicking the activity you will be doing in them. The best shoes are not always the most expensive ones, but you should aim to purchase the highest-quality footwear you can afford. Ask for assistance from a knowledgeable salesperson—let him or her know what activities you are planning to pursue, and ask which shoes would be most appropriate for your plans.

Clothing for exercise can be very simple (e.g., shorts and a T-shirt) or very technical (e.g., clothing with wicking fibers or special treatments for protection against harsh weather). The most important thing is to dress appropriately for your chosen activity. Make sure that your clothing is comfortable and does not restrict your range of motion. Women may wish to wear supportive athletic

casestudy

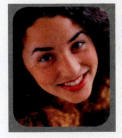

LILY

"I've started jogging again! I'm back to jogging 30 minutes twice a week and thinking of bumping things up to three times a week. I'm hoping to eventually work my way up to jogging for 45 minutes straight, each time I go out. I'm not tempted to run a 10k again any time soon, but if I can keep this new routine going, maybe I will be ready for a 5k—without hurting my knees this time."

THINK! What kinds of things would you advise Lily to do, in order to reduce her chances of injury?

ACT NOW! Today, describe Lily's exercise routine, using the FITT formula. This week, figure out what you might do the same or different from her. In two weeks, figure out what system you will use for tracking your physical activities (journal, log, smart phone, etc.).

HEAR IT! ONLINE

---

bras, and men may want to consider wearing supportive compression shorts or undergarments. If you are planning to exercise outdoors, take temperature into consideration and dress accordingly. The longer you plan to exercise, the more carefully you should think about what to wear for a successful workout.

What Individual Factors Should I Consider When Designing a Fitness Program?

There is no such thing as a "one-size-fits-all" physical fitness program. Different individuals have different needs, and general recommendations often need to be adapted to fit those individual needs. Your age, weight, current fitness level, and any disabilities and special health concerns are all factors that should be considered when designing a safe and effective exercise routine.

Age

Healthy individuals of all ages can become more active; however, older adults may require additional precautions in order to prevent injury while exercising. Men over age 45 and women over age 55 should look closely at their health and cardiovascular risks before initiating a vigorous exercise program.[15] Moderate aerobic activity, muscle-strengthening exercises, and flexibility work are all recommended activities for older adults. In addition, balance exercises should be included to help prevent the risk of falls and injury.

Weight

Overweight individuals are at higher risk of musculoskeletal injuries due to increased stress on their muscles and joints, and they should take precautions to ensure safe workouts. If you are overweight, consider a cross-training routine with a mix of moderate weight-bearing (e.g., walking and stair-climbing) and non-weight-bearing (e.g., bicycling and water exercise) activities. If you feel pain in your lower-body joints during exercise, shift to more non-weight-bearing activities during your workout.

Underweight individuals, on the other hand, should perform more strength-training and weight-bearing activities to ensure proper muscle and bone maintenance.

Current Fitness Level

Design a program that suits your current fitness level. If you already exercise regularly, consider gradually increasing the frequency or intensity of your workouts to realize more fitness gains. If you are currently sedentary and are just beginning to think about starting an exercise routine, do not just suddenly attempt to participate in a triathlon! Pick an activity that you find enjoyable, start at a level that is comfortable for you, and proceed from there.

Disabilities

If you have mobility restrictions, poor balance, dizziness, or other physically limiting conditions, you can still incorporate activity into your daily life with alternative or adaptive exercises. Many colleges, community centers, parks and recreation facilities, and fitness centers offer adaptive courses, equipment, and specially trained instructors to help you meet your fitness goals. After obtaining medical clearance, seek out such facilities; your physician or a physical therapist may have good recommendations. The box Physical Activity and Sport for Everyone on page 42 provides additional suggestions.

Special Health Concerns

Certain medical conditions may require you to exercise under medical supervision. Anyone with symptoms of diagnosed metabolic, cardiovascular, renal, or pulmonary disease (including asthma) needs to obtain medical clearance before beginning an exercise program.[16] If you have special health concerns, seek out the advice of a qualified medical professional on how to exercise safely.

Individuals with significant bone or joint problems can benefit from selecting lower-impact activities such as swimming, water exercise, bicycling, walking, or low-impact aerobics. They can also benefit from resistance training exercises that can strengthen muscles and joint structures and contribute to bone-density maintenance and improvement (if their joint limitations will allow it).

If you are taking any prescription medications, ask your doctor whether there are side effects that you should consider before exercising. In addition, beware of over-the-counter medications and other products that may cause drowsiness (e.g., antihistamines, certain cough/cold medicines, and alcohol), as this will decrease your reaction time, coordination, and balance.

(If you are pregnant, the box Can I Exercise While I'm Pregnant? in Chapter 15 offers advice on exercising safely while expecting.)

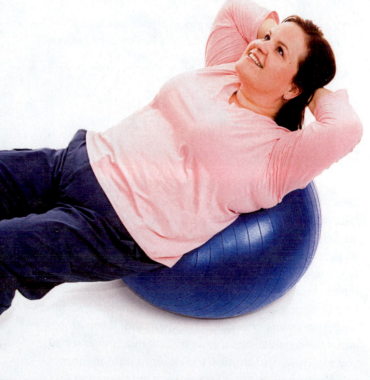

DIVeRSiTY
Physical Activity and Sport for Everyone

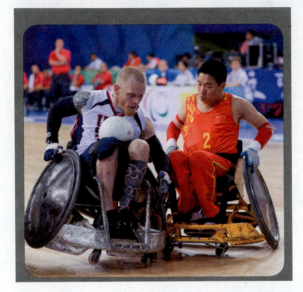

In the summer of 2012 the Paralympic Games were held in London after the Summer Olympic Games. There were over 4,000 athletes from 164 countries competing in 20 different sports.[1] Whether it was archery, judo, swimming, tennis, powerlifting, or one of the other sports, the athletes' stories are an inspiration to persons of all abilities across the globe. The athleticism displayed at the games demonstrates that physical limitations do not have to hinder the achievement of even the highest levels of physical fitness.

With personal motivation, support from friends and family, and assistance from medical and fitness professionals, persons with disability can make exercise part of their daily routine and live physically active lives. In fact, the U.S. Department of Health and Human Services recommends that adults with disabilities follow the 2008 Physical Activity Guidelines for Americans, adjusting as necessary for varying abilities and physician recommendations.[2] Unfortunately, only about 10 percent of persons with disabilities meet the recommended guidelines.[3]

There are various options available for modifying physical activities and helping all people achieve their health and fitness goals. For example, most strength-training machines are used from a seated position and can be operated by people in wheelchairs. Rubber exercise bands, meanwhile, can serve as alternative strength-building aids. Many companies offer modified sports equipment for people with disabilities: Handcycles allow people to ride bikes using arm power, and wakeboards and flotation devices enable waterskiing and swimming activities. Several kinds of seated skis make downhill skiing accessible to those with physical handicaps. And as witnessed in the Paralympic Games, persons with physical limitations can play a long list of sports, including volleyball, tennis, golf, soccer, basketball, bowling, bocci, archery, tai chi, and karate.

1. Official website of the Paralympic Movement, March 2013, www.paralympic.org
2. Office of Disease Prevention and Health Promotion, U.S. Department of Health and Human Services, *2008 Physical Activity Guidelines for Americans: Be Active, Healthy, and Happy!* ODPHP Publication no. U0036 (Washington, DC: U.S. Department of Health and Human Services, 2008).
3. J. S. Schiller, J. W. Lucas, and J. A. Peregoy, "Summary health statistics for U.S. adults: National Health Interview Survey, 2011," *National Center for Health Statistics, Vital Health Stat*, no. 256 (2012).

How Can I Get Started Improving My Fitness Behaviors?

You know that exercise is good for you, but starting a fitness program and sticking with it over the long term can be a real challenge! Worldwide, over 31 percent of adults are physically inactive and that number rises to over 43 percent in the United States.[17] Despite the statistics, making fitness part of your daily life is within your reach—and can be tremendously fun and rewarding. However, preparing to exercise for the first time (or after a long sedentary period) can be daunting. If you are unsure how to start, what to do, or how much to exercise, you may have the impulse to just jump right in, do something your friends are doing, or try something you saw on TV or in a magazine. This haphazard approach often leads to disappointment and frustration—not to mention muscle soreness and even injury. A better approach is to think carefully about your exercise motivations, goals, and needs; select activities that will meet those needs (and that you enjoy!); apply the FITT formula to each of those activities, and then make a conscious long-term commitment to your exercise program.

As you plan your fitness program, ask yourself: What motivates me? What obstacles are in my way? What are reasonable fitness goals I can set for myself? Am I prepared to commit to a fitness program? To begin, fill out **Lab 2.1** to assess your current readiness for a physical activity behavior change and to determine whether you should see a health care provider before beginning to exercise.

DO IT! ONLINE

Understand Your Motivations for Beginning a Fitness Program

If you understand your motivations for participating in a fitness program, you can plan activities in a way that makes you more likely to stick with the program. Below are some of the most common reasons people decide to exercise, along with tips for how to maximize your chances of long-term fitness success.

- *I want to gain health benefits.* If this is your main motivation, try to design a program centered on physical activities that you find *enjoyable* and *easy to incorporate* in your day-to-day life. If you don't like gyms, don't sign up for one! Instead, select an activity in which you genuinely take pleasure, such as walking with a friend or family member.

- *I want to have fun.* If your main motivation is fun, consider joining an intramural sports team on campus, or going on regular outdoor trips with friends. Seek out activities that, first and foremost, you know you will enjoy, and that have the beneficial "side effect" of fitness.

- *I want to meet new people or exercise with friends.* Participating in a fitness program can be a great way to socialize. Even if you do not consider this one of your main reasons to start exercising, social motivations can often keep you coming back. Look for activity classes, clubs, or teams that you can join with friends or where you can meet new people with similar interests.

- *I like the challenge of setting goals and doing well in competition.* If this sounds like you, regardless of what activity you choose, be sure to set realistic, attainable goals. You may find a clearly defined target—such as an upcoming 5K race—to be just what you need to get started, so sign up!

- *I want to lose some weight.* If weight loss is your main motivation, you will need to consider your nutrition and diet plan along with your fitness plan. Choose fitness activities that burn plenty of calories and that you will enjoy doing often.

- *I would like to have a stronger, more toned body.* If this is your primary reason for exercise, select your favorite aerobic activity, begin strength training, or take a sport-specific class regularly. Regular exercise will help your brain, too, as you can see in the GetFitGraphic on page 47.

Anticipate and Overcome Obstacles to Exercise

If you are not currently physically active, why not? Are you too busy? Do you simply dislike exercise?

You can probably immediately identify several things that keep you from being as active as you want to be. Obstacles, or **barriers to physical activity**, can be categorized as either environmental or personal. *Environmental barriers* include both external/physical factors and social/interpersonal factors that may make it harder or easier for you to exercise. Do you feel safe exercising on the streets around your campus? Is the weather conducive to exercising? Are facilities open during the hours that you need them? Do you have friends who exercise and who might be interested in exercising with you? These external factors can greatly affect your exercise habits.

Likewise, *personal barriers* can play a role in whether you are successful in sticking to an exercise plan. Typical personal barriers include lack of self-motivation, injury, starting fitness levels and weight, disability, relationship difficulties, or psychological problems such as depression or anxiety. Older-than-average students, students with children, and those who work long hours while attending school often face unique challenges as they work to improve their fitness levels. The box Overcoming Common Obstacles to Exercise provides strategies for overcoming specific obstacles. **Lab 2.2** helps you assess your motivations for exercise and identify your obstacles to beginning a fitness program.

DO IT! ONLINE

> **barriers to physical activity** Personal or environmental issues that hinder your participation in regular physical activity

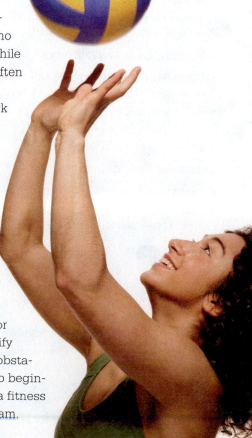

TOOLS FOR CHANGE

Overcoming Common Obstacles to Exercise

Below are lists of strategies for overcoming common obstacles to exercise.

Obstacle: Lack of Time

- Monitor your daily activities for one week. Identify at least three 30-minute time slots you could use for physical activity.
- Add physical activity to your daily routine. For example, walk or ride your bike to work or shopping, walk the dog, exercise while you watch TV, and so on.
- Select activities requiring minimal time, such as walking, jogging, or stair-climbing.

Obstacle: Lack of Social Support

- Explain your interest in physical activity to friends and family. Ask them to support your efforts.
- Invite friends and family members to exercise with you. Plan social activities involving exercise.
- Develop new friendships with physically active people. Join a group, such as the YMCA or a hiking club.

Obstacle: Lack of Energy

- Schedule physical activity for times in the day or week when you feel energetic.
- Convince yourself that if you give it a chance, physical activity will increase your energy level; then try it.

Obstacle: Lack of Willpower

- Plan ahead. Make physical activity a regular part of your schedule and write it on your calendar.
- Invite a friend to exercise with you on a regular basis and write it on your calendar.
- Join an exercise group or class.

Obstacle: Fear of Injury

- Learn how to warm up and cool down to prevent injury.
- Learn how to exercise appropriately considering your age, fitness level, skill level, and health status.
- Choose activities involving minimum risk.

Obstacle: Lack of Skill

- Select activities requiring no new skills, such as walking, climbing stairs, or jogging.
- Exercise with friends who are at your skill level.
- Find a friend who is willing to teach you some new skills.
- Take a class to develop new skills.

Obstacle: Lack of Resources

- Select activities that require minimal facilities or equipment, such as walking, jogging, jumping rope, or calisthenics.
- Identify inexpensive, convenient resources available in your community (community education programs, park and recreation programs, worksite programs, etc.).

Obstacle: Weather Conditions

- Develop a set of regular activities that are always available regardless of weather (indoor cycling, aerobic dance, indoor swimming, stair-climbing, mall-walking, dancing, gymnasium games, etc.).

Obstacle: Travel

- Put a jump rope and resistance bands in your suitcase.
- Walk the halls and climb the stairs in hotels.
- Stay in places with swimming pools or exercise facilities.
- Join the YMCA or YWCA.
- Visit the local shopping mall and walk for half an hour or more.
- Pack your favorite aerobic exercise DVD.

Obstacle: Family Obligations

- Trade babysitting time with a friend, neighbor, or family member who also has small children.
- Exercise with the kids—go for a walk together, play tag or other running games, get an aerobic dance or exercise video for kids, and exercise together.
- Hire a babysitter and look at the cost as a worthwhile investment in your health.
- Jump rope, do calisthenics, ride a stationary bicycle, or use other home gymnasium equipment while the kids are busy playing or sleeping.
- Try to exercise when the kids are not around (e.g., during school hours or their nap time).

THINK! What obstacles to exercise do you anticipate?

ACT NOW! Today, for each obstacle, write down how you will get around it. This week, post reminders around your home and work to help you "stick" to your plan. In two weeks, try a different motivational strategy than you have tried in the past.

Source: Adapted from Centers for Disease Control and Prevention, "Physical Activity for Everyone: Overcoming Barriers to Physical Activity," March 2013, www.cdc.gov and U.S. Department of Health and Human Services, *Promoting Physical Activity: A Guide For Community Action*, 2nd Edition, 1999.

Make Time for Exercise

People often state that they don't exercise because they don't have enough time. That might be the case—or they may simply be assigning exercise a lesser priority in their life than other activities, such as watching TV or text-messaging friends. While socializing and scheduling downtime in a busy life *are* important, consider how much time you spend in your life on sedentary activities. Then consider the benefits to your health and sense of well-being that would result if you replaced some of that sedentary time with physical activity.

To successfully stick with a fitness program, you need to prioritize exercise the same way that you prioritize your classes, homework, job, and social life. Schedule your exercise sessions into your calendar. Prove to yourself that you are serious about getting fit by *making* the time for exercise. Get started by completing **Lab 2.3**, where you will make a plan to incorporate more physical activity into your daily life.

DO IT! ONLINE

Select Fun and Convenient Activities

Even if you have committed to set aside time to exercise, you may not always *want* to. If you are accustomed to a sedentary lifestyle, it can be difficult to tear yourself away from the computer or to get off the couch. One way to counter a lack of motivation is to choose fun activities. If your workout is a form of play, you will look forward to it time and time again.

Choosing the best type of exercise is often also about convenience. Despite your good intentions and high level of motivation when starting a new activity, if it's not convenient for your existing lifestyle and commitments, you will have a hard time sticking with it. Look for activities, facilities, and workout times that make sense for your schedule.

Activities can be classified into three general categories or types: lifestyle physical activities, exercise training options, and sports and recreational activities. **Figure 2.5** illustrates sample moderate to vigorous lifestyle, exercise, and sports activities that you can choose from to meet activity guidelines and increase your fitness level.

Lifestyle Physical Activities Lifestyle physical activities are those that you perform during daily life. These include things such as walking the dog and bicycling to class. Lifestyle physical activities can be light, moderate, or vigorous, depending on what the task is and how long it takes you. For instance, watering your garden for 15 minutes may be a light activity, but raking leaves for four hours can be vigorous.

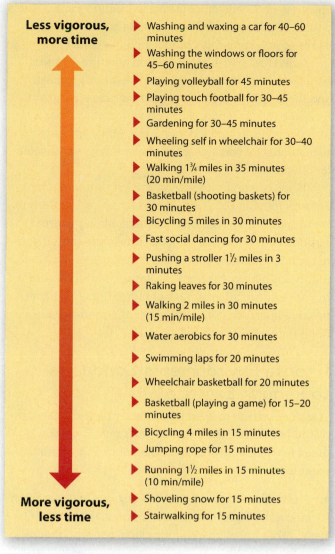

Less vigorous, more time

- Washing and waxing a car for 40–60 minutes
- Washing the windows or floors for 45–60 minutes
- Playing volleyball for 45 minutes
- Playing touch football for 30–45 minutes
- Gardening for 30–45 minutes
- Wheeling self in wheelchair for 30–40 minutes
- Walking 1¾ miles in 35 minutes (20 min/mile)
- Basketball (shooting baskets) for 30 minutes
- Bicycling 5 miles in 30 minutes
- Fast social dancing for 30 minutes
- Pushing a stroller 1½ miles in 3 minutes
- Raking leaves for 30 minutes
- Walking 2 miles in 30 minutes (15 min/mile)
- Water aerobics for 30 minutes
- Swimming laps for 20 minutes
- Wheelchair basketball for 20 minutes
- Basketball (playing a game) for 15–20 minutes
- Bicycling 4 miles in 15 minutes
- Jumping rope for 15 minutes
- Running 1½ miles in 15 minutes (10 min/mile)
- Shoveling snow for 15 minutes
- Stairwalking for 15 minutes

More vigorous, less time

FIGURE **2.5** Sample moderate to vigorous physical activities.

Source: Data from Centers for Disease Control and Prevention, "A Report of the Surgeon General: Physical Activity and Health At-A-Glance, 1996," Accessed May 2013, www.cdc.gov

Exercise Training Options Most people think of typical exercise options when asked how they will increase their fitness. These include aerobics classes, jogging or running, weight training, indoor cardio workouts, yoga, tai chi, lap swimming, and water aerobics. These activities are great for specifically increasing your fitness. However, consider including a variety of activities to counter the boredom that may come from doing the same exercise week after week. Add a few sports and recreational activities every now and then to keep yourself motivated and your body challenged.

Sports and Recreational Activities Traditional team sports offer a great deal of fun, motivation, and fitness. Most cities have sports leagues for adult soccer, softball, basketball, ultimate Frisbee, and other team sports. If you like the camaraderie of working with a team and enjoy the challenge of team sports, strongly consider this option. You may be able to find team sports classes on campus, at community centers, and in sports clubs.

Individual sports activities can offer great fitness benefits as well. Court sports such as tennis, squash, and racquetball will increase your cardiorespiratory fitness and muscle endurance and will improve your agility, coordination, and reaction time. Many sports are recreational for some people but a competitive pastime for others.

If you are going to rely on a sport or recreational activity for your regular fitness routine, just make sure that it really is regular. For instance, skiing is great, but does not constitute a good fitness program if you get to the mountain only a few times a year. Golf, mountain biking, hiking, ice skating, and rock climbing are additional examples of recreational and competitive sports that can maintain or increase fitness if done regularly.

Choose Environments Conducive to Regular Exercise

A major obstacle to exercise for many people is having a suitable, convenient place to work out. The following are some factors to consider when deciding where to exercise.

Exercise Facility Options Exercise facilities are often located at colleges, community centers, health and fitness clubs, athletic and tennis clubs, parks and recreation facilities, YMCAs, corporate fitness centers, and schools. Choosing a facility based upon its location is a good idea because the farther away a facility is from your home, the less likely you are to use it. Other factors to consider when choosing a basic exercise facility are variety of classes, quality of cardio and weight equipment, hours that are compatible with your schedule, and ease of parking (if you drive) or bus access. Additionally, you may be interested in facilities with a swimming pool, basketball and racquetball courts, locker rooms, showers, and spa.

Cost can be a big factor. Larger facilities with more offerings will likely be more expensive per month than a basic fitness center. Community centers and parks facilities often offer reasonable day use or multiday use fees. Almost all facilities offer day use passes for a fee, or even one-time free passes to check out the facility. Be sure to try the facility for several days to see whether you like the atmosphere, the equipment, and the instructors, and whether you feel safe and comfortable using the facility.

If you have not taken advantage of your college facilities yet, you may be missing out on a good deal. As a student, you can typically get access to classes, courts, leagues, equipment, and even personal trainers. College is the perfect time to try out new sports and activities.

Neighborhood When people live in safe neighborhoods where it is easy to exercise, they are more likely to be active.[18] This is becoming a bigger issue as growing cities and suburbs lead to a dramatic increase in urban sprawl. Some experts even suggest that urban sprawl is partially to blame for the rise in obesity in the United States in recent years. For example, researchers in New Jersey found that residents of sprawling counties were less likely to walk during leisure time, weighed more, and had high blood pressure more often than residents living in compact urban areas.[19] Living near streets that are conducive to physical activity (with sidewalks, bike lanes, street lights, slower traffic) and parks with bike and walking paths might make the difference between whether you stay regularly active.

Weather If you are an outside exerciser, the weather can create obstacles to regular physical activity. The impact of weather will, of course, depend on where you live and the time of year. If you are prepared, you can exercise in most weather conditions. Pay attention to your body. If you feel too hot when exercising outside, slow down, move into the shade, and consider suspending your workout for the day. Limit your exercise time in the rain if you become too wet and cold.

Safety Do you feel safe walking to the local gym to exercise? Do you feel comfortable jogging around your neighborhood? The box Exercising Safely in Any Setting on page 48 presents tips for exercising safely in different environments.

Set Reasonable Goals for Increased Fitness

Setting appropriate, realistic goals can mean the difference between success and failure in fitness programming. People often start a fitness program and think they can train to run a 10k in three weeks—an unrealistic goal for a beginning exerciser. Make sure your goals are realistic; you may want to start with the sample plans in Activate, Motivate, & Advance Your Fitness: A Walking Program in this chapter (page 61). As you begin a fitness program, your progress may initially be slow, while your body adjusts to the new activity. Setting reasonable

CAN EXERCISE MAKE YOU SMARTER?

IT'S TEST DAY! You have a big math midterm at 10:00am. What would be the best thing for you to do at 7:00am?

A
Wake up, drink coffee, and study until you have to leave for the test

B
Sleep longer to make sure you are fully rested

C
Get up, eat a candy bar, and head to the test

D
Get out of bed and exercise vigorously for 30 minutes to an hour

If your answer was D, you're setting yourself up for success on that math test! Exercise stimulates the brain, enhances attention, and increases your ability to concentrate. It may even improve your test scores![1]

REGULAR EXERCISE = HIGHER COGNITIVE FUNCTIONING

Exercise doesn't just help your brain that day either. A recent review of studies relating exercise to brain function confirmed **a positive association between physical activity and brain function** in both children and adults.[2]

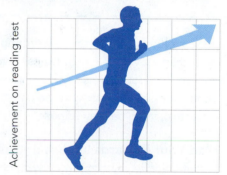

Achievement on math test — Aerobic fitness

Achievement on reading test — Aerobic fitness

"A" IS FOR ACTIVE

In one study, college students who exercised[3]

30 MINUTES about **3½ times per week** were more likely to earn **A grades**

LESS THAN 30 MINUTES and less than **3 times per week** were more likely to earn **C, D, or F grades**

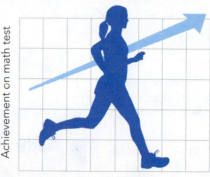

BENEFITS OF EXERCISE ON THE BRAIN
Exercise improves[4]
- memory
- mood
- energy and productivity
- attention span
- response time
- decision-making
- problem solving
- ability to learn new skills

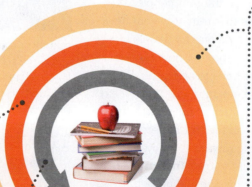

TAKE A BRAIN BREAK AND JOG YOUR MEMORY!
Get up from your chair and pretend you are jumping rope for 5 minutes, jog in place for 5-10 minutes, or head outside for a 10-15 minute walk.

TOOLS FOR # CHANGE

Exercising Safely in Any Setting

In order to maintain a regular exercise routine, you need to feel safe and comfortable in your surroundings. Below are some suggestions for exercising safely in different environments:

- If your neighborhood is not safe, consider exercising with a friend or training group, or consider driving to a different nearby neighborhood to exercise.

- If you are exercising where there are many cars, wear bright clothing and face traffic when walking or running. Seek out areas that are less busy and where speed limits are lower.

- If you are heading into a wilderness area for a hike, trail run, or mountain-bike ride, plan your outing with a friend, or at least let someone know specifically where you are going and when you will return. Know your route and carry a map, a cell phone, a spare tube (if you're biking), and basic safety supplies, including food and water for at least a day, a flashlight or headlamp, first-aid supplies, a pocketknife, and a space or emergency blanket.

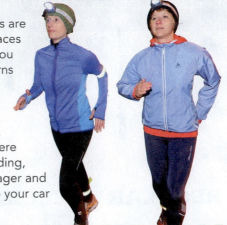

- Exercise facilities are typically safe places to work out. If you have any concerns for your safety in the locker room, workout areas, parking areas, or anywhere around the building, talk to the manager and get an escort to your car at night.

goals includes considering everything that you have assessed about yourself: your fitness level when you begin, your reasons for exercise, your motivations and attitudes about physical activity, and the constraints that other aspects of your life may impose.

Plan Your Rewards If you find yourself unmotivated to become active, try coming up with goal-related rewards to motivate yourself. Rewards can be highly individual; after all, different things motivate different people. The key is to come up with rewards that reinforce your new, more active lifestyle. A common reward for people trying to lose weight, for example, is to shop for new clothes. But rewards do not necessarily have to be material. If competition or personal challenges motivate you, for example, you may find the exhilaration of finishing a half-marathon or completing a race in the top 10 percent of contenders to be a considerable reward of its own.

Rewards can be internal or external. **Internal exercise rewards** commonly involve feeling better about yourself, feeling healthier, and having better life satisfaction from exercising. Long-term exercisers often report that internal exercise rewards

---

internal exercise rewards
Rewards for exercise that are based upon how one is feeling physically and mentally (sense of accomplishment, relaxation, increased self-esteem)

---

casestudy

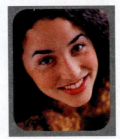

LILY

"I've been following my new jogging routine for three weeks, but now the weather is cold and I cannot get motivated to run! I don't want to give up running but I don't live close to a gym and cannot afford a home treadmill. I just heard about a running group that uses the local track once a week and I know my school has a jogging and running class. Maybe I should try one of those to keep my motivation up and my running program on track? Perhaps I will meet someone I can run with who is just my speed."

THINK! What is Lily doing to increase her chances of sticking to her new exercise plans?

ACT NOW! Today, write down three things you can do to make exercise a regular part of your life. This week, write an answer to the question that Lily asked at the beginning of the chapter". . . *what does it actually mean to be fit?"* In two weeks, ask two other people in your life that same question and compare your answer to theirs.

HEAR IT! ONLINE

are their primary motivation. Studies have shown that exercise releases endorphins in your body that can fill you with a sense of well-being.[20] For many long-term exercisers, the physical activity itself is truly its own reward. New exercisers, however, often rely on **external exercise rewards**—at least initially. External exercise rewards can be anything from a new workout wardrobe to a celebratory dinner to the admiration and praise of your peers or fitness instructor.

As you incorporate regular physical activity and exercise into your lifestyle, you may find that just having fun and feeling good while exercising is reward enough. If this switch to an internal reward motivation does not happen right away, keep setting external rewards to keep yourself motivated until it does. Don't be surprised if the switch happens faster than you think.

Make a Personal Commitment to Regular Exercise

Deciding that you are going to lead a more physically active lifestyle is the first step to changing your exercise behaviors. The harder step is to commit to that decision. Examine what a more active lifestyle would mean to you and write out your personal commitment statement: a list of reasons to commit to fitness. Review this list regularly until your new behaviors become routine.

Remember that changing behavior takes perseverance. If you feel your commitment flagging, reread your personal commitment statement and remind yourself of the reasons you began your program in the first place.

external exercise rewards Rewards for exercise that come from outside of a person (trophy, compliment, day at the spa)

CHAPTER IN REVIEW

MasteringHealth™

Build your knowledge—and wellness!—in the Study Area of MasteringHealth with a variety of study tools.

audio tools

HEAR IT! ONLINE

Audio case study
MP3 chapter review

chapter review

REVIEW IT! ONLINE

Chapter reading quizzes
Glossary flashcards

LIVE IT! ONLINE

programs & behavior change

Customizable four-week starter walking programs

Take Charge of Your Health! Worksheets:
Worksheet 26 How Much Do I Move?

Behavior Change Log Book and Wellness Journal

DO IT! ONLINE

labs

Lab 2.1 Assess Your Physical Activity Readiness

Lab 2.2 Identify Your Physical Activity Motivations and Obstacles

Lab 2.3 Changing Your Sedentary Time into Active Time

reviewquestions

1. Examples of moderate physical activity include
   a. yard work, housework, and leisurely walking.
   b. cycling, weight training, and brisk walking.
   c. hard physical labor, jogging, and aerobics classes.
   d. playing competitive sports, cycling up a steep hill, and running.

2. Which health-related component of fitness involves moving your joints through a full range of motion?
   a. Cardiorespiratory fitness
   b. Muscular endurance
   c. Flexibility
   d. Body composition

3. Which skill-related component of fitness is most involved in braking quickly when a car in front of you stops suddenly?
   a. Agility
   b. Power
   c. Coordination
   d. Reaction time

4. The principle of individuality with respect to fitness states that
   a. adaptations to training overload may vary widely from person to person.
   b. all individuals respond the same way to exercise.
   c. genetic makeup has nothing to do with individual responses to exercise.
   d. nonresponders are individuals who do not benefit from exercise.

5. The 2008 Physical Activity Guidelines for Americans emphasize
   a. vigorous physical activity every day of the week.
   b. moderate physical activity for 150 minutes per week or vigorous physical activity for 75 minutes per week.
   c. resistance training for 300 minutes per week.
   d. limiting the amount of time you spend walking.

6. A proper warm-up consists of
   a. a few quick side bends.
   b. stretches that you hold for one minute or more.
   c. quick stair climbing.
   d. a gradual increase in body temperature and easy movements in the muscles and joints.

7. Experiencing knee pain can be categorized as having a(n) _____ barrier to physical activity.
   a. social
   b. scheduling
   c. environmental
   d. personal

8. Which of the following is an example of an internal exercise reward?
   a. Buying new workout clothing
   b. Having fun while exercising
   c. Placing third in your age group in the local 5K race
   d. Taking a celebratory trip after meeting an exercise goal

9. Enlisting a friend, classmate, or co-worker to be your workout buddy and hold you accountable is a good strategy for which common exercise obstacle below?
   a. Lack of time
   b. Travel
   c. Weather conditions
   d. Lack of willpower

10. Which fitness principle refers to subjecting the body or body system to more physical activity than it is accustomed to?
    a. Overload
    b. Adaptation
    c. Dose-response
    d. Specificity

critical thinkingquestions

1. Give an example of how a training overload can lead to adaptations and training effects.
2. Describe the similarities and differences between the principle of diminished returns and the principle of progression.
3. Imagine you are about to begin a fitness program centered on bicycling. Apply the FITT formula to describe how you might set up your program.
4. If you are reluctant to increase your activity level due to fear of injury, what are five strategies that will help you overcome those fears and avoid injury?
5. Exercise options include lifestyle physical activities, exercise training options, and sports/recreational activities. Think of at least one activity in each category that you can incorporate into your weekly schedule.

references

1. R. Vigen et al., "Association of Cardiorespiratory Fitness with Total, Cardiovascular, and Noncardiovascular Mortality Across 3 Decades of Follow-Up in Men and Women," *Circulation. Cardiovascular Quality Outcomes* 5, no. 3 (2012): 358–64.
2. H. Suominen, "Muscle Training for Bone Strength," *Aging Clinical and Experimental Research* 18, no. 2 (2006): 85–93.
3. K. Small, L. McNaughton, and M. Matthews, "A Systematic Review into the Efficacy of Static Stretching as Part of a Warm-Up for the Prevention of Exercise-Related Injury," *Research in Sports Medicine* 16, no. 3 (2008): 213–31.
4. L. O. Mikkelsson et al., "Adolescent Flexibility, Endurance Strength, and Physical Activity as Predictors of Adult Tension Neck, Low Back Pain, and Knee Injury: A 25 Year Follow Up Study," *British Journal of Sports Medicine* 40, no. 2 (2006): 107–13; M. J. Spink et al., "Foot and Ankle Strength, Range of Motion, Posture, and Deformity Are Associated with Balance and Functional Ability in Older Adults," *Archives of Physical Medicine and Rehabilitation* 92, no. 1 (2011): 68–75.
5. T. D. Brutsaert and E. J. Parra, "What Makes a Champion? Explaining Variation

in Human Athletic Performance," *Respiratory Physiology and Neurobiology* 151, no. 2–3 (2006): 109–23.

6. W. D. McArdle, F. I. Katch, and V. L. Katch, *Exercise Physiology: Energy, Nutrition, and Human Performance*, 7th edition (Baltimore: Lippincott Williams & Wilkins, 2010); K. Kubo et al., "Time Course of Changes in Muscle and Tendon Properties During Strength Training and Detraining," *Journal of Strength and Conditioning Research* 24, no. 2 (2010): 322–31.

7. E. S. George, R. R. Rosenkranz, and G. S. Kolt, "Chronic Disease and Sitting Time in Middle-Aged Australian Males: Findings from the 45 and Up Study," *International Journal of Behavioral Nutrition and Physical Activity* 10, no. 20 (2013), www.ijbnpa.org

8. Office of Disease Prevention and Health Promotion, U.S. Department of Health and Human Services, *2008 Physical Activity Guidelines for Americans: Be Active, Healthy, and Happy!* ODPHP Publication no. U0036 (Washington, DC: U.S. Department of Health and Human Services, 2008).

9. World Health Organization, "Global Recommendations on Physical Activity for Health," Global Strategy on Diet, Physical Activity and Health, www.who.int; C. E. Garner et al., "American College of Sports Medicine Position Stand: Quantity and Quality of Exercise for Developing and Maintaining Cardiorespiratory, Musculoskeletal, and Neuromotor Fitness in Apparently Healthy Adults: Guidance for Prescribing Exercise," *Medicine and Science in Sports and Exercise* 43, no. 7 (2011): 1334–59.

10. B. W. Ward, J. S. Schiller, and G. Freeman, "Early release of selected estimates based on data from the January–June 2012 National Health Interview Survey," National Center for Health Statistics, December 2012, Available from www.cdc.gov

11. Office of Disease Prevention and Health Promotion, U.S. Department of Health and Human Services, Healthy People 2020, "2020 Objectives and Goals: Physical Activity," http://healthypeople.gov

12. J. M. Conn, J. L. Annest, and J. Gilchrist, "Sports and Recreation Related Injury Episodes in the U.S. Population, 1997–99," *Injury Prevention* 9, no. 2 (2003): 117–23.

13. M. N. Sawka et al., "American College of Sports Medicine Position Stand: Exercise and Fluid Replacement," *Medicine and Science in Sports and Exercise* 39, no. 2 (2007): 377–90.

14. H. H. Fink, A. E. Mikesky, and L. A. Burgoon, *Practical Applications in Sports Nutrition*, 3rd edition (Sudbury, MA: Jones and Bartlett Publishers, 2011).

15. American College of Sports Medicine, *ACSM's Guidelines for Exercise Testing and Prescription*, 9th edition (Baltimore: Lippincott Williams & Wilkins, 2014).

16. Ibid.

17. P. C. Hallal et al., "Global Physical Activity Levels: Surveillance Progress, Pitfalls, and Prospects," *Lancet* 380, no. 9838 (2012): 247–57.

18. J. F. Sallis and K. Glanz, "The Role of Built Environments in Physical Activity, Eating, and Obesity in Childhood," *The Future of Children* 16, no. 1 (2006): 89–108; H. M. Grow et al., "Where Are Youth Active? Roles of Proximity, Active Transport, and Built Environment," *Medicine and Science in Sports and Exercise* 40, no. 12 (2008): 2071–9.

19. R. Ewing et al., "Relationship between Urban Sprawl and Physical Activity, Obesity, and Morbidity," *American Journal of Health Promotion* 18, no. 1 (2003): 47–57.

20. L. Carrasco, C. Villaverde, and C. M. Oltras, "Endorphin Responses to Stress Induced by Competitive Swimming Event," *The Journal of Sports Medicine and Physical Fitness* 47, no. 2 (2007): 239–45.

getfitgraphic references

1. M. C. Gallotta et al., "Effects of Varying Type of Exertion on Children's Attention Capacity," *Medicine and Science in Sports and Exercise* 44, no. 3 (2012): 550-5, doi: 10.1249/MSS.0b013e3182305552.

2. C. H. Hillman, K. I. Erickson, and A. F. Kramer, "Be Smart, Exercise Your Heart: Exercise Effects on Brain And Cognition, Nature Reviews," *Neuroscience* 9, no. 1 (2008): 58-65.

3. K. D.Keating, D. Castelli, and S. F. Ayers, "Strength Exercise Frequency, Body Mass Index, and Academic Performance among University Students," Journal of Strength and Conditioning Research 27, no. 7 (2013): 1988-93, doi: 10.1519/JSC.0b013e318276bb4c.

4. J.E. Ahlskog et al., "Physical Exercise as a Preventive or Disease-Modifying Treatment of Dementia and Brain Aging," *Mayo Clinic Proceedings* 86, no. 9 (2011): 876-884, doi: 10.4065/mcp.2011.0252; J. J. Ratey, *Spark: The Revolutionary New Science of Exercise and the Brain* (New York, NY: Little, Brown and Company, 2008).

Name: _____   Date: _____

Instructor: _____   Section: _____

SECTION I: THE PHYSICAL ACTIVITY READINESS QUESTIONNAIRE

Physical Activity Readiness
Questionnaire - PAR-Q
(revised 2002)

PAR-Q & YOU

(A Questionnaire for People Aged 15 to 69)

Regular physical activity is fun and healthy, and increasingly more people are starting to become more active every day. Being more active is very safe for most people. However, some people should check with their doctor before they start becoming much more physically active.

If you are planning to become much more physically active than you are now, start by answering the seven questions in the box below. If you are between the ages of 15 and 69, the PAR-Q will tell you if you should check with your doctor before you start. If you are over 69 years of age, and you are not used to being very active, check with your doctor.

Common sense is your best guide when you answer these questions. Please read the questions carefully and answer each one honestly: check YES or NO.

YES	NO		
☐	☐	1.	Has your doctor ever said that you have a heart condition <u>and</u> that you should only do physical activity recommended by a doctor?
☐	☐	2.	Do you feel pain in your chest when you do physical activity?
☐	☐	3.	In the past month, have you had chest pain when you were not doing physical activity?
☐	☐	4.	Do you lose your balance because of dizziness or do you ever lose consciousness?
☐	☐	5.	Do you have a bone or joint problem (for example, back, knee or hip) that could be made worse by a change in your physical activity?
☐	☐	6.	Is your doctor currently prescribing drugs (for example, water pills) for your blood pressure or heart condition?
☐	☐	7.	Do you know of <u>any other reason</u> why you should not do physical activity?

If

you

answered

YES to one or more questions

Talk with your doctor by phone or in person BEFORE you start becoming much more physically active or BEFORE you have a fitness appraisal. Tell your doctor about the PAR-Q and which questions you answered YES.

- You may be able to do any activity you want —— as long as you start slowly and build up gradually. Or, you may need to restrict your activities to those which are safe for you. Talk with your doctor about the kinds of activities you wish to participate in and follow his/her advice.
- Find out which community programs are safe and helpful for you.

NO to all questions

If you answered NO honestly to <u>all</u> PAR-Q questions, you can be reasonably sure that you can:
- start becoming much more physically active – begin slowly and build up gradually. This is the safest and easiest way to go.
- take part in a fitness appraisal – this is an excellent way to determine your basic fitness so that you can plan the best way for you to live actively. It is also highly recommended that you have your blood pressure evaluated. If your reading is over 144/94, talk with your doctor before you start becoming much more physically active.

DELAY BECOMING MUCH MORE ACTIVE:
- if you are not feeling well because of a temporary illness such as a cold or a fever – wait until you feel better; or
- if you are or may be pregnant – talk to your doctor before you start becoming more active.

PLEASE NOTE: If your health changes so that you then answer YES to any of the above questions, tell your fitness or health professional. Ask whether you should change your physical activity plan.

<u>Informed Use of the PAR-Q</u>: The Canadian Society for Exercise Physiology, Health Canada, and their agents assume no liability for persons who undertake physical activity, and if in doubt after completing this questionnaire, consult your doctor prior to physical activity.

No changes permitted. You are encouraged to photocopy the PAR-Q but only if you use the entire form.

NOTE: If the PAR-Q is being given to a person before he or she participates in a physical activity program or a fitness appraisal, this section may be used for legal or administrative purposes.
"I have read, understood and completed this questionnaire. Any questions I had were answered to my full satisfaction."

NAME _____

SIGNATURE _____   DATE_____

SIGNATURE OF PARENT _____   WITNESS _____
or GUARDIAN (for participants under the age of majority)

Note: This physical activity clearance is valid for a maximum of 12 months from the date it is completed and becomes invalid if your condition changes so that you would answer YES to any of the seven questions.

CSEP
SCPE   © Canadian Society for Exercise Physiology   Supported by: 🇨🇦   Health   Santé
Canada   Canada

SECTION II: PRE-EXERCISE SCREENING QUESTIONNAIRE

Fill out the following questionnaire about your health and fitness history and current status. Alert your instructor to any medical issues that may affect your ability to participate in physical activity.

Age: _____   Weight: _____   Blood Pressure (if known):

Sex: _____   Height: _____   _____ / _____

Cholesterol (if known): Total - _____ **LDL** - _____ **HDL** - _____

Current **smoker**? **YES** or **NO** If yes, how many packs/day?

_____

Past smoker? **YES** or **NO** If yes, how long since you last smoked?

_____

Any **family history** of heart disease or diabetes? **YES** or **NO**

If yes, explain:

_____

Please indicate whether you have any of the following conditions:

Asthma	**YES**	**NO**
Heart disease	**YES**	**NO**
Diabetes	**YES**	**NO**
Pregnant	**YES**	**NO**
Musculoskeletal disease/disorder	**YES**	**NO**
Currently receiving medical care	**YES**	**NO**

Please **explain any YES condition/symptom** from Section I (PAR-Q) or from above:

_____

_____

List **medications** that you regularly take: _____

_____

Any **other health issues** your fitness instructor should know about? **YES** or **NO** If yes, explain:

_____

NOTE: If you have diagnosed cardiac, peripheral vascular, or cerebrovascular disease, COPD, asthma, interstitial lung disease, cystic fibrosis, diabetes, renal disease, or symptoms of these or other disorders (chest pain, shortness of breath at rest, dizziness, fainting, difficulty breathing while sleeping, ankle swelling, fast heart beat at rest, claudication leg pain, heart murmur, or unusual fatigue at rest) notify your fitness instructor and **seek medical clearance** before beginning an exercise program.[1]

Source:
1. American College of Sports Medicine, *ACSM's Guidelines for Exercise Testing and Prescription*, 9th edition (Baltimore: Lippincott Williams & Wilkins, 2014), 28.

SECTION III: PHYSICAL ACTIVITY STAGES OF CHANGE QUESTIONNAIRE

1. After carefully reading each of the following statements, please answer **YES** or **NO**.

(1)	I am currently physically active.*	YES	NO
(2)	I intend to become more physically active in the next six months.	YES	NO
(3)	I currently engage in regular** physical activity.	YES	NO
(4)	I have been regularly physically active for the past six months.	YES	NO

*Physical activity or exercise: Activities such as walking briskly, jogging, bicycling, swimming, or any other activity in which the exertion is at least as intense as these activities.
**Regular activity: Activity that adds up to a total of 30 minutes or more per day and is done at least five days per week.

2. Identify your physical activity stage of change (circle your stage):

→ If you answered NO to questions 1 and 2, you are in **PRECONTEMPLATION.**

(To move toward behavior change, it is important at this stage to start thinking about physical activity and its benefits.)

→ If you answered NO to question 1 and YES to question 2, you are in **CONTEMPLATION.**

(In order to move into preparation, you must gain information about how to get started moving toward your goal.)

→ If you answered YES to question 1 and NO to question 3, you are in **PREPARATION.**

(In this stage, it is important to remove barriers that are preventing regular physical activity.)

→ If you answered YES to questions 1 and 3, but NO to question 4, you are in **ACTION.**

(In order to maintain your new behavior, in this stage you need to track your progress, maintain your motivation, and head off potential relapses before they occur.)

→ If you answered YES to questions 1, 3, and 4, you are in **MAINTENANCE.**

(To keep your active lifestyle habits, try new activities and cross-training, make it fun, and strive to keep a consistent program despite life's obstacles.)

Source: B. H. Marcus and B. A. Lewis, "Physical Activity and the Stages of Motivational Readiness for Change Model," *President's Council on Physical Fitness and Sports Research Digest* 4, no.1 (2003): 1–8.

SECTION IV: REFLECTION

1. After reviewing your answers to the questions in Sections I–III, do you feel ready to begin an exercise program? Why or why not?

_____

_____

_____

2. If you already exercise, what are you currently doing?

_____

_____

_____

3. If you have exercised in the past but have since stopped, what exercise did you do? Why did you stop?

_____

_____

_____

Name: _____   Date: _____

Instructor: _____   Section: _____

Purpose: To identify your motivations for starting a physical activity, exercise, or sport (or maintaining your current fitness routine) and your obstacles to exercise, plus learn how to set up exercise-specific rewards to overcome those obstacles.

SECTION I: WHAT MOTIVATES YOU?

Assign a rating of 1–7 for each of the motivations listed below, using the following scale: 1 = not at all true for me, 7 = very true for me

I participate (or want to participate) in my physical activity or sport because:

_____ **1.** I want to be physically fit.

_____ **2.** It's fun.

_____ **3.** I like engaging in activities that physically challenge me.

_____ **4.** I want to obtain new skills.

_____ **5.** I want to maintain my weight and/or look better.

_____ **6.** I want to be with my friends.

_____ **7.** I like to do this activity.

_____ **8.** I want to improve existing skills.

_____ **9.** I like the challenge.

_____ **10.** I want to define my muscles so that I look better.

_____ **11.** It makes me happy.

_____ **12.** I want to keep up my current skill level.

_____ **13.** I want to have more energy.

_____ **14.** I like activities which are physically challenging.

_____ **15.** I like to be with others who are interested in this activity.

_____ **16.** I want to improve my cardiovascular fitness.

_____ **17.** I want to improve my appearance.

_____ **18.** I think it's interesting.

_____ **19.** I want to maintain my physical strength to live a healthy life.

_____ **20.** I want to be attractive to others.

_____ **21.** I want to meet new people.

_____ **22.** I enjoy this activity.

_____ **23.** I want to maintain my physical health and well-being.

_____ **24.** I want to improve my body shape.

_____ **25.** I want to get better at my activity.

_____ **26.** I find this activity stimulating.

_____ **27.** I will feel physically unattractive if I don't.

_____ **28.** My friends want me to.

_____ **29.** I like the excitement of participation.

_____ **30.** I enjoy spending time with others doing this activity.

SECTION II: SCORING MOTIVATIONS

The following table lists the motivation categories for each question above. Fill in your scores for the questions above in the appropriate boxes (for example, in the box for "Q 2," enter the numerical value you answered for question #2). Then add the totals for each type of motivation. Your total scores reflect which category motivates you the most.

Interest/Enjoyment	Competence	Appearance	Fitness	Social
Q 2:	Q 3:	Q 5:	Q 1:	Q 6:
Q 7:	Q 4:	Q 10:	Q 13:	Q 15:
Q 11:	Q 8:	Q 17:	Q 16:	Q 21:
Q 18:	Q 9:	Q 20:	Q 19:	Q 28:
Q 22:	Q 12:	Q 24:	Q 23:	Q 30:
Q 26:	Q 14:	Q 27:		
Q 29:	Q 25:			
Total:	Total:	Total:	Total:	Total:

Source: Based on R. M. Ryan and C. M. Frederick, "Intrinsic Motivation and Exercise Adherence," *International Journal of Sport Psychology* 28 (1997) and C. M. Frederick and R. M. Ryan, "Differences in Motivation for Sport and Exercise and Their Relationships with Participation and Mental Health," *Journal of Sport Behavior* 16 (1993).

SECTION III: MOTIVATION REFLECTION

1. What were your highest and lowest motivators for physical activity or sport?

Highest: _____   Lowest: _____

2. Were you surprised by these results? Explain why or why not.

_____

3. How can you use your motivation preferences to increase your level of activity? (See the *Understand Your Motivations for Beginning a Fitness Program* section on page 43 in this chapter.)

_____

SECTION IV: WHAT KEEPS YOU FROM BEING ACTIVE?

Listed below are common reasons that people give to describe why they do not get as much physical activity as they would like. Read each statement and indicate how likely you are to state the same reason.

How likely are you to say:	Very likely	Somewhat likely	Somewhat unlikely	Very unlikely
1. My day is so busy now, I just don't think I can make the time to include physical activity in my regular schedule.	3	2	1	0
2. None of my family members or friends like to do anything active, so I don't have a chance to exercise.	3	2	1	0
3. I'm just too tired after work to get any exercise.	3	2	1	0
4. I've been thinking about getting more exercise, but I just can't seem to get started.	3	2	1	0
5. I'm getting older, so exercise can be risky.	3	2	1	0
6. I don't get enough exercise because I have never learned the skills for any sport.	3	2	1	0
7. I don't have access to jogging trails, swimming pools, bike paths, etc.	3	2	1	0
8. Physical activity takes too much time away from other commitments—work, family, etc.	3	2	1	0
9. I'm embarrassed about how I will look when I exercise with others.	3	2	1	0
10. I don't get enough sleep as it is. I just couldn't get up early or stay up late to get some exercise.	3	2	1	0
11. It's easier for me to find excuses not to exercise than to go out to do something.	3	2	1	0
12. I know of too many people who have hurt themselves by overdoing it with exercise.	3	2	1	0
13. I really can't see learning a new sport at my age.	3	2	1	0
14. Exercise is just too expensive. You have to take a class or join a club or buy the right equipment.	3	2	1	0
15. My free periods during the day are too short to include exercise.	3	2	1	0
16. My usual social activities with family or friends do not include physical activity.	3	2	1	0
17. I'm too tired during the week, and I need the weekend to catch up on my rest.	3	2	1	0
18. I want to get more exercise, but I just can't seem to make myself stick to anything.	3	2	1	0
19. I'm afraid I might injure myself or have a heart attack.	3	2	1	0
20. I'm not good enough at any physical activity to make it fun.	3	2	1	0
21. If we had exercise facilities and showers at work, then I would be more likely to exercise.	3	2	1	0

Source: Centers for Disease Control and Prevention, "Barriers to Being Active Quiz," 2013, www.cdc.gov

SECTION V: SCORING OBSTACLES

Follow these instructions to score your answers in Section III:

- Enter the circled number in the spaces provided, putting together the number for statement 1 on line 1, statement 2 on line 2, and so on.
- Add the three scores on each line. Your obstacles to physical activity fall into one or more of seven categories below. Circle any physical activity obstacles category with a score of 5 or above, because this is an important obstacle for you to overcome.

_____ +	_____ +	_____ =	_____
1	8	15	**Lack of time**
_____ +	_____ +	_____ =	_____
2	9	16	**Social influence**
_____ +	_____ +	_____ =	_____
3	10	17	**Lack of energy**
_____ +	_____ +	_____ =	_____
4	11	18	**Lack of willpower**
_____ +	_____ +	_____ =	_____
5	12	19	**Fear of injury**
_____ +	_____ +	_____ =	_____
6	13	20	**Lack of skill**
_____ +	_____ +	_____ =	_____
7	14	21	**Lack of resources**

SECTION VI: OVERCOME OBSTACLES TO EXERCISE

List two of your biggest personal obstacles to exercise. Next, come up with TWO strategies to overcome each one (see the Tools for Change Box: Overcoming Common Obstacles to Exercise on page 44 for ideas).

Obstacle #1: _____

Strategy for Obstacle #1: _____

_____

_____

Strategy for Obstacle #1: _____

_____

_____

Obstacle #2: _____

Strategy for Obstacle #2: _____

_____

_____

Strategy for Obstacle #2: _____

_____

_____

LAB 2.3

CHANGING YOUR SEDENTARY TIME INTO ACTIVE TIME

MasteringHealth™

Name: _____ **Date:** _____

Instructor: _____ **Section:** _____

Purpose: To create a plan for reducing your sedentary time and replacing it with active time.

Directions:

1. On Worksheet A, list your typical activity for each hour of your day in the column labeled "Activity."

Worksheet A

Time of Day	Activity	Revised Activity
6:00 AM		
7:00 AM		
8:00 AM		
9:00 AM		
10:00 AM		
11:00 AM		
12:00 PM		
1:00 PM		
2:00 PM		
3:00 PM		
4:00 PM		
5:00 PM		
6:00 PM		
7:00 PM		
8:00 PM		
9:00 PM		
10:00 PM		
11:00 PM		

2. Now examine your list. What are your major sedentary activities? Highlight or circle them on Worksheet A.

3. List three physical activities that you would like to do but typically don't have time to do:

_____

_____

_____

4. Go back to Worksheet A and examine the sedentary activities you highlighted or circled in #2. Can you replace some of these sedentary activities with any of the physical activities you listed in #3? If so, write in the revised activity (in the "Revised Activity" column) next to the sedentary activity it is replacing.

5. If the physical activities you'd like to add to your schedule won't work in the time slots you have allotted for sedentary activity (e.g., it may not be possible or safe to go out running at 11:30 PM), what are alternative physical activities you can safely pursue? Write them in.

6. How likely are you to follow this plan? What can you do to increase your success at carrying out this new more active schedule?

_____

_____

_____

_____

Activate, Motivate,
& ADVANCE YOUR FITNESS

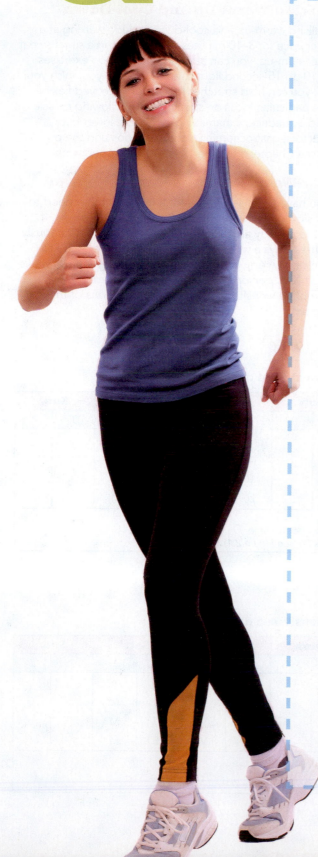

SCAN TO SEE IT
ONLINE!

A WALKING PROGRAM

ACTIVATE!

Walking is the most popular fitness activity in the United States and worldwide. If you are not currently active, walking is one of the best ways to start; you can participate at your own level, minimal equipment is required, and you can do the activity just about anywhere!

What Do I Need for Walking?

SHOES: Obtain good-quality shoes. Visit a local running and walking store to get fitted for walking shoes or running shoes (which also work well for walking). A good fit is one of the most important determinants of the right shoe for you.

CLOTHING: Wear comfortable, nonrestrictive clothing and cushioned socks that prevent blisters (avoid all-cotton socks). If you are walking outside, wear the right clothing for the weather, be it light clothing in the heat, waterproof clothing in the rain and snow, or warm clothing in the winter; dressing in layers is always a good idea. During the daytime, wear sunscreen, sunglasses, and a hat; if you are walking outside at sunrise, dusk, or dark, wear reflective clothing and/or vest and lights.

How Do I Start a Walking Program?

HEALTH WALKING TECHNIQUE AND SKILLS: Walking for *health* involves a basic walking stride with a focus on posture. Keep your head up and look straight ahead. Make sure that your shoulders are over your hips and you are not leaning too far forward or backward. Swing your arms easily at your sides, keeping your shoulders down and relaxed. Take natural strides and avoid overstriding (stepping out too far). Focus on being "light" on your feet; particularly avoid slapping your toes down. Instead, control your feet and roll your foot forward.

FITNESS WALKING TECHNIQUE AND SKILLS: Increasing your walking pace for *fitness* involves a few adjustments to your walking stride. Follow the basic posture and foot recommendations above but add the following changes. Bend your elbows at 90 degrees and swing your arms in time with your stride. Avoid letting your elbows "chicken-wing" out to the side; instead, keep your elbows close to you. Your hands (in a loose fist) should swing from your lower chest back to your hips. Remember that the faster you swing your arms, the faster your legs will go to keep up! Shorten your stride and take faster steps instead of longer steps. Keep your light heel strike but exaggerate the roll through your foot even more. Forcefully press off your toes with each stride to propel you forward.

Walking Tips

STREET AND TRAIL WALKING: Plan safe and interesting walking routes considering traffic and available walking paths. You can use an online mapping program to figure out your distance or to create a new route and calculate the distance. Carry a cell phone, ID, a few dollars, and a water bottle. Walk with a partner, if possible, and avoid wearing headphones or wear only one earpiece at a time. Always be aware of your surroundings and walk on the left facing traffic if possible. Follow traffic laws and do not assume that a car or bike operator has seen you.

TRACK WALKING: Walking on a track provides a nice flat, stable surface with a measured distance to walk. If you have a track near you, ensure that it is safe and that you have access to it. Most tracks are 400 meters around, with four laps being equal to a mile (on the innermost lane). When on the track, follow track etiquette by utilizing outside lanes for most of your training and leaving the inside lane (lane 1) for runners and sprinters or for timing yourself on a distance. If you are using the inside lane and a faster individual approaches behind you, move out to lane 2 or 3 to allow the person to pass on the inside.

TREADMILL WALKING: Walking inside on a treadmill can be a great option when the weather outside prohibits safe walking. When using the treadmill, be sure to familiarize yourself with the controls before starting out. Learn to use the shut-off button (usually a large red button) and as a back-up wear the emergency shut-off clip on your clothing. Keep your body upright and avoid using the handrails or leaning forward too much. Keep your body in the center of the treadmill near the console. Most treadmills have preprogrammed workouts but you can also adjust the speed and incline manually. Start and stop by gradually increasing and decreasing the speed. When you finish, be careful exiting the treadmill; your legs may feel strange on the "non-moving" ground.

Walking Warm-Up and Cool-Down

A walking warm-up and cool-down include walking at a slower pace for 3–10 minutes. After breaking a slight sweat in the warm-up, you can add range-of-motion exercises and 10- to 15-second light stretches. When you finish your walk, you can hold stretches longer for improved flexibility. In particular, focus on stretching the following muscle groups: quadriceps, hamstrings, gluteals, lower back, abductors, gastrocnemius, tibialis anterior, and the pectorals (see Chapter 5 for specific stretches to perform).

Four-Week Starter Walking Program

If you have been sedentary for a long time and need to start slowly, start with the Beginner Program below. If you are already able to walk 10–15 minutes continuously on three days a week, start with the Intermediate Program below. *Adjust time, intensity, and days of the walks to suit your personal fitness level and schedule; visit the mobile website for customizable versions of these programs.*

BEGINNER

PROGRAM **GOAL:** To walk 15–20 minutes continuously, 3–4 days a week

	Mon.		Tue.		Wed.		Thurs.		Fri.		Sat.		Sun.	
	T	I	T	I	T	I	T	I	T	I	T	I	T	I
Week 1	5	L			5	L			8	M				
Week 2	5	L			8	M			10	M	8	M		
Week 3	10	M			12	M			10	M	12	M		
Week 4	15	M			15	M			20	M	15	M		

T = Time. Total time is listed in minutes. Time does not include warm-up or cool-down time.
I = Intensity. Intensity is listed as Light/Lifestyle (L), Moderate (M), or Vigorous (V) (see Figure 2.1).

INTERMEDIATE

PROGRAM **GOAL:** To walk 25–30 minutes continuously, 4–5 days a week

	Mon.		Tue.		Wed.		Thurs.		Fri.		Sat.		Sun.	
	T	I	T	I	T	I	T	I	T	I	T	I	T	I
Week 1	15	M			15	M			20	M				
Week 2	18	M			20	M			22	V	20	M		
Week 3	22	M	20	M	18	M			25	V	20	M		
Week 4	25	M	22	V	28	M			30	V	25	M		

T = Time. Total time is listed in minutes. Time does not include warm-up or cool-down time.
I = Intensity. Intensity is listed as Light/Lifestyle (L), Moderate (M), or Vigorous (V) (see Figure 2.1).

MOTIVATE!

Creating a plan and monitoring your progress are key motivators for any fitness program or behavior change project. Use an exercise log to track your walking program—make note of dates, times, distances, and intensity. Depending on your personal goals and the equipment available to you, you may also choose to keep track of heart rate, steps taken, or calories burned.

Sticking to a fitness plan can be tough, but there are plenty of things you can do to motivate yourself and overcome the obstacles that prevent you from achieving your goals. Here are a few; see the Tools for Change box Overcoming Common Obstacles to Exercise on page 44 for more ideas.

- **Is lack of time an obstacle for you?** If so, monitor your daily activities for one week to identify time slots of 15 minutes to half an hour that you could use for walking. Can you incorporate walking into any of your daily activities, such as walking between classes or when running errands? Figure out the timing in advance, and write your walking "appointments" into your schedule.

- **Do you need concrete numbers and immediate targets to keep you motivated?** If so, purchase a pedometer and start keeping track of the number of steps you take. Challenge yourself with mini-goals to increase your step count.

- **Is lack of willpower an obstacle for you?** If so, enlist a friend to join you on your walks, and schedule it into both of your calendars. Committing to another person can be a great motivator.

- **Is boredom an obstacle for you?** If so, look for ways to switch up your route or walk in places that offer sensory stimulation, such as a shopping mall or a wilderness trail. If you are walking on a treadmill, plan your walks to coincide with a favorite radio or television program (if your treadmill has a TV monitor) or download podcasts or audiobooks to listen to while you walk.

- **Is lack of energy or dislike of exertion an obstacle for you?** If so, create a special playlist of music to listen to while you walk, choosing up-tempo songs that will energize you, distract you from the minor discomforts of physical exertion, and help you keep pace.

- **Do you feel a need for more challenge or a long-term goal?** If so, sign up for an upcoming charity walk and join a group that is training for it.

ADVANCE!

Ready for the next step? Once you have established your walking program, you may want to challenge yourself to try something new or take your activities to the next level. Below is a more advanced four-week program you can follow; visit the mobile website to personalize this or any of the programs in this book.

ADVANCED

PROGRAM   GOAL: To walk 40–45 minutes continuously, 5 days a week

	Mon.		Tue.		Wed.		Thurs.		Fri.		Sat.		Sun.	
	T	I	T	I	T	I	T	I	T	I	T	I	T	I
Week 1	20	M			25	M			25	M				
Week 2	28	M			25	V			30	M	28	M		
Week 3	30	V	28	M	35	M			38	M	35	V		
Week 4	40	M	30	V	42	M			45	V	40	M		

T = Time. Total time is listed in minutes. Time does not include warm-up or cool-down time.
I = Intensity. Intensity is listed as Light/Lifestyle (L), Moderate (M), or Vigorous (V) (see Figure 2.1).

Disclaimer: These programs are designed for beginners and assume that all participants have been medically cleared for exercise via the procedures outlined in this chapter. Please also be sure that you have read and understood the basic fitness principles and procedures for starting a fitness program outlined in this chapter. This program is focused on the cardiorespiratory component of fitness, but remember that a well-rounded program will also include muscle strength, muscle endurance, flexibility, and back health components.

3 Conditioning Your Cardiorespiratory System

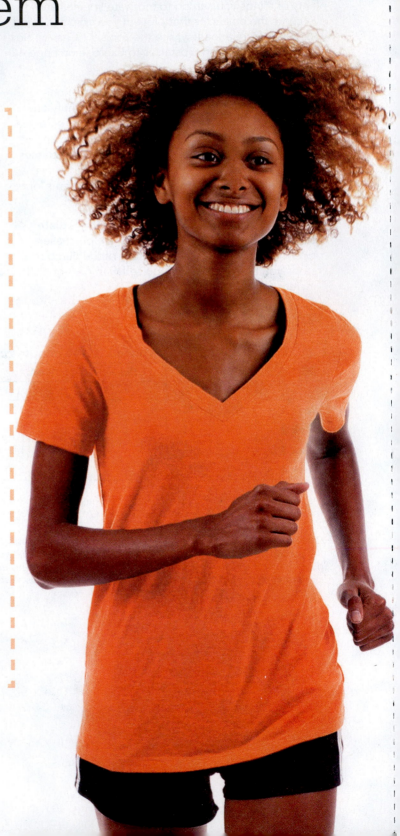

LEARNINGoutcomes

1 Explain how cardiorespiratory fitness is a key component of your overall fitness and wellness. Identify the key structures of the cardiorespiratory system and state how they work together to provide oxygen to the body.

2 Outline how the three metabolic systems provide energy for exercise.

3 Describe the fitness and wellness benefits you can get from cardiorespiratory training.

4 Assess your cardiorespiratory fitness level on a regular basis using a variety of methods.

5 Set and work toward appropriate cardiorespiratory fitness goals.

6 Implement a cardiorespiratory exercise plan compatible with your goals and lifestyle.

7 Incorporate strategies to prevent injuries during cardiorespiratory training.

MasteringHealth™

Go online for chapter quizzes, interactive assessments, videos, and more!

casestudy

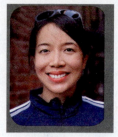

ANGELA

"Hi, I'm Angela. In high school, I was on the varsity tennis team; I played #2 singles and was pretty competitive! After high school, I spent a few years working and saving up money for college, so I'm a little older than most of my classmates. Unfortunately, I got out of shape during that time, too. Our coach used to have us do all kinds of cardio and cross-training drills. I want to start playing tennis again, but without a coach or a team, I'm not sure how to go about getting in shape for it. Should I just find a partner and dive right back in?"

HEAR IT! ONLINE

Cardiorespiratory fitness is the ability of your cardiovascular and respiratory systems to supply oxygen and nutrients to large muscle groups to sustain continuous activity. It is a key component of your overall fitness and wellness. A healthy cardiorespiratory system can be the difference between having adequate energy to sustain daily, recreational, and sports activities and becoming tired out by performing simple physical tasks.

When people decide to "get in shape," they often choose cardiorespiratory activities such as walking, jogging, or running. It is convenient to just put on a pair of athletic shoes and head out the door, but remember you need to consider many things to ensure that your cardiorespiratory fitness activities are safe and effective. In this chapter we provide a brief overview of how the cardiorespiratory system works. We also discuss the benefits of regular cardiorespiratory training. We then cover how to set goals for cardiorespiratory fitness and how to design a cardiorespiratory exercise program that is personalized for your needs.

cardiorespiratory fitness The ability of your cardiovascular and respiratory systems to supply oxygen and nutrients to large muscle groups in order to sustain dynamic activity

respiratory system The body system responsible for the exchange of gases between the body and the air

cardiovascular system The body system responsible for the delivery of oxygen and nutrients to body tissues and the delivery of carbon dioxide and other wastes back to the heart and lungs

How Does My Cardiorespiratory System Work?

The cardiorespiratory system is made up of the cardiovascular system and the respiratory system. Together, these systems deliver essential oxygen and nutrients to your body's cells and tissues and remove carbon dioxide and wastes.

An Overview of the Cardiorespiratory System

The **respiratory system** (also called the *pulmonary system*) consists of the air passageways and the lungs; the **cardiovascular system** consists of the heart and blood vessels (see **Figure 3.1**).

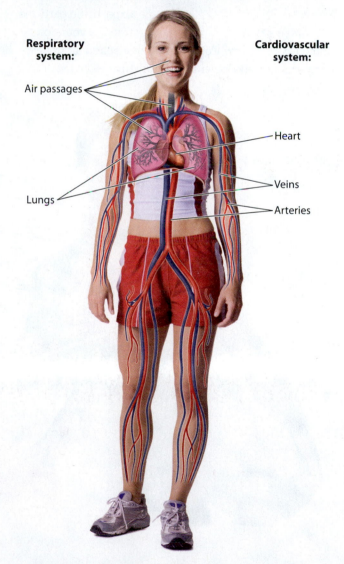

Respiratory system:

Air passages

Lungs

Cardiovascular system:

Heart

Veins

Arteries

FIGURE **3.1** The cardiorespiratory system consists of the cardiovascular and respiratory systems.

respiration The exchange of gases in the lungs or in the tissues

atria Upper chambers of the heart that collect blood from the body

ventricles Lower chambers of the heart that pump blood to the body

pulmonary circulation Blood circulation from the heart to the lungs and back

systemic circulation Blood circulation from the heart to the rest of the body and back

pulmonary artery The artery that carries blood from the right ventricle to the lungs

aorta The artery that carries blood from the left ventricle to the rest of the body

Air Passageways

Air enters your body via your nose and mouth. It then continues through your throat (*pharynx*), voice box (*larynx*), and windpipe (*trachea*) (see **Figure 3.2**). These upper respiratory passageways warm, humidify, and filter the air, promoting optimal gas exchange. Mucus and small, hairlike projections called *cilia* filter out unwanted particles in the air; you expel these particles through your nose or mouth, or you swallow them. The inspired air travels down through the lower respiratory tract—the lower trachea, *bronchi*, and *bronchioles*—eventually reaching air sacs (*alveoli*) in the lungs, where gas exchange (i.e., the delivery of oxygen and the removal of carbon dioxide) occurs.

Lungs The air passageways in the lungs have extensive branching, similar to the branches on a large tree. At the very ends of the smallest branches (the bronchioles) are alveoli, which are surrounded by small blood vessels called *capillaries*. Because the walls of the alveoli and capillaries are very thin, oxygen moves easily from the alveolar sacs into the capillary blood. Vessels then transport oxygen to the heart and the rest of the body. Meanwhile, carbon dioxide moves from the capillaries into the alveoli and exits the body when you exhale. This exchange of oxygen and carbon dioxide is called **respiration**.

Heart The heart is a fist-sized pump consisting of four chambers: the *right atrium*, the *right ventricle*, the *left atrium*, and the *left ventricle* (**Figure 3.3** on page 67). Small *valves* regulate the steady, rhythmic flow of blood between chambers and prevent the blood from flowing backward. The two **atria** are collecting chambers that receive blood from the body. The two **ventricles** pump blood out again. With each beat of the heart, the atria and ventricles fill and contract. The heart pumps blood through two different circulatory systems: in **pulmonary circulation**, blood circulates from the heart to the lungs and back; in **systemic circulation**, blood circulates from the heart to the rest of the body and back.

Blood returning to the heart from the body enters the heart through the right atrium. The right atrium pumps blood into the right ventricle. The right ventricle pumps blood through the **pulmonary artery** into the lungs. Blood returning from the lungs enters the heart through the left atrium. The left atrium pumps blood into the left ventricle. The left ventricle fills and contracts, pumping the blood out of the heart via the **aorta** and transporting it to the cells of the heart, brain, and body.

Contraction of the ventricle chambers must be forceful enough to send blood out of the heart. In order

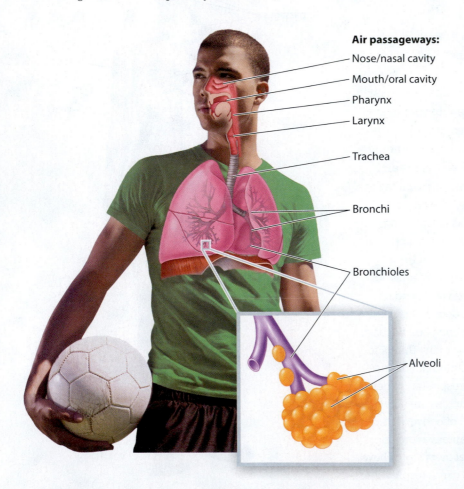

Air passageways:
- Nose/nasal cavity
- Mouth/oral cavity
- Pharynx
- Larynx
- Trachea
- Bronchi
- Bronchioles
- Alveoli

FIGURE **3.2** The respiratory system consists of the air passageways and the lungs.

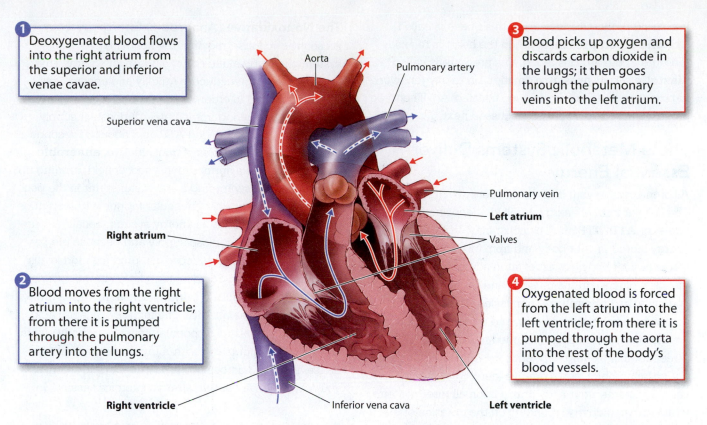

1 Deoxygenated blood flows into the right atrium from the superior and inferior venae cavae.

3 Blood picks up oxygen and discards carbon dioxide in the lungs; it then goes through the pulmonary veins into the left atrium.

Aorta

Pulmonary artery

Superior vena cava

Pulmonary vein

Left atrium

Right atrium

Valves

2 Blood moves from the right atrium into the right ventricle; from there it is pumped through the pulmonary artery into the lungs.

4 Oxygenated blood is forced from the left atrium into the left ventricle; from there it is pumped through the aorta into the rest of the body's blood vessels.

Right ventricle

Inferior vena cava

Left ventricle

FIGURE **3.3** The heart is a four-chambered pump. The right atrium and left atrium collect blood from the body. The right and left ventricles pump blood back out. In pulmonary circulation, blood circulates from the heart to the lungs and back. In systemic circulation, blood circulates from the heart to the rest of the body and back.

to accomplish this task the ventricles are more muscular than the atria. The left ventricle is the most muscular chamber, because it must contract forcefully enough to send blood to the entire body.

The heart cycle consists of two phases: systole and diastole. During **systole**, the ventricles contract and blood is pumped out of the heart. During **diastole**, the ventricles relax and fill back up with blood from the right and left atria. Specialized heart tissue involuntarily and automatically starts the heart cycle. This tissue, located in the right atrium, is called the *pacemaker;* it determines how fast your heart beats. One "beat" of your heart consists of a full heart cycle. Through a stethoscope, you can hear your heartbeat as a "lub dub." The "lub" signals the end of the diastole phase (ventricular relaxation), and the "dub" signals the end of the systole phase (ventricular contraction). The number of times your heart beats in one minute is your **heart rate**.

Blood Vessels Blood vessels transport blood throughout your body. There are two types of blood vessels: **arteries**, which carry blood away from the heart, and **veins**, which carry blood back toward the heart. As arteries branch off from the heart, they divide into smaller blood vessels called

arterioles, and then into even smaller blood vessels known as capillaries. As mentioned earlier, capillaries have thin walls that permit the exchange of substances between cells and the blood. Oxygen and nutrients move from the blood to body cells, while carbon dioxide and waste products move from body cells to the blood for transport to the lungs and kidneys through veins and *venules* (small veins).

The pressure that blood exerts on the walls of blood vessels is called **blood pressure**. The blood pressure in arteries must be high in order to drive the flow of blood to all your cells. (In veins, blood pressure is close to zero.) Due to the strength of the heart contraction, pressure in the arteries is higher during systole. The pressure

systole The contraction phase of the heart cycle

diastole The relaxation phase of the heart cycle

heart rate The number of beats of the heart in one minute

arteries High-pressure blood vessels that carry blood away from the heart to the lungs or cells

veins Low-pressure blood vessels that carry blood from the cells or lungs back to the heart

blood pressure The pressure that blood in the arteries exerts on the arterial walls

measured in the arteries during this phase is called **systolic blood pressure**. When the heart is relaxed, pressure in the arteries drops; this pressure is called **diastolic blood pressure**. In addition to oxygen, working muscles need energy to keep contracting. The three primary energy systems are discussed next.

Three Metabolic Systems Deliver Essential Energy

All of the cells in your body need energy to function. The cellular form of energy is called *adenosine triphosphate,* or **ATP**. ATP must be constantly regenerated from energy stored in your body and from food. The energy stores in your body consist of fat in adipose tissues and muscles, glucose in the muscles and liver, and protein and **creatine phosphate** in muscles. The energy in food comes from fat, carbohydrates, and protein. Your body breaks down stored and consumed nutrients to ATP via three metabolic energy systems: the *immediate, nonoxidative* (anaerobic), and *oxidative* (aerobic) systems. To varying extents, your body draws upon all three systems while you are active, depending on the duration of the activity. Let's examine each of these systems in detail.

The Immediate Energy System When it needs quick, immediate access to energy, your body first draws upon the ATP stored in your muscles. "Explosive" activities such as a basketball jump shot, a 50-meter sprint, or a dive off a diving board are all examples of actions fueled by this immediate energy system. However, your body depletes energy stored in your muscles within a matter of seconds: ATP in muscle cells is typically used up in less than 10 seconds, and creatine phosphate (which is used to make more ATP) is typically gone within 30 seconds. As a result, your body must rely on other energy systems in order to sustain longer activities.

systolic blood pressure
Blood pressure during the systole phase of the heart cycle

diastolic blood pressure
Blood pressure during the diastole phase of the heart cycle

ATP Adenosine triphosphate; the cellular form of energy

creatine phosphate A molecule that is stored in muscle cells and used in the immediate energy system to donate a phosphate to make ATP

anaerobic Without oxygen (nonoxidative)

lactic acid An end product of the nonoxidative breakdown of glucose that can increase acidity in muscles and the blood and contribute to muscular fatigue

The Nonoxidative (Anaerobic) Energy System

As soon as you start moving, the nonoxidative energy system begins breaking down glucose for energy. This system breaks down glucose quickly and *anaerobically* (without oxygen) in order to produce ATP. Although this system starts working immediately, it does not supply the majority of your needed ATP until about 30 seconds into an activity. Examples of nonoxidative, **anaerobic** activities include a sprint down a soccer field, running up a steep hill, and swimming a 100-meter sprint in the pool.

You may experience muscular fatigue with activities that use the nonoxidative energy system, because your body has a limited glucose supply and because the process of breaking down glucose can produce high levels of **lactic acid**. Lactic acid accumulation in the muscles and blood can produce a burning sensation in the muscles during intense activity. The increase in lactic acid is temporary; contrary to popular belief, your body clears lactic acid from muscles within minutes or hours of exercise. Lactic acid does *not* cause the muscle soreness you may feel a day or two after an exercise session. In

casestudy

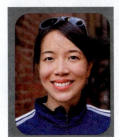

ANGELA

"I thought I would kick-start my plan to get back into shape by doing one of the workouts my tennis coach had us do in high school. I jogged for a mile, did some calisthenics on the court, and then played two sets of tennis with a friend. That was a mistake. My friend has a killer serve—it's like a bullet coming at you. She won every point she served because I couldn't move fast enough to return the ball. Also, I was surprised at how much that jog tired me out. I used to run a mile with no problem at all! By the end of the first set, I was completely exhausted. My friend won 6-1, 6-1."

THINK! Which energy system do you think Angela's friend relied on most while hitting her serves?

ACT NOW! Today, write out activities you would do for a 10-minute cardiorespiratory warm-up. This week, try your 10-minute warm-up and think about how the three energy systems are providing fuel to keep your muscles moving. In two weeks, log an entire workout session and outline the energy systems you are using.

HEAR IT! ONLINE

fact, during and after exercise, lactic acid cleared from the muscles and blood is reused for energy.

The nonoxidative energy system supplies your body with most of its needed ATP until about three minutes into an activity. At that point, the oxidative energy system becomes the primary provider of ATP.

The Oxidative (Aerobic) Energy System During the first three minutes of activity (when the immediate and nonoxidative systems are supplying most of the ATP you need), your body is also gradually increasing its *oxidative* production of ATP using oxygen in the **mitochondria** of your cells. The oxidative energy system is also called the **aerobic** energy system (*aerobic* means "with oxygen"). Mitochondria are often referred to as the "powerhouses of the cell," because most energy production occurs in these structures. The complete breakdown of fat, glucose, and protein occurs only in the mitochondria and the oxidative energy system yields more ATP from each energy source than any other system.

Aerobic activities are low- to moderate-intensity activities that are usually sustained for 20 minutes or longer. Examples of aerobic activities include cycling, treadmill walking, jogging, and water aerobics.

Figure 3.4 illustrates how the proportion of each energy system's contribution of ATP changes, depending on the duration of a given activity.

The Cardiorespiratory System at Rest and during Exercise

Your cardiorespiratory system must adapt in order to meet your body's needs during exercise.

Resting Conditions At rest, your body works to maintain **homeostasis**, a stable, constant internal environment. If you're healthy, your resting heart rate is between 50 and 90 beats per minute, your breathing rate is around 12 to 20 breaths per minute, and your resting blood pressure is below 120 systolic and below 80 diastolic. During homeostasis, your oxygen and nutrient delivery matches the needs of your cells. Your body breaks down fat via the oxidative energy system in order to supply ATP to the body. Although you "burn" fat for energy, your total energy expenditure is low.

Response to Exercise Physical activity disrupts your body's homeostasis. During exercise, your body must increase blood flow to working muscles in order to maintain adequate oxygen and nutrient delivery.

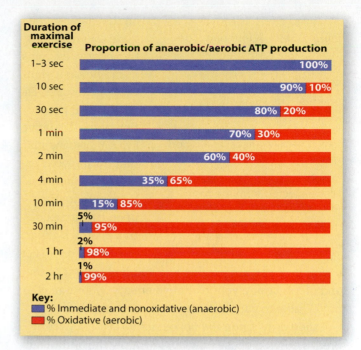

FIGURE **3.4** In the first two minutes of exercise, a body primarily uses ATP generated by the two nonoxidative (anaerobic) energy systems. After about three minutes into the exercise, a body begins to primarily use ATP generated by the oxidative (aerobic) energy system.

Your heart rate increases, and stronger heart contractions result in an increase in **cardiac output**—the amount of blood exiting your heart in one minute. Your breathing rate also increases to ensure that adequate oxygen is transferred into the blood for working muscles.

The increased volume of blood moving from your heart into your blood vessels in exercise results in an increase in systolic blood pressure. The body directs this increased blood to contracting muscles and the vessels *dilate* (open up wider) to accommodate the increased blood flow. This arterial dilation allows diastolic blood pressure to stay the same or even decrease during aerobic exercise. In addition, capillaries that were not open at rest open up to allow for oxygen and nutrient exchange with muscles.

When you begin to exercise, it takes a few minutes for your body to increase blood flow and to fully engage the oxidative energy system. This is why your body must rely

mitochondria Cellular structures where oxidative energy production takes place

aerobic Dependent on oxygen (oxidative)

homeostasis A stable, constant internal environment

cardiac output The volume of blood ejected from the heart in one minute; expressed in liters or milliliters per minute

hemoglobin A four-part globular, iron-containing protein that carries oxygen in red blood cells

plasma The yellow-colored fluid portion of blood that contains water, proteins, hormones, ions, energy sources, and blood gases

stroke volume The volume of blood ejected from the heart in one heartbeat; expressed in liters or milliliters per beat

on the faster immediate and nonoxidative energy systems in the first few minutes of exercise. The slower ATP production of the oxidative system also means that during your exercise session, you may have to draw upon the nonoxidative energy system more than once. For example, if you are jogging and suddenly sprint to the end of the street, your oxidative energy system may not be able to supply ATP quickly enough. Your body will then draw upon the nonoxidative system (which breaks down glucose quickly) to supply the additional ATP you need.

How Does Aerobic Training Condition My Cardiorespiratory System?

Recall that aerobic activities are low- to moderate-intensity activities performed for an extended period of time (i.e., 20 minutes or longer). Regular aerobic training conditions your cardiorespiratory system by improving your body's ability to (1) deliver large amounts of oxygen to working muscles, (2) transfer and use oxygen efficiently in the muscles, and (3) use energy sources for sustained muscular contractions. **Figure 3.5** on the following page summarizes these and other adaptations that occur over time with aerobic training.

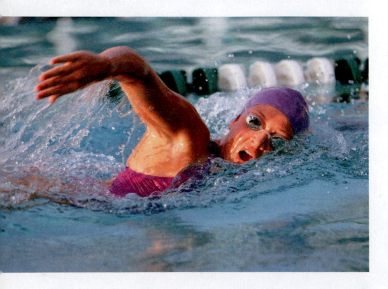

Aerobic Training Increases Oxygen Delivery to Your Muscles

With regular aerobic training, your body gets better at delivering oxygen to working muscles. Your respiratory muscles become more efficient and you experience less fatigue in an extended workout. You can carry more oxygen in your blood, due to an increase in **hemoglobin**, the oxygen-carrying protein. Since the fluid portion of your blood, the **plasma**, also increases with aerobic training, you will see an increase in your total blood volume. Your heart will adapt to this greater volume by increasing the blood-holding capacity of your left ventricle. The ventricle will not only hold more blood, but (with training) it will also have stronger contractions. All of this will allow you to pump more blood out of your heart with every heartbeat, thus increasing your heart's **stroke volume**.

Aerobic Training Improves the Transfer and Use of Oxygen

Delivering oxygen to working muscles is only part of the picture. Your body also needs to transfer oxygen into the muscles and use it efficiently. With consistent aerobic training, your body increases the number of capillaries in the muscles that you train. This enables increased blood flow to these muscles and improves oxygen transfer from the blood into the muscles. Once inside the muscle cells, the oxygen is transported to mitochondria for use in the oxidative energy system. Mitochondria numbers increase within each muscle cell, improving oxygen use by muscles and subsequently improving oxidative production of ATP as well.

Aerobic Training Improves Your Body's Ability to Use Energy Efficiently

Regular aerobic training enhances your ability to store glycogen within muscles. When needed, glycogen can be broken down into glucose and used for energy during exercise. In fact, a minimal amount of glucose is needed during exercise to keep the oxidative energy system running efficiently.

Since fat breakdown for energy is accomplished within the mitochondria, an increase in the number of mitochondria will improve your body's ability to use

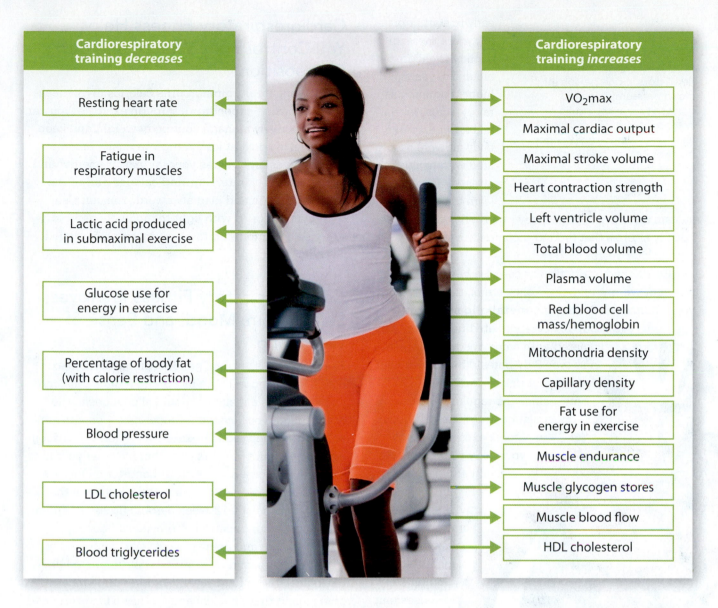

Cardiorespiratory training *decreases*	Cardiorespiratory training *increases*
Resting heart rate	VO$_2$max
Fatigue in respiratory muscles	Maximal cardiac output
Lactic acid produced in submaximal exercise	Maximal stroke volume
Glucose use for energy in exercise	Heart contraction strength
Percentage of body fat (with calorie restriction)	Left ventricle volume
Blood pressure	Total blood volume
LDL cholesterol	Plasma volume
Blood triglycerides	Red blood cell mass/hemoglobin
	Mitochondria density
	Capillary density
	Fat use for energy in exercise
	Muscle endurance
	Muscle glycogen stores
	Muscle blood flow
	HDL cholesterol

FIGURE **3.5** Regular cardiorespiratory training results in numerous adaptations to the cardiovascular, respiratory, and muscle systems and an increase in overall health and wellness.

fat for energy, sparing glucose and glycogen stores. Improving your body's ability to burn fat may allow you to have some glucose "left over" for that last-minute sprint to the finish! Less use of glucose and the nonoxidative energy system also means less lactic acid production during exercise and a delaying of fatigue.

What Are the Benefits of Improving My Cardiorespiratory Fitness?

There are many health-related reasons to improve your cardiorespiratory fitness.

Cardiorespiratory Fitness Decreases Your Risk of Disease

Having a low fitness level can put you at higher risk for disease and early death. The good news is that you don't need to increase your fitness to extremely high levels in order to see risk-reducing health benefits. Having an intermediate fitness level (being able to walk about three–four miles per hour) can significantly reduce early mortality from cardiovascular diseases, and it can lower heart disease risk factors as well.[1] An increase in cardiorespiratory fitness can decrease your resting heart rate, decrease your blood levels of "bad" (LDL) cholesterol, and help prevent blood clots—all of which can lower your risk of heart attack and stroke. And it is never too early to start improving your fitness: in a study of children around 10 years old, higher cardiorespiratory fitness levels and lower amounts of body fat were associated with healthier arteries.[2] If children learn to be active and sustain an active lifestyle, they can avoid the stiffer, less healthy arteries that tend to accompany a sedentary lifestyle in later years.[3]

Cardiorespiratory fitness can also help you manage your weight and blood cholesterol, thus reducing your chances of developing **metabolic syndrome** (a group of obesity-related risk factors associated with cardiovascular disease and type 2 diabetes).[4] It can also help lessen your risk of developing diabetes, since the regular rhythmic muscular contractions that occur in aerobic exercise improve your body's ability to use insulin and glucose.[5]

Regular physical activity stimulates hormones, anti-inflammatory agents, and immune responses that help protect against many forms of cancer. Studies have shown that regular physical activity and increased cardiorespiratory fitness can lower mortality rates in some of the most common cancers, including lung, colon, breast, and prostate.[6]

Cardiorespiratory Fitness Helps You Control Body Weight and Body Composition

Cardiorespiratory training burns calories. By increasing your calorie expenditure through exercise, you can more effectively manage your body weight and keep your level of body fat low. A high-intensity aerobic exercise session elevates your fat use for energy[7] and overall metabolic rate,[8] burning calories during the exercise session and long afterward. You can also burn many calories with light to moderate aerobic exercise by performing the activity for an extended period of time.

Cardiorespiratory Fitness Improves Self-Esteem, Mood, and Sense of Well-Being

Exercise makes you feel good! A single aerobic exercise session can improve mood and reduce tension and anxiety as a result of chemical changes in the brain and nervous system.[9] Since these benefits are primarily seen in regular exercisers,[10] don't be discouraged if you don't feel instantly "happy" after your first exercise session—stick with it! Long-term changes are even more dramatic. One study has shown that over the course of a 12-week aerobic fitness program, men and women reported improved self-concept, anxiety, mood, and depression scores, compared to a control group, and maintained their improved psychological health for a year.[11] Another more recent study found that physical activity has a long-term association with happiness.[12] Inactive people were more than twice as likely to be unhappy as those who were active over a two-year period, and if active people became inactive, they increased their chances of becoming unhappy. Not surprisingly, numerous studies point to the importance of exercise in reducing symptoms of depression.[13]

Cardiorespiratory Fitness Improves Immune Function

Light to moderate exercise can boost your immune system.[14] Regular, moderate aerobic exercise can reduce stress and improve the quality of your sleep (stress and sleep are both tied to immune system health). Research has also shown that regularly participating in aerobic exercise can slow the reduction in immune system function that tends to occur as you get older.[15]

Cardiorespiratory Fitness Improves Long-Term Quality of Life

Cardiorespiratory fitness has a protective effect against age-related cognitive declines.[16] Research even suggests that aerobic exercise training can increase brain volume and thus *improve* cognitive function and memory as you age.[17]

Increased cardiorespiratory fitness can also improve the quality of life for individuals with chronic diseases or other medical conditions. Research has shown that after a six-month exercise program, men living with HIV improved their scores in cardiorespiratory fitness and in cognitive function and overall health.[18] Cardiorespiratory fitness has also been linked to better quality of life for survivors of breast cancer,[19] heart attacks,[20] and strokes.[21] Of course, the best time to incorporate a cardiorespiratory program into your life is before you show signs of disease.

How Can I Assess My Cardiorespiratory Fitness?

How fit is your cardiorespiratory system? Chances are you already have a general idea. If you get easily winded after walking up a short flight of stairs or have trouble walking quickly for more than 10 minutes or so, you likely have a low cardiorespiratory fitness level.

Monitoring your **resting heart rate** is one way to keep track of general changes in your fitness level. Recall that your heart rate is the number of times your heart beats in one minute. Your resting heart rate decreases as your cardiorespiratory system becomes more conditioned. With an increase in stroke volume, your heart does not have to beat as many times per minute to deliver the same amount of blood to the body; at rest, your heart can slow down and still deliver adequate oxygen to all your cells.

When the heart contracts and pushes blood out, that wave of blood can be felt moving through the arteries. This is your **pulse**. To determine your heart rate, feel for your pulse at specific arteries around the body. The most common arteries to use for checking an exercise pulse are the *carotid* and the *radial* arteries (see **Figure 3.6**). Press your index and middle fingers gently against your skin and count the number of beats that you feel. Avoid using your thumb when taking your pulse, because the pulse in your thumb can interfere with your ability to count accurately. **Lab 3.1** walks

DO IT! ONLINE

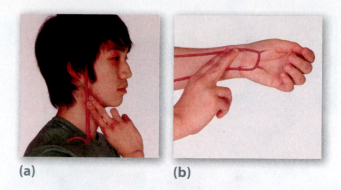

(a)   **(b)**

FIGURE **3.6** To determine your heart rate, feel for your pulse at either (a) the carotid artery or (b) the radial artery.

you through how to take an accurate heart rate reading at rest and during exercise.

Understand Your Maximal Oxygen Consumption

Your body's maximal ability to utilize oxygen during exercise is called **maximal oxygen consumption** or **VO$_2$max**. Your VO$_2$max is the measure of your body's ability to deliver oxygen to the muscles and the muscles' ability to consume or use the oxygen. VO$_2$max numbers range from 20 to 94 ml/kg·min, with male athletes typically ranging from 50 to 70 ml/kg·min and female athletes ranging from 40 to 60 ml/kg·min. Your maximal oxygen consumption is largely determined by genetics and tends to decrease as you get older. That said, you can typically improve your VO$_2$max an average of 15 to 20 percent with training. The more deconditioned you are before beginning a training program, the more dramatic an improvement you can achieve with training.

The most accurate measurements of VO$_2$max are performed in a laboratory setting (see **Figure 3.7**). The test is usually completed on a treadmill or stationary bike and requires specialized equipment and technicians to ensure safety. The technicians measure the precise amount of oxygen that enters and exits the body during a maximal exercise session.

resting heart rate The number of times your heart beats in a minute while the body is at rest; typically 50 to 90 beats per minute

pulse The pressure wave felt in the arteries due to blood ejection with each heartbeat

maximal oxygen consumption (VO$_2$max) The highest rate of oxygen consumption your body is capable of during maximal exercise; expressed in either liters per minute (L/min) or milliliters per minute per kilogram of body weight (ml/kg·min)

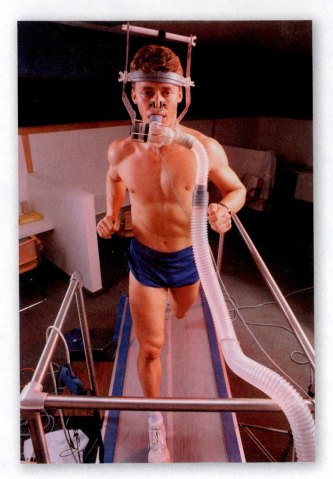

FIGURE **3.7** VO$_2$max can be most accurately measured in a laboratory setting, where direct gas analysis can determine the volume of oxygen a person's body is using while exercising at maximum capacity.

Test Your Submaximal Heart Rate Responses

An alternative to testing your true maximal oxygen consumption is to perform a *submaximal* test. Submaximal tests do not test your body's maximal oxygen consumption but rather test for submaximal values that can be compared against norm charts or used to predict maximal values. Submaximal tests are safer, require less equipment and expertise, and are performed either in a laboratory or in a field/classroom setting.

Submaximal tests in the laboratory are usually performed on a stationary bike or treadmill. These tests predict your maximal effort level and oxygen consumption by assessing your heart rate response. A higher heart rate means higher oxygen consumption. By testing your heart rate response to different exercise intensities, an exercise technician can use your predicted **maximal heart rate (HRmax)** to estimate

maximal heart rate (HRmax) The highest heart rate you can achieve during maximal exercise

your maximal exercise intensity and oxygen consumption. Your maximal heart rate is the fastest your heart will beat in exhaustive exercise (a number that will decrease as you get older). One way to predict your HRmax is to subtract your age from the number 220. For example, if you are 18 years old, your predicted HRmax would be $220 - 18 = 202$ beats per minute. This formula is not as accurate as maximal laboratory tests, but it is used in many submaximal tests and heart rate training equations.

Test Your Cardiorespiratory Fitness in the Field/Classroom

Most classes in health and fitness enroll too many students to perform laboratory testing. More appropriate for these classes is classroom or field tests of cardiorespiratory fitness. Like laboratory tests, these tests either predict your maximal oxygen consumption from submaximal test results or allow you to compare your results with norm tables. In **Lab 3.2** you will perform three different assessments of cardiorespiratory fitness: the Queen's College step test, the 1-mile walking test, and the 1.5-mile running test. **DO IT! ONLINE**

Queen's College Step Test In this test, you will step up and down on a 16.25-inch-high step bench. At the end of three minutes, take your recovery heart rate for 15 seconds. Use your results to calculate an estimated VO$_2$max and determine your fitness level for your age and sex. The faster your heart recovers from exercise, the better conditioned you are.

One-Mile Walking Test In this test, you will walk as fast as you can for one mile. Record your finish time and your heart rate at the end of the one mile. Use your results to calculate an estimated VO$_2$max and determine your fitness level for your age and sex. A faster time and lower heart rate indicate a higher level of fitness.

1.5-Mile Running Test In this test, you will run 1.5 miles as fast as you can. If you cannot run the entire course, you may take walking breaks. Use your finish time to calculate your estimated VO$_2$max and determine your fitness level for your age and sex. A faster time indicates a higher level of fitness.

How Can I Create My Own Cardiorespiratory Fitness Program?

Having a plan is one of the most important things you can do before beginning a personalized cardiorespiratory fitness program. Careful planning will help you reach your goals, prevent injuries, and ensure that you have fun while exercising!

Set Appropriate Cardiorespiratory Fitness Goals

Goal-setting for cardiorespiratory fitness should follow the SMART goal-setting guidelines (first introduced in Chapter 1). Recall that SMART goals are *specific*, *measurable*, *action-oriented*, *realistic*, and *time-oriented*. Setting a vague goal such as "Build a stronger cardiorespiratory system" is not as useful as setting a specific goal that follows the SMART guidelines, such as "Improve my cardiorespiratory fitness from a 'fair' rating on my three-minute step test to a 'good' rating, by exercising on the elliptical machine three days a week for 30 minutes for the next two months."

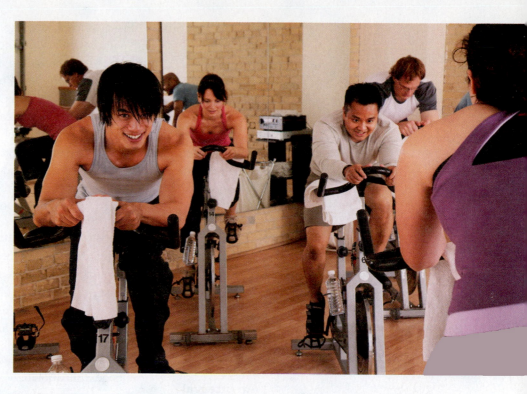

In **Lab 3.3** you will set your own short- and long-term goals for cardiorespiratory fitness. Review the training adaptations and benefits of cardiorespiratory training discussed earlier to guide your goal-setting. Be realistic: If your goal is to run a marathon but you hate running, you will likely be setting yourself up for failure (unless your attitude toward running changes!). Choose goals that you can achieve, doing the types of activities that you enjoy most.

DO IT! ONLINE

Learn about Cardiorespiratory Training Options

A wide variety of cardiorespiratory training options are available to you.

Classes If you enjoy the company of other people and like the motivating aspect of an instructor leading a workout, consider enrolling in a group exercise class. Classes that incorporate a continuous, rhythmic activity lasting more than 20 minutes will help you maintain or improve your cardiorespiratory fitness. Such classes can be found in colleges, recreational centers, and fitness centers in almost every community. Class formats and instructors can vary widely, so consider sampling a few different classes and instructors before deciding on a regular class. Choose classes where the instructors are not only motivating, but also experienced, certified, and knowledgeable about your current health/fitness levels.

Indoor Workouts If you are not sure about working out in a group or with an instructor, you can design your own cardiorespiratory workout using indoor cardio equipment. You can find cardio equipment at most gyms or fitness centers or purchase it for home use. Indoor cardio workout equipment includes stationary bicycles, treadmills, elliptical trainers, stair-climbing machines, recumbent bikes, arm cycle ergometers, rowing machines, and jump ropes. If you are using a machine in a fitness facility, get an introduction to the features, use, and safety from a facility employee. In addition, consider running on an indoor track, swimming in a pool, deep-water jogging, or participating in a racquet sport.

Outdoor Workouts If you like to be outside, explore outdoor options for a cardiorespiratory workout. It is not uncommon to pursue a combination of indoor and outdoor exercise routines, depending on the weather and the facility options available to you. Exercising outdoors can be very rewarding if you live in an area with interesting sights, safe routes, and beautiful trails. The options for outdoor cardio workouts are endless. Here are just a few ideas: walking, jogging, running, cycling, track workouts, trail running, hiking, tennis, cross-country skiing, open-water swimming, and inline skating.

interval workout A workout that alternates periods of higher-intensity exercise with periods of lower-intensity exercise or rest

circuit-training workout A workout where exercisers move from one exercise station to another after a certain number of repetitions or amount of time

perceived exertion A subjective assessment of exercise intensity

talk test A method of measuring exercise intensity based on assessing your ability to speak during exercise

target heart rate The heart rate you are aiming for during an exercise session; often a range with high and low heart rates called your *training zone*

Differing Workout Formats (Continuous, Interval, Circuit)

Aerobic training is a type of *continuous* training—that is, you perform a rhythmic activity and sustain it for a period of time (ideally 20 minutes or more). While aerobic training should be the cornerstone of your cardiorespiratory training program, other workout formats can add variety, intensity, and other fitness benefits.

An **interval workout** alternates periods of higher-intensity exercise with periods of lower-intensity exercise or rest. An interval workout method allows you to increase the intensity of your workout to a level that you might not otherwise be able to sustain for a long period of time. If done correctly, this type of workout can further develop your body's aerobic training adaptations. High-intensity anaerobic intervals improve anaerobic conditioning but also have a greater injury potential.

A **circuit-training workout** involves moving from location to location in a circuit-training room and exercising for a certain amount of time (or number of repetitions) at each "station." You can enroll in a circuit-training class or circuit-train on your own. The circuit can contain alternating aerobic and weight-training activities, just weight stations, or just aerobic stations. The best circuit for cardiorespiratory conditioning is one with all aerobic exercise stations.

Apply FITT Principles to Cardiorespiratory Fitness

After setting goals and selecting the types of cardiorespiratory exercise that you want to do, you must decide how much, how hard, and how long to exercise. Recall the FITT principles (introduced in Chapter 2): *frequency, intensity, time,* and *type*. Let's look at how each of these principles applies to a cardiorespiratory fitness program.

Frequency According to the American College of Sports Medicine, you should spend three to five days per week on cardiorespiratory conditioning. If you are exercising at higher-intensity levels, you can improve or maintain your VO_2max by working out only three days per week. If you are exercising at lower-intensity levels, you may need more than three days per week (five is recommended) to improve cardiorespiratory fitness.

If your goals include weight loss or disease prevention, you will benefit from exercising more often but at a lower intensity to prevent injuries and overtraining.

Intensity Your workouts should be intense enough to tax your cardiorespiratory system, but not so difficult as to discourage you or increase your chances of injury. You can measure the intensity of your exercise by various methods, including determining your heart rate, assessing your **perceived exertion**, and self-administering a **talk test**.

Determining Your Heart Rate Your heart rate provides a good indication of how hard your cardiorespiratory system is working, since it is related to the amount of oxygen that your body is consuming. You can determine your heart rate by using a heart rate monitor or (as we discussed earlier) by counting your pulse.

Heart rate monitors can be found on cardio equipment and merely require you to place your hands on the receiving pads for a few seconds. Personal heart rate monitors, which consist of a chest strap transmitter and a wrist receiver, are also widely available.

Counting your pulse while you are exercising is an easy and low-cost way to measure your heart rate. Your heart rate decreases rapidly after stopping exercise, especially after 15 seconds; therefore, count your pulse for only 10 seconds, and try to keep moving as you count. Then multiply your 10-second count by six to convert to the number of beats per minute (bpm).

What **target heart rate** should you aim for in a workout? The answer depends on your goals and fitness level. As you can see in **Table 3.1** on the following page, the American College of Sports Medicine's recommendations for exercise intensity level cites a wide range of target heart rates: 64 to 95 percent of HRmax. Use the following guidelines to determine where within this range you should aim:

- If your fitness level is low, you should follow the guidelines for moderate cardiorespiratory exercise or 64–75 percent of your HRmax. Start below or at the low end of this range if you are very deconditioned or brand new to exercise.

- If your fitness level is moderate, aim for the vigorous exercise guidelines or 76–95 percent of your HRmax or choose to do a mix of moderate and vigorous exercise.

TABLE 3.1 ACSM's Training Guidelines for Cardiorespiratory Fitness

Recommendations for the General Adult Population

Frequency (days/week)	Moderate: 5 Vigorous: 3
Intensity (how hard)	Moderate: 64–75% of HRmax Vigorous: 76–95% of HRmax
Time (how long)	Moderate: 30–60 min (150 min/week) Vigorous: 20–60 min (75 min/week)
Type (exercises)	Rhythmic, aerobic, large muscle group activity

Data from: American College of Sports Medicine, *ACSM's Guidelines for Exercise Testing and Prescription*, 9th Edition (Baltimore: Lippincott Williams & Wilkins, 2014).

Table 3.2 also provides target heart rate guidelines for exercise, using the HRmax method based on your age. Another method of determining your target heart rate is to measure your **heart rate reserve (HRR)**, the difference between your resting and maximum heart rates. **Lab 3.1** walks you through how to determine your HRR.

DO IT! ONLINE

Perceived Exertion Another way to assess the intensity of your workout is by determining your perceived exertion: your perception of how hard you are working during exercise. One of the most well-known perceived exertion scales was developed by Gunnar Borg in 1970. His Rating of Perceived Exertion (RPE) scale is a subjective 15-point scale, from 6 through 20, that is related to heart rate responses to exercise.[22] The Borg RPE Scale can be a very valuable tool when it is not easy or appropriate to use heart rate monitoring to check your workout intensity. For example, if you participate in a water sport such as swimming, heart rate monitoring can be misleading; heart rates tend to slow down while you exercise in water due to increased hydrostatic pressure and decreased temperature. For this reason, you may prefer to use RPE to determine your exercise intensity.

Another perceived exertion scale is the OMNI Scale of Perceived Exertion. Although originally developed for children, adult versions now exist and these provide a simple way to assess workout intensity on a 1–10 scale (see **Figure 3.8**). The OMNI Scale is correlated with the Borg RPE scale and heart rate responses.[23] As you become more experienced with a particular cardiorespiratory activity and become more attuned to how your body feels during exercise, your ability to use the perceived exertion scales accurately will improve.

The Talk Test The talk test method of measuring exercise intensity is based on assessing how easily you can talk during exercise. While exercising at a *light* intensity, you should be able to talk easily and continuously. If you are exercising at a *moderate* intensity, you should be able to talk easily, but not continuously, during the activity. If you are too out of breath to carry on a conversation easily, you are working at a high or *vigorous* intensity. If you cannot talk at all, you are probably doing an anaerobic interval or sprinting.

TABLE 3.2 Target Heart Rate Guidelines*

Age	Target HR Range (bpm)	10-Sec Count
18–24	139–179	23–30
25–29	135–174	22–29
30–34	132–169	22–28
35–39	129–165	21–28
40–44	125–160	21–27
45–49	122–156	20–26
50–54	118–151	20–25
55–59	114–147	19–25
60–64	110–142	18–24
65+	108–140	18–23

*Based upon the HRmax method, where 220 − age = HRmax and the training zone is 70 to 90% of HRmax (moderate to vigorous). Individuals with low fitness levels should start below or at the low end of these ranges.

heart rate reserve (HRR)
The number of beats per minute available or in reserve for exercise heart rate increases; maximal heart rate minus resting heart rate

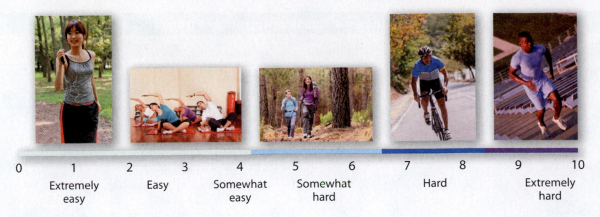

0	1	2	3	4	5	6	7	8	9	10
Extremely easy		Easy		Somewhat easy		Somewhat hard		Hard		Extremely hard

FIGURE **3.8** Determine your exercise intensity on a 1–10 scale by assessing how you feel when exercising. Aim for ratings of 5, 6, 7, or 8 for most cardiorespiratory activities.

Source: Based on A. C. Utter et al., "Validation of the Adult OMNI Scale of Perceived Exertion for Walking/Running Exercise," *Medicine & Science in Sports & Exercise* 36, no. 10 (2004): 1776–80.

To increase cardiorespiratory fitness, aim for at least a moderate intensity level for most of your workout or the highest level you can comfortably sustain for 20 to 30 minutes. You can incorporate short periods of light and vigorous activity for workout variety or interval training. **Table 3.3** summarizes the most common intensity scales for cardiorespiratory endurance exercise. Use the one that works best for you and the type of exercise you have chosen.

Time For optimal cardiorespiratory conditioning, your exercise sessions should be 20 to 30 minutes long. If you are just starting out, exercise continuously for as long as you can, and then work your way up to the minimum guideline of 20 minutes. The GetFitGraphic Are Short Workouts Worth My Time? on the following page examines how workouts as short as 10 to 15 minutes can benefit health.

TABLE **3.3** Cardiorespiratory Intensity Scales*					
General	Talk Test	OMNI	Borg RPE	% HRR	% HRmax
Light	Easy conversation	0	6	30	57
		1	7	35	60
		2	8		
			9		
		3	10		
		4	11	39	63
Moderate	Brief sentences and words	5	12	40	64
			13		
		6	14	59	75
Vigorous	A few words	7	15	60	76
			16		
		8	17	89	95
Anaerobic	Barely or not able to talk	9	18	90	96
			19		
		10	20	100	100

*The various methods to quantify exercise intensity in this table may not be equivalent to one another.

Data are from: American College of Sports Medicine, *ACSM's Guidelines for Exercise Testing and Prescription*, 9th Edition (Baltimore, MD: Lippincott Williams & Wilkins, 2014); Office of Disease Prevention and Health Promotion, U.S. Department of Health and Human Services, 2008 Physical Activity Guidelines for Americans: Be Active, Healthy, and Happy! ODPHP Publication no. U0036 (Washington, DC: U.S. Department of Health and Human Services, 2008), Available at www.health.gov; R. J. Robertson et al., "Validation of the Adult OMNI Scale of Perceived Exertion for Cycle Ergometer Exercise," *Medicine & Science in Sports & Exercise* 36, no. 1 (2004): 102–8; A. C. Utter et al., "Validation of the Adult OMNI Scale of Perceived Exertion for Walking/Running Exercise," *Medicine & Science in Sports & Exercise* 36, no. 10 (2004): 1776–80; G. Borg, Borg's *Perceived Exertion and Pain Scales* (Champaign, IL: Human Kinetics, 1998): 27–38.

ARE SHORT WORKOUTS WORTH MY TIME?

IN SHORT, YES! Experts once believed that long aerobic workouts were more effective than short workouts for your health. Recent research shows that: (1) you don't have to exercise a long time to get benefits, and (2) a short but a *high intensity* training can have a major impact on your health.

What are the BENEFITS of MULTIPLE SHORT WORKOUTS during the day?

Short workouts are better than one continuous workout at

- Lowering fats in the bloodstream.[1]

- Burning calories and balancing blood glucose/insulin levels (because metabolism increases after 10 minutes of exercise and persists for 60 minutes).[2]

What is HIGH-INTENSITY INTERVAL TRAINING (HIIT)?

HIIT is a workout strategy that alternates high intensity quick bursts of exercise activity with recovery periods of lower intensity exercise.

- 4 minutes of HITT can lead to similar improvements in VO_2max and greater improvements in muscular endurance than 30 minutes of traditional endurance training.[3]

HOW DO YOU HIIT?

1 GET READY

Because of the **HIGHER INTENSITY** of some **HIIT PROTOCOLS, GO SLOW** if you aren't fit.

2 GET SET

CHOOSE AN INTERVAL that you can perform for 15 seconds to 4 minutes at 80-95% of your maximum heart rate or a rating of 8-10 on the perceived exertion scale. Here are some common interval recommendations:

JUST STARTING
1:3 ratio — 30 sec high-intensity : 90 sec recovery

MODERATE FITNESS
1:2 ratio — 40 sec high-intensity : 80 sec recovery

ALREADY FIT
1:1 ratio — 60 sec high-intensity : 60 sec recovery

3 GO

OUTSIDE?

Interval: running/walking sprints or hills

Recovery: jog/walk

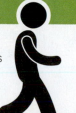

INSIDE?

Interval: jumping jacks, jump rope, jump squats, jump lunges, burpees

Recovery: walk/jog in place

Type For optimal motivation, training adaptation, and injury prevention, choose activities that you enjoy. Alternate your participation in these activities by the day or week for a **cross-training** effect. Cross-training can help you maintain muscle balance by working different muscle groups.

Include a Warm-Up and Cool-Down Phase in Your Workout Session

A cardiorespiratory workout session should consist of three components: the **warm-up** phase, the main cardiorespiratory endurance conditioning set, and the **cool-down** phase. **Figure 3.9** illustrates a sample 60-minute workout showing each of these components. Remember that your warm-up should ideally consist of light physical activity that mimics the movements of your main exercise set. For example, if your main exercise set is jogging, an ideal warm-up would be to walk briskly. Likewise, your cool-down should ideally be a less-vigorous version of your main exercise set. (Review Chapter 2 for more guidelines on warming up and cooling down.) Keep in mind that when you are starting an exercise program, you should generally perform longer warm-up (10 to 15 minutes) and cool-down (10 minutes or more) segments.

cross-training The practice of using different exercise modes or types in your cardiorespiratory training program

warm-up The initial 5-to 10-minute preparation phase of a workout

cool-down The ending phase of a workout where the body is brought gradually back to rest

Plan for Proper Progression of Your Program

When you are starting a new exercise program, it is easy to attempt to do too much too soon. A fitness program needs to be *progressive* in order for you to achieve results and avoid injury. As you begin a fitness program, your progress may initially be slow, while your body adjusts to the new activity. Eventually, consistent exercise will result in noticeable improvement.

In order to avoid injuring yourself, increase your workout by no more than 10 percent per week (the *10 percent rule*). That means that your weekly increases in frequency, intensity, and/or time should not total more than 10 percent. For example, if you are jogging for 30 minutes per exercise session, next week you could safely increase each session to 33 minutes (10 percent increase in time).

How Can I Maintain My Cardiorespiratory Program?

How many times have you started a fitness program only to quit after a few weeks? For many people, the biggest challenge to improving cardiorespiratory fitness is not beginning a program, but keeping it up. Next we discuss the stages of progression and the importance of tracking your progress and reassessing your needs.

Understand the Stages of Progression

Start-up In the *start-up* phase of a cardiorespiratory program, you will be adjusting to the new activity in your weekly routine. During this stage, it is important to pay attention to how you feel during exercise so that you can make adjustments if necessary. Do you prefer exercising in the morning or in the evening? Is that aerobics class really right for you? In this first stage, your main concern should be fine-tuning your program until you settle on an activity and routine that is comfortable for you. Depending on your fitness level and exercise experience, this stage can last anywhere from two to four weeks.

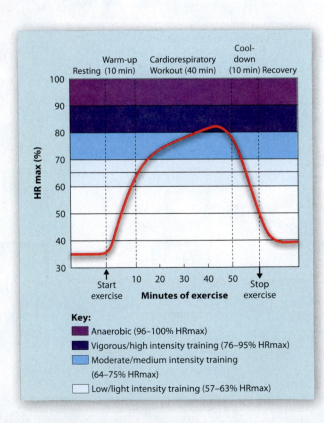

FIGURE **3.9** This graph charts a sample 60-minute cardiorespiratory workout, including a warm-up, cardiorespiratory fitness workout, and a cool-down.

casestudy

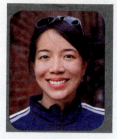

ANGELA

"After practically killing myself on the tennis court last week, I did some research into exactly what it means to 'get in shape.' I was really interested to learn about things like target heart rates and the different ways to measure cardiorespiratory fitness. I took the 1.5-mile run test and found out that my current fitness rating is only 'fair.' So my plan is to design a cardio workout that will get my rating up to 'good' or 'excellent' before challenging my friend to another match!"

THINK! Pretend you are Angela's fitness trainer and decide on an appropriate target goal for Angela. Does the goal you outlined for Angela follow the SMART guidelines?

ACT NOW! Today, become your own personal fitness trainer and write yourself a target cardiorespiratory goal incorporating the SMART guidelines. This week, get started working toward your cardiorespiratory goal. Put the first workout in your schedule. In two weeks, reevaluate your SMART cardiorespiratory goal. Does it seem realistic or too easy? How can you modify it, if needed?

HEAR IT! ONLINE

Improvement Once you have the "kinks" worked out of your program, you are ready to move into the *improvement* phase. In this stage, your body starts adapting to the cardiorespiratory exercise. Some of these changes will be evident to you; some will not (refer to Figure 3.5). You should, however, start feeling better during exercise, have more energy when not exercising, and feel that you can exercise for longer periods of time without fatigue. As in the initial stage, listen to your body so that you can make changes as needed. The improvement stage can last anywhere from three to eight months, depending on your program and goals.

Maintenance After months of hard work you are at the fitness level you desire and you feel great! You have reached the *maintenance* stage. The key to this stage is to keep your program consistent. If you stop exercising, you can lose your newly achieved fitness level in only half the time it took you to acquire it. In fact, athletes can start losing cardiorespiratory fitness within just two weeks of inactivity. If you need to cut back but don't want to lose your hard-earned improvements, cut back on exercise time but not intensity level. It is easier to maintain cardiorespiratory fitness with shorter but more intense workouts. The maintenance stage lasts for as long as you continue your program.

Record and Track Your Fitness Progress

Do you remember how you felt during that spinning workout three weeks ago? What was the speed and incline of your treadmill workout last week? One of the best ways to make sure that you stay on track with your fitness program is to record your activity and track your progress over time. Keeping a workout journal or log will encourage you to write down things such as the FITT components of your workout, how you felt during the workout, the time of day, and any other information that may be relevant. Record your successes as well as your setbacks—this will remind you of the progress you have made since beginning the program and help determine if your goals or workouts should be adjusted over time. The box Technology to Track Your Fitness on page 82 explains some of the technology and websites you can use to assess and log your fitness progress.

Troubleshoot Problems Right Away

Everyone will experience obstacles or problems when starting an exercise program. You may not have enough time in your day to work out, it may be difficult for you to physically get to your workout facility, you may be feeling pain in your knee, and so on. While these issues may set you back temporarily, they should not keep you from reaching your goals. Address the problems right away and brainstorm solutions; the sooner you acknowledge a problem and address it, the sooner you can get back on track.

Periodically Reassess Your Cardiorespiratory Fitness Level

Although you will certainly feel your progress by how your body responds to exercise, it is always nice to have quantitative measures of your progress as well. Complete the assessments in **Lab 3.2** at least twice—once after three months of your new program and again at six months. Keep in mind that you will see the most improvements in assessments that are similar to your chosen workout activity (e.g., if you are doing step aerobics, you will probably see more improvement in the step test than in the 1.5-mile run test). If you have

DO IT! ONLINE

CHANGE

Technology to Track Your Fitness

There are countless technology tools out there for tracking exercise, diet, and fitness goals. **Wearable monitors** containing tiny motion sensors (such as pedometers) can track your activity levels and workouts. A **wrist-watch GPS** can track miles, time, and pace and may even include a heart rate monitor to track your intensity levels. The latest **smartphone apps** and **online tracking programs** can track your workouts and progress toward your goals.

Get started with the *Get Fit, Stay Well* Activate, Motivate, Advance Website, an online tracking program and smartphone mobile website that integrates fitness programs available in this book. To access the site, visit the Study Area in MasteringHealth or scan the QR codes for each program in the book.

Here are a few additional suggestions for fitness apps and tracking programs:

My Fitness Pal www.myfitnesspal.com

An online tracking program and smartphone app for diet and exercise.

MapMyRun www.mapmyrun.com

Uses the built-in GPS of your mobile device to track all of your fitness activities, including duration, distance, pace, speed, elevation, calories burned, and route traveled on an interactive map.

Zombies-Run www.zombiesrungame.com

An ultra-immersive running game and audio adventure.

Fitness Builder www.fitnessbuilder.com

Offers 750+ workouts and 5,600+ exercise images and videos, access to a personal trainer, performance tracking, and sharing tools.

Lose It! www.loseit.com

Helps you set a daily calorie budget, track your food and exercise, and stay motivated to achieve your goals.

USDA SuperTracker www.supertracker.usda.gov

Get nutrition and fitness plans and track your food intake and exercise in this comprehensive website.

When you search for fitness apps or online tracking programs, make sure to consider if the source is reputable, if the program is easy-to-use, if it will adequately track your goals, and if it is motivating and appealing to you. While nothing can substitute for your own motivation and adherence, new technology can enhance your motivation and provide support via social media.

---

not improved, look at your program again and figure out whether you need to redesign it.

Reassess Your Goals and Program as Needed

Once a target date arrives, review your goals for that date. Did you achieve what you set out to do? If not, list the reasons why. You may need to set more realistic goals with more realistic target dates, or select a different activity. If you need more motivation, consider finding a workout partner or working with a personal trainer. If you did reach your goal, set a new goal for maintenance or a more challenging goal to improve your fitness level even more. The sample running, cycling, and swimming programs in Activate, Motivate, & Advance Your Fitness at the end of this chapter (pages 102–111) can help you set new goals and develop new fitness plans.

How Can I Avoid Injury during Cardiorespiratory Exercise?

The fastest way to disrupt a training program is to get injured. Reduce your injury risk by understanding and following common exercise injury prevention methods.

Design a Personalized, Balanced Cardiorespiratory Program

The most common injuries from cardiorespiratory fitness programs are from overuse, such as strains and tendonitis, particularly in the lower body. If you attempt to do too much too soon, you put yourself at risk for such injuries. Make sure your exercise program considers your current level of fitness and make your FITT targets realistic and achievable. You may also want to consider incorporating cross-training into your program, since doing one activity exclusively can result in uneven muscle development, making you more vulnerable to injury.

Wear Appropriate Clothing and Footwear

Use common sense when you are dressing for your chosen cardiorespiratory activity. If you are cycling, a helmet and bright clothing are essential. If you are running, walking, taking a group fitness class, or participating in a racquet sport, pay particularly close attention to your footwear. You need shoes that will protect your feet and provide the right amount of support and cushioning. See **Figure 3.10** for tips to help you find the right shoes.

What about those people you see running in bare feet, or with minimalist shoes? The box Barefoot Running: Is It Safe for Me? on page 84 provides an overview of this style of running.

Pay Attention to Your Exercise Environment

Prevent Heat-Related Illness

When exercising indoors, be sure the exercise room is well ventilated and cool enough to prevent your body from overheating. When exercising outdoors in hot weather, take precautions to avoid heat-related illnesses such as **heat cramps**, **heat exhaustion**, or **heat stroke**. Your risk of heat-related illness

heat cramps Severe cramping in the large muscle groups and abdomen caused by high fluid and electrolyte loss in sustained exertion in the heat

heat exhaustion An elevated core body temperature, headache, fatigue, profuse sweating, nausea, and clammy skin brought on by sustained exertion in the heat with dehydration and electrolyte losses

heat stroke A core body temperature above 104°F, headache, nausea, vomiting, diarrhea, rapid pulse, cessation of sweating, and disorientation resulting from extreme exertion in very hot conditions

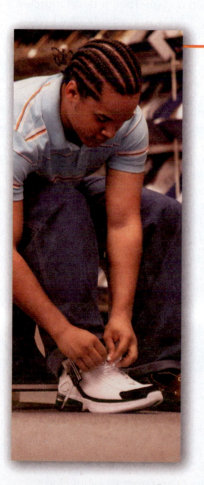

How do I choose the right exercise shoe?

Shop for shoes after a workout or at the end of the day when your feet are their biggest

Wear socks you will wear when exercising

Be sure you can freely wiggle all of your toes

Lace shoes up correctly and walk/run around the store

Make sure your heel doesn't slide up and down as you walk/run

Shoes should feel comfortable as soon as you try them on

Choose a sport specific shoe if you participate in a sport 3 or more times a week or will be doing high-intensity workouts

FIGURE **3.10** Use these tips to find the right exercise shoes.

Source: Based on the American Academy of Orthopaedic Surgeons, "Your Orthopaedic Connection: Athletic Shoes," Reviewed August 2012, http://orthoinfo.aaos.org

Q&A Is Barefoot Running Safe for Me?

Have you noticed people out on the street running without shoes or wearing "FiveFingers"—those funny-looking shoes with toes? What are these people up to? They are part of a new and growing trend: barefoot running. What's behind this trend? And should you be running barefoot?

Advocates of barefoot running point out that humans have been running without shoes or with minimal shoes since they stood up on two legs and indicate several perceived advantages to doing so. One claimed benefit is that the shorter stride in barefoot running is more natural from an evolutionary standpoint and it can reduce running injuries.[1] Advocates say the less support you give to your arch, the stronger your arch becomes—barefoot activity builds up the muscles of the foot. And, they say, running barefoot makes you more aware of the terrain you are running through, encouraging a connection with the environment.[2] Researchers have shown that runners who run barefoot tend to strike the ground with their forefoot or midfoot rather than their heel;[3] there is anecdotal evidence that forefoot or midfoot striking can help avoid and/or mitigate repetitive stress injuries, especially stress fractures, plantar fasciitis, and runner's knee.[4]

Critics of the trend, though, point out that this is still a theory. As yet, there is no evidence that barefoot or minimalist running reduces injuries. Critics concede there is no evidence that running shoes reduce injuries either.[5] More research is needed before conclusions can be drawn about any of these opinions, pro or con. However, critics do point out that, unlike running in shoes, barefoot running can result in puncture wounds from sharp objects on the ground.

So, where does that leave you? Scientists do say that some barefoot running as a part of an overall training plan can be beneficial in strengthening the bones, ligaments,

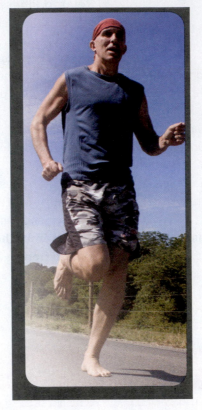

muscles, and tendons in the feet. And, using a barefoot *style* of running—striking the ground with the midfoot rather than the heel even when you're wearing running shoes—may also be beneficial.[6] The benefits of barefoot running in the sand or grass, for example, have been noted as a training tool, but not for every run. There is some validity to letting your foot move in a more natural way and steering away from shoes that don't allow your foot to move at all. Increasing the actual strength of your foot muscles is another benefit.

If you want to incorporate barefoot or "barefoot-like" running into your workout, some solid advice is to make the change slowly. Don't just throw out your running shoes and do a five-mile run! Start out by doing activities around the house barefoot, and walking barefoot to build up your foot and calf muscles slowly. Check with your doctor before adding barefoot running to your exercise program; people who have circulatory or nerve issues should not attempt to run barefoot, as they are at increased risk for injury. If your doctor clears you for incorporating barefoot running, you may want to try shoes with more flexibility and less cushioning and then gradually work your way to minimalist shoes for part of your weekly workout time. Then, do a portion of your running in bare feet to allow your feet to develop calluses for running on rough surfaces. As your muscles strengthen, you can build on the time you spend running barefoot.[7]

Sources:
1. D. E. Lieberman, "What We Can Learn About Running from Barefoot Running: An Evolutionary Medical Perspective," *Exercise and Sport Science Reviews* 40, no. 2 (2012): 63–72, doi: 10.1097/JES.0b013e31824ab210.
2. R. Collier, "The Rise of Barefoot Running," *Canadian Medical Association Journal* 183, no. 1 (2011): E37–38, doi: 10.1503/cmaj.109-3745.
3. D. E. Lieberman et al., "Foot Strike Patterns and Collision Forces in Habitually Barefoot Versus Shod Runners," *Nature* 463, no. 7280 (2010): 531–35, doi:10.1038/nature08723.
4. D. E. Lieberman et al., "Running Barefoot, Forefoot Striking and Training Tips," Biomechanics of Foot Strikes & Applications to Running Barefoot or in Minimal Footwear, www.barefootrunning.fas.harvard.edu
5. R. Collier, "The Rise of Barefoot Running," 2011.
6. D. E. Lieberman et al., "Foot Strike Patterns and Collision Forces," 2010.
7. C. Pauls and L. Kravitz, "Barefoot Running," *IDEA Fitness Journal* 7, no. 5 (2010): 14–17.

increases if you (1) exercise too hard for your fitness level, (2) exercise in high heat, humidity, and sunshine, (3) have a low fitness level overall, (4) are lacking in adequate sleep, (5) are not accustomed to the environment, (6) have an underlying infection, or (7) are overweight.[24] You can decrease your risk by being more fit, wearing

light, sweat-wicking clothing, picking cooler times of the day to exercise, avoiding hazardous conditions, letting your body gradually become accustomed to the environment, and increasing your workout slowly.

If you suspect you are developing a heat-related illness, act immediately. For heat cramps, cease activity, seek a cool environment, and restore your body's fluid and electrolyte balances by drinking water or a sports drink. For heat exhaustion, rest in a cool environment, apply cold packs to your head and neck, drink water or a sports drink, and seek medical attention. If you suspect heatstroke, you will need medical attention immediately; untreated heatstroke is very serious and can lead to death. In heatstroke illness the body can no longer cool itself and ice-water immersion and IV fluids may be necessary right away. Because exercise increases your core body temperature, your risk of heat illness is greater when you are active, even in lower temperatures. Take extra precautions during difficult workouts to take breaks and drink fluids.

Prevent Cold-Related Illness Exercising in extreme cold also presents risks. If you like to ski, hike in the mountains, swim in cold water, or just exercise in snowy, windy, rainy environments, you should take precautions to prevent **hypothermia**, a condition in which the body's internal temperature drops so low that it can no longer warm itself back up. If untreated, hypothermia leads to death. To avoid hypothermia, (1) minimize heat loss by wearing a warm hat and clothing, (2) keep yourself dry by wearing sweat-wicking clothing and changing out of wet clothes as quickly as possible, (3) exercise with a workout partner who can help recognize early warning signs of cold-related illness, (4) avoid exercising in poor weather conditions, (5) warm up thoroughly, (6) drink fluids to stay hydrated, and (7) get out of the cold and warm up if you start shivering.

The early warning signs of hypothermia include shivering, goose bumps, and fast, shallow breathing. The next stage involves violent shivering, muscle incoordination, mild confusion, pale skin, and potentially blue lips, ears, fingers, and toes. In the most dangerous and potentially fatal stage of hypothermia, shivering will stop and the person will have trouble thinking, speaking, walking, and using his or her hands. If you suspect you are at risk of hypothermia, get dry and warm as soon as possible. If you are in an advanced stage of hypothermia, you will need medical attention immediately.

Be Aware of the Impact of Air Quality Air pollution can irritate your air passageways and lungs, particularly if you have asthma, allergies, bronchitis, or other pulmonary disorders. If you experience a disruption in your breathing pattern, irritated eyes, or a headache, stop exercising and go indoors. Avoid exercising outdoors when the air quality is poor,

particularly if you have a smog or air-quality alert in your city that day. If you exercise outside on a regular basis, take measures to reduce your intake of air pollution. Exercise in wilderness areas, in parks, or on low-traffic streets. Try to exercise at times when the air quality is better, such as early in the morning and on weekends.

Watch for Hazards Watch for hazards in your exercise environment that may cause you to trip and fall. When exercising indoors, seek out a space with a well-maintained floor and where you can work out without obstructions. When exercising outdoors, seek out lower-impact surfaces such as a school track, running or bike path, or a dirt trail. Use your common sense: Avoid slippery or muddy surfaces and areas with heavy vehicle traffic. If you exercise outdoors at night, wear reflective clothing and clip a light somewhere on your body so that drivers can easily see you.

hypothermia A condition where the core temperature of the body drops below the level required for sustaining normal bodily functions

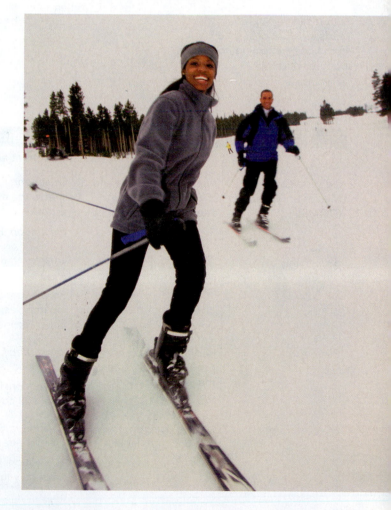

THINK! What hazards do you face in your exercise routine? Can cars really see you when you are running on the road at night? Do your shoes have decent soles, so you don't slip?

ACT! List three things about your workout routine, your clothing, or your environment that might put you at risk for injury or illness. For each risky item or behavior, list what steps you need to take to reduce your risk.

Drink Enough Water

If you sweat profusely and do not replace the lost fluid, you will become dehydrated. Your body needs a certain amount of water in order to function. Loss of body water will decrease your blood volume and will subsequently decrease the blood flow to muscles, lowering exercise performance. **Dehydration** will also slow your sweat rate and significantly increase your susceptibility for heat-related illness.

According to the ACSM, you should lose no more than 2 percent of your body weight in fluid during an exercise session.[25] A loss of fluid equivalent to 1 percent of your body weight will cause you to feel thirsty; losses over

dehydration A process that leads to a lack of sufficient fluid in the body, affecting normal body functioning

3 percent may start to affect your exercise performance. Weigh yourself before and after exercise to determine how much water weight you have lost and adjust your fluid intake accordingly. Water loss is an individual issue. Everyone sweats at different rates in response to exercise. To decrease water loss, start drinking additional fluid several hours before an exercise session and drink during exercise as well. If you are exercising for more than an hour, you may benefit from drinking fluid with sugars and electrolytes (salts) in it, such as a sports drink.

Understand How to Prevent and Treat Common Injuries

The following are some of the most common exercise injuries, as well as guidelines for how to prevent and treat them. See also **Table 3.4** for a summary of these and other common exercise injuries.

Delayed-Onset Muscle Soreness *Delayed-onset muscle soreness* (DOMS) is the muscle tightness and tenderness you may feel a day or two after a hard workout session. This soreness is due to microscopic tears in your muscle fibers and connective tissues; it occurs when the body sustains excessive overloads. Most people experience DOMS at one point or another and typically recover quickly. DOMS is a sign that you did too much too soon. If you experience DOMS (especially common when starting an exercise program),

TABLE 3.4 Common Exercise Injuries, Treatments, and Prevention

Injury	Description	Treatment and Prevention
Delayed-Onset Muscle Soreness (DOMS)	Muscle tenderness and stiffness 24–48 hours after strenuous exercise	*Treatment:* Reduce exercise to light activity until the pain stops, gently stretch the area; for some, heat and anti-inflammatory medications help as well *Prevention:* Follow proper exercise programming guidelines
Back Pain	Sharp or dull pain and stiffness in the mid to lower back	*Treatment:* Reduce exercise until the acute pain stops; gently stretch the area; use ice, heat, anti-inflammatory medications *Prevention:* Strengthen abdominal and back muscles, stretch back and hip muscles, maintain a healthy body weight, have good posture and lifting techniques
Blisters	Red, fluid- or blood-filled pockets of skin, often on the feet after a long exercise session	*Treatment:* Change shoes that may have caused the blister, keep the area clean, and cover if needed; do not purposefully pop blisters *Prevention:* Use comfortable shoes that fit well and sweat-wicking socks (avoid all-cotton socks)
Muscle Cramps	Muscle pain, tightness, and uncontrollable spasms	*Treatment:* Stop activity; massage and stretch the affected area until the cramp releases *Prevention:* Follow warm-up, cool-down, and general exercise guidelines; stay fully hydrated for exercise

(Continued)

TABLE **3.4** (*Continued*)

Injury	Description	Treatment and Prevention
Muscle Strain	Damage to the muscle or tendon fibers due to injury or overtraining resulting in pain, swelling, and decreased function; varying levels of severity	*Treatment:* Reduce painful activity; use ice as needed; apply ice and/or heat after a few days; use anti-inflammatory medications if desired; stretching *Prevention:* Follow warm-up, cool-down, and general exercise guidelines; reduce or stop activity if muscles feel overly weak and fatigued
Joint Sprain	Damage to ligaments or joint structures; the result of an acute injury resulting in pain, swelling, and loss of function; varying levels of severity	*Treatment:* Stop activity; use ice, compression, elevation; seek medical attention *Prevention:* Avoid high joint-stress activities, strengthen joint-supporting muscles, wear supportive bracing if necessary
Dislocation	Separation of bones in a joint causing structural alterations and potential ligament and nerve damage	*Treatment:* Stop activity; use ice, immobilization; seek medical treatment *Prevention:* Avoid high joint-stress activities, strengthen joint-supporting muscles, wear supportive bracing if necessary
Tendonitis	Chronic pain and swelling in tendons as a result of overuse	*Treatment:* Reduce exercise to light activity until the pain stops; apply ice, gently stretch the area; anti-inflammatory medications may help *Prevention:* Follow proper exercise programming guidelines, work for muscle balance in strength and flexibility
Plantar Fasciitis	Irritation, pain, and swelling of the fascia under the foot	*Treatment:* Reduce painful activities, gently stretch the area; for some people, ice, heat, and/or anti-inflammatory medications help *Prevention:* Wear good athletic shoes with adequate arch support and cushioning; warm up and stretch the plantar fascia prior to exercise
Runner's Knee	Patella-femoral pain syndrome where there is chronic pain behind or around the kneecap	*Treatment:* Reduce exercises that cause pain; use ice, anti-inflammatory medications if needed for pain and swelling *Prevention:* Work for balance in strength and flexibility in all of the knee-supporting muscles; wear good athletic shoes with support and foot control; exercise on softer surfaces; control weight
Shin Splints	Chronic pain in the front of the lower leg (the shins); can also occur as pain on the sides of the lower leg	*Treatment:* Reduce painful exercise; apply ice, gently stretch the area, switch to less weight-bearing activities *Prevention:* Work for balance in strength and flexibility in the lower-leg muscles, wear good athletic shoes with support and cushioning, exercise on softer surfaces
Stress Fracture	Small crack or breaks in the bone in overused areas of the body causing chronic pain; must be medically diagnosed via X-ray	*Treatment:* Perform non-weight-bearing exercise until the acute pain stops, seek medical attention, rest *Prevention:* Follow proper exercise programming guidelines to avoid overtraining, wear good athletic shoes with support and cushioning, exercise on softer surfaces

examine your program design. Find ways to decrease the time, intensity, resistance, or repetitions of the exercise.

Muscle and Tendon Strains A muscle or tendon strain is a soft-tissue injury that can be acute or chronic. An acute, sudden strain occurs due to a trauma or sudden movement/force that you are not accustomed to. A chronic, perpetual strain occurs from overstressed muscles that are worked in the same way over and over. Muscle strains involve damage to the muscle fibers; tendon strains involve damage to the tissue that connects muscles to bones. The primary symptoms of a strain are muscle pain, spasms, and weakness. In addition, there may be swelling of the area, cramping, and difficulty moving the muscle involved. Commonly strained areas of the body are the lower back and the back of the thighs (hamstrings).

Ligament and Joint Sprains A sudden movement or trauma can cause a sprain (damage to joint structures). A *mild* or *first-degree sprain* involves overstretching or slight tearing of the ligament(s), resulting in some pain and swelling but little or no decrease in joint stability. In a *moderate* or *second-degree sprain,* ligaments are partially torn, and the area is painful, swollen, and bruised. In this level of sprain, mobility is limited and medical attention should be sought to determine the true severity of the injury. A *severe* or *third-degree sprain* involves a complete tearing or rupturing of the ligament or joint structures. Excessive pain, swelling, bruising, and an inability to move or put any weight on the joint are symptoms of a third-degree sprain. Immediate medical attention is necessary to determine whether bones were broken during the injury process. The most common sprains occur in the ankle while landing from a jump, in the knee from a fall or a blow to the side, and in the wrist during a fall.

Overuse Injuries Overuse injuries are due to repetitive use. You are at an increased risk of an overuse injury if you are new to sports and exercise, if you dramatically change your exercise routine, or if you do the same type of activity day in and day out.

Tendonitis is a typical overuse injury that can result from overusing the lower- or upper-body muscles. The repetitive contractions of skeletal muscles can cause pain and swelling in the tendons near joints. Common tendonitis

RICE Acronym for *rest, ice,* compression, and elevation; a method of treating common exercise injuries

locations are the elbow, ankle, and shoulder; these often result from tennis ("tennis elbow"), running, and weight-lifting, respectively.

A frequent overuse injury in runners and walkers is *plantar fasciitis,* or inflammation in the fascia on the underside of the foot. Pain in the arch and the heel of the foot, particularly when you are not warmed up (stepping out of bed in the morning), is the hallmark of this overuse injury.

Another injury common in runners is "runner's knee," or *patella-femoral pain syndrome*. Pain behind the kneecap (patella), inflammation, and tenderness can result from an imbalance in knee-stabilizing muscles that will cause the patella to get "off track" with your other knee joint structures. Women tend to have more problems with this syndrome than men due to the greater dynamic flexibility of their hips and knees.

Shin splints is the general term used to describe any pain that occurs in the front or sides of the lower legs. It may be tendonitis, a muscle strain, connective tissue inflammation, or a stress fracture. In response to repetitive stresses on hard surfaces, the muscles, tendons, and connective tissues of your lower leg muscles become inflamed and painful. Shin splints are common in runners and high-mileage walkers. Over time, repeated stress to the lower leg can lead to a *stress fracture*, a small crack or break in a bone. If you think you have shin splints but the pain won't go away with rest, ice, and therapy, you should get medical attention to rule out a stress fracture.

Treating Injuries with RICE The **RICE** treatment for injuries involves *rest, ice,* compression, and elevation. After an injury, you should *rest* or stop using that body part and allow for treatment and recovery. Most injuries will require *ice* immediately to reduce blood flow, acute inflammation, and pain. Apply ice or an ice pack for 10 to 30 minutes at a time, three to five times a day until symptoms lessen. *Compression* or applying pressure to the injury can be helpful for injuries that are bleeding or swelling. Using an elastic bandage around the injury will reduce swelling but still allow for adequate blood flow to the area. Tingling or discolored skin can be a sign that your wrapping is too tight. In order to promote blood flow back to the heart and lower the amount of swelling, *elevate* the injury above heart level. Following the RICE treatment is a good start for most exercise and sports-related injuries. Seek further medical attention if you are unsure how injured you are or if symptoms do not cease within a few hours.

CHAPTER IN REVIEW

MasteringHealth™

Build your knowledge—and wellness!—in the Study Area of MasteringHealth with a variety of study tools.

SEE IT! ONLINE

videos

Heart Rate: Radial Pulse
Heart Rate: Carotid Pulse

HEAR IT! ONLINE

audio tools

Audio case study
MP3 chapter review

REVIEW IT! ONLINE

chapter review

Chapter reading quizzes
Glossary flashcards

LIVE IT! ONLINE

programs & behavior change

Customizable four-week running programs
Customizable four-week biking programs
Customizable four-week swimming programs
Take Charge of Your Health! Worksheets
Behavior Change Log Book and Wellness Journal

DO IT! ONLINE

labs

Lab 3.1 Monitoring Intensity during a Workout
Lab 3.2 Assessing Your Cardiorespiratory Fitness Level
Lab 3.3 Plan Your Cardiorespiratory Fitness Goals and Program
Alternate Aerobic Fitness Assessments

reviewquestions

1. Cardiorespiratory fitness would be most improved by which of the following?
   a. Stretching your leg muscles every day
   b. A 90-minute yoga class, three times per week
   c. Vigorously riding your bicycle every day for 30 minutes
   d. Walking to and from classes across campus

2. Regular cardiorespiratory fitness activities reduce your chance of developing
   a. metabolic syndrome.
   b. HIV.
   c. athlete's foot.
   d. dehydration.

3. Which circulation delivers blood to the lungs?
   a. Pulmonary
   b. Systemic
   c. Hepatic
   d. Cardiac

4. Which energy system will provide most of the ATP during an hour-long bicycle ride?
   a. The immediate energy system
   b. The nonoxidative energy system
   c. The creatine phosphate energy system
   d. The oxidative energy system

5. Which of the following will decrease with regular aerobic training?
   a. Muscle cell size
   b. Blood volume
   c. Resting heart rate
   d. Maximal cardiac output

6. Which of the following is the *best* example of vigorous exercise?
   a. Weight training
   b. Cycling up a steep hill
   c. Cleaning the house
   d. Hiking on a flat trail

7. Which OMNI Scale of Perceived Exertion value is associated with training in your target heart rate range?
   a. 1
   b. 3
   c. 7
   d. 9

8. Which of the following is the *best* way to plan for cardiorespiratory program progression?
   a. Follow the 10 percent rule
   b. Increase your exercise duration each time you work out
   c. Schedule reassessments of your cardiorespiratory fitness every four weeks
   d. Increase your exercise intensity with every workout session

9. Which of the following is a good strategy to stay on track with your cardio fitness program?
   a. Read articles online about fitness topics
   b. Post pictures around your house of being active
   c. Attend motivational talks about fitness and health
   d. Record your activities and track your progress over time

10. What is the most common type of injury or illness in cardiorespiratory exercisers?
   a. Heat illness
   b. Hypothermia
   c. Overuse injuries
   d. Head injuries

critical thinkingquestions

1. Name three benefits of having a high level of cardiorespiratory fitness and explain how each impacts your overall health and wellness.

2. What are the pros and cons of each method of intensity monitoring: target heart rate, perceived exertion, and the talk test?

references

1. S. Kodama et al., "Cardiorespiratory Fitness as a Quantitative Predictor of All-Cause Mortality and Cardiovascular Events in Healthy Men and Women," *Journal of the American Medical Association* 301, no. 19 (2009): 2024–35, doi: 10.1001/jama.2009.681.

2. S. Sakuragi, "Influence of Adiposity and Physical Activity on Arterial Stiffness in Healthy Children," *Hypertension* 53, (2009): 611–16, doi: 10.1161/HYPERTENSIONAHA.108.123364.

3. Y. Zhang et al., "Characteristics of Pulse Wave Velocity in Elastic and Muscular Arteries: A Mismatch Beyond Age," *Journal of Hypertension* 31, no. 3 (2013): 554–59.

4. C. P. Earnest et al., "Maximal Estimated Cardiorespiratory Fitness, Cardiometabolic Risk Factors, and Metabolic Syndrome in the Aerobics Center Longitudinal Study," *Mayo Clinic Proceedings* 88, no. 3 (2013): 259–70, doi: 10.1016/j.mayocp.2012.11.006.

5. J. W. Van Dijk et al., "Exercise and 24-h Glycemic Control: Equal Effects for All Type. 2 Diabetes Patients?," *Medicine and Science in Sports and Exercise* 45, no. 4 (2013): 628–35, doi: 10.1249/MSS.0b013e31827ad8b4.

6. X. Sui et al., "Influence of Cardiorespiratory Fitness on Lung Cancer Mortality," *Medicine and Science in Sports and Exercise* 42, no. 5 (2010): 872–8; S. W. Farrell et al., "Cardiorespiratory Fitness, Different Measures of Adiposity, and Total Cancer Mortality in Women," *Obesity (Silver Spring)* 19, no. 11 (2011): 2261–7, doi: 10.1038/oby.2010.345.

7. J. R. Trombold et al., "Acute High-Intensity Endurance Exercise Is More Effective Than Moderate Intensity Exercise for Attenuation of Postprandial Triglyceride Elevation," *Journal of Applied Physiology* 114, no. 6 (2013): 792–800, doi: 10.1152/japplphysiol.01028.2012.

8. G. R. Hunter et al., "Increased Resting Energy Expenditure After 40 Minutes of Aerobic but Not Resistance Exercise," *Obesity (Silver Spring)* 14, no. 11 (2006): 2018–25.

9. S. M. Markowitz and S. M. Arent, "The Exercise and Affect Relationship: Evidence for the Dual-Mode Model and a Modified Opponent Process Theory," *Journal of Sport & Exercise Psychology* 32, no. 5 (2010): 711–30.

10. M. D. Hoffman and D. R. Hoffman, "Exercisers Achieve Greater Acute Exercise-Induced Mood Enhancement Than Nonexercisers," *Archives of Physical Medicine and Rehabilitation* 89, no. 2 (2008): 358–63, doi: 10.1016/j.apmr.2007.09.026; M. E. Hopkins et al., "Differential Effects of Acute and Regular Physical Exercise on Cognition and Affect," *Neuroscience* 215 (2012): 59–68, doi: 10.1016/j.neuroscience.2012.04.056.

11. T. M. DiLorenzo et al., "Long-Term Effects of Aerobic Exercise on Psychological Outcomes," *Preventative Medicine* 28, no. 1 (1999): 75–85.

12. F. Wang et al., "Long-Term Association Between Leisure-time Physical Activity and Changes in Happiness: Analysis of the Prospective National Population Health Survey," *American Journal of Epidemiology* 176, no. 12 (2012): 1095–1100, doi: 10.1093/aje/kws199.

13. P. J. Carek, S. E. Laibstain, and S. M. Carek, "Exercise for the Treatment of Depression and Anxiety," *International Journal of Psychiatry in Medicine* 41, no. 1 (2011): 15–28; V. S. Conn, "Depressive Symptom Outcomes of Physical Activity Interventions: Meta-Analysis Findings," *Annals of Behavioral Medicine* 39, no. 2 (2010): 128–38, doi: 10.1007/s12160-010-9172-x.

14. J. Romeo et al., "Physical Activity, Immunity and Infection," *The Proceedings of the Nutrition Society* 69, no. 3 (2010): 390–99.

15. M. H. Arai, A. J. Duarte, and V. M. Natale, "The Effects of Long-Term Endurance Training on the Immune and Endocrine Systems of Elderly Men: The Role of Cytokines and Anabolic Steroid Hormones," *Immunity and Aging* 3 (2006): 9.

16. J. E. Ahlskog et al., "Physical Exercise as a Preventive or Disease-Modifying Treatment of Dementia and Brain Aging," *Mayo Clinic Proceedings* 86, no. 9 (2011): 876–84, doi: 10.4065/mcp.2011.0252; R. J. Simpson et al., "Exercise and the Aging Immune system," *Ageing Research Reviews* 11, no. 3 (2012): 404–20.

17. K. I. Erickson et al., "Aerobic Fitness Is Associated with Hippocampal Volume in Elderly Humans," *Hippocampus* 19 (2009): 1030–9, doi: 10.1002/hipo.20547; K. I. Erickson et al., "Exercise Training Increases Size of Hippocampus and Improves Memory," *Proceedings of the National Academy of Sciences U.S.A.*, 108, no. 7 (2011): 3017–22, doi: 10.1073/pnas.1015950108.

18. S. Fillipas et al., "A Six-Month, Supervised, Aerobic and Resistance Exercise Program Improves Self-Efficacy in People with Human Immunodeficiency Virus: A Randomized Controlled Trial," *Australian Journal of Physiotherap* 52, no. 3 (2006): 185–90.

19. L. P. Forsythe et al., "Pain in Long-Term Breast Cancer Survivors: The Role of Body Mass Index, Physical Activity, and Sedentary Behavior," *Breast Cancer Research and Treatment* 137, no. 2 (2013): 617–30, doi: 10.1007/s10549-012-2335-7.

20. M. Benetti, C. L. Araujo, and R. Z.Santos, "Cardiorespiratory Fitness and Quality of Life at Different Exercise Intensities After Myocardial Infarction," *Arquivos Brasileiros de Cardiologia* 95, no. 3 (2010): 399–404.

21. S. Marzolini et al., "The Effects of an Aerobic and Resistance Exercise Training Program on Cognition Following Stroke,"*Neurorehabilitation & Neural Repair* 27, no. 5 (2013): 392–402, doi: 10.1177/1545968312465192.

22. G. Borg, *Borg's Perceived Exertion and Pain Scales* (Champaign: Human Kinetics, 1998): 27–38.

23. R. J. Robertson et al., "Validation of the Adult OMNI Scale of Perceived Exertion for Cycle Ergometer Exercise," *Medicine & Science in Sports & Exercise* 36, no. 1 (2004): 102–8; A. C. Utter et al., "Validation of the Adult OMNI Scale of Perceived Exertion for Walking/Running Exercise," *Medicine & Science in Sports & Exercise* 36, no. 10 (2004): 1776–80.

24. Centers for Disease Control and Prevention (CDC), The National Center for Environmental Health's Health Studies Branch (HSB), "Frequently Asked Questions (FAQs) About Extreme Heat," Reviewed June 2012, www.bt.cdc.gov

25. M. N. Sawka et al., "American College of Sports Medicine Position Stand. Exercise and Fluid Replacement," *Medicine & Science in Sports & Exercise* 39, no. 2 (2007): 377–90, doi: 10.1249/mss.0b013e31802ca597.

getfitgraphic references

1. M. Miyashita, S.F. Burns, and D.J. Stensel, "An Update on Accumulating Exercise and Postprandial Lipaemia: Translating Theory Into Practice," *Journal of Preventive Medicine & Public Health* 46, (2013): S3–S11, doi: 10.3961/jpmph.2013.46.S.S3.

2. G.D. Lewis et al., "Metabolic Signatures of Exercise in Human Plasma," *Scientific Translational Medicine* 2, no. 33 (2010): 33–7, doi: 10.1126/scitranslmed.3001006.

3. G. McRae et al., "Extremely Low Volume, Whole-Body Aerobic-Resistance Training Improves Aerobic Fitness and Muscular Endurance in Females," *Applied Physiology Nutrition and Metabolism* 37, no. 6 (2012): 1124–31, doi: 10.1139/h2012-093.

LAB 3.1 LEARN A SKILL
MONITORING INTENSITY DURING A WORKOUT

MasteringHealth™

Name: _____ Date: _____

Instructor: _____ Section: _____

Materials: Calculator and a stopwatch

Purpose: (1) To measure your resting heart rate (RHR); (2) to calculate your personal target heart rate range for exercise; and (3) to assess the intensity of your workout.

SECTION I: COUNTING YOUR HEART RATE

1. **Practice Taking Your Pulse** Take a *radial pulse* (a) by placing your middle and index fingers at the thumb side of your wrist. You can also press your middle and index fingers gently on the side of your throat to take your *carotid pulse* (b). Practice taking resting heart rate (RHR) measurement by counting your pulse for 60 seconds. Record your count below.

(a)

SCAN TO SEE IT ONLINE!

Resting Pulse Rate (60 sec) _____ **1 full minute RHR**

Practice taking an exercise heart rate (EHR) measurement by jogging in place for two minutes and counting your pulse for 10 seconds. Record your count below and convert to a heart rate by multiplying by six.

(b)

SCAN TO SEE IT ONLINE!

Exercise Pulse Rate (10 sec) _____ × 6 = _____ **Calculated 1-minute EHR**

2. **Determine Your True Resting Heart Rate** Take your pulse first thing in the morning on four different days. Record and average the results below. For an accurate resting heart rate, always count your pulse for a full minute. Ideally, you should take your pulse after waking up *without an alarm* and after a good night's rest.

	Resting Heart Rate (RHR)	Time of Day
Day 1		
Day 2		
Day 3		
Day 4		

Average RHR = _____

SECTION II: CALCULATE YOUR TARGET HEART RATE RANGE FOR EXERCISE

Calculate your personal target heart rate range for exercise using two methods: the maximum heart rate (HRmax) method and the heart rate reserve (HRR) method. Your target heart rate will provide a guideline for how many beats per minute (bpm) your heart should be beating during exercise, in order to achieve improvements in cardiorespiratory fitness. Note that you must count your pulse within 15 seconds of stopping exercise in order for your heart rate to reflect the exercise rate. Thus, if you take five seconds to find your pulse and start counting, that leaves you 10 seconds to take an exercise heart rate.

Method #1: Maximum Heart Rate (HRmax)

1. Find your predicted HRmax = 220 − _____ = _____
                                      (age)   (predicted HRmax)

2. Find your low HR target = _____ × .70 = _____ bpm ÷ 6 = _____
                       (predicted HRmax)   ***Low HR target***   ***Low 10 sec target***

3. Find your high HR target = _____ × .90 = _____ bpm ÷ 6 = _____
                       (predicted HRmax)   ***High HR target***   ***High 10 sec target***

Method #2: Heart Rate Reserve (HRR)

1. Find your HRR = _____ – _____ = _____
                           (predicted HRmax)   RHR   HRR
                           (from Section I)

2. Find 50% of HRR = (_____ × .50) + _____ = _____ bpm ÷ 6 = _____
                                 HRR   RHR   ***Low HR target***   ***Low 10 sec target***

3. Find 80% of HRR = (_____ × .80) + _____ = _____ bpm ÷ 6 = _____
                                 HRR   RHR   ***High HR target***   ***High 10 sec target***

SECTION III: MONITOR YOUR WORKOUT INTENSITY LEVEL

Practice monitoring your workout intensity during a 30-minute exercise session. You can choose any form of individual exercise that allows you to easily monitor your heart rate via a pulse check.

1. Calculate your estimated heart rate goal as a 10-second count for each time interval in the chart below.

2. Conduct your exercise session. Take your pulse and record your actual exercise heart rates.

3. In the last column of the chart, write your perceived exertion scores (1–10 OMNI Scale) 30 seconds before the end of the time period indicated on the workout schedule.

Time	Planned Intensity	Calculated HR 10 sec Count	Actual 10 sec HR	Perceived Exertion (1–10)
5 min warm-up	Slowly up to 55% HRmax	Predicted HRmax × .55 = _____ ÷ 6 = _____		
5 min	65% HRmax	Predicted HRmax × .65 = _____ ÷ 6 = _____		
4 min	75% HRmax	Predicted HRmax × .75 = _____ ÷ 6 = _____		
3 min	85% HRmax	Predicted HRmax × .85 = _____ ÷ 6 = _____		
4 min	75% HRmax	Predicted HRmax × .75 = _____ ÷ 6 = _____		
5 min	65% HRmax	Predicted HRmax × .65 = _____ ÷ 6 = _____		
4 min cool-down	55% HRmax	Predicted HRmax × .55 = _____ ÷ 6 = _____.		

SECTION IV: REFLECTION

1. How close were your calculated and actual heart rates during your 30-minute exercise session?

_____

_____

2. Did the intensity levels feel higher or lower than you thought they would at each percentage of HRmax?

_____

_____

LAB 3.2

ASSESS YOURSELF

ASSESSING YOUR CARDIORESPIRATORY FITNESS LEVEL

Name: _____ **Date:** _____

Instructor: _____ **Section:** _____

Materials: Calculator, 16.25-inch step or bleacher bench, stopwatch, metronome

Purpose: To measure (1) recovery from physical activity, (2) walking speed, and (3) current level of cardiorespiratory fitness.

SECTION I: THE QUEEN'S COLLEGE STEP TEST

For this test, you will be stepping on a 16.25-inch-high step bench for three minutes and then measuring your recovery pulse for 15 seconds.

1. Setup and preparation. Set up a 16.25-inch-high step bench or bleacher bench (a typical gym bleacher bench is 16.25 inches high) in a place that will be safe to perform the test. Warm-up prior to the assessment with walking and range of motion exercises. Set the metronome to a pace of 96 beats per minute for men (24 steps/min) and 88 bpm for women (22 steps/min). Listen to the metronome and do a couple of practice steps to ensure that you can step with the right cadence ("up, up, down, down"). One foot will be stepping up or down with each beat of the metronome. Have a stopwatch available to time your three minutes on the step and your 15 second recovery heart rate (HR) afterward.

2. Step up and down for three minutes. Start the metronome and march in place to the beat. Start stepping up on the bench and down to the floor after starting the stopwatch. Maintain this exact pace for the entire three minutes.

3. Stop and count your pulse for 15 seconds. At the end of three minutes, stop stepping, turn off the metronome, and immediately find your carotid or radial pulse. Within five seconds of stopping the exercise, start counting your recovery pulse and count for 15 seconds.

4. Record your results and calculate your estimated maximal oxygen consumption (VO$_2$max). Record your 15-second recovery HR below and then use the appropriate formula (men or women) to calculate your estimated VO$_2$max. This number will more accurately reflect your fitness level if you followed the test instructions carefully.

5. Find the cardiorespiratory fitness level that corresponds to your predicted VO$_2$max. Use the chart at the end of Section III (page 96) to determine your cardiorespiratory fitness level, as determined by the Queen's College Step Test.

The Queen's College Step Test Results

15 Sec Recovery HR: _____ (bpm)

Estimated VO$_2$max: Plug in your HR from above, compute the number in parentheses first, and complete the calculation (based on your gender) to find your estimated VO$_2$max.

Men:

- VO$_2$max = 111.33 − [0.42 × HR (bpm)]
- VO$_2$max = 111.33 − [0.42 × _____ (bpm)]
- VO$_2$max = 111.33 − _____

VO$_2$max = _____ Fitness Rating: _____

Women:

- $VO_2max = 65.81 - [0.1847 \times HR \text{ (bpm)}]$
- $VO_2max = 65.81 - [0.1847 \times$ _____ $\text{(bpm)}]$
- $VO_2max = 65.81 -$ _____

VO$_2$max = _____ **Fitness Rating:** _____

Source: Based on W.D. McArdle et al., "Reliability and Interrelationships Between Maximal Oxygen Update, Physical Work Capacity and Step-Test Scores in College Women," *Medicine and Science in Sports and Exercise* 4, (1972): 182–6.

SECTION II: THE ONE-MILE WALK TEST

You will walk one mile and determine your heart rate response to the exercise immediately after. IMPORTANT REMINDERS: The accuracy of this test depends on three things: (1) Walk during this test. Do not run. (2) Walk the mile as fast as you can. (3) Keep a steady pace throughout the mile. Do not "sprint" at the end.

1. **Preparation and warm-up.** Make sure that you have an accurate one-mile course to complete (four laps around a standard track) and a stopwatch. Warm up with three to five minutes of light walking and range-of-motion activities.

2. **Walk one full mile as fast as you can.** After completing the one mile, record your finish time (from your watch, stopwatch, or someone calling out the time) below. Convert the time from minutes and seconds to minutes with a decimal fraction.

3. **Immediately take an exercise heart rate and cool-down.** Within five seconds of finishing the walk, find your carotid or radial pulse and count your pulse for 10 seconds. Multiply the number by 6 and record your HR below. After recording your finish time and your HR, cool down by walking slowly for another five minutes and doing some light stretching.

4. **Calculate your estimated maximal oxygen consumption (VO$_2$max).** Use the formula below to calculate your estimated VO$_2$max. This number will more accurately reflect your fitness level if you followed the test instructions carefully.

5. **Find the cardiorespiratory fitness level that corresponds to your predicted VO$_2$max.** Use the chart at the end of Section III to determine your cardiorespiratory fitness level, as determined by this one-mile walking test.

The One-Mile Walk Test Results

One-Mile Walk Time: _____ (min:sec); divide sec by 60 = _____ (min w/decimal)

Exercise HR: _____ (beats) $\times$ 6 = _____ (bpm)
(10 sec count)

Estimated VO$_2$max: Use the following equation to estimate VO$_2$max, where gender = 0 for female and 1 for male; time = walk time to the nearest hundredth of a minute; and HR = heart rate (bpm) at the end of the walking test. Plug in your weight and numbers from above and calculate the numbers in parentheses first. Complete the calculation to find your estimated VO$_2$max.

- $VO_2max = 132.853 - [0.0769 \times \text{body weight (lb)}] - [0.3877 \times \text{age (yr)}] + [6.3150 \times \text{gender}] - [3.2649 \times \text{time (min)}] - [0.1565 \times HR \text{ (bpm)}]$
- $VO_2max = 132.853 - [0.0769 \times$ _____ $\text{(lb)}] - [0.3877 \times$ _____ $\text{(yr)}] + [6.3150 \times$ _____ $\text{(gender)}] - [3.2649 \times$ _____ $\text{(min)}] - [0.1565 \times$ _____ $\text{(bpm)}]$
- $VO_2max = 132.853 -$ _____ $-$ _____ $+$ _____ $-$ _____ $-$ _____
- $VO_2max =$ _____ (ml/kg·min)

Walk Test VO$_2$max Fitness Rating: _____

SECTION III: 1.5-MILE RUN TEST

1. **Preparation and warm-up.** Make sure that you have an accurate 1.5-mile course to complete (six laps around a standard track) and a stopwatch. Warm up with 5 to 10 minutes of walking/jogging and range-of-motion activities.

2. **Run (with walk breaks if needed) 1.5 miles as fast as you can.** After reaching 1.5 miles, mark your finish time (from your watch, stopwatch, or someone calling out the time) below. Convert the time from minutes and seconds to minutes with a decimal fraction.

3. **Cool down.** After recording your finish time, cool down by walking for five minutes and doing some light stretching.

4. **Calculate your estimated maximal oxygen consumption (VO$_2$max).** Use the formula below to calculate your estimated VO$_2$max.

5. **Find your cardiorespiratory fitness level that corresponds to your predicted VO$_2$max.** Use the chart at the end of this section to determine your cardiorespiratory fitness level, as determined by this 1.5-mile running test.

The 1.5-Mile Run Test Results

1.5-Mile Run Time: _____ (min:sec); divide sec by 60 = _____ (min w/decimal)

Estimated VO$_2$max: You will use the following equation to estimate VO$_2$max, where time = run time to the nearest hundredth of a minute. Plug in your time from above, compute the number in parentheses first, and complete the calculation to find your estimated VO$_2$max.

- VO$_2$max = [483 ÷ time (min)] + 3.5
- VO$_2$max = [483 ÷ _____ (min)] + 3.5
- VO$_2$max = _____ + 3.5
- VO$_2$max = _____ (ml/kg·min)

Run Test VO$_2$max Fitness Rating: _____

Estimated VO$_2$max Fitness Ratings (ml/kg·min)						
Men	**Superior**	**Excellent**	**Good**	**Fair**	**Poor**	**Very Poor**
18–29 yrs	>56.1	51.1–56.1	45.7–51.0	42.2–45.6	38.1–42.1	<38.1
30–39 yrs	>54.2	48.9–54.2	44.4–48.8	41.0–44.3	36.7–40.9	<36.7
40–49 yrs	>52.8	46.8–52.8	42.4–46.7	38.4–42.3	34.6–38.3	<34.6
50–59 yrs	>49.6	43.3–49.6	38.3–43.2	35.2–38.2	31.1–35.1	<31.1
60–69 yrs	>46.0	39.5–46.0	35.0–39.4	31.4–34.9	27.4–31.3	<27.4

Women	**Superior**	**Excellent**	**Good**	**Fair**	**Poor**	**Very Poor**
18–29 yrs	>50.1	44.0–50.1	39.5–43.9	35.5–39.4	31.6–35.4	<31.6
30–39 yrs	>46.8	41.0–46.8	36.8–40.9	33.8–36.7	29.9–33.7	<29.9
40–49 yrs	>45.1	38.9–45.1	35.1–38.8	31.6–35.0	28.0–31.5	<28.0
50–59 yrs	>39.8	35.2–39.8	31.4–35.1	28.7–31.3	25.5–28.6	<25.5
60–69 yrs	>36.8	32.3–36.8	29.1–32.2	26.6–29.0	23.7–26.5	<23.7

You may also use the chart below to estimate your fitness level using only your run time.

Estimated Run Time Ratings				
Men	Excellent	Good	Fair	Poor
Ages 20–29	<10:10	10:10–11:29	11:30–12:38	>12:38
Ages 30–39	<10:47	10:47–11:54	11:55–12:58	>12:58
Ages 40–49	<11:16	11:16–12:24	12:25–13:50	>13:50
Ages 50–59	<12:09	12:09–13:35	13:36–15:06	>15:06
Ages 60–69	<13:24	13:24–15:04	15:05–16:46	>16:46

Women	Excellent	Good	Fair	Poor
Ages 20–29	<11:59	11:59–13:24	13:25–14:50	>14:50
Ages 30–39	<12:25	12:25–14:08	14:09–15:43	>15:43
Ages 40–49	<13:24	13:24–14:53	14:54–16:31	>16:31
Ages 50–59	<14:35	14:35–16:35	16:36–18:18	>18:18
Ages 60–69	<16:34	16:34–18:27	18:28–20:16	>20:16

Reprinted with permission from The Cooper Institute, Dallas, Texas, from *Physical Fitness Assessments and Norms for Adults and Law Enforcement*, Copyright ©2007, available online at www.CooperInstitute.org.

SECTION IV: REFLECTION

1. Were you surprised by your fitness assessment results or were they in line with what you were expecting? Explain why or why not.

_____

_____

_____

_____

_____

_____

_____

Name: _____   Date: _____

Instructor: _____   Section: _____

Materials: Results from cardiorespiratory fitness assessments, calculator, lab pages.

Purpose: To learn how to set appropriate cardiorespiratory fitness goals and create a personal cardiorespiratory fitness program designed to meet those goals.

SECTION I: SHORT- AND LONG-TERM GOALS

Create short- and long-term goals for cardiorespiratory fitness. Be sure to use SMART goal-setting guidelines (specific, measurable, action-oriented, realistic, time-oriented). Select appropriate target dates and rewards for completing your goals.

Short-Term Goal (3–6 Months)

_____

_____

Target Date: _____

Reward: _____

Long-Term Goal (12+ Months)

_____

_____

Target Date: _____

Reward: _____

SECTION II: CARDIORESPIRATORY FITNESS OBSTACLES AND STRATEGIES

1. What barriers or obstacles might hinder your plan to improve your cardiorespiratory fitness? Indicate your top three obstacles below:

a. _____

b. _____

c. _____

2. Overcoming these barriers/obstacles to change will be an important step in reaching your goals. Write down three **strategies** for overcoming the obstacles listed above:

a. _____

b. _____

c. _____

SECTION III: GETTING SUPPORT

1. List resources you will use to help you change your cardiorespiratory fitness:

Friend/partner/relative: _____

School-based resource: _____

Community-based resource: _____

Other: _____

2. How will you use these supportive resources to help you meet your cardiorespiratory fitness goals?

_____

_____

_____

_____

_____

_____

_____

SECTION IV: CARDIORESPIRATORY FITNESS PROGRAM REFLECTIONS

1. How realistic are the short- and long-term target dates you have set for achieving your cardiorespiratory fitness goals?

_____

_____

_____

2. How many days per week are you planning to work on your cardiorespiratory fitness program?

_____

3. What types of workouts are you planning to try?

_____

_____

_____

4. Do you have a workout partner? Do you plan to work with a workout partner, personal trainer, or instructor to help get you started?

_____

_____

_____

SECTION V: CARDIORESPIRATORY TRAINING PROGRAM DESIGN

Plan a four-week cardiorespiratory training program, using resources available to you (facility, instructor, text) and completing the following training calendar (A = activity, I = intensity, T = time).

Four-Week Cardiorespiratory Training Program						
Sun	Mon	Tues	Wed	Thurs	Fri	Sat
Date: _____	Date: _____	Date: _____	Date: _____	Date: _____	Date: _____	Date: _____
A:	A:	A:	A:	A:	A:	A:
I:	I:	I:	I:	I:	I:	I:
T:	T:	T:	T:	T:	T:	T:
Date: _____	Date: _____	Date: _____	Date: _____	Date: _____	Date: _____	Date: _____
A:	A:	A:	A:	A:	A:	A:
I:	I:	I:	I:	I:	I:	I:
T:	T:	T:	T:	T:	T:	T:
Date: _____	Date: _____	Date: _____	Date: _____	Date: _____	Date: _____	Date: _____
A:	A:	A:	A:	A:	A:	A:
I:	I:	I:	I:	I:	I:	I:
T:	T:	T:	T:	T:	T:	T:
Date: _____	Date: _____	Date: _____	Date: _____	Date: _____	Date: _____	Date: _____
A:	A:	A:	A:	A:	A:	A:
I:	I:	I:	I:	I:	I:	I:
T:	T:	T:	T:	T:	T:	T:

SECTION VI: TRACKING YOUR PROGRAM AND FOLLOWING THROUGH

1. **Goal and Program Tracking:** Use the following chart to monitor your progress. Change the activity, intensity, or time of your workout plan to reflect your progress as needed.

2. **Goal and Program Follow-Up:** At the end of the course or at your short-term goal target date, reevaluate your cardiorespiratory fitness and ask yourself the following questions:

a. Did you meet your short-term goal or your goal for the course? If so, what positive behavioral changes contributed to your success? If not, which obstacles blocked your success?

_____

b. Was your short-term goal realistic? What would you change about your goals or training plan?

_____

Four-Week Cardiorespiratory Training Log					
Dates	Activity	Time	Av. HR	RPE	Comments
Week 1					
Week 2					
Week 3					
Week 4					

Activate, Motivate, & ADVANCE YOUR FITNESS

A RUNNING PROGRAM

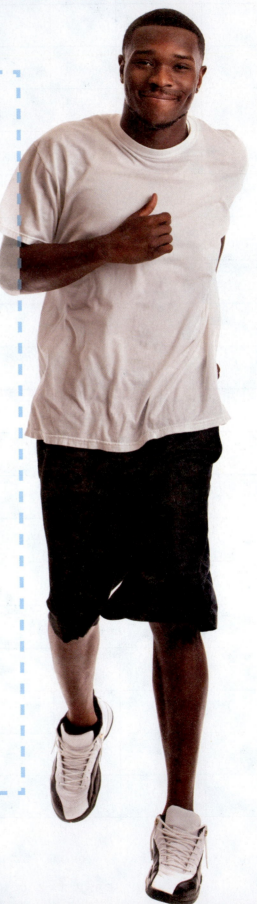

SCAN TO SEE IT ONLINE!

ACTIVATE!

Whether this is your first attempt at running or you want to take your current run workouts to the next level, there is a program built just for you.

Running Program Preparation and Safety

Going too far or too fast right away is the number-one cause of injury among new runners. Focus on the minutes instead of miles, and use these programs to gradually increase your run time.

What Do I Need for Running?

SHOES: Visit your local running store to find your most important running tool, your shoes! The employees are generally experienced runners who can assist you in finding a good fit for your foot, running style, gait, running surface and, of course, your goals.

CLOTHING: Wear comfortable and supportive clothing. Choose materials that wick moisture away from your skin. In cold weather, wear layers. In the sun, wear sunscreen, sunglasses, and a hat or visor. At sunrise, dusk, or night, wear reflective clothing and/or a vest and lights.

How Do I Start a Running Program?

TECHNIQUE: Relax your shoulders and gently swing your arms (90-degree elbow) up to your chest and down to your hips. Keep hands loose and relaxed. Look forward, rather than down at the ground. Stay light on your feet and use shorter, quicker steps. Land on the mid-foot or balls of your feet and push off. Aim for a stride rate (your turnover) of 180 steps per minute. Count the number of times your right foot strikes the ground in a minute and multiply that by two.

ETIQUETTE: Follow a few basic guidelines whether you are running alone or with a group, especially if you run in a high-traffic area. On a sidewalk or a multi-use path or trail, run on the right and pass on the left, after alerting others you are passing. Say, "On your left" as you approach. No matter where you run, remember to never run more than two abreast. If you need to stop, step off to the right to allow others to get by.

Running Tips

ROAD RUNNING: Plan safe and interesting routes that consider both traffic and available running paths. Check with your local running store or club for routes and running partners. Let someone know where you are going and when you will return. Carry a cell phone, ID, a few dollars, and a water bottle. Stay aware of your surroundings by wearing only one piece of your earphones. Run facing traffic and pay attention to traffic signals and signs.

TRACK RUNNING: A track will give you a stable and soft running surface. Other benefits? Tracks are usually well lit and you won't have to plan a route. Plus, you may have access to a rest room and a place to keep your water bottle and phone nearby. On a track, you can test pacing, adjust your run/walk ratios, and retest your cardiorespiratory fitness level regularly. Most tracks are 400 meters; four laps on the inner lane equal a mile. Follow track etiquette by utilizing outside lanes for most of your training and leave the inside lane (lane 1) for faster runners and sprinters and for timing yourself on a specific distance. If you are using the inside lane and a faster individual approaches behind you, move out to lane 2 or 3 to allow the person to pass. Finally, try to change your running direction every few runs to vary the stresses on your body of going around turns.

TREADMILL RUNNING: Treadmills offer convenience, efficiency, and a safe environment when the weather is less than ideal. Be sure to familiarize yourself with the controls before starting out. Remember to maintain good form and avoid both the handrails and the back of the treadmill belt.

TRAIL RUNNING: Take a break from the asphalt jungle to run in nature. Ease into trail running by starting with flat, soft, easy-to-navigate trails (dirt, bark dust, pine needles, wood chips) and work your way up to more challenging ones. Take smaller steps, slow down, and constantly scan the trail to find the best footing. If possible, trail run with a buddy. If not, be sure that you know your route, take water, and tell someone of your location, start time, and anticipated end time.

Running Warm-Up and Cool-Down

Walk or jog at a slower pace for 5–10 minutes to warm-up or cool-down. After breaking a light sweat in your warm-up, you may want to add dynamic range-of-motion exercises. After you finish your cool-down, you can hold static stretches longer for improved flexibility.

Four-Week Running Programs

If you are new to running, if you want to transition from walking to running, or if you have taken a break from running for six months or more, then build your run program gradually and start with the Beginner Program. If you are already running 15 minutes continuously on two days a week, start with the Intermediate Program. Adjust time, intensity, and training days to suit your personal fitness level and schedule; visit the mobile website for more options.

BEGINNER: RUNNING

PROGRAM **GOAL:** Transition from walking to running. Increase run minutes while maintaining a moderate intensity level three to four days a week.

	Mon		Tue		Wed		Thurs		Fri		Sat		Sun	
	T	I	T	I	T	I	T	I	T	I	T	I	T	I
Week 1	20 1/4	L			20 1/4	L			20 1/4	L–M				
Week 2	24 1/5	M			24 1/5	M			24 1/5	M				
Week 3	32 1/7	M			32 1/7	M			32 1/7	M				
Week 4	24 2/10	M			24 2/10	M			24 2/10	M	24 2/10	M		

T = Time. Total time is listed in minutes with the Walk/Run minute ratio below.
I = Intensity. Intensity is listed as Light/Lifestyle (L), Moderate (M), or Vigorous (V). (See Table 3.3.)
Workouts do not include warm-up or cool-down time.

INTENSITY LEVEL L — Light   M — Moderate   V — Vigorous

PROGRAM **GOAL:** Run at a moderate to vigorous intensity level three to five days a week, complete a 30-minute continuous run, and incorporate vigorous interval training sessions.

	Mon		Tue		Wed		Thurs		Fri		Sat		Sun	
	T	I	T	I	T	I	T	I	T	I	T	I	T	I
Week 1	20	L–M 3–5	20	M 5–6	20	M 5–6			20	L–M 3–5				
Week 2	20	M 5–6			25	M 5–6			20	M 5–6	25	L–M 3–5		
Week 3	25	M 5–6			20	M 5–6	Interval	L–M–V			30	M 5–6		
Week 4	25	M 5–6	Interval	L–M–V	20	L–M 3–5	Interval	L–M–V			30	L–M 3–5		

T = Time. Total time is listed in minutes.
I = Intensity. Intensity is listed as Light/Lifestyle (L), Moderate (M), or Vigorous (V) and the OMNI scale of 0–10. (See Figure 3.8 and Table 3.3.)
Workouts do not include warm-up or cool-down time.

INTENSITY LEVEL   Light   Moderate   Vigorous

Intermediate Program Interval Workout—Three Miles

800m (.5 mile) at 7–8 on the OMNI scale (V)
800m (.5 mile) recovery (easy jog or walk/jog) at 2–5 on the OMNI scale (L–M)
**REPEAT this 1:1 ratio two more times for a total of 4800m or 3 miles.

MOTIVATE!

Create your own exercise log to track your running program—make note of dates, times, distances, intensity level—or use the one on the mobile website. Here are a few tips to keep you running:

MORNING WORKOUTS: Try running first thing in the morning. That way, you can check it off your to-do list, and nothing can push your run off your day's schedule. Tip for success: Organize your running clothes, shoes, gear, water bottle, and breakfast the night before.

DON'T PUT AWAY YOUR GEAR: Place your workout log, shoes, workout clothes, water bottle, and stretching mat in plain sight, in your work bag, or your car. Visual cues can help you remember your goals and prioritize your run.

DO IT FOR CHARITY: Need a reason or just more support? Name your cause and chances are there is a local run or race to raise awareness and funds for it. Committing to run for worthy causes reminds you that you are fortunate to be healthy and able to run. Fuel your motivation by knowing you're doing good for more than just yourself.

ADVANCE!

Now that you have established your running program, challenge yourself to try something new or take your running to the next level. How about participating in your first 5k? If you've been there, done that, how about actually racing (picking up your pace to set a new personal record)? On the next page is a more advanced four-week program you can follow; visit the mobile website to find more options or simply to personalize this or any of the programs in this book.

ADVANCED: RUNNING

PROGRAM **GOAL:** Run 5k/3.1miles!

	Mon		Tue		Wed		Thurs		Fri		Sat		Sun	
	T/D	I	T/D	I	T/D	I	T/D	I	T/D	I	T/D	I	T/D	I
Week 1	25	L–M 3–5 62–70	25	L–M 3–5 62–70			25	M 5–6 65–85	25	M 5–6 65–85				
Week 2	25	M 5–6 65–85			Interval	L–M–V			2 miles	M 5–6 65–85	30	M 5–6 65–85		
Week 3	25	M 5–6 65–85	Interval	L–M–V	2.5 miles	L–M 3–5 62–70	Interval	L–M–V	3 miles	M 5–6 65–85				
Week 4	30	M 5–6 65–85			35	L–M 3–5 62–70					Goal 5k Run!			

T/D = Time/Distance. Total time/distance is listed in minutes or miles.
I = Intensity. Intensity is listed as Light/Lifestyle (L), Moderate (M), or Vigorous (V),
the OMNI scale of 0–10, and % of HRmax. (See Figure 3.8 and Table 3.3.)
Workouts do not include warm-up or cool-down time.

INTENSITY LEVEL
Light   Moderate   Vigorous

Advanced Program Interval Workout

Alternate two minutes hard and two minutes easy for one mile:
2 minutes at 85% HRmax or 7–8 on the OMNI scale (V)
2 minutes at <60% HRmax or 2–3 on the OMNI scale (L)
5 minutes at 65–84% HRmax or 5–6 on the OMNI scale (M)
**REPEAT twice more (total of three sets)

Activate, Motivate, & ADVANCE YOUR FITNESS

A CYCLING PROGRAM

SCAN TO SEE IT
ONLINE!

ACTIVATE!

Whether you cycle indoors or take your bike out on the road or trail, you can get a fun and amazing workout.

Cycling Program Preparation and Safety

Sure, cycling can be an intense, calorie-burning workout, but it can also be a simple way to take care of errands, commute, meet up with friends, or just enjoy the great outdoors. Follow the programs below to get started. As you get stronger, you can increase your mileage and speed.

What Do I Need for Cycling?

GEAR: Safe cycling requires quite a bit of equipment (helmet, padded cycling shorts, gloves, shoes, reflective gear, racks) and, of course, the bike. You can start on almost any style of bicycle, but most importantly, you need a bike that fits. Visit your local bike shop to get the right bike for you. When indoor cycling, adjust both seat and handlebar height to create a comfortable and safe fit. If you are new to indoor cycling or unfamiliar with the stationary bikes at your facility, be sure to ask a trained instructor to assist you with proper bike setup.

How Do I Start a Cycling Program?

TECHNIQUE: Work on developing a smooth and efficient pedaling technique. Lighten up, pedal in a smooth circle, and pull through the back of the stroke. *Cadence* is pedaling speed in revolutions per minute (RPM). A cadence of 60 RPM means that one pedal makes a complete revolution 60 times in one minute. Monitor your cadence with periodic cadence checks. Count the revolution of one leg for 15 seconds and then multiply by four. The cadence range is 80–110 RPM for cycling on a flat road and 60–80 RPM for climbing hills.

ETIQUETTE: Participating in group rides will teach you the etiquette for road cycling and mountain biking. Inquire about weekly rides or a beginners' cycling group at your local bike shop.

Cycling Tips

INDOOR CYCLING: Weather, traffic, flat tires ... with indoor cycling you won't have these excuses for missing your workout. Indoor cycling also allows you to precisely control your workout and mix periods of higher-intensity cycling with resting pedal strokes.

OUTDOOR CYCLING: Whether you choose streets, bike paths, or trails, plan safe routes that consider both traffic and terrain.

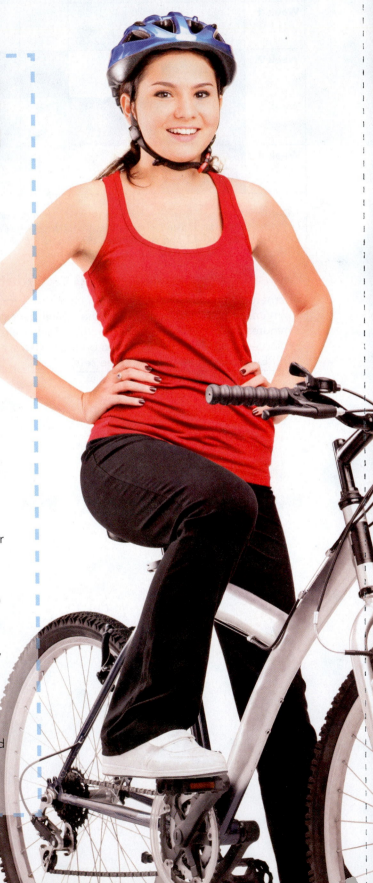

Try using a mapping program or stop by your local bike shop to learn more about the routes and popular riding areas in your neighborhood. Safety tips: Brush up on your cycling skills, have proper reflective equipment, learn how to use a bike repair kit (fixing flat tires), and know local traffic laws and trail usage rules.

Cycling Warm-Up and Cool-Down

Cycle at a slow cadence for 5 to 15 minutes to warm up or cool down. After the cool-down portion of your ride, perform a few light stretches that focus on your low back muscles, hamstrings, quadriceps, and calves.

Four-Week Cycling Programs

If you are new to cycling or are coming back after time off, start with the Beginner Program to build your cardiorespiratory fitness base. If you are already riding for 15 or more continuous minutes at least twice a week, then start with the Intermediate Program. Adjust time, intensity, and training days to suit your personal fitness level and schedule; visit the mobile website for more options.

BEGINNER: CYCLING

PROGRAM GOAL: Increase cycling minutes while maintaining a moderate intensity level three to four days a week, building to 100 total minutes by week four.

	Mon		Tue		Wed		Thurs		Fri		Sat		Sun	
	T	I	T	I	T	I	T	I	T	I	T	I	T	I
Week 1	20	L			20	L			20	L–M				
Week 2	25	M			25	M			25	M				
Week 3	20	M			25	M			15	M	30	L–M		
Week 4	25	M			25	M			25	M	25	L–M		

T = Time. Total time is listed in minutes.
I = Intensity. Intensity is listed as Light/Lifestyle (L), Moderate (M), or Vigorous (V).
(See Table 3.3.)
Workouts do not include warm-up or cool-down time.

INTENSITY LEVEL
Light Moderate Vigorous

INTERMEDIATE: CYCLING

PROGRAM GOAL: Cycle at a moderate intensity level three to five days a week, build to a 40-minute ride, and incorporate vigorous interval training sessions each week.

	Mon		Tue		Wed		Thurs		Fri		Sat		Sun	
	T	I	T	I	T	I	T	I	T	I	T	I	T	I
Week 1	25	L–M 3–5			25	L–M 3–5			25	M 5–6	25	M 5–6		
Week 2	25	M 5–6			30	M 5–6			25	L–M 3–5	35	M 5–6		
Week 3	30	M 5–6	Interval	L–M–V	20	L–M 3–5	Interval	L–M–V	30	M 5–6				
Week 4	30	M 5–6	Interval	L–M–V	25	M 5–6	30	M 5–6			40	L–M 3–5		

T = Time. Total time is listed in minutes.
I = Intensity. Intensity is listed as Light/Lifestyle (L), Moderate (M), or Vigorous (V) and the OMNI scale of 0–10. (See Figure 3.8 and Table 3.3.)
Workouts do not include warm-up or cool-down time.

INTENSITY LEVEL
Light Moderate Vigorous

Intermediate Program Interval Workout—25 Minutes

2 minutes of flat cycling (cadence 80–110 RPM) at 7–8 on the OMNI scale (V)
1 minute of recovery (pedal easy, below 80 RPM) at 3 on the OMNI scale (L)
**REPEAT this 2:1 ratio four more times for a total of 15 minutes
30 seconds of hill work (increase tension and drop cadence to 60–80 RPM) at 7–8 on the OMNI scale (V)
90 seconds of recovery (pedal easy, below 80 RPM with little or no resistance) at 3 on the OMNI scale (L)
**REPEAT this 1:3 ratio four more times for a total of 10 minutes

MOTIVATE!

Create your own exercise log to track your cycling program—note dates, times, distances, cadence, intensity level—or use the one on the mobile website. Here are a few tips to keep you cycling:

RIDE FOR 10: If you lack energy or motivation for a spin, give yourself 10 minutes. Tell yourself that you can quit after 10 minutes if you still don't feel like riding. Chances are that once you have made the effort to start, you'll complete your workout. If not, at least you managed a solid 10 minutes and you can feel good about listening to your body and taking a rest day.

REWARD YOURSELF: Promise yourself a healthy treat or fun experience at week's end if you stick to your cycling program. Maybe a pedicure or a massage or a scoop of frozen yogurt; hard work makes a reward that much more satisfying.

INDOOR GROUP RIDE: Sometimes just knowing that others are expecting you is enough to help you show up for your workout. Try an indoor cycling class at your gym. You'll develop new friendships with other physically active people and increase your cardiorespiratory fitness. Win-Win!

ADVANCE!

Ready to be challenged in your cycling program or try a new approach? Below is a more advanced four-week program you can follow. Visit the mobile website to find more options or to personalize this or any of the programs in this book.

ADVANCED: CYCLING

PROGRAM GOAL: Ride 20k/12.4mi in ≤ 60 minutes (indoors or out)!

	Mon		Tue		Wed		Thurs		Fri		Sat		Sun	
	T/D	I	T/D	I	T/D	I	T/D	I	T/D	I	T/D	I	T/D	I
Week 1	25	L–M 3–5 62–70	25	M 5–6 65–85	25	L–M 3–5 62–70	25	M 5–6 65–85			35	M 5–6 65–85		
Week 2	30	M 5–6 65–85	20	V 7–8 85–94	6 miles	L–M 3–5 62–70	30	M 5–6 65–85			40	M 5–6 65–85		
Week 3	35	M 5–6 65–85	Interval	L–M–V			Interval	L–M–V	35	L–M 3–5 62–70	45	M 5–6 65–85		
Week 4	40	M 5–6 65–85	20	L–M 3–5 62–70	40	M 5–6 65–85	Interval	L–M–V			Goal 20k Ride!	M 5–6 65–85		

T/D = Time/Distance. Total time/distance is listed in minutes or miles.
I = Intensity. Intensity is listed as Light/Lifestyle (L), Moderate (M), or Vigorous (V), the OMNI scale of 0–10, and % of HRmax. (See Figure 3.8 and Table 3.3.)
Workouts do not include warm-up or cool-down time.

INTENSITY LEVEL
Light Moderate Vigorous

Advanced Program Interval Workout—30 Minutes

3 minutes of flat cycling (cadence 80–110 RPM) at 85% HRmax or 7–8 on the OMNI scale (V)
1 minute of recovery (pedal easy, below 80 RPM) at 3 on the OMNI scale (L)
**REPEAT this 3:1 ratio four more times for a total of 20 minutes
1 minute of hill work (increase tension and drop cadence to 60–80 RPM) at 85% HRmax or 7–8 on the OMNI scale (V)
1 minute of recovery (pedal easy, below 80 RPM with little or no resistance) at 3 on the OMNI scale (L)
**REPEAT this 1:1 ratio four more times for a total of 10 minutes

Activate, Motivate,
& ADVANCE YOUR FITNESS

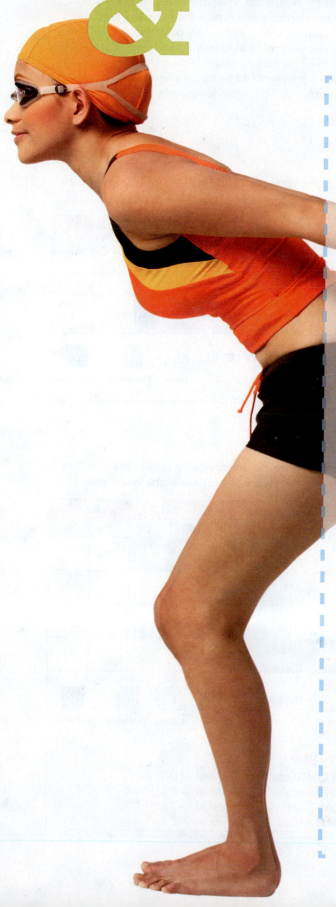

A SWIMMING PROGRAM

SCAN TO SEE IT
ONLINE!

ACTIVATE

Low impact and fun, swimming is an excellent way to improve your overall fitness!

Swimming Program Preparation and Safety:

If you have access to a pool, all you really need are two key items—swimsuit and goggles—and you're set to hit the water. Start and build slowly, focusing on minutes, not laps, and, as you gain strength, you will swim further and faster.

What Do I Need for Swimming?

GEAR: Look for a swimsuit that stays in place and moves with you, and be sure to try on goggles to ensure a good fit. You may want a swim cap to keep your hair out of your face. In addition, various pieces of equipment are commonly used to help swimmers improve technique and performance: kickboards, pull buoys, fins, and a stopwatch or the pool's pace clock. Lastly, don't forget your shatter-proof water bottle.

How Do I Start a Swimming Program?

TECHNIQUE: Taking a lesson is the best way to become more comfortable in the water and develop a more efficient technique. Inquire at your local college or American Red Cross chapter about adult swim classes or private swim coaches in your area.

ETIQUETTE: Pools are busy at open swim times and you will rarely get a lane to yourself. Aim to share a lane with other swimmers close to your same speed. You will most likely encounter *circle swimming* (swimming in a counter clockwise direction in the pool lane). Allow faster swimmers to take the lead, make sure there is a five-second gap between you and the person in front of you, and avoid swimming in the middle of the lane. If you need to take a break at the wall, keep to the side of the lane so that others can turn or rest as well.

Swimming Tips

OPEN WATER: Although it takes strong skills, open-water swimming can be exciting and invigorating! Check with your local swim store or a swim or triathlon club to find swim partners and learn more about safe open water swim areas. Remember, the water temperature is generally much cooler than a pool; many open-water swimmers wear neoprene wetsuits to stay warm. Practice "sighting" (looking up to see where you are in relation to land, buoys, docks) and swimming in a straight line before heading out.

Swimming Warm-Up and Cool-Down

A swimming warm-up and cool-down consists of slow water walking, water jogging, or swimming at a slower pace for 5–10 minutes. You can also warm up on deck with light, dynamic full range movements. After your cool-down, you can hold basic stretches for 10–30 seconds to improve flexibility.

Four-Week Swimming Programs

As you start a new swimming program, rest often, use resting swim strokes (elementary backstroke, sidestroke) as needed, and monitor your intensity periodically.

Heart rates are typically 10–13 beats per minute lower when swimming than when performing exercise on land, so evaluate intensity using perceived exertion level. If even one length of the pool is tiring for you, start with Beginner Program and focus on swim time, not distance or number of laps. If you are already able to swim comfortably at a moderate intensity level for close to 15 minutes (continuously or with minimum rest) and you are swimming at least twice a week, then start with the Intermediate Program. Adjust time, intensity, and days of the swims to suit your personal fitness level and schedule; visit the mobile website for more options.

BEGINNER: SWIMMING

PROGRAM **GOAL:** Increase continuous swim minutes at a light- to moderate-intensity level three to four days a week, building to 100 total minutes by week four.

	Mon		Tue		Wed		Thurs		Fri		Sat		Sun	
	T	I	T	I	T	I	T	I	T	I	T	I	T	I
Week 1	15	L			20	L			20	M				
Week 2	20	M			25	M			25	M				
Week 3	25	M			20	M			15	M	25	M		
Week 4	25	M			25	M			25	M	25	M		

T = Time. Total time is listed in minutes.
I = Intensity. Intensity is listed as Light/Lifestyle (L), Moderate (M), or Vigorous (V). (See Table 3.3.)
Workouts do not include warm-up or cool-down time.

INTENSITY LEVEL

Light   Moderate   Vigorous

INTERMEDIATE: SWIMMING

PROGRAM **GOAL:** Increase continuous swim minutes at a moderate intensity level three to five days a week, build to a 30-minute swim, and incorporate vigorous interval training sessions each week.

	Mon		Tue		Wed		Thurs		Fri		Sat		Sun	
	T	I	T	I	T	I	T	I	T	I	T	I	T	I
Week 1	25	L–M 3–5			25	M 5–6			25	M 5–6	25	M 5–6		
Week 2	25	M 5–6			Intervals	L–M–V			25	M 5–6				
Week 3	20	M 5–6			25	M 5–6			20	M 5–6	30	L–M 3–5		
Week 4	25	M 5–6	Intervals	L–M–V	30	M 5–6	Intervals	L–M–V	25	M 5–6				

T = Time. Total time is listed in minutes.
I = Intensity. Intensity is listed as Light/Lifestyle (L), Moderate (M), or Vigorous (V) and the OMNI scale of 0–10. (See Figure 3.8 and Table 3.3.)
Workouts do not include warm-up or cool-down time.

INTENSITY LEVEL

Light   Moderate   Vigorous

Intermediate Program Interval Workout—700 m/yds

3 × 100 m/yds with 60 seconds of rest between [100s at 7–8 on the OMNI scale (V) and rest at 0–2 (L)]
2 × 75 m/yds with 45 seconds of rest between [75s at 7–8 on the OMNI scale (V) and rest at 0–2 (L)]
3 × 50 m/yds with 30 seconds of rest between [50s at 7–8 on the OMNI scale (V) and rest at 0–2 (L)]
4 × 25 m/yds with 15 seconds of rest between [25s at 7–8 on the OMNI scale (V) and rest at 0–2 (L)]

MOTIVATE!

Create your own exercise log to track your swimming program—note dates, times, laps, intensity level—or use the one on the mobile website. Here are a few tips to keep you swimming:

LEARN SOMETHING NEW: Taking a lesson can help you develop confidence, which leads to more efficient swimming and increased enjoyment. The more you enjoy your workout, the better the results will be and the more likely you are to stick with it.

JOIN A TEAM: Lacking the support you need to swim regularly? Masters Swimming is a national program where adults 18 and older can swim in a team setting. You can swim at your own pace and be competitive or noncompetitive—your choice! There are teams and clubs in communities across the country and all of them offer multiple practice options, workouts, and coaching; you will gain a new group of friends who will be expecting you at the pool.

Try a water exercise class: Getting bored? Mix things up, make new friends, and take a break from swimming laps while still getting a great workout in the water. Most pools have different types of group water exercise classes; chances are one will be right for you.

ADVANCE!

Congratulations! You have established your swim fitness program. Are you ready to challenge yourself with a new goal and take your swimming to the next level? Below is a more advanced four-week program that you can follow; visit the mobile website to find more options or to personalize this or any of the programs in this book.

ADVANCED: SWIMMING

PROGRAM   **GOAL:** Swim a mile, continuous (or with minimum rest)! (1650 yards/1508 meters)

	Mon T/D	Mon I	Tue T/D	Tue I	Wed T/D	Wed I	Thurs T/D	Thurs I	Fri T/D	Fri I	Sat T/D	Sat I	Sun T/D	Sun I
Week 1	25	L–M 3–5 62–70	700	M 5–6 65–85	25	L–M 3–5 62–70	700	M 5–6 65–85	25	M 5–6 65–85				
Week 2	30	M 5–6 65–85	1000	M 5–6 65–85	Interval	L–M–V	1000	M 5-6 65–85	30	L–M 3–5 62–70				
Week 3	25	M 5–6 65–85	Interval	L–M–V	30	L–M 3–5 62–70	Interval	L–M–V			35	M 5–6 65–85		
Week 4	30	M 5–6 65–85	1500	M 5–6 65–85	Interval	L–M–V	20	L–M 3–5 62–70			Goal Mile Swim!			

T/D = Time/Distance. Total time/distance is listed in minutes or yards/meters.
I = Intensity. Intensity is listed as Light/Lifestyle (L), Moderate (M), or Vigorous (V), the OMNI scale of 0–10, and % of HRmax. (See Figure 2.1, Figure 3.8, and Table 3.3.)
Workouts do not include warm-up or cool-down time.
Heart rates are typically 10–13 beats per minute lower when swimming than when performing exercise on land. Adjust heart rate targets accordingly.

INTENSITY LEVEL
Light   Moderate   Vigorous

Advanced Program Interval Workout—1200 m/yds

3 × 100 m/yds with 60 seconds of rest between [100s at 65–84% HRmax, 5–6 on the OMNI scale (M), and rest at 0–2 (L)]
2 × 200 m/yds with 2 minutes of rest between [200s at 85% HRmax, 7–8 on the OMNI scale (V), and rest at 0–2 (L)]
1 × 500 m/yds [at 65–84% HRmax, 5–6 on the OMNI scale (M)]

4 Building Muscular Strength & Endurance

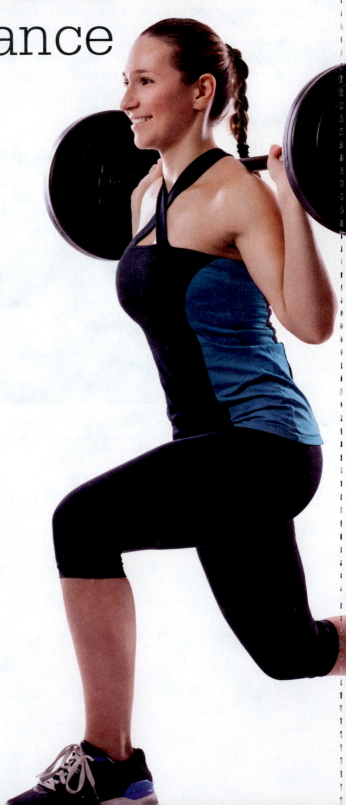

LEARNINGoutcomes

1. Explain how muscular strength and muscular endurance relate to life-long fitness and wellness.

2. Identify key skeletal muscle structures and explain how they work together to allow for basic muscle function.

3. Articulate the fitness and wellness improvements you can make with regular resistance training.

4. Evaluate your changes in muscle fitness over time by assessing your muscular strength and muscular endurance at regular intervals.

5. Set and work toward appropriate muscular fitness goals.

6. Implement a safe and effective resistance-training exercise program compatible with your goals and lifestyle.

7. Observe safety precautions when resistance training.

8. Incorporate strategies to avoid the risks associated with supplement use.

MasteringHealth™

Go online for chapter quizzes, interactive assessments, videos, and more!

casestudy

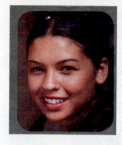

GINA

"Hi, I'm Gina. I'm from San Francisco and I'm a sophomore majoring in economics. I'm taking a fitness and wellness class this semester, and this week we're starting the section on muscular fitness. I'm curious about it because I've never lifted weights before! I like to go hiking and I take yoga classes from time to time, but I wouldn't call myself an athlete. Does it really make sense for someone like me to start a strength-training program?"

HEAR IT! ONLINE

Whether you're a beginner like Gina or an athlete interested in conditioning, this chapter answers common questions about muscular fitness, explains the benefits of resistance training, and gives you the tools for designing a program that is custom-made for you.

Muscular fitness is the ability of your musculoskeletal system to perform daily and recreational activities without undue fatigue and injury. Muscular fitness involves having adequate muscular strength and endurance. **Muscular strength** is the ability of a muscle or group of muscles to contract with maximal force. It describes how strong a muscle is or how much force it can exert. Exercise professionals often measure muscular strength by determining the maximum weight a person can lift at one time. **Muscular endurance** is the ability of a muscle to contract repeatedly over an extended period of time. It describes how long you can sustain a given type of muscular exertion. One way that fitness professionals measure muscular endurance is by determining the maximum weight a person can lift 20 times consecutively.

You can build better muscular strength and endurance through resistance training. **Resistance training** is also referred to as *weight training* or *strength training* and can be done with measured weights, body weight, or other resistive equipment (i.e., exercise bands or exercise balls). Resistance exercises stress the body's musculoskeletal system, which enlarges muscle fibers and improves neural control of muscle function, resulting in greater muscular strength and endurance.

Are you already participating in a resistance-training program? If so, you are not alone. In 2011, 24.2 percent of adults over the age of 18 reported regular participation in muscular strength and endurance activities.[1] The numbers are up from 2008, when 21.9 percent of adults reported participating in muscle strengthening activities on two or more days of the week.[2] The increase in Americans who participate in strength training meets the *Healthy People 2020* target, which is great news![3] However, it still leaves 76 percent of the population not doing strengthening exercises at the recommended level. If you are not participating, now may be the perfect time to start because facilities and classes are readily available at most colleges and universities and you may have a group of peers who want to support one another in getting fit and healthy.

Resistance training offers such varied benefits that exercise professionals recommend it in nearly all health-related fitness programs. Regular resistance training can make daily activities easier: Carrying around a backpack full of heavy textbooks won't tire you as much; bringing in a bag of groceries will be less taxing; and taking the stairs will seem natural and feel better than riding in an elevator. No matter what your age or goals, resistance training is an important part of staying healthy and functional throughout your life.

How Do My Muscles Work?

The human body contains hundreds of muscles, each of which belongs to one of three basic types: (1) voluntary *skeletal muscle,* which allows movement of the skeleton and generates body heat; (2) involuntary *cardiac muscle,* which exists only in the heart and facilitates the pumping of blood through the body; and (3) involuntary *smooth muscle,* which lines some internal organs and

muscular fitness The ability of your musculoskeletal system to perform daily and recreational activities without undue fatigue and injury

muscular strength The ability of a muscle to contract with maximal force

muscular endurance The ability of a muscle to contract repeatedly over an extended period of time

resistance training Controlled and progressive stressing of the body's musculoskeletal system using resistance (i.e., weights, resistance bands, body weight) exercises to build and maintain muscular fitness

tendons The connective tissues attaching muscle to bone

muscle fibers The cells of the muscular system

myofibrils Thin strands within a single muscle fiber that bundle the skeletal muscle protein filaments and span the length of the fiber

sarcomeres Basic functional contractile units within skeletal and cardiac muscle that contain both thin actin and thick myosin protein filaments

moves food through the stomach and intestines. Resistance training and cardiorespiratory exercises benefit your skeletal and cardiac muscles. Here we focus on skeletal muscles and the signals from the nervous system that coordinate and control their contraction.

An Overview of Skeletal Muscle

Each skeletal muscle is surrounded by a sheet of connective tissue that draws together at the ends of the muscle, forming the **tendons** (see **Figure 4.1**). Muscular contractions allow for skeletal movement because muscles are attached to bones via tendons. These attached muscles pull the bones, which pivot at joints, creating a specific body movement.

Within each skeletal muscle are individual muscle cells called **muscle fibers**. Bundles of muscle fibers

are called *fascicles*. Each muscle fiber extends the full length of the muscle. Within each muscle fiber are many **myofibrils**, each containing contractile protein filaments. These filaments are primarily made up of two kinds of protein—*actin* and *myosin*—which partially overlap at rest and give the whole cell a striped appearance. Actin and myosin filaments exist in repeating units called **sarcomeres**. *Sarcomere* is a term for the smallest area in a muscle fiber where everything required for muscle contraction exists. Sarcomeres repeat along the length of the myofibril, and one muscle can have over 100,000 sarcomeres along its length. The microscopic structure and function of actin and myosin allow them to slide across each other, which shortens the sarcomere, myofibril, and muscle fiber. You can picture this sliding and shortening as similar to the way your forearms can slide past each other inside the front pocket of a hooded sweatshirt, pulling your elbows closer together. Simultaneous shortening of the many fibers within a whole muscle causes the pattern of muscular tension we call *contraction*. It is this whole-muscle contraction that moves bones and surrounding body parts.

Every muscle fiber can be categorized as either *slow* or *fast,* depending on how quickly it can contract. **Slow-twitch muscle fibers** (Type I) depend on oxygen and contract relatively slowly, but can contract for

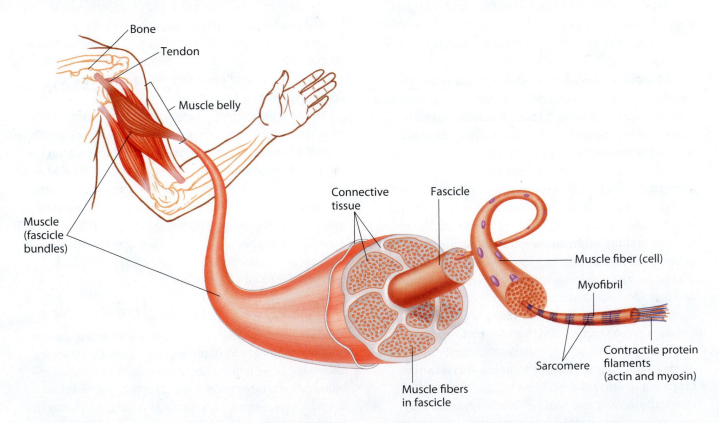

FIGURE **4.1** Muscle is attached to bones via tendons. Tendons are a continuation of the connective tissue that surrounds the entire muscle as well as each muscle bundle (fascicle). A fascicle is made up of many muscle cells (muscle fibers). Within each muscle fiber, myofibril strands contain actin and myosin proteins.

longer periods of time without fatigue. In slow-twitch fibers, the energy for contraction primarily comes from the breakdown of fat from the blood, muscle cells, and adipose tissue. For efficient fat breakdown, oxygen and minimal levels of glucose breakdown are required. **Fast-twitch muscle fibers** (Type II) are not oxygen-dependent and contract more rapidly than slow-twitch fibers, but tire relatively quickly (they also produce greater muscle power). In fast-twitch fibers, the energy for contraction primarily comes from phosphocreatine and glycogen reserves within the muscles, glycogen stored within the liver, and glucose in the blood.

All fiber types exist in skeletal muscles, but some muscles within the body (e.g., postural trunk muscles) have more slow-twitch fibers, while other muscles (such as those in the calves) have more fast-twitch fibers. The proportion of muscle fiber types varies from person to person based on both genetics and training. Elite athletes have muscle fiber compositions that complement their sport. Marathoners, for instance, have higher levels of slow-twitch fibers that supply them with optimal muscular endurance. Power weight lifters, on the other hand, have more fast-twitch fibers that allow feats of enormous muscular strength over short periods of time. Sedentary individuals and people who do general resistance training typically have 50 percent slow-twitch and 50 percent fast-twitch fiber composition.

Muscle Contraction Requires Stimulation

For a voluntary skeletal muscle to contract, the nervous system must send a signal directly to the muscle. When you want to move any part of your body—for example, a finger on your right hand—your brain sends a signal down the spinal cord and through motor nerves to the skeletal muscle fibers in that finger. One motor nerve stimulates many skeletal muscle fibers, together creating a functional unit called a **motor unit** (**Figure 4.2**). A motor unit can be small or large, depending on the number of muscle fibers that the motor nerve stimulates. Motor units are made up of one type of muscle fiber or the other, either slow-twitch or fast-twitch. In general, small motor units comprise slow-twitch fibers and larger motor units comprise fast-twitch fibers. The strength of a muscle contraction depends upon the intensity of the nervous system stimulus, the number and size of motor units activated, and the types of muscle fibers that are stimulated. For example, if you are getting ready to lift a heavy weight, your central nervous system sends a stronger signal. This activates a greater number of large, fast motor units, resulting in a more forceful muscle contraction than if you were merely picking up an apple.

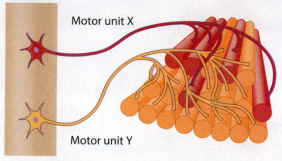

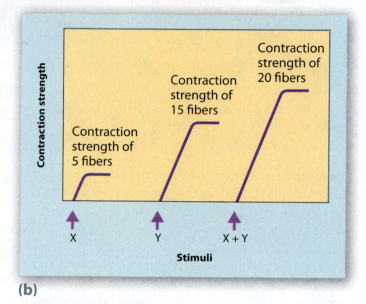

FIGURE **4.2** Motor units and muscle contraction strength. (a) Motor unit X is smaller (5 fibers) than motor unit Y (15 fibers). (b) The strength of a muscular contraction increases with increased fibers per motor unit (X vs. Y) and with more motor units activated (X + Y).

Three Primary Types of Muscle Contractions

Muscle contractions all result in an increase in tension or force within the muscle, but some contractions move body parts while others do not. There are three primary types of contractions: isotonic, isometric, and isokinetic.

Isotonic contractions are characterized by a consistent muscle tension as the contraction proceeds and a resulting movement of body parts (**Figure 4.3a**, page 116). An arm curl with a 10-pound hand weight involves isotonic contractions throughout your arm.

slow-twitch muscle fibers Muscle fiber type that is oxygen dependent and can contract over long periods of time

fast-twitch muscle fibers Muscle fiber type that contracts with greater force and speed but also fatigues quickly

motor unit A motor nerve and all the muscle fibers it controls

isotonic A muscle contraction with relatively constant tension

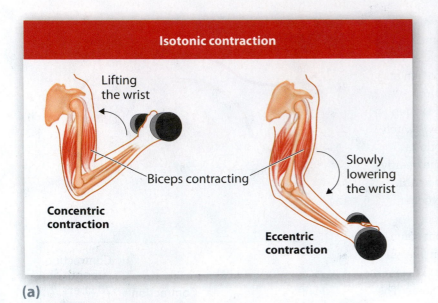

Isotonic contraction

Lifting the wrist

Biceps contracting

Concentric contraction

Slowly lowering the wrist

Eccentric contraction

(a)

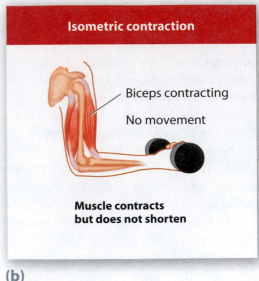

Isometric contraction

Biceps contracting

No movement

Muscle contracts but does not shorten

(b)

FIGURE 4.3 (a) Isotonic contractions include concentric (shortening) and eccentric (lengthening) contractions. (b) Isometric contractions produce force in the muscle with no movement.

Isometric contractions are characterized by a consistent muscle length throughout the contraction with no visible movement of body parts. An example of an isometric contraction occurs when you hold a hand weight at arm's length in front of you; your arm is not moving, but you feel tension in your arm muscles (**Figure 4.3b**). **Isokinetic** contractions are characterized by a consistent muscle contraction speed within a moving body part. In order to perform isokinetic contractions, you need specialized equipment that holds the speed of movement constant as your arm, leg, or other muscles contract with varying forces.

Isotonic contractions are the most common in exercise programs. Lifting free weights, working on machines, and doing push-ups are all examples of isotonic contractions. Isotonic contractions can be either concentric or eccentric. **Concentric** contractions occur when force is developed in the muscle as the muscle is shortening—for example, when you curl a free weight up toward your shoulder. In **eccentric** muscle contractions, force remains in the muscle while the muscle is lengthening. This occurs as you lower a free weight back to its original position. Figure 4.3a

isometric A muscle contraction with no change in muscle length

isokinetic A muscle contraction with a constant speed of contraction

concentric A muscle contraction with overall muscle shortening

eccentric A muscle contraction with overall muscle lengthening

case study

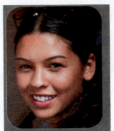

GINA

"I love to go on short hikes. There are some gorgeous trails in the San Francisco Bay Area. Some of them are hilly but I don't mind—the views from the top are always worth it. My calves definitely get a workout! I'd like to be able to do longer hikes, but the truth is that I usually get tired after about three miles. I know there are some longer hikes with spectacular views, but I don't feel ready for them yet."

THINK! Given what you've learned so far, what would you tell Gina about how resistance training can benefit her? Which type of muscle fibers would you guess that Gina has more of: slow-twitch fibers or fast-twitch fibers?

ACT NOW! Today, go outside and enjoy a favorite activity. During the activity, name the muscle fiber types you are using most (slow-twitch or fast-twitch). This week, try isometric contractions by doing wall sits. Sit with your back against a wall, feet out in front of you, and your knees bent at 90 degrees or more (but not less than 90 degrees). Hold this position for 30 seconds to one minute. Repeat one to two more times. In two weeks, name the concentric and eccentric portions of each exercise you perform during a resistance-training session. Write this down in your workout log.

HEAR IT! ONLINE

illustrates these muscular contractions, using a bicep-curl exercise as an example.

How Can Regular Resistance Training Improve My Fitness and Wellness?

People used to think that weight lifting was solely a means of improving body shape and producing bigger muscles. We now know that, in addition to improving physical appearance, resistance training can result in specific physiological changes that have significant fitness and wellness benefits. **Figure 4.4** summarizes these changes. We discuss the benefits of resistance training in detail in the following section.

Regular Resistance Training Increases Your Strength

Regular resistance training with an adequate load, or amount of weight lifted, will result in an increase in muscle strength. Although men have larger muscles due to higher testosterone levels, men and women improve relative strength with resistance training at similar rates.[4] Stronger lower- and upper-body muscles benefit both men and women.

Neural Improvements When you start a resistance-training program, you will gain muscular strength before noticing any increase in muscle size. This is because internal physiological adaptations to training take place before muscle enlargement. The strength of a muscular contraction depends, in large part, on effective recruitment of the motor units needed for that contraction. The better your body is at recruiting the necessary motor units through voluntary neural signaling, the stronger your muscles will be. In the first few weeks or months of a resistance-training program, most of the adaptation involves an increased ability to recruit motor units, which causes more muscle fibers to contract.

Increased Muscle Size With consistent resistance training, the amount of actin and myosin within your muscle fibers increases. This results in **hypertrophy**, an increase in the size or cross-sectional area of the protein filaments. With more contractile proteins, a muscle can contract more forcefully; in other words, larger muscles are stronger muscles. While both slow- and fast-twitch muscles will increase in size with resistance training, greater increases in strength will result from hypertrophy of fast-twitch muscle fibers.

hypertrophy An increase in muscle cross-sectional area

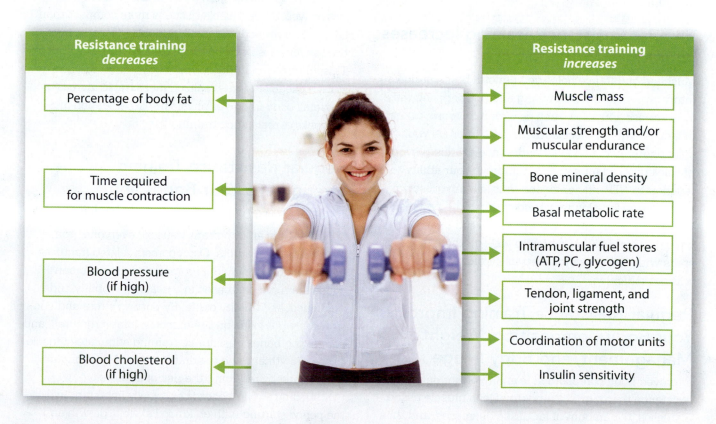

Resistance training *decreases*	Resistance training *increases*
Percentage of body fat	Muscle mass
Time required for muscle contraction	Muscular strength and/or muscular endurance
Blood pressure (if high)	Bone mineral density
Blood cholesterol (if high)	Basal metabolic rate
	Intramuscular fuel stores (ATP, PC, glycogen)
	Tendon, ligament, and joint strength
	Coordination of motor units
	Insulin sensitivity

FIGURE **4.4** Physiological changes from resistance training.

Muscle hypertrophy in response to resistance training takes longer than neural improvements, but is the most important contributor to strength gains over time. The degree of hypertrophy or enlargement you can expect with weight training depends upon your gender, age, genetics, and how you design your training program. Some individuals will develop larger muscles more quickly than others; some will experience only limited hypertrophy. In particular, women and men with smaller builds will realize less muscle development than those with larger builds, even with identical training programs (see the GetFitGraphic Pumping Up Women to Strength Train on the following page). Older individuals will also have slower progress and overall less muscle development, though they can still see significant improvements.

A program with heavier weights, longer durations, or more frequent training can produce greater gains than a more standard fitness-training program. People who stop resistance training will experience some degree of **atrophy**, a shrinking of the muscle to its pretraining size and strength. To avoid atrophy, you need to make a long-term commitment to resistance training.

Regular Resistance Training Increases Your Muscular Endurance

Muscular endurance helps you perform both cardiorespiratory activities, such as hiking and running, and muscular fitness activities, such as circuit or sports training. In fact, just doing these activities will improve your muscular endurance. Muscular endurance exercises trigger physiological adaptations that improve your ability to regenerate ATP efficiently and thus sustain muscular contractions for a longer period of time. The end result will be the ability to snowboard a long run instead of having to rest halfway down, to walk up three flights of stairs with ease, or to rake leaves vigorously for an hour without difficulty.

Regular Resistance Training Improves Your Body Composition, Weight Management, and Body Image

Improved body composition is an important outcome of resistance training: The amount of lean muscle tissue increases, the amount of fat tissue decreases, and thus the ratio of lean to fat improves. Research has demonstrated that such higher lean-to-fat ratios improve your overall health profile and reduce your risk of heart attack, diabetes, and death from cardiovascular diseases.[5] Fat does not turn into muscle or vice versa; the number of fat and muscle cells remains the same, with cells merely enlarging or shrinking depending on food intake and activity levels.

More muscle means a faster metabolic rate; pound for pound, muscle tissue expends more energy than fat tissue.[6] With more total calories being expended during the day, weight control becomes easier and more effective.[7] Resistance training should be combined with aerobic exercise for overall weight loss,[8] but resistance training during weight loss helps ensure that you will lose fat and not precious muscle tissue;[9] your body can be lighter, stronger, and leaner (i.e., more toned) instead of just lighter (and potentially still flabby), as often happens with traditional diet-only weight-loss methods.

When you begin a resistance-training program, you may experience a slight initial weight gain as muscle tissue grows. If you focus only on the scale, this can be discouraging. It is better to focus on how much stronger and more toned your muscles feel. With a consistent fitness and nutrition program, fat loss will eventually "catch up" to muscle gain and will be reflected in weight loss as well. Since muscle tissue is more compact than fat tissue, your body size will gradually decrease over time as muscles become toned and fat tissues shrink. This, in turn, can improve your body image. In one study, college students realized measurable increases in overall body image or physical self-perception after 12 weeks of resistance training.[10]

Regular Resistance Training Strengthens Your Bones and Protects Your Body from Injuries

Bone health is an important issue for everyone, from children to older adults. Osteoporosis-related fractures are common among older women and men and can cause dramatic decreases in a person's mobility, independence, and quality of life. By putting stress and controlled-weight loads on the muscles, joint structures, and supporting bones, resistance training stimulates muscle tissue growth and the generation of harder, stronger bones, thereby reducing the risk of fracture.

Building strong bones is especially important in the period starting with childhood skeletal growth and

PUMPING UP WOMEN TO STRENGTH TRAIN

With fewer than 18% of college age American women meeting the CDC's strength training recommendations,[1] some women may need a boost to start strength training.

WHO DIDN'T PARTICIPATE IN ANY STRENGTH TRAINING OVER THE LAST WEEK?[2]

61% of undergraduate **WOMEN**

45% of undergraduate **MEN**

ARE THESE MYTHS STOPPING WOMEN FROM STRENGTH TRAINING?

MYTH	FACT
Women who **LIFT WEIGHTS** will develop bulky muscles.	It's **physiologically impossible** for most women to bulk up. Women don't have enough testosterone, the "muscle-bulking" hormone.
Women are **NOT AS STRONG** as men.	While technically true in most cases, it's because men (on average) have more muscle mass than women. Compared pound for pound, **women can be equally strong**.
Weight training will **REDUCE** your flexibility.	Resistance training can actually **enhance** your joint range of motion/flexibility.[3]
If you build muscle and then **STOP EXERCISING**, your muscle will turn to fat.	**Not possible!** Fat and muscle are two different substances; you can't turn one into the other.
The weight room is an **INTIMIDATING PLACE** full of men.	After an orientation to the gym, fellow exercisers and the gym equipment will be **familiar and welcoming**. Still intimidated? Try women-specific facilities and/or strength training classes.

STRENGTH TRAINING
benefits women by

- ▶ **INCREASING** self-confidence and body image.
- ▶ **BUILDING BONES** to reduce the risk of osteoporosis.[4]
- ▶ **SLOWING** the 8-10% loss of muscle mass that women experience each decade after age 40.[5]

TO JUMP INTO
Strength Training
RIGHT NOW

 LEARN good technique to get the maximum benefit and to avoid injury.

 START SLOWLY with the number of repetitions, the amount of resistance, and the number of workouts per week.

 USE THE PROPER weight, where you can just barely finish the last 12-15 repetitions.

development and ending at about age 30. The "reservoir" of bone tissue you lay down in those years and then maintain throughout life will help prevent weak, brittle bones as you age. Even the bones of older individuals can benefit from strength training; in one study, eight months of resistance training positively affected hip bone density in older women, whereas no change occurred with moderate-impact aerobic exercise over the same time period.[11]

Getting hurt will put you on the sidelines. Whether you exercise for fun, fitness, or competition, preventing injuries is a key to continued participation. Injury prevention tips are often specific to your chosen activity; however, strong muscles, bones, and connective tissues are the common denominator for preventing injury in any activity. Regular resistance training improves not only muscular strength and endurance, but also the strength of tendons, ligaments, and other supporting structures around each joint. As they grow stronger, the joints themselves are better protected from injury. A stronger body can handle the physical stresses of everyday life (carrying heavy books or groceries, lifting laundry baskets, moving furniture, etc.) with less chance of injury.

A strong, pain-free back and proper posture are crucial to daily functioning without injury. Individuals who participate in regular resistance-training exercise have stronger postural muscles and report less low back pain.

Imbalanced muscles around a joint may result in a change in joint alignment with subsequent pain or injury. Muscular balance will reduce this risk. A well-designed muscle fitness program will work toward improving strength and muscle endurance in opposing muscular groups, promoting overall muscle balance.

Regular Resistance Training Helps Maintain Your Physical Function with Aging

Starting between the ages of 25 and 30, men and women begin to lose muscle mass. As they age, they lose up to one-third of their muscle mass due to changes in hormones, activity levels, and nutrition. Injury and chronic diseases can cause people to exercise less and accelerate typical muscle loss. **Sarcopenia**, literally "poverty of flesh," is the term applied to this age-related loss in skeletal muscle (see **Figure 4.5**). Sarcopenia reduces overall physical functioning by decreasing muscular strength and endurance and causing losses in **muscle power**, or the capacity to exert force rapidly. While no one is immune from the aging process, resistance training throughout one's life can

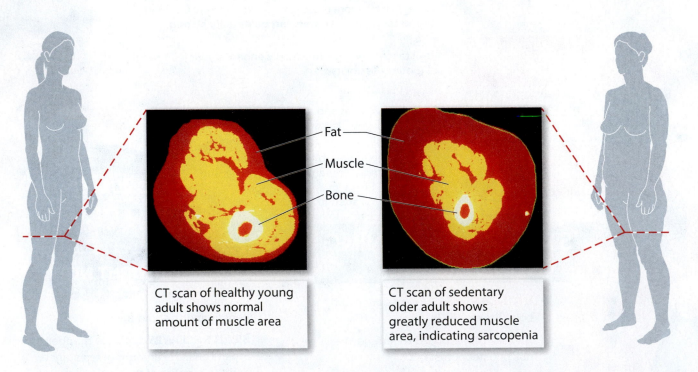

Fat

Muscle

Bone

CT scan of healthy young adult shows normal amount of muscle area

CT scan of sedentary older adult shows greatly reduced muscle area, indicating sarcopenia

FIGURE **4.5** CT scans showing the difference in muscle mass in a healthy young adult vs. an older adult with sarcopenia. Age-related muscle loss can be slowed down with resistance training.

significantly slow natural muscle loss. In fact, older individuals who do resistance training can retain strength at or above that of untrained younger people.[12] The increase in muscular fitness and the improvements it brings to everyday physical functioning help individuals live independently for a longer portion of their lives.[13]

Regular Resistance Training Helps Reduce Your Cardiovascular Disease Risk

Regular resistance training can lower your risk of cardiovascular disease by increasing blood flow to working muscles and vital tissues throughout your body. In fact, research studies in numerous populations have shown performing regular resistance-training exercise can lower

blood pressure and blood cholesterol.[14] Since being overfat (having a higher than recommended percentage of body fat) increases your risk of cardiovascular disease and adult-onset diabetes, an improved body composition achieved through resistance training can help you lower your risk of both of these diseases.

Regular Resistance Training Enhances Your Performance in Sports and Activities

Achieving muscular fitness through resistance training has yet another benefit: A stronger body is more resistant to fatigue, moves more quickly, and recovers more quickly from illness or injury. All of these traits contribute to better performance in sports, recreational activities, and other fitness pursuits. Resistance training is often the common denominator among training programs for different sports and activities. Because of these benefits, physically active adults often incorporate some form of resistance training that builds strength and endurance in the muscle groups most crucial to their sport.

case study

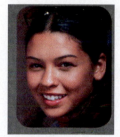

GINA

"I've always wanted to hike to the top of Nevada Falls in Yosemite National Park. I'm told that it can be done as a day hike, but it is about seven miles round trip. There is also a steep section of rocks near another waterfall along the way—apparently you get completely soaked while hiking that part of the trail! Even on dry trails, I'm always extra careful hiking downhill, because I once sprained my ankle on a hike, which was not fun.

If resistance training can help me take on Nevada Falls, I'm interested. I've also always wished I had better muscle tone, but to be honest, I don't want to 'bulk up' . . ."

THINK! What are two ways that resistance training can help Gina realize her goal of safely hiking to the top of Nevada Falls? How would you respond to Gina's concerns about "bulking up"?

ACT NOW! Today, think about your "Nevada Falls." That is, what is something you have always wanted to do, if only you were in better physical shape? Write down your ideas and post the note somewhere you can see it each day for motivation. This week, start an action plan to reach your goal with written measurable steps to be completed this week and next! In two weeks, share your plan with a close friend or family member and enlist additional ideas to help you reach your "Nevada Falls."

HEAR IT! ONLINE

How Can I Assess My Muscular Strength and Endurance?

Before you can plan an appropriate resistance-training program, it is important to assess your current muscular strength and endurance. You can then compare the results to norm charts for your age and gender, or simply use them as a starting point for designing your program. After you've followed your program for a while, follow-up assessments will help you evaluate your progress and make adjustments to stay on track.

Test Your Muscular Strength

Tests of muscular strength gauge the maximum amount of force you can generate in a muscle. People usually carry out these tests in a weight room where measured weights of all sizes are readily available.

1 RM Tests One repetition maximum (1 RM) tests are the most common tool fitness instructors and personal trainers use to assess their clients' muscular strength. To participate in the tests safely, you must be medically cleared to lift heavier weights than you have in the past, have detailed instructions for the test procedure, know general weight-training guidelines, have a few weeks of weight-training experience, and have qualified **spotters** standing nearby to watch and assist if necessary. If you are weight training on campus or at a gym, an instructor will be able to help you through these preliminary steps.

These 1 RM tests are performed by discovering the maximum amount of weight you can lift one time on a particular exercise. You must accurately determine your 1 RM within three to five trials so that muscle fatigue from repetitions does not change your result. In general health and fitness classes or beginning weight-training programs, instructors often tell students to predict their 1 RM instead of actually attempting a maximum lift. This is particularly true when students are new to resistance training and are unfamiliar with weight-training guidelines. To predict your 1 RM, you will lift, press, or pull a weight that will fully fatigue your upper- or lower-body muscles in 2 to 10 repetitions. You can then use a formula that converts actual weight lifted and real number of repetitions to predict your 1 RM capacity for that exercise. In **Lab 4.1** (at the end of this chapter), you will use chest-press and leg-press exercises to determine your predicted 1 RM. You can perform these tests for any weight-training exercise and then convert to the predicted 1 RM value. Many weight-training programs use a percentage of your 1 RM or predicted 1 RM to determine a safe starting level for weight lifting.

DO IT! ONLINE

Grip Strength Test
Another common test of muscle strength is the hand grip strength test using a piece of equipment called a *grip strength dynamometer*. As you squeeze the dynamometer (with one hand at a time), it measures the static or isometric strength of your grip-squeezing muscles in pounds or kilograms (kg). If you have a grip strength dynamometer available to use, assess your grip strength with the online Alternate Lab: Assessing Grip Strength.

Test Your Muscular Endurance
Muscular endurance tests evaluate a muscle's ability to contract for an extended period of time. Some of these tests must be performed in a weight room, whereas others require only your body weight for resistance and can be performed anywhere.

20 RM Tests You can use any weight-training exercise to find your **20 repetition maximum (20 RM)**. This test determines the maximal amount of weight you can lift exactly 20 times in a row before the muscle becomes too fatigued to continue. The 20 RM tests are particularly useful for setting muscular endurance goals and then tracking your progress. Try to discover your 20 RM within one to three tries to avoid fatiguing your muscles and altering your results. **Lab 4.2** walks you through the steps of finding your 20 RM for the chest-press and leg-press exercises.

DO IT! ONLINE

Calisthenic Tests **Calisthenics** are conditioning exercises that use your body weight for resistance. Calisthenic tests use sit-ups, curl-ups, pull-ups, push-ups, and flexed arm support/hang exercises to assess muscular endurance. The procedures for these tests vary. You will learn how to perform curl-up and push-up assessments in Lab 4.2. Calisthenic tests allow you to test yourself outside of a weight-training facility and to compare your results to well-established physical fitness norms.

How Can I Design My Own Resistance-Training Program?

Designing an effective resistance-training program requires some knowledge, and many people enlist the help of a personal trainer or fitness professional. You can become your own personal trainer, however, by using the guidelines in this section to plan a safe and effective muscular fitness program.

Set Appropriate Muscular Fitness Goals
Remember to use SMART goal-setting guidelines: Goals should be *s*pecific, *m*easurable, *a*ction-oriented, and *r*ealistic and should have a *t*imeline. Your goals may be appearance-based, function-based, or a combination of the two.

Appearance-Based Goals Many people have appearance-based goals for muscular fitness: They want larger muscles, or muscles that are more toned and less flabby. "Spot reduction" (i.e., trimming down just one area of the body) is another often-voiced goal. Researchers have proven spot reduction to be a myth, showing that fat doesn't disappear through repeated exercise to one area.[15]

In order to judge your progress toward appearance-based goals, be sure to include some sort of measure of progress in your resistance-training plan. For muscle size, measure the circumference of your biceps or calves, for example, and then set a goal to increase or decrease this number. For overall body size, your goal may be to increase lean tissue weight but decrease fat tissue and percentage of body fat. If your goal is to become more "toned," quantify this in some way. Look in the mirror and make notes about the way your body looks and moves. After you reach the target date for your plan, reread your notes, look in the mirror, and then reevaluate whether your muscle tone has improved.

Function-Based Goals Include some specific goals for improving muscle function in your fitness plan. Function-based goals focus on your muscular capabilities and include gaining better muscular strength, greater muscular endurance, or both. **Lab 4.3** will guide you in setting goals for realistic changes in muscle function and then help you assess your improvements.

DO IT! ONLINE

Explore Your Equipment Options

Should you use weight machines in your resistance-training program? Free weights? Other equipment? No equipment at all? These are important decisions, and they will be determined by your fitness goals, the type of equipment available to you, your experience with weight-training exercises, and your preferences.

Machines If you are new to resistance training, weight machines can be very useful. Systems such as Cybex®, Nautilus®, Life Fitness®, and many others allow you to isolate and strengthen specific muscle groups as well as to train without a spotting partner.

Free Weights Personal trainers and exercise physiologists consider free-weight exercises to be a more advanced approach to weight training than machine-weight exercises. Free-weight exercises use **dumbbells**; **barbells**; incline, flat, or decline benches; squat racks; and related equipment. Free-weight exercises allow your body to move through its natural range of motion instead of the path predetermined by a weight machine. This both requires and promotes development of more muscle control. Some athletes prefer free-weight exercises because the balance and movement patterns needed to successfully lift free weights are closer to their sport movement patterns, whether that be tossing a football, putting a shot, or doing the breaststroke. Since workout facilities often have both free weights and weight machines, many people start their resistance-training program exclusively with machine-weight exercises and then progress to free weights within the first few months. **Table 4.1** on page 124 compares machine-weight training and free-weight training.

Alternate Equipment You can increase resistance on your body with equipment other than machines or free weights. Resistance bands made of tubing or flat strips of rubber allow you to simultaneously increase resistance throughout a range of motion and to improve muscular endurance. You can perform many different exercises with these bands. They fold up and pack perfectly in a suitcase or gym bag for a portable workout. Stability balls (also called Swiss, fitness, or exercise balls) are 18-inch to 30-inch diameter vinyl balls that have various uses for muscular fitness, endurance, and balance. Ball routines involve performing exercises while sitting, lying, and/or balancing on the ball. The ball exerciser must use core trunk muscles to counteract the natural instability of the ball, which enhances overall body function. People sometimes use heavily weighted balls called medicine balls to increase resistance, either individually, with a partner, or in a group. You can hold a medicine ball while doing calisthenic or free-weight exercises or pass a ball from partner to partner for a functional increase in muscle endurance.

No-Equipment Training Calisthenics such as push-ups, pull-ups, lunges, squats, leg lifts, and curl-ups do not involve equipment. Instead, they use your body weight to provide the resistance. Like resistance bands, these exercises are perfect for maintaining muscular strength and endurance while traveling.

Understand the Different Types of Resistance-Training Programs

You can plan a resistance-training program with various types of equipment and numerous exercise routines. The right program for you will be determined by your goals, experience, and personal preference.

Traditional Weight Training Traditional weight training takes place in a weight room and usually includes a combination of machine-weight, free-weight, and calisthenic exercises. Individuals may work alone or with a partner and will usually perform multiple **sets** and **repetitions** of a particular exercise

> **dumbbells** Weights intended for use by one hand; typically one uses a dumbbell in each hand
>
> **barbells** Long bars with weight plates on each end
>
> **sets** Single attempts at an exercise that include a fixed number of repetitions
>
> **repetitions** The number of times an exercise is performed within one set

TABLE 4.1 Machine-Weight vs. Free-Weight Training

Machine Weights	Free Weights
PROS	**PROS**
Safe and less intimidating for beginners	Can be tailored for individual workouts
Quicker to set up and use	Range of motion set by lifter, not machine
Spotters not typically needed	Some exercises can be done anywhere
Support of standing posture not needed	Standing and sitting postural muscles worked
Adaptable for those with limitations	Movements can transfer to daily activities
Variable resistance is possible	Good for strength and power building
Good isolation of specific muscle groups	Additional stabilizer muscles worked
Only good option for some muscle groups	Lower cost and more available for home use
CONS	**CONS**
Machine sets range of motion	More difficult to learn
May not fit every body size and type	A spotter may be needed
Some people lack access to weight machines	Incorrect form may lead to injuries
Posture supporting muscles used less	More time may be needed to change weights
Limited number of exercises/machines	More training needed to create program

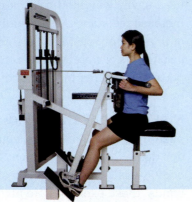

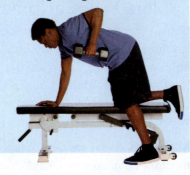

before moving on to the next exercise. Guidelines for setting up your traditional weight-training program are outlined in the next section and sample traditional weight-training programs are available at the end of this chapter.

Circuit Weight Training Circuit weight training is done in a specialized circuit-training room, a general workout room, or a weight room. Exercisers move from one station to another in a set pattern (the "circuit") after a certain amount of time at a station or after performing a certain number of repetitions of an exercise such as a biceps curl, leg press, or chest press. Some circuits include only resistance-training exercises and have the single goal of improving muscular fitness. Some circuits involve cardiorespiratory or aerobic training equipment, such as stair-steppers or stationary bicycles, mixed in with the resistance exercises to improve both cardiorespiratory and muscular fitness.

In circuit training, it is important to remember the specificity training principle: In order to get optimal muscle fitness benefits, you must focus on the resistance exercises; in order to realize added cardiorespiratory benefits, you must spend a minimal amount of time on the cardio machines (20 to 30 minutes total per exercise session).

Circuit exercises should be organized properly in order to ensure a safe and effective exercise session. For example, multi-joint exercises (bench press, leg press) are often performed before single-joint exercises (biceps curl, leg extension) and muscle groups worked are spread out to allow recovery between sets. Exercises that stress the core postural muscles are reserved for the end of the workout because these muscles provide important trunk support during seated and standing exercises.

Plyometrics and Sports Training Resistance-training programs designed to support specific sports can be quite different from general resistance training. Athletes may use many of the general weight-training exercises illustrated in this chapter, but they usually also perform exercises or exercise methods that specifically benefit their sports performance. Plyometrics, power lifts, and speed and agility drills are examples.

A **plyometric exercise** program incorporates explosive exercises that mimic the quick transition movements needed in many sports (e.g., basketball, wrestling, and gymnastics). These exercises are characterized by a landing and slowing down of the body mass followed immediately by a rapid movement in the opposite direction (e.g., jumping down off a box and then immediately jumping back up as high as you can). Plyometrics is a highly specialized training method that should be performed under proper direction and only by individuals who have achieved a high level of muscular fitness.

Power lifting is a type of resistance training that incorporates fast and forceful actions to improve strength and speed. Lifting for **power** stresses the nervous system to act quickly and the tendons, ligaments, and joint structures to become more stable. Sports that require high levels of explosive movement and power (football, wrestling, gymnastics, and track-and-field events) may require power-lifting training to build strength with speed. Power lifting is a competitive sport in itself. Competitive power lifts include the bench press, the squat, the dead lift, and the Olympic lifts (the clean and jerk and the snatch). Like plyometrics, power lifting should be practiced only by experienced athletes or those with comparable weight-training experience.

The training regimens for certain athletes may include **speed** and **agility** drills. These drills are making their way into mainstream sports training and boot-camp-style group exercise classes. Speed and agility drills improve muscle responsiveness, speed, footwork, and coordination. Typical speed and agility drills include line sprints, high-knee runs, fast-foot-turnover running, and hopping quickly through varying foot patterns (using agility dots or other markers). Speed and agility drills can be performed by anyone who is physically fit enough to learn and perform the skills. Proper instruction and modification of the drills for differing ability levels is essential to prevent injuries.

Whole-Body Exercise Programs The increasing popularity of "functional" training, training that carries over to life activities, has given rise to exercise programs that focus on whole-body exercises. These programs, such as Cross-Fit and kettlebell, focus on exercises that integrate various muscle groups into one exercise rather than isolate a muscle group, as do some traditional weight-room exercises. The exercises aim to address three planes of movement (forward and back, side to side, and rotational) for increased cross-over into daily activities and enhanced sports and recreation performance. There has been initial evidence that this type of training can reduce neck and back pain.[16] It's not necessary to join a special gym or exercise class (although those are available) to take advantage of this type of training. Take the concepts presented in the previous section on plyometrics and sports training, think about your current resistance-training program, and integrate the concepts to add more whole-body and functional exercises. For instance, instead of limiting yourself to stationary lunges, add a walking forward movement with a twist to the opposite side to every lunge step.

plyometric exercise An exercise that is characterized by a rapid deceleration of the body followed by a rapid acceleration of the body in the opposite direction

power The ability to produce force quickly

speed The ability to rapidly accelerate; exercises for speed will increase stride length and frequency

agility The ability to rapidly change body position or body direction without losing speed, balance, or body control

THINK! Many people find group exercise classes to be motivating. Do you?

ACT! Today, find classes that will help you meet your muscular fitness goals (e.g., Pilates, fitness "boot camp," or muscle pump). Some classes are designed solely for muscular fitness, while others address both muscular fitness and cardiovascular training. Either way, be sure to use enough resistance or weight to elicit a muscle training response.

Learn and Apply FITT Principles

FITT stands for *f*requency, *i*ntensity, *t*ime, and *t*ype. The acronym represents a checklist for determining how often, how hard, and how long to exercise, and what types of exercise to choose at your current level of muscular fitness.

Frequency of Training Your goals and your schedule determine how often you will train each week. At a minimum, you should work each muscle group twice per week. A full-body muscle workout means two sessions in the weight room each week. If you split your muscle workouts (e.g., into upper body and lower body), then you would go to the weight room four times per week. **Table 4.2** on page 126 presents American College of Sports Medicine (ACSM) guidelines for muscular fitness programs.

It is important to let each muscle group rest for 48 hours before taxing it again with resistance training. Especially when you are just beginning, schedule your workouts so that they are at least two days apart.

When you perform an intense weight-training session, micro-damage occurs within the muscle cells and rest time is needed for muscle repair and adaptation. Your muscles will adapt by constructing new actin and myosin

TABLE 4.2 ACSM's Guidelines for Resistance Training in Healthy Adults

Goal	Level	Intensity (% 1 RM)	Repetitions	Sets	Rest (min between sets)[a]	Frequency (days/week)[b]	Number and Types of Exercises
Improve Muscular Fitness[c]	Beginner/novice	40–70	8–12	1–3	2–3	2–3	8–10+ emphasizing multiple-joint exercises for opposing muscle groups in the lower body, upper body, and trunk; add single-joint exercises as needed for muscle balance
	Intermediate/advanced	60–80	8–12	2–4	2–3	2–3	
Increase Muscular Endurance	All levels	<50	15–25	1–2	1–2	2–3	
Further Increase Muscular Strength	Intermediate	70–80	1–12	2–4	2–3	2–5	
	Advanced	>80	1–6	2–4	2–3	2–5	

[a]Decrease rest between sets for endurance and increase for strength; rest a particular muscle group 48 hours between workout sessions.
[b]2–3 days/week = total body workouts, 4–5 days/week = split routine to train each major muscle group twice per week.
[c]Muscular strength, mass, and to some extent, muscular endurance.

Data are from: American College of Sports Medicine, *ACSM's Guidelines for Exercise Testing and Prescription*. 9th edition. (Baltimore, MD: Lippincott Williams & Wilkins, 2014); and N. A. Ratamess et al., "ACSM Position Stand: Progression Models in Resistance Training for Healthy Adults," *Medicine and Science in Sports and Exercise* 341, no. 3 (2009): 687–708; C. E. Garber et al., "American College of Sports Medicine Position Stand: Quantity and Quality of Exercise for Developing and Maintaining Cardiorespiratory, Musculoskeletal, and Neuromotor Fitness in Apparently Healthy Adults: Guidance for Prescribing Exercise," *Medicine and Science in Sports and Exercise* 43, no. 7 (2011): 1334–59, doi: 10.1249/MSS.0b013e318213fefb.

resistance The amount of effort or force required to complete the exercise

contractile proteins and other supporting structures. Over time, this adaptation results in stronger, leaner, larger muscles. Intense workouts of the same muscle group on subsequent days will disrupt the repair and adaptation process. Rather than faster muscle development, this overtraining is more likely to cause injuries, muscle fatigue, and weakening. An exception can be made for lower intensity muscular fitness classes or calisthenics, which can be done daily as long as they are not overly fatiguing.

Muscle soreness that sets in within a day or two is called delayed-onset muscle soreness (DOMS); it is a sign that your body was not ready for the amount of overload you applied. Contrary to popular belief, it is not lactic acid that causes DOMS; accumulated lactic acid is cleared from the muscle cells within hours of exercise. If you choose weight amounts correctly, your muscles will sustain small amounts of micro-damage that does not result in soreness and that your body can repair within 48 hours after the workout.

Intensity of Training The intensity of a weight-training program

refers to the amount of **resistance** you apply through any given exercise. For each exercise, the intensity you choose will depend on your fitness goals for that particular muscle group or your body as a whole. The ACSM guidelines in Table 4.2 for muscular fitness can help you choose weight-training intensities (shown as a percentage of your 1 RM or percentage of predicted 1 RM).

The intensity or weight chosen for each exercise should be enough to overload the muscle group you are working; that means you should feel slight discomfort or muscle fatigue near the end of your exercise set. If you feel no fatigue during the entire set of repetitions and feel you could lift the weight another 3 to 10 times, then the intensity is too low. Aim for muscle fatigue but not complete exhaustion.

Resting between sets will affect your weight-training intensity and performance on subsequent exercises. The greater the weight you lift for strength building, the longer the rest period you may want between sets. Resting periods can be shorter for muscular endurance-building exercises. In fact, shorter rests may help build better muscular endurance.

Time: Sets and Repetitions
Choosing the appropriate number of repetitions or lifts within

each set is yet another important part of setting up your resistance-training program. Once again, your fitness goals help determine the number of sets you will execute for each exercise and the number of repetitions within each set. Your weight-training experience and the time you have available to work out will affect your planning as well. ACSM recommends that you perform two to four sets of each exercise during a given workout session (see Table 4.2). However, if you are new to resistance training, you will see progress with just one set per muscle group. As you progress in your resistance-training program, you can increase your sets from one to two, and eventually to three or more. You can execute two, three, or four sets for all your exercises, or perform two sets of certain exercises, three of others, and so on. Keep in mind, however, that overtraining one particular muscle group can lead to muscle imbalance and injury.

Intensity and repetitions have an inverse relationship relative to muscular strength and endurance (see **Figure 4.6**): For muscular strength development, you will lift heavier weights and do fewer repetitions; for muscular endurance, you will lift lighter weights with more repetitions.

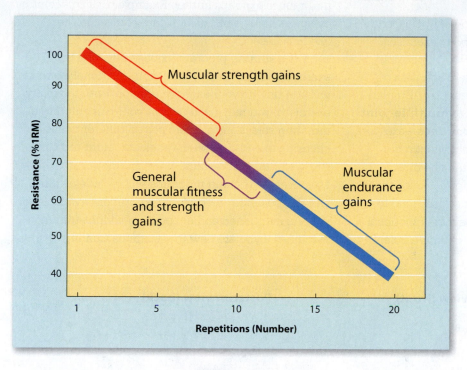

FIGURE **4.6** Fewer repetitions with higher resistance will produce gains in muscular strength. More repetitions with lower resistance will produce gains in muscular endurance.

Type: Choosing Appropriate Exercises

Which exercises should you do during each workout session? The final part of designing a muscular fitness program is choosing exercises that will help you achieve your goals and muscle balance. Create your own muscular fitness goals in Lab 4.3 and use **Figure 4.7** to start planning your resistance-training program. Next, decide which specific exercises will help you attain your muscular

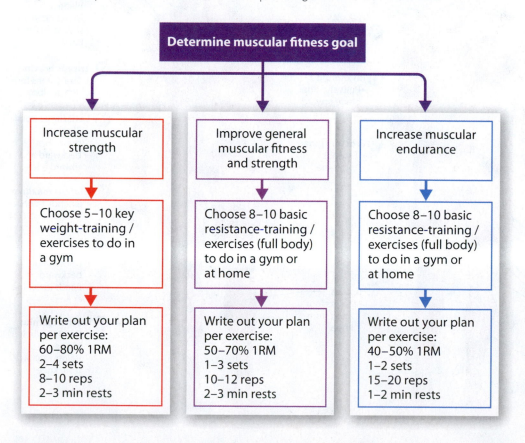

Determine muscular fitness goal

Increase muscular strength	Improve general muscular fitness and strength	Increase muscular endurance
Choose 5–10 key weight-training / exercises to do in a gym	Choose 8–10 basic resistance-training / exercises (full body) to do in a gym or at home	Choose 8–10 basic resistance-training / exercises (full body) to do in a gym or at home
Write out your plan per exercise: 60–80% 1RM 2–4 sets 8–10 reps 2–3 min rests	Write out your plan per exercise: 50–70% 1RM 1–3 sets 10–12 reps 2–3 min rests	Write out your plan per exercise: 40–50% 1RM 1–2 sets 15–20 reps 1–2 min rests

FIGURE **4.7** Use this flowchart as you design your muscular fitness program. Just starting? Begin at the lower end of all recommended ranges (for rest periods, begin at the upper end).

fitness goals: Complete **Lab 4.4** to plan a muscular fitness program using **Figures 4.8** and **4.9** (starting on page 136) to assist you in exercise selection.

DO IT! ONLINE

Muscle balance requires a selection of upper-body exercises, trunk exercises, and lower-body exercises. Choose exercises from Figure 4.9 that work *opposing muscle groups,* muscles on both the front and back of your body. Emphasize **multiple-joint exercises**—exercises that affect more than one muscle group—since these exercises tend to be more functional and time-efficient.

Examples of multiple-joint exercises include chest press, overhead press, leg press, and lunges. **Single-joint exercises** can be added as needed to target major muscle groups further. Examples of single-joint exercises include biceps curl, lateral raise, leg curl, and heel raise.

For a starting program, choose between 8 and 10 exercises, remembering that each additional exercise will add time to your exercise session; with too many exercises, you may need to split your workout into alternating selections of exercises on different days. In choosing exercises, you may select weight machines, free weights, calisthenics, or a combination of all three. Most weight-training programs will include all three and will be determined by the equipment available to you. As mentioned earlier, focus on weight-training machines if you are new to resistance training. See

> **multiple-joint exercises** Exercises that involve multiple joints and muscle groups to achieve an overall movement
>
> **single-joint exercises** Exercises that involve a single joint and typically focus on one muscle group

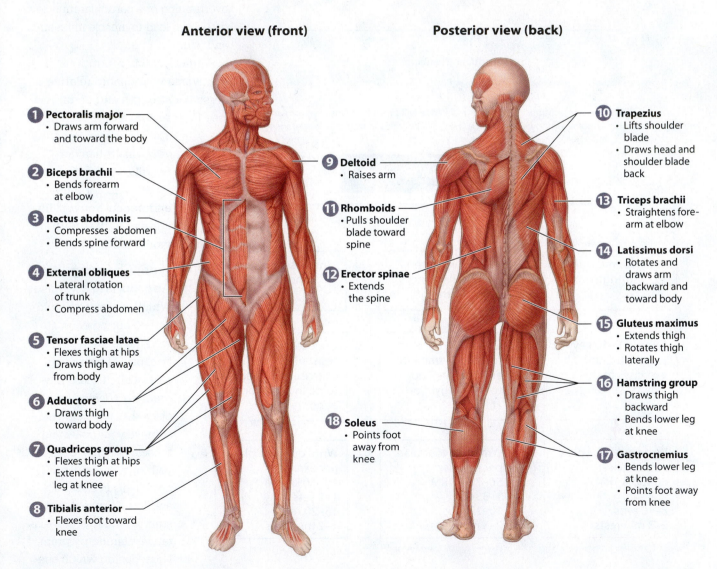

Anterior view (front)

1 Pectoralis major
- Draws arm forward and toward the body

2 Biceps brachii
- Bends forearm at elbow

3 Rectus abdominis
- Compresses abdomen
- Bends spine forward

4 External obliques
- Lateral rotation of trunk
- Compress abdomen

5 Tensor fasciae latae
- Flexes thigh at hips
- Draws thigh away from body

6 Adductors
- Draws thigh toward body

7 Quadriceps group
- Flexes thigh at hips
- Extends lower leg at knee

8 Tibialis anterior
- Flexes foot toward knee

9 Deltoid
- Raises arm

11 Rhomboids
- Pulls shoulder blade toward spine

12 Erector spinae
- Extends the spine

18 Soleus
- Points foot away from knee

Posterior view (back)

10 Trapezius
- Lifts shoulder blade
- Draws head and shoulder blade back

13 Triceps brachii
- Straightens forearm at elbow

14 Latissimus dorsi
- Rotates and draws arm backward and toward body

15 Gluteus maximus
- Extends thigh
- Rotates thigh laterally

16 Hamstring group
- Draws thigh backward
- Bends lower leg at knee

17 Gastrocnemius
- Bends lower leg at knee
- Points foot away from knee

FIGURE **4.8** These muscles or muscle groups are commonly used in resistance-training exercises. On pages 136–149, Figure 4.9 illustrates exercises you can use to work the muscle groups shown.

Activate, Motivate, & Advance Your Fitness: A Resistance-Training Program at the end of this chapter (page 164) for sample resistance-training programs to help you get started.

What If I Don't Reach My Goals?

Once you've applied FITT principles, chosen training levels, designed a program, and set target dates, you may find that your muscular development is not keeping up with your ambitions or that you cannot follow through consistently with training sessions. What other steps can you take to ensure success in your muscular fitness program?

Track Your Progress Use a weight-training log, notebook, online program, or smart phone application to track your progress. Lab 4.4 provides you with a log that allows you to (1) see your week-to-week progress, (2) stay motivated, (3) detect problems with your program design or goals, and (4) know where to redesign your program if needed.

Evaluate and Redesign Your Program as Needed Periodically reevaluate your muscular fitness program. Common times to reassess are at your target completion date, when you feel you aren't making progress, when your improvement rate is faster than anticipated, and when you feel overtraining fatigue or injury. First, retake the initial tests for muscular strength and endurance. Second, reassess your goals: accomplished or not? Third, evaluate your overall program and write out what you like and don't like about it. If you have met your goals and enjoy your program, continue but set more challenging goals based on FITT parameters. If you have not met your goals or don't like your program, rewrite the goals and target dates, redesigning to solve your issues. Get help from an exercise professional if needed. Evaluating and redesigning should allow you, once again, to move toward your muscular fitness goals successfully. Lab 4.4 provides practice at evaluation and redesign.

What Precautions Should I Take to Avoid Resistance-Training Injuries?

Greater muscular fitness achieved through resistance training helps prevent general injury during sports or daily activity. However, weight training itself can cause injuries such as muscle or tendon strains, ligament sprains, fractures, dislocations, and other joint problems. This is especially true if the lifter pushes for an unrealistic overload. You can prevent injuries by getting proper instruction and guidance and by heeding a few basic suggestions.

Follow Basic Weight-Training Guidelines

When starting your resistance-training program, be conservative. Resist the temptation to begin with too many exercises or sets or with too much weight! Before increasing your resistance-training intensity or duration, observe how your body responds to the training over a few weeks. After that, you can safely increase the number of repetitions and/or the amount of weight. The safest approach is to follow the "10 percent rule." Limit increases in exercise frequency, intensity, or time to no more than 10 percent per week. Gentle increases will help prevent injury, overtraining, or soreness. Break this rule only if the initial intensity you selected was very low or a certified fitness professional instructs you to do otherwise.

casestudy

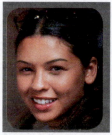

GINA

"My main goals in resistance training are to improve my muscle endurance so that I can go on longer hikes and to strengthen my muscles and joints so that I can reduce the chance I'll be injured on the trail. I live close to campus and there is a gym with weight equipment available, but how do I decide what equipment to use and what exercises to focus on?"

THINK! What would you say to Gina about the benefits of using free weights versus machines? What would you tell her about the differences between traditional weight-training, circuit weight-training, and plyometrics programs? Which would you advise her to begin with?

ACT NOW! Today, verbalize your own resistance-training goals. Are they appearance based or function based? This week, write out your initial ideas for applying the FITT principles to your goals. In two weeks, choose five key resistance-training exercises and perform them at least two days during the week (1–3 sets of 10). Did you choose traditional weight training or another style of resistance training?

HEAR IT! ONLINE

Be Sure to Warm Up and Cool Down Properly

Weight-training guidelines include a warm-up and a cool-down before and after training sessions. A proper weight-training warm-up includes a general warm-up and a specific warm-up. The general warm-up consists of 5 to 10 minutes of cardiorespiratory exercises—walking, jogging (on or off a treadmill), biking, stationary biking, elliptical trainer use, or any activity that increases body temperature (breaking a light sweat) and blood flow to muscles. The specific warm-up should include range-of-motion exercises that mimic (without weight added) the resistance exercises you'll be performing. Move your limbs through a full range of motion before using a given weight machine or lifting free weights. Then, do a warm-up set with very light resistance. Now you are ready to perform your serious sets.

Some people also like to stretch before weight training. If you want to add stretching to your warm-up, do so only after a general warm-up to be sure your body has been adequately warmed up in preparation for stretching. Pre-exercise stretching should be light, and you should hold each stretch no more than 10 to 15 seconds. (See Chapter 5 for more about the timing of your stretches within the warm-up and cool-down.) A proper cool-down for resistance training includes general range-of-motion exercises and stretches for the muscle groups applied during the weight-training session.

Know How to Train with Weights Safely

Get a proper introduction to weight training before you begin. Learn the proper grips and postures; the right way to isolate some muscle groups and stabilize others; the correct way to adjust machines for your height; and the safe way to sit, stand, and move during weight lifting to prevent injury. Learn the proper use of weights and weight machines. Use safety collars at the ends of weight bars to secure the weights on the bar.

When lifting free weights, use a spotter to watch, guide, and assist you. Perform all exercises in a slow and controlled manner. Some personal trainers recommend using a count of two up and four down to control the weight-lowering phase. Ask the spotter to watch your control and to make sure you are lifting safely and can return the bar safely after the lift. The objective is to avoid fast, jerky, or bouncy motions that can injure your muscles or allow the weight to get away from you and cause injury.

Spotters typically assist when a weight lifter is attempting to lift a weight near his or her maximal fatigue level and the lift requires full-body balance. Exercises such as squats and the bench press require the weight to be lifted over the head or in a position that could present a danger to the lifter. When performing these free-weight exercises, always enlist the help of a spotter.

Perform all exercises through a full range of motion. With free weights, you must determine the range yourself. Be sure to request extra training and attention if you need help.

Stay balanced: Set up in a relaxed, balanced position and maintain that position after a lift or set of lifts. Lifting while off balance is an easy way to create strain on one side and to pull or tear a muscle. Balance your exercise to build equal strength on both sides and from front to back.

Breathe continuously as you contract your muscles to lift and lower weights or perform resistive movements. Some weight lifters use a **Valsalva maneuver** (i.e., they exhale forcibly with a closed throat so no air exits) as a way to stabilize the trunk during a lift. However, holding your breath this way can cause an unhealthy blood pressure increase and slow blood flow to the heart, lungs, and brain. Breathe out during the push or pull part of a lift, particularly while lifting heavy weights, to avoid a Valsalva maneuver.

Use lighter weights when attempting new lifts or after taking time off from your routine. You can build up by 3 to 5 percent per session or 10 percent per week. Don't assume you can pick up where you left off before a break in your training; that's asking for muscle strain or injury.

Do not continue resistance training if you are in pain. Learn to differentiate the effort of lifting from the pain of an injury, particularly to a joint.

Muscle strains are common among people who use improper lifting techniques and machine setups. Quick or heavy eccentric contractions, in particular, tend to cause microtears in the muscle fibers and connective tissue within and surrounding the muscles. Eccentric contractions are responsible for the

Valsalva maneuver The process of holding one's breath while lifting heavy weight; this practice can increase chest cavity pressure and result in light-headedness during the lift; excessively increased blood pressure can result after the lift and breath are released

lowering of a weight, so it is important not to "drop" a weight to its starting position, whether lifting free weights or using a machine. Wear gym shoes to protect your feet and wear gloves to improve your grip and protect your hands.

Get Advice from a Qualified Exercise Professional

A qualified trainer can help you learn the proper head and body position for lifting each type of weight (with or without the help of a spotter) and for using weight machines of each type. Learning to adjust the machines properly is part of this training. Seek out people qualified to provide accurate resistance-training information, especially if you are just getting started or before significantly changing aspects of your routine, such as amount of weight, number of repetitions, speed of movement, or body posture.

How can you recognize a qualified exercise professional? Ask any potential personal trainer or instructor questions such as the following:

- Are you certified as a personal trainer or fitness instructor by a reputable, nationally recognized organization such as ACSM, National Strength and Conditioning Association (NSCA), the American Council on Exercise (ACE), and the National Academy of Sports Medicine (NASM)?

- Do you have a certificate or degree in exercise science from an accredited two- or four-year college?

- What types of experience have you had as an instructor or personal trainer?

- How long have you been working in the field of fitness and wellness?

- What are your references from employers and past/present clients?

- How current are you with the changing guidelines and emerging trends in exercise and fitness, and how can you demonstrate this currency?

You'll want to look at practical details such as how much the personal trainer charges, whether he or she has liability insurance, and how well his or her schedule will accommodate yours. Intangibles are equally important: How well do you get along with this potential trainer, and how motivated does he or she help you feel?

Consider enrolling in a specific weight-training class at your college or university. Instructors in such courses are already screened for the qualifications listed here, and the cost will be significantly lower than hiring your own personal trainer.

Persons with Disabilities May Have Different Weight-Training Guidelines

Weight-training programs benefit virtually everyone, including people with some limitations or disabilities. Resistance training can decrease pain and increase mobility in people with joint and muscle disabilities and orthopedic conditions such as arthritis, multiple sclerosis, or osteoarthritis.

Safety guidelines and appropriate exercises will vary and will be determined by the disability or limitation of each person. Everyone will need medical clearance before beginning a resistance-training program, and those with certain chronic conditions and muscle disorders may need specific exercise recommendations and directions from a physician. If your gym lacks specialized equipment, look for a trainer who can help you perform modified exercises on the available machines. Wheelchair exercisers can perform many seated resistance-training exercises in the gym or at home. Visit this book's website to view demonstrations of easily adaptable resistance-training exercises for people of all abilities.

Is It Risky to Use Supplements for Muscular Fitness?

Dietary supplements marketed as promoters of muscle conditioning are called performance aids or dietary **ergogenic aids**. Some supplements are safe but ineffective; some are both unsafe and ineffective. Few, if any, are worth the risk and expense. Manufacturers of nutritional supplements need not prove their products are safe or effective before offering them for sale on the open market. The Food and Drug Administration (FDA) may remove unsafe products, but this occurs after the product is "tested" on the buying public. To avoid being an inadvertent subject in an uncontrolled experiment, look into the risks of a supplement very carefully before considering its use.

ergogenic aids Any nutritional, physical, mechanical, psychological, or pharmacological procedure or aid used to improve athletic performance

Some ergogenic aids, such as anabolic steroids, are controlled substances. This means they require a prescription for legal use and should not be used for nonprescription purposes. Their use can get you banned from athletic competitions.

Anabolic Steroids

Anabolic steroids are synthetic drugs that are chemically related to the hormone testosterone. Physicians sometimes prescribe small doses within a medical setting for people with muscle diseases, burns, some cancers, and pituitary disorders. Some athletes and recreational weight trainers take anabolic steroids—illegally, outside of a medical setting, and without a prescription—to increase muscle mass, strength, and power. Anabolic steroids can produce some of these results in some users, but with overwhelmingly negative side effects that far outweigh the benefits. Besides being illegal, steroids increase the risk of liver and heart disease, cancer, acne, breast development in men, and masculinization in women. Because dramatically stronger muscles may exert more force than the body can handle, anabolic steroid use can also promote connective tissue and bone injuries. Steroid use can also be habit forming, lead to other drug addictions, and even cause death, as explained in the box Why Are Steroids Dangerous? the following page.

Creatine

Creatine is a legal nutritional supplement containing amino acids. It is most often sold as creatine monohydrate in powder, tablet, capsule, or liquid form. The body's natural form of creatine (phosphocreatine) is generated by the kidneys and stored in muscle cells. You can also consume creatine in the diet by eating meat products.

Creatine taken at recommended levels can improve performance by temporarily increasing the body's normal muscle stores of phosphocreatine. Since this natural energy substance powers bursts of activity lasting less than 60 seconds, creatine users sometimes find they can train more effectively in power activities and may be able to maintain higher forces during lifting. This can result in increased training adaptations such as strength and muscle size.[17] Creatine intake also causes a temporary retention of water in muscle tissue that produces a small temporary increase in size, strength, and ability to generate power. Creatine has no effect on performance of aerobic endurance exercise.

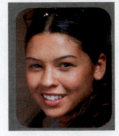

So far, there have been few serious side effects reported in studies of people using creatine for up to four years. Since the long-term effects of creatine use are unknown, however, potential users should proceed with caution.

Adrenal Androgens (DHEA, Androstenedione)

Dehydroepiandrosterone (DHEA) is the body's most common hormone; it occurs naturally in the body and acts as a weak steroid chemical messenger (a conveyor of internal control signals and information). Discovered in the 1930s, DHEA was banned by the U.S. FDA in 1985 and then brought back in 1994 as an approved nutritional supplement. Manufacturers produce and sell it in a synthetic concentrated form despite the lack of definitive proof of its safety or effectiveness.[18] DHEA proponents claim that it increases muscle mass and strength, lowers body fat, alters natural hormone levels, slows down aging, and boosts immune functions. However, research studies have produced conflicting results on DHEA and overall do not provide strong evidence of a large positive effect on muscle mass and strength or on body fat levels.[19]

Q&A Why Are Steroids Dangerous?

Why are government drug regulators—not to mention parents, educators, and coaches—so worried about steroid use in young people? Steroid use in teens and young adults is a problem for several major reasons:

1. Steroid use can lead to the abuse of other drugs. Some of the side effects of steroid use are so disruptive that people turn to opiate drugs such as cocaine and heroin to relieve their distress.

2. Anabolic steroids can permanently disrupt normal development. A person's body and brain are still developing during adolescence and into their early twenties. Steroids interfere with the normal effects of sex hormones. Most of these changes are irreversible.

3. Steroid use can lead to behavioral changes, including irritability, hostility, aggression, and depression. These changes can continue even after the user stops using steroids.[1]

4. Steroids promote heart disease, heart attacks, and strokes, even in athletes younger than 30. The drugs also cause blood-filled cysts in the liver that can burst and cause serious internal bleeding.

5. Injecting steroids and sharing needles with other users can lead to the transmission of dangerous infections. The disease risks include hepatitis, HIV, and endocarditis, a bacterial infection of the heart.

6. Long-term anabolic steroid use can cause cognitive deficits. In one study, greater lifetime exposure to steroids was related to greater losses in visual-spatial memory.[2]

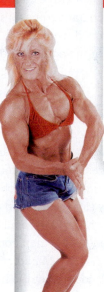

Problems in men	Problems in both	Problems in women
• Baldness	• Strokes and blood clots	• Increase in facial and body hair
• Headaches	• Aggressive behavior	• Deepened voice
• Development of breasts	• Mood swings	• Reduced breast size
• Shrinkage of testicles	• Severe acne on face and back	• Menstrual problems
• Enlarged prostate	• High blood pressure and heart disease	• Enlarged clitoris
• Reduced sperm count	• Liver damage	
	• Nausea	
	• Bloating	
	• Urinary and bowel problems	
	• Impotence	
	• Increased risk of tendon injuries	
	• Aching joints	

Sources:
1. R. L. Cunningham et al., "Androgenic Anabolic Steroid Exposure During Adolescence: Ramification for Brain Development and Behavior," *Hormones and Behavior* (2013), doi: 10.1016/j.yhbeh.2012.12.009. [Epub ahead of print].
2. G. Kanayama et al., "Cognitive Deficits in Long-Term Anabolic-Androgenic Steroid User," *Drug and Alcohol Dependence* 130 (2013): 208–14, doi: 10.1016/j.drugalcdep.2012.11.008.

Androstenedione (nickname "andro") is another naturally occurring steroid hormone with a structure related to both DHEA and testosterone. It is found naturally in meats and some plants. Even though manufacturers used to claim that "andro" increased testosterone levels, one pivotal study found that it actually lowered the body's natural production of testosterone, did not increase the body's adaptations to resistance training, and increased heart disease risk in men.[20]

Although DHEA and androstenedione were banned from athletic competition by the International Olympic Committee (IOC) in 1996 and 1997, respectively, only androstenedione was included in the Anabolic Steroids Control Act of 2004 prohibiting its sale without a prescription. It is now a "controlled substance," along with anabolic steroids. DHEA was given an exemption due to supporters advocating its purported "natural anti-aging" properties. Since androstenedione was ordered off the market by the FDA, its use is dwindling. Both DHEA and androstenedione may lower your "good cholesterol" (HDL-C, high-density lipoprotein cholesterol), which increases cardiovascular disease risk. Both can increase your risk of estrogen-sensitive cancers (breast, ovarian, uterine), and could be dangerous for individuals with endocrine, liver, or mood disorders.[21] These serious side effects strongly argue against the use of DHEA or "andro."

Growth Hormone (GH)

Your body's pituitary gland produces human growth hormone (GH), which promotes bone growth and muscle growth and decreases fat stores. Drug manufacturers produce GH synthetically for medical use in children and young adults with abnormally slow or reduced growth and related disorders. Although the FDA regulates GH, athletes wanting to gain an edge over their competitors sometimes obtain and use it illegally. Marketers claim that GH supplementation will counteract the muscle mass lost with disuse and aging, among other alleged benefits. However, GH side effects include irreversible

bone growth (acromegaly/gigantism), increased risk of cardiovascular disease and diabetes, and decreased sexual desire, among others.

Marketers of oral GH supplements claim the same positive benefits to lean muscle mass and fat mass, but this is not borne out in tests or actual use. Oral GH, in fact, cannot even be absorbed from your digestive tract into your bloodstream! Exercise is a far better way to increase natural levels of GH. In particular, regular aerobic exercise can result in a two-fold increase in 24-hour GH release in young women.[22] Interestingly, one 30-minute session and three 10-minute sessions of exercise are both effective for stimulating GH increases.[23]

Amino Acid and Protein Supplements

Many bodybuilders and weight lifters take amino acid supplements because they believe that consuming protein or its building blocks (amino acids) will lead to enhanced muscle development. However, evidence is mixed that high intake of protein or taking protein-based supplements will improve training or exercise performance or build muscle mass beyond the levels achieved through normal dietary protein. When combined with resistance training, moderate increases in protein intake via supplementation lead to increases in lean muscle mass and strength beyond resistance training alone.[24] In contrast, supplementing with the building blocks of protein, amino acids (e.g., glutamine), seems to produce no real benefit above and beyond resistance training itself.[25] Taking moderate doses of these supplements has no dramatic side effects, but large doses of either the supplements or protein itself can create amino acid imbalances, alter protein and bone metabolism, and increase risk of cardiovascular diseases.[26] See the box Should I Increase My Protein Intake Immediately After Resistance Training? on the following page for more on protein supplementation.

Q&A Should I Increase My Protein Intake Immediately After Resistance Training?

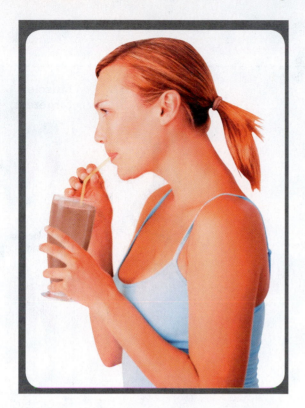

If you are looking to increase muscle strength and size, then definitely YES! Even if your goals are health and muscle maintenance, a balanced recovery meal or drink is beneficial. After resistance training, the muscles worked are depleted of nutrients and are in a state of muscle breakdown from the exercise. Providing muscles with nutrients and correcting protein imbalances helps repair breakdown damage and promotes recovery. Eating protein after exercise, particularly essential amino acids, promotes protein synthesis. Protein synthesis is even more pronounced when protein consumption is accompanied by easily digestible carbohydrates.[1] Carbohydrates will increase the release of insulin into the blood, which will in turn enhance protein storage in cells.

Timing is important. Immediately after resistance training the muscles are receptive to bringing protein into cells. That increased protein helps with repair and recovery and promotes increases in the strength and size of the muscle.[2] Increasing your intake a little bit right *before* exercise can also help.[3] In one study, subjects who took protein supplements immediately before and after resistance training had 86 percent greater increase in lean tissue mass and 30 percent greater overall strength after 10 weeks of resistance training than those who had the same supplements in the morning and night (not close to the exercise session).[4]

How much protein should you take in? Recent evidence found that ingesting 20g of protein every three hours after resistance exercise stimulates protein synthesis better than smaller doses more frequently or larger doses less frequently.[5] Follow these tips for enhancing your post–resistance-training nutrition:

- Consume 100–500 calories—depending upon your body size, workout length and intensity, and goals.
- Consume something that is digested rapidly—a liquid source is great!
- Drink or eat something with essential amino acids for your protein source—whey protein is a great source and you can get this in milk and chocolate milk.
- Make sure your snack is easily digested and has high-glycemic load carbohydrates—again, chocolate milk fills the bill!
- Consume about two parts carbohydrate to one part protein. Healthy fats can also be included.
- For the greatest effect, consume your post-exercise drink or snack within an hour, preferably within 30 minutes, of stopping your exercise session.
- After an hour or later in the day, eat a full recovery meal with a balance of protein, carbohydrates, and healthy fats.

Sources:
1. M. Beelen et al., "Nutritional Strategies to Promote Postexercise Recovery," *International Journal of Sports Nutrition and Exercise Metabolism* 20, no. 6 (2010): 515–32.
2. T. A. Churchward-Venne et al., "Role of Protein and Amino Acids in Promoting Lean Mass Accretion with Resistance Exercise and Attenuating Lean Mass Loss During Energy Deficit in Humans," *Amino Acids* (2013). [Epub ahead of print].
3. C. Kerksick et al., "International Society of Sports Nutrition Position Stand: Nutrient Timing," *Journal of the International Society of Sports Nutrition* 5 (2008): 17, doi: 10.1186/1550-2783-5-17.
4. P. J. Cribb and A. Hayes, "Effects of Supplement Timing and Resistance Exercise on Skeletal Muscle Hypertrophy," *Medicine and Science in Sports and Exercise* 38, no. 11 (2006): 1918–25.
5. J. L. Areta et al., "Timing and Distribution of Protein Ingestion During Prolonged Recovery from Resistance Exercise Alters Myofibrillar Protein Synthesis," *The Journal of Physiology* (2013). [Epub ahead of print].

FIGURE 4.9 **RESISTANCE-TRAINING EXERCISES**

Videos for these exercises and more are available online in MasteringHealth.

LOWER-BODY EXERCISES

1 Squat

(a) **Free weight squat** and

(b) **Machine squat:** Place the barbell or pad on your upper back and shoulders. Stand with feet shoulder-width apart, toes pointing forward, hips and shoulders lined up, abdominals pulled in. Looking forward and keeping your chest open, bend your knees and press your hips back. Lower until the angle created between your thigh and calf is between 45 degrees and 90 degrees. Keep your knees behind the front of your toes. To return to the start position, contract your abdominals, press hips forward, and extend your legs until they are straight.

(c) **Ball squat:** Place the ball between your mid-back and a smooth wall. Your feet should be 6 to 12 inches in front of your hips, shoulder-width apart, and toes pointing forward. Contract your abdominals, look forward, and keep your shoulders and hips lined up as you lower your torso. Lower until the angle created between your thigh and calf is about 90 degrees. Your knees should be just above your toes (but not in front of them) or directly above your ankles depending upon your starting position, strength, and ankle flexibility. If not, reposition your feet before the next repetition. Return to the starting position by contracting your legs and pushing the ball into and back up the wall.

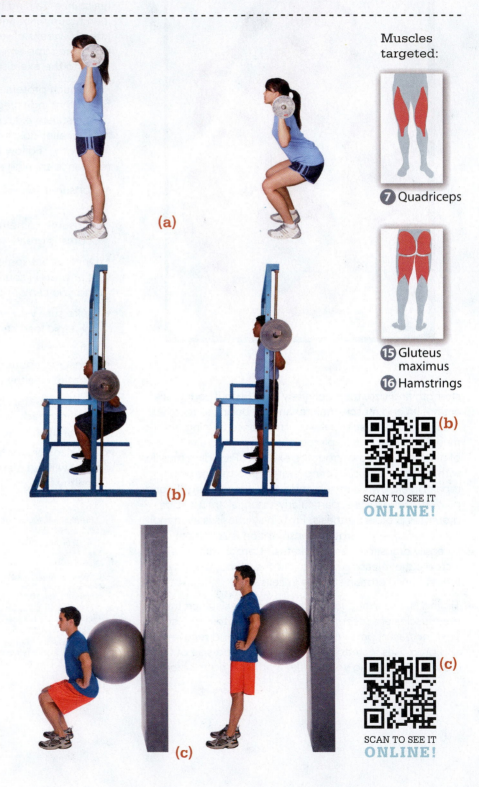

(a)

(b)

(c)

Muscles targeted:

7 Quadriceps

15 Gluteus maximus
16 Hamstrings

(b)

SCAN TO SEE IT
ONLINE!

(c)

SCAN TO SEE IT
ONLINE!

❷ Leg Press

Sit with your back straight or firmly against the backrest. Place your feet on the foot pads so that your knees create a 60- to 90-degree angle. Stabilize your torso by contracting your abdominals and holding the hand grips or seat pad. Press the weight by extending your legs slowly outward to a straight position without locking your knees. Return the weight slowly back to the starting position. If your buttocks rise up off of the seat pad, you may be lifting too much weight.

SCAN TO SEE IT
ONLINE!

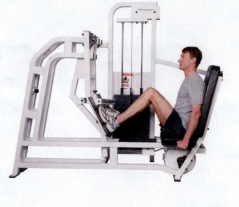

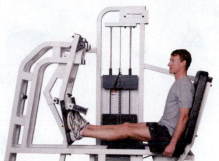

Muscles targeted:

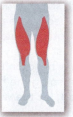

❼ Quadriceps

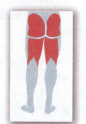

⓯ Gluteus maximus
⓰ Hamstrings

---

❸ Lunge

Stand with feet shoulder-width apart. Step forward and transfer weight to the forward leg. Lower your body straight down with your weight evenly distributed between the front and back legs.

SCAN TO SEE IT
ONLINE!

Keep your front knee in line with your ankle by striding out far enough. Make sure the front knee does not extend over your toes. Repeat with the other leg.

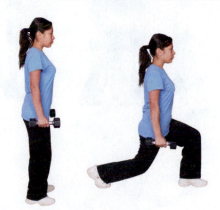

Muscles targeted:

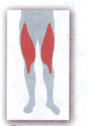

❼ Quadriceps

⓯ Gluteus maximus
⓰ Hamstrings

---

❹ Leg Extension

Sit with your back straight or firmly against the backrest and place your legs under the foot pad. Stabilize your torso by contracting your abdominals and holding the handgrips or seat

SCAN TO SEE IT
ONLINE!

pad. Lift the weight by extending your legs slowly upward to a straight position without locking your knees. Return the weight slowly to the starting position. If your buttocks rise up off the seat pad, you may be lifting too much weight.

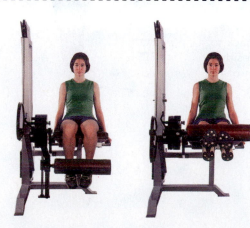

Muscles targeted:

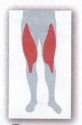

❼ Quadriceps

5 Leg Curl

(a) Machine: Lie on your stomach so that your knees are placed at the machine's axis of rotation and the roller pad is just above your heel. Keep your head on the machine pad. Grasping the hand grips for support, lift the weight by contracting your hamstrings and pulling your heels toward your buttocks. Slowly lower the weight back to the start position.

(b) Calisthenics with ball: Lie on your stomach with knees bent and place the ball between your feet. Keep your head on the mat. Lower the ball to the ground and lift it back up by contracting your hamstrings and pulling your heels toward your buttocks.

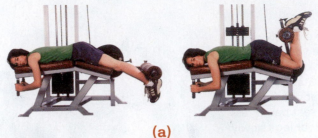

(a)

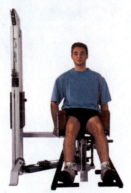

(b)

Muscles targeted:

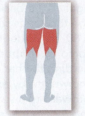

16 Hamstrings

(b)

SCAN TO SEE IT
ONLINE!

---

6 Hip Abduction

(a) Machine: Sit with your back straight or firmly against the backrest and place your legs against the pads. Grasping the hand grips or seat pad for support, press your legs outward slowly by contracting your outer thighs or hip abductors. Be careful not to extend the legs further than your normal range of motion. Slowly lower the machine weight by bringing your legs back together.

(b) Calisthenics with resistance band: Connect the resistance band to a low point on a machine and attach the free end to your outside leg. Stand with good posture and hold onto a wall or machine for support. Contract your hip abductors and extend your leg out to the side of your body. Slowly release the outside leg back to the starting position beside or crossed slightly in front of the standing leg.

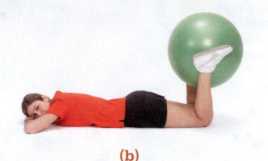

(a)

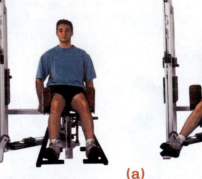

(b)

Muscles targeted:

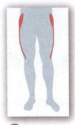

5 Tensor fasciae latae

(b)

SCAN TO SEE IT
ONLINE!

7 Hip Extension

(a) **Machine:** Stand tall with your working leg extended in front of you and connected to the cable machine. Support yourself by contracting your abdominals and holding on to the machine or handrails. Press the working leg behind you, contracting the gluteals and hamstrings. Hold the end position for one to three seconds before slowly returning to the starting position.

(b) **Calisthenics with resistance band:** Connect the resistance band to a low point on a machine and attach the free end to your lower leg. Stand with good posture and hold on to a wall or machine for support. Contract your gluteals and hamstrings and extend the working leg behind your body. Slowly release the leg back to the starting position slightly in front of the standing leg.

SCAN TO SEE IT
ONLINE!

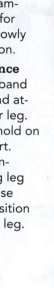 (a)

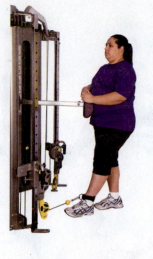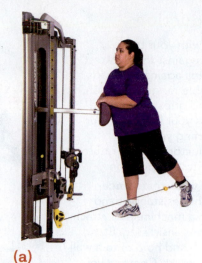

(a)

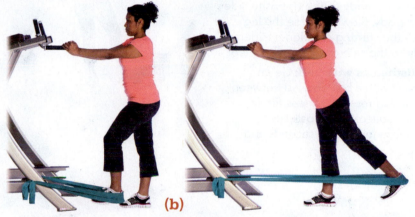

(b)

Muscles targeted:

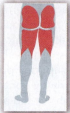

15 Gluteus maximus
16 Hamstrings

8 Heel Raise

(a) **Straight-leg:** Stand tall with good posture and place your heels lower than the toes. (You should feel just a slight stretch in the calf muscle.) Looking forward and contracting your trunk muscles for balance and support, lift your heels up by contracting your gastrocnemius muscle. Be sure to do a full range of motion and slow, controlled repetitions.

(b) **Bent-leg:** Place your body in the machine with your heels lower than the toes and the weight pad placed comfortably on your thighs. Lift your heels up slightly and release the weight support bar with your hand. Slowly lower and lift the weight by contracting your soleus calf muscle through its full range of motion.

SCAN TO SEE IT
ONLINE!

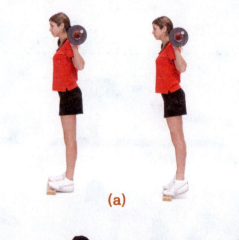

(a)

(a)

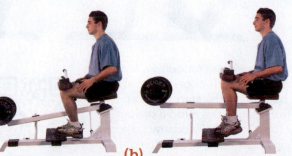

(b)

Muscles targeted:

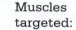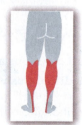

17 Gastrocnemius

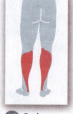

18 Soleus

9 Hip Adduction

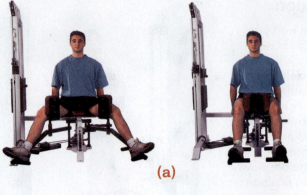

(a) **Machine:** Sit with your back straight or firmly against the backrest and place your legs against the pads set at a comfortable range of motion. Grasping the hand grips or seat pad for support, press your legs together slowly by contracting your inner thighs or hip adductors. Slowly return your legs to the starting position.

(a)

(b) **Calisthenics with resistance band:** Connect the resistance band to a low point on a machine and attach the free end to your inside leg. Stand with good posture and hold onto a wall or machine for support. Contract your hip adductors and cross your leg in front of your body to the opposite side of your body. Slowly release the leg back to the starting position beside or slightly to the side of the standing leg.

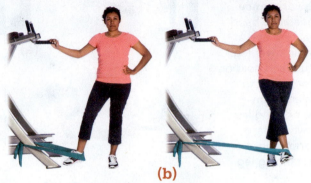

(b)

(c) **Calisthenics with ball:** Lie on your back with a ball pressed between your knees. Press your knees firmly together, squeezing the ball. Hold the squeeze for 3 to 10 seconds and release.

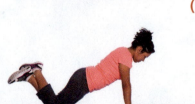

(c)

Muscles targeted:

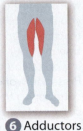

6 Adductors

(b)

SCAN TO SEE IT
ONLINE!

(c)

SCAN TO SEE IT
ONLINE!

UPPER-BODY EXERCISES

10 Push-Up

(a) **Full push-ups** and

(b) **Modified push-ups:** Support yourself in push-up position (from the knees or feet) by contracting your trunk muscles so that your neck, back, and hips are completely straight. Place hands slightly wider than shoulder-width apart. Slowly lower your body toward the floor, being careful to keep a straight body position. Your elbows will press out and back as you lower to a 90-degree elbow joint angle. Press yourself back up to the start position. Be careful not to let your trunk sag in the middle or your hips lift up during the exercise. Continually contract the abdominals to keep a strong, straight body position.

(a)

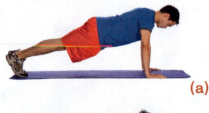

(b)

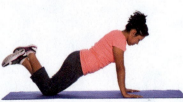

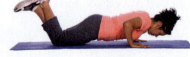 (a)

 (b)

SCAN TO SEE IT
ONLINE!

SCAN TO SEE IT
ONLINE!

Muscles targeted:

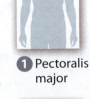

1 Pectoralis major

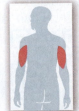

13 Triceps brachii

140 GET FIT, STAY WELL!

11 Chest Press

(a) Free weight: Lie down on the bench and position yourself with the weight bar directly above your chest. Stabilize your legs and back by placing your feet firmly on the ground and keeping your lower back flat. Grasp the bar with your hands slightly wider than shoulder-width apart and lift the bar off the rack. Slowly lower the bar to just above your chest. Press the weight up to a straight arm position and return the bar to the rack when your set of repetitions is complete. Use a spotter when lifting heavier free weights.

(b) Machine: Place yourself on the chest press machine and adjust the seat height so that the hand grips are at chest height. Stabilize your torso by firmly pressing your upper back against the seat back and planting your feet on the ground or foot supports. Press the hand grips away from the body until the arms are straight. Slowly return your hands to the starting position.

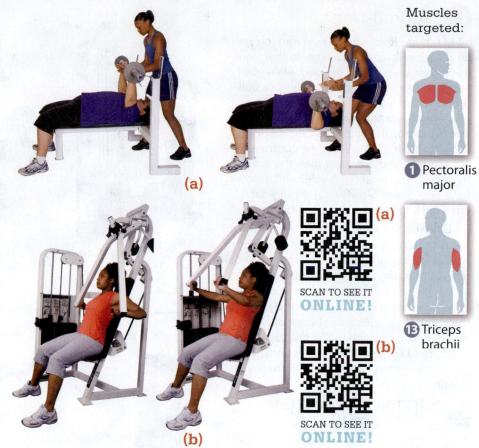

(a)

(b)

(a)

SCAN TO SEE IT
ONLINE!

(b)

SCAN TO SEE IT
ONLINE!

Muscles targeted:

1 Pectoralis major

13 Triceps brachii

---

12 Chest Fly

(a) Machine: Sit with your back straight or firmly against the back-rest, plant your feet on the ground or place on the foot pads, and grab the handles or place your arms behind the machine pads. Your arms should be directly to the side but not behind your body. Press your arms together slowly by contracting your chest and shoulder muscles. Slowly return your arms to the starting position.

(b) Bench chest flys: Lie down on the bench and position yourself with the dumbbells directly above your chest. Stabilize your legs and back by placing your feet firmly on the ground and keeping your lower back flat against the bench. Holding the dumbbells with a slight bend in the elbow joint, slowly lower them out to the side until your upper arms are parallel with the floor. Don't extend the arms beyond this position. Return your arms to the starting position by contracting your chest and shoulder muscles.

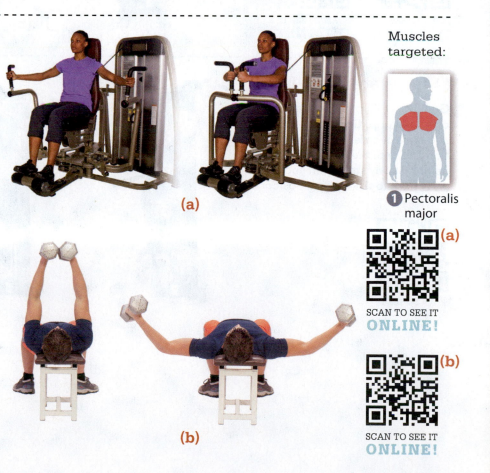

(a)

(b)

(a)

SCAN TO SEE IT
ONLINE!

(b)

SCAN TO SEE IT
ONLINE!

Muscles targeted:

1 Pectoralis major

13 Lat Pull-Down

(a) Machine: Position the seat and leg pad on the lat pull-down machine so that your thighs are snug under the pad while your feet are flat on the ground. Grab the pull-down bar with a wide overhand grip on your way down to a seated position. Sitting directly under the cable, pull the bar down to your upper chest. Focus on contracting the mid-back first and then the arms by pulling the shoulder blades and elbows back and down. Slowly straighten your arms back to the starting position.

(b) Calisthenics with resistance band: Hold the resistance band above your head with your arms straight up and your hands shoulder-width apart. Pull down and outward with your hands. Focus on contracting the mid-back first and then the arms by pulling the shoulder blades and elbows back and down. End with the band at the top of your chest, hold for one to three seconds, then slowly straighten your arms back to the starting position.

(a) SCAN TO SEE IT ONLINE! **(b)** SCAN TO SEE IT ONLINE!

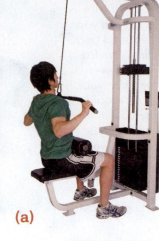 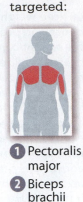 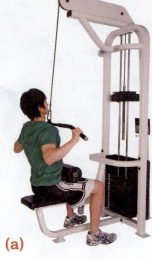

(a)

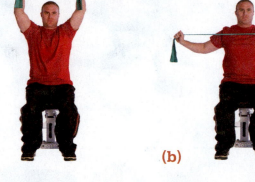

(b)

Muscles targeted:

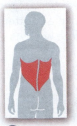

❶ Pectoralis major
❷ Biceps brachii

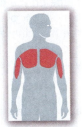

⓮ Latissimus dorsi

---

14 Assisted Pull-Up

Grab the pull-up bar with a wide overhead grip. Contract the back and arms in order to pull your body up until the bar is at chin height. Slowly straighten your arms back to the starting position.

SCAN TO SEE IT ONLINE!

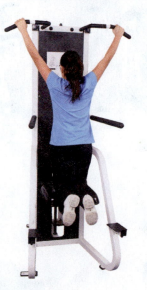 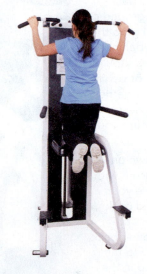

Muscles targeted:

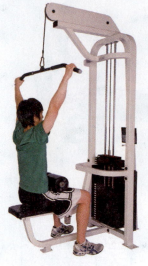

❶ Pectoralis major
❷ Biceps brachii

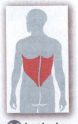

⓮ Latissimus dorsi

15 Row

(a) Machine compound row: Position the seat height until the handles are at the level of your shoulders. Sit upright and place your feet on the ground or foot pads. Grab the handgrips and pull your elbows back. Hold this position for one to three seconds, then slowly return to the starting position.

(b) Row on cable machine: Grab the cable machine handles, ropes, or bar. Make sure that you are seated so that your arms and shoulders are fully extended forward. Position your feet on foot pedals or firmly on the ground with your heels. Make sure there is a slight bend in your knees. Pull your shoulder blades and elbows back until your hands are just in front of your chest. Hold this position for one to three seconds, then slowly return to the starting position.

(c) Free weight dumbbell: Position right hand and right knee on bench as shown. Keep your back flat and head in a straight line. Pull dumbbell up to the side of your chest with your left hand, contracting your mid-back and leading with your elbow. Return to starting position and repeat on other side.

(d) Calisthenics with resistance band: Wrap the resistance band low around a weight machine or around your feet in the seated position. Hold the resistance band with your arms straight out and initial tension on the band. Pull back with your hands, focusing on contracting the mid-back first. Pull the shoulder blades and elbows back until your hands are at the lower chest, hold for one to three seconds, then slowly straighten your arms back to the starting position.

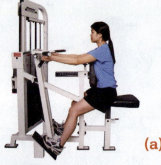
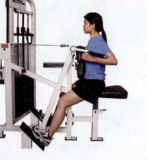
(a)

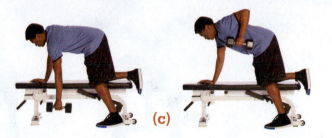
(b)

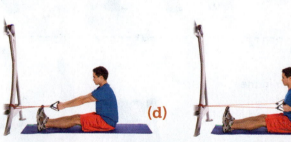
(c)

(d)

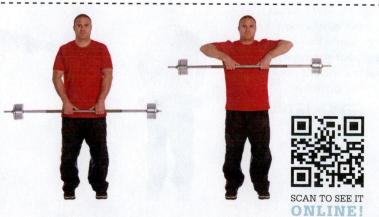

(a) SCAN TO SEE IT ONLINE!

(c) SCAN TO SEE IT ONLINE!

(d) SCAN TO SEE IT ONLINE!

Muscles targeted:

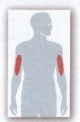

2 Biceps brachii

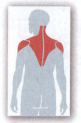

9 Deltoids (posterior)
10 Trapezius

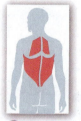

11 Rhomboids
14 Latissimus dorsi

16 Upright Row

Stand with your feet in a shoulder-width position. Keep your hips and shoulders aligned and your abdominals pulled in. Hold a barbell (or dumbbells) down in front of the body with straight arms and your hands positioned shoulder-width apart. Lift the weight to chest height keeping your elbows out, wrists straight, shoulders down. Return slowly to the starting position and repeat.

SCAN TO SEE IT ONLINE!

Muscles targeted:

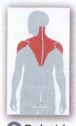

9 Deltoids (posterior)
10 Trapezius

17 Overhead Press

(a) Machine and

(b) Free weight dumbbell: Sit with your back straight or firmly against the backrest, plant your feet firmly on the ground, and pull in your abdominals. Position your hands just wider than shoulder-width and just above the shoulders. Carefully press the weight over your head until your arms are straight but your elbows are not locked out. Slowly return the weight to the starting position and repeat.

 (a)
SCAN TO SEE IT
ONLINE!

 (b)
SCAN TO SEE IT
ONLINE!

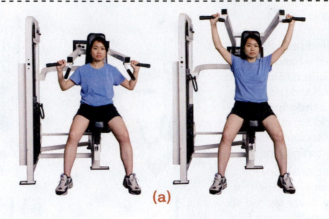
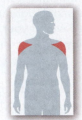

(a)

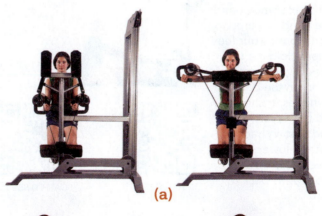

(b)

Muscles targeted:

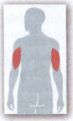
9 Deltoids (anterior and medial)

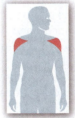
13 Triceps brachii

18 Lateral Raise

(a) Machine: Position yourself in the machine and sit with a tall, straight back. Contract your shoulders and lift your arms out to the side until they are parallel with the ground. Slowly lower your arms back down to your sides.

(b) Free weight dumbbell: Stand with your feet shoulder-width apart. Hold the dumbbells to your sides or slightly in front of you. Lift your arms out to the side until they are parallel with the ground. While lifting, your elbows should have a slight bent to avoid overextension of the elbow joint. Keep the weights at the same height as your elbows and keep your shoulders down. Slowly return the dumbbells back down to the starting position.

 (a)
SCAN TO SEE IT
ONLINE!

 (b)
SCAN TO SEE IT
ONLINE!

(a)

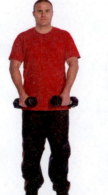
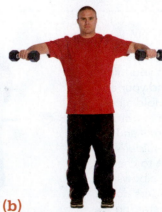

(b)

Muscles targeted:

9 Deltoids (anterior and medial)

19 Biceps Curl

(a) **Machine:** Position yourself in the machine so that your feet are on the ground and your elbows are placed at the axis of rotation for the exercise. Grab the hand grips with an underhand grip and start with your arms straight but not overextended. Lift your hands toward your head until your biceps are fully contracted. Slowly lower the weight back down to the starting position.

(b) **Free weight barbell:** Stand with your feet either in a stride or a shoulder-width position and your knees slightly bent. Keep your hips and shoulders aligned and your abdominals pulled in. Hold a barbell down in front of the body with an underhand grip, straight arms, and your hands at shoulder-width. Lift the weight up to your shoulders while keeping your back straight and abdominal muscles tight. If you are leaning back to perform the lift, you may be lifting too much weight. Return the weight to the starting position slowly and repeat.

(c) **Free weight dumbbell:** For one-arm concentration curls, sit on a bench and hold a dumbbell in one hand. Start with the working arm extended toward the ground and your elbow pressed into your inner thigh. Lift the dumbbell up to the shoulder and then return slowly to the starting position.

(d) **Alternating free weight dumbbell:** Sit on a bench or chair with a dumbbell in each hand. Sit with good posture (ears and shoulders over hips and abdominals contracted) and your feet planted on the ground for balance. Lift one dumbbell up to your shoulder turning your palm toward your shoulder as you lift. Slowly lower the dumbbell to the starting position as you lift the dumbbell in your other hand.

(e) **Calisthenics with resistance band:** Place the center of a resistance band under one foot and grab the free ends of the band with a straight arm on the same side. Stand tall with your feet either in a stride or a side-to-side position and your knees soft. Keep your hips and shoulders aligned and your abdominals pulled in. Lift the resisted hand toward your shoulder until the biceps are fully contracted. Slowly lower the hand back to the starting position and repeat.

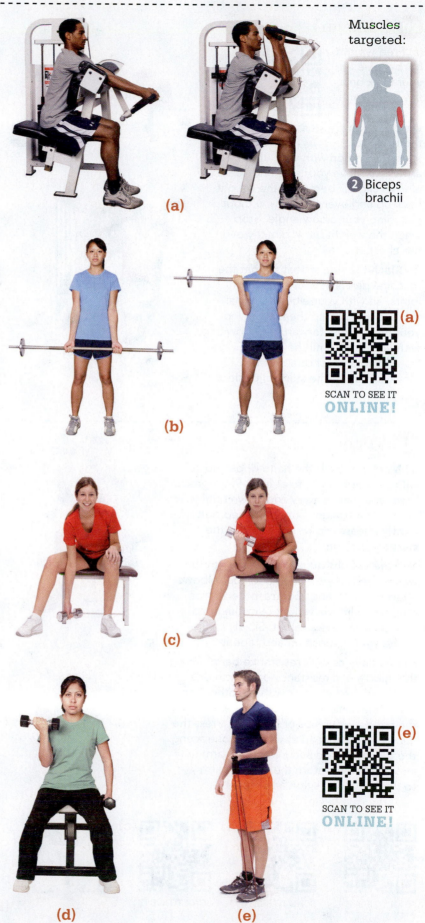

Muscles targeted:

2 Biceps brachii

(a)

(b)

SCAN TO SEE IT
ONLINE!

(c)

(d)

(e)

SCAN TO SEE IT
ONLINE!

20 Pullover

(a) Free weight barbell: Lie on your back on a flat bench with your feet on the floor. Move the bar to the starting position with your upper arms just above your ears and your elbows slightly bent. Pull the weight back up and over the body without changing your elbow angle. Stop when the weight bar is directly over the chest.

(b) Machine: Adjust seat so that the machine pivots at your shoulder joints. Sit with your elbows against the pads and grasp the bar behind your head. Press forward and down with your arms until the bar is in front of your chest or abdomen. Slowly return to the starting position.

SCAN TO SEE IT **ONLINE!**

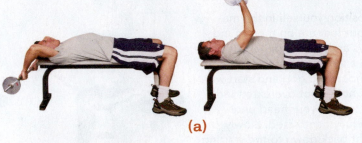

(a)

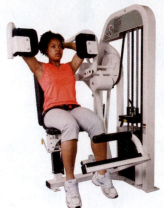
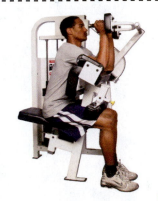

(b)

Muscles targeted:

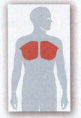

1 Pectoralis major

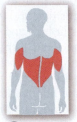

13 Triceps brachii
14 Latissimus dorsi

---

21 Triceps Extension

(a) Machine: Grab the hand grips and start with your arms bent to at least 90 degrees. Press your hands away and down until your elbows are straight but not locked out. Slowly release the weight back to the starting position.

(b) Free weight dumbbell: Start with the weight behind your head and your elbows lifted to the ceiling. Contract the triceps muscles to lift the weight over the head until the arms are straight. Slowly return to the starting position and repeat.

(c) Calisthenics with resistance band: Grasp the middle of a resistance band with one hand and the free ends with the other hand. Place one hand behind you and "anchor" the band at your hips or low back. Press the hand near your head upward by contracting the triceps muscle and extend the arm until straight. Slowly return the working arm to the starting position and repeat.

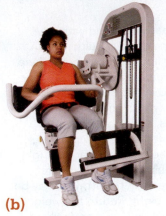
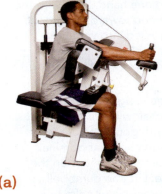

(a)

Muscles targeted:

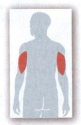

13 Triceps brachii

(a) (b) (c)

SCAN TO SEE IT **ONLINE!**   SCAN TO SEE IT **ONLINE!**   SCAN TO SEE IT **ONLINE!**

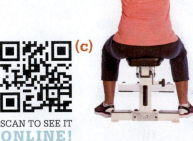
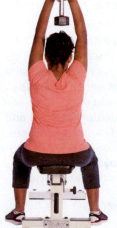
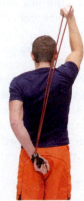

(b)   (c)

TRUNK EXERCISES

22 Back Extension

(a) **Machine:** Position yourself in the machine so that your hips are pressed all the way back, the back pad is on your mid to upper back, and your back is rounded over. Stabilize with your legs but try to refrain from pushing with the legs and hips during the exercise. Contract your back extensors and straighten out your back until you are in an upright position.

(b) **Calisthenics on a mat:** Start in a prone position with arms and legs extended and your forehead on the mat. Lift and further extend your arms and legs using your back and hip muscles. If you are free of low-back problems, you can lift a little further up for increased intensity. Hold the position for three to five seconds and then slowly lower to the mat.

(c) **Calisthenics on a ball:** Lie with your stomach over the ball, anchoring your feet and knees on the ground. Place your hands behind your head or extend the arms out straight for increased exercise intensity. Lift the head, shoulders, arms, and upper back until you have a slight curve in the back. Hold this position for three to five seconds and then lower to the ball.

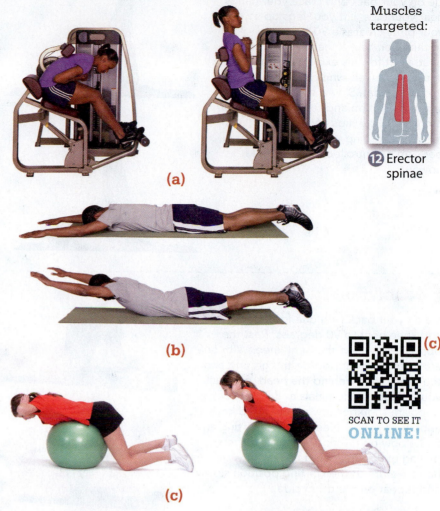

(a)

(b)

(c)

Muscles targeted:

12 Erector spinae

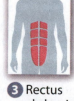

SCAN TO SEE IT
ONLINE!

(c)

23 Abdominal Curl

(a) **Machine:** Place yourself in the sitting or lying abdominal machine according to the machine instructions. Place your feet on the ground or foot pads and grab the hand grips and/or place your arms or chest behind the machine pads. Contract your abdominals while flexing your upper torso forward. Slowly return to the starting position and repeat.

(b) **Calisthenics on a ball:** Lie back with the ball placed at your low- to mid-back region. Place your feet shoulder-width apart on the ground so that your knees are bent at about 90 degrees. Cross your hands at your chest or place them lightly behind your head. Contract your abdominals while flexing your upper torso forward. Slowly return to the starting position and repeat.

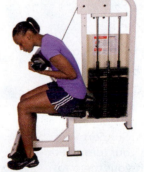

(a)

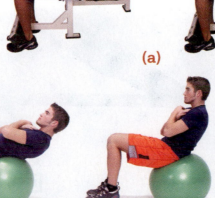

(b)

Muscles targeted:

3 Rectus abdominis

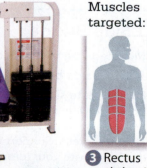

(a)

(b)

SCAN TO SEE IT
ONLINE!

SCAN TO SEE IT
ONLINE!

24 Reverse Curl

Lie on your back and place your hands near your hips. Lift your legs up so that your body creates a 90-degree angle to the floor. Your knees may be bent or straight for this exercise. Contract your abdominals while lifting your hips up off the mat. Slowly return to the starting position and repeat. Be careful not to rock the hips and legs back and forth when doing this exercise; instead, perform a controlled lifting of the hips upward.

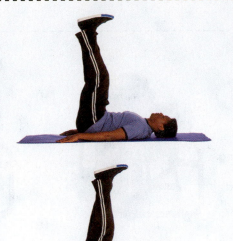

SCAN TO SEE IT
ONLINE!

Muscles targeted:

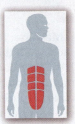

3 Rectus abdominis

25 Oblique Curl

Lie on your back with one foot on the mat and knee bent to 90 degrees. Rest the opposite ankle on the bent knee. With one arm providing support on the ground and the other hand behind the head, contract your oblique abdominals and lift your opposite shoulder toward the lifted knee (elbow stays out). Keep the supporting arm and elbow on the floor and refrain from pulling on the head and neck with your hand. Return to the starting position slowly and repeat on the other side.

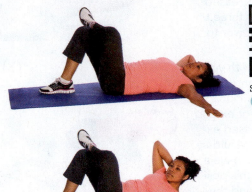

SCAN TO SEE IT
ONLINE!

Muscles targeted:

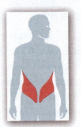

4 External obliques

26 Side Bridge

(a) **Modified side bridge** and

(b) **Forearm side bridge** and

(c) **Intermediate side bridge:** Lie on your side with your legs together and straight or bent behind you at 90 degrees. Support your body weight with your forearm or a straight arm. Lift your torso to a straight body position by contracting your abdominal and back muscles. Hold this position for a number of seconds or slowly drop the hip to the mat and lift back up for repeated repetitions.

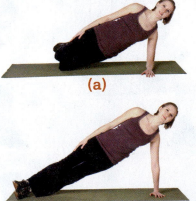

(a)

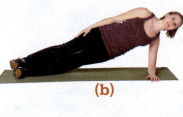

(b)

(c)

Muscles targeted:

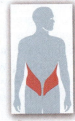

4 External obliques

 (a)

 (b)

 (c)

SCAN TO SEE IT
ONLINE!

SCAN TO SEE IT
ONLINE!

SCAN TO SEE IT
ONLINE!

27 Plank

(a) **Modified plank** and

(b) **Forearm plank** and

(c) **Push-up position plank:** Lie on your stomach and support yourself in plank position (from the forearms or hands) by contracting your trunk muscles so that your neck, back, and hips are completely straight. Your forearms or hands should be under your chest and placed slightly wider than shoulder-width apart. Hold this position for 5 to 60 seconds, increasing duration as you gain muscular endurance.

(b)
SCAN TO SEE IT
ONLINE!

(c)
SCAN TO SEE IT
ONLINE!

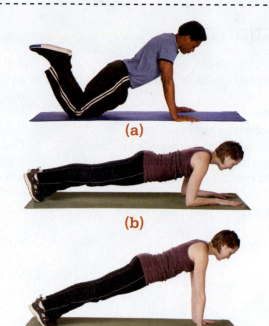
(a)

(b)

(c)

Muscles targeted:

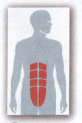
❸ Rectus abdominis

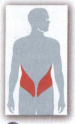
❹ External obliques

CHAPTER IN REVIEW

MasteringHealth™

Build your knowledge—and wellness!—in the Study Area of MasteringHealth with a variety of study tools.

SEE IT! ONLINE

videos
Free-Weight Exercises
Resistance Band Exercises
Stability Ball Exercises
Strength Exercises Requiring No Equipment
Machine Exercises
Assessments
Sports Drinks Science: Is It Hype?

HEAR IT! ONLINE

audio tools
Audio case study
MP3 chapter review

REVIEW IT! ONLINE

chapter review
Chapter reading quizzes
Glossary flashcards

LIVE IT! ONLINE

programs & behavior change
Customizable four-week resistance-training programs
Behavior Change Log Book and Wellness Journal

DO IT! ONLINE

labs
Lab 4.1 Assessing Your Muscular Strength
Lab 4.2 Assessing Your Muscular Endurance
Lab 4.3 Setting Muscular Fitness Goals
Lab 4.4 Your Resistance-Training Workout Plan
Alternate Strength Assessments

1. Muscular strength is the ability to
   a. contract your muscles repeatedly over time.
   b. run a six-minute mile.
   c. look "toned" in a swimsuit.
   d. contract your muscle with maximal force.

2. Which of the following benefits of resistance training will reduce your risk of cardiovascular diseases?
   a. Increased bone density
   b. Increased muscle power
   c. Reduced body fat levels
   d. Better sports recovery

3. What is a single muscle cell called?
   a. Muscle fiber
   b. Muscle fascia
   c. Fascicle
   d. Contractile bundle

4. Which of the following will result in a stronger muscle contraction?
   a. Eating more protein before your workout
   b. Activating slow, smaller motor units
   c. Taking DHEA before your workout
   d. Activating more motor units overall

5. Sitting down in a chair and standing up again is an example of which type of exercise?
   a. Isotonic
   b. Isokinetic
   c. Isometric
   d. Isostatic

6. Muscle strength improvements in the first few weeks of a program are due to
   a. increased size of muscle fibers.
   b. increased activation and coordination of motor units.
   c. increased ability of muscles to move through a full range of motion.
   d. increased blood flow to working muscles.

7. A test of muscular endurance includes
   a. a 1 RM test.
   b. a grip-strength test.
   c. a 20 RM test.
   d. a sit-n-reach test.

8. One disadvantage of using machines for resistance-training exercises is
   a. it takes time to adjust the machine for your height and desired resistance level.
   b. the machine does not promote the use of postural and stabilizing muscles during the exercise.
   c. spotters are needed.
   d. it can be hard to isolate specific muscle groups.

9. Which of the following is part of the criteria you should use when selecting a personal trainer?
   a. Certified by ACSM, NSCA, NASM, or ACE
   b. Looks like someone who works out a lot
   c. Recommended by a friend who was sore after a workout with the trainer
   d. Able to provide dietary supplements at a reduced cost

10. Which of the following supplements/drugs promotes irreversible bone growth, cardiovascular disease, diabetes, and decreased sexual desire?
    a. Anabolic steroids
    b. Creatine
    c. Growth hormone
    d. Androstenedione

critical thinking questions

1. Why is weight training a popular activity among college students and adults of all ages?

2. Define sarcopenia and discuss how it can be reversed through exercise. How are sarcopenia and atrophy different?

3. What is the predominant fiber type in the postural trunk muscles and why does this make sense?

4. Discuss the role of resistance training in preventing injuries.

5. In your opinion, do any of the supplements discussed have benefits that outweigh the risks or side effects?

references

1. Office of Disease Prevention and Health Promotion, U.S. Department of Health and Human Services, "Healthy People 2020 Topics and Objectives: Physical Activity," Updated April 2013, www.healthypeople.gov

2. Ibid.

3. Ibid.

4. D. R. Claflin et al., "Effects of High- and Low-Velocity Resistance Training on the Contractile Properties of Skeletal Muscle Fibers from Young and Older Humans," *Journal of Applied Physiology* 111, no. 4 (2011): 1021–30, doi: 10.1152/japplphysiol.01119.2010.

5. K. Davison et al., "Relationships Between Obesity, Cardiorespiratory Fitness, and Cardiovascular Function," *Journal of Obesity* 2010 (2010), doi: 10.1155/2010/191253; M. Fogelholm, "Physical Activity, Fitness and Fatness: Relations to Mortality, Morbidity and Disease Risk Factors. A Systematic Review," *Obesity Reviews* 11, no. 3 (2010): 202–21, doi: 10.1111/j.1467-789X.2009.00653.x; J. G. Stegger et al., "Body Composition and Body Fat Distribution in Relation to Later Risk of Acute Myocardial Infarction: A Danish Follow-up Study," *International Journal of Obesity* 35, no. 11 (2011): 1433–41, doi: 10.1038/ijo.2010.278.

6. Z. Wang et al., "Specific Metabolic Rates of Major Organs and Tissues Across Adulthood: Evaluation by Mechanistic Model of Resting Energy Expenditure," *American Journal of Clinical Nutrition* 92, no. 6 (2010): 1369–77, doi: 10.3945/ajcn.2010.29885.

7. S. M. Fernando et al., "Myocyte Androgen Receptors Increase Metabolic Rate and Improve Body Composition by Reducing Fat Mass," *Endocrinology* 151, no. 7 (2010): 3125–32, doi: 10.1210/en.2010-0018; R. R. Wolfe, "The Underappreciated Role of Muscle in Health and Disease," *American Journal of Clinical Nutrition* 84, no. 3 (2006): 475–82.

8. J. E. Donnelly et al., "American College of Sports Medicine Position Stand: Appropriate Physical Activity Intervention Strategies for Weight Loss and Prevention of Weight Regain for Adults," *Medicine and Science in Sports and Exercise* 41, no. 2 (2009): 459–71, doi: 10.1249/MSS.0b013e3181949333.

9. A. Figueroa et al., "Effects of Diet and/or Low-Intensity Resistance Exercise Training on Arterial Stiffness, Adiposity, and Lean Mass in Obese Postmenopausal Women," *American Journal of Hypertension* 26, no. 3 (2013): 416–23, doi: 10.1093/ajh/hps050.

10. J. B Moore et al., "Effects of a 12-Week Resistance Exercise Program on Physical Self-Perceptions in College Students," *Research Quarterly for Exercise and Sport* 82, no. 2 (2011): 291–301.

11. E. A. Marques et al., "Effects of Resistance and Aerobic Exercise on Physical Function, Bone Mineral Density, OPG, and RANKL in Older Women," *Experimental Gerontology* 46, no. 7 (2011): 524–32, doi: 10.1016/j.exger.2011.02.005.

12. C. S. Bickel, J. M. Cross, and M. M. Bamman, "Exercise Dosing to Retain Resistance Training Adaptations in Young and Older Adults," *Medicine and Science in Sports and Exercise* 43, no. 7 (2011): 1777–87, doi: 10.1249/MSS.0b013e318207c15d.

13. J. Holviala et al., "Effects of Prolonged and Maintenance Strength Training on Force Production, Walking, and Balance in Aging Women and Men," *Scandinavian Journal of Medicine and Science in Sport* (2012), doi: 10.1111/j.1600-0838.2012.01470.x. [Epub ahead of print].

14. V. A. Cornelissen et al., "Impact of Resistance Training on Blood Pressure and Other Cardiovascular Risk Factors: A Meta-Analysis of Randomized, Controlled Trials," *Hypertension* 58, no. 5 (2011): 950–8, doi: 10.1161/HYPERTENSIONAHA.111.177071; N. Gelecek et al., "The Effects of Resistance Training on Cardiovascular Disease Risk Factors in Postmenopausal Women: A Randomized-Controlled Trial," *Health Care for Women International* 33, no. 12 (2012): 1072–85, doi: 10.1080/07399332.2011.645960; D. Sheikholeslami Vatani et al., "Changes in Cardiovascular Risk Factors and Inflammatory Markers of Young, Healthy, Men After Six Weeks of Moderate or High Intensity Resistance Training," *Journal of Sports Medicine and Physical Fitness* 51, no. 4 (2011): 695–700.

15. M. A. Kostek et al., "Subcutaneous Fat Alterations Resulting from an Upper-Body Resistance Training Program," *Medicine and Science in Sports and Exercise* 39, no. 7 (2007): 1177–85.

16. K. Jay et al., "Kettlebell Training for Musculoskeletal and Cardiovascular Health: A Randomized Controlled Trial," *Scandinavian Journal of Work, Environment, and Health* 37, no. 3 (2010): 196–203, doi: 10.5271/sjweh.3136.

17. D. G. Candow et al., "Effect of Different Frequencies of Creatine Supplementation on Muscles Size and Strength in Young Adults," *Journal of Strength and Conditioning Research* 25, no. 7 (2011): 1831–38, doi: 10.1519/JSC.0b013e3181e7419a.

18. National Institutes of Health, Medline Plus, "DHEA," Updated March 2013, www.nlm.nih.gov

19. W. L. Baker, S. Karan, and A. M. Kenny, "Effect of Dehydroepiandrosterone on Muscle Strength and Physical Function in Older Adults: A Systematic Review," *Journal of the American Geriatrics Society* 59, no. 6 (2011): 997–1002, doi: 10.1111/j.1532-5415.2011.03410.x.

20. C. E. Brodeur et al., "The Andro Project: Physiological and Hormonal Influences of Androstenedione Supplementation in Men 35–65 Years Old Participating in a High-Intensity Resistance Training Program," *Archives of Internal Medicine* 160, no. 20, (2000): 3093–104.

21. S. Basaria, "Androgen Abuse in Athletes: Detection and Consequences," *Journal of Clinical Endocrinology & Metabolism* 95, no. 4 (2010): 1533–43, doi: 10.1210/jc.2009-1579.

22. L. Wideman et al., "Growth Hormone Release During Acute and Chronic Aerobic and Resistance Exercise: Recent Findings," *Sports Medicine* 32, no. 15 (2002): 987–1004.

23. A. Weltman et al., "Effects of Continuous Versus Intermittent Exercise, Obesity, and Gender on Growth Hormone Secretion," *The Journal of Clinical Endocrinology and Metabolism* 93, no. 12 (2008): 4711–920, doi: 10.1210/jc.2008-0998.

24. N. M. Cermak et al., "Protein Supplementation Augments the Adaptive Response of Skeletal Muscle to Resistance-Type Exercise Training: A Meta-Analysis," *The American Journal of Clinical Nutrition* 96, no. 6 (2012): 1454–64, doi: 10.3945/ajcn.112.037556.

25. M. Williams, "Dietary Supplements and Sports Performance: Amino Acids," *Journal of the International Society of Sports Nutrition* 2, no. 2 (2005): 63–7.

26. P. Lagiou et al., "Low Carbohydrate-High Protein Diet and Incidence of Cardiovascular Diseases in Swedish Women: Prospective Cohort Study," *BMJ* 344 (2012): e4026, doi: http://dx.doi.org/10.1136/bmj.e4026.

getfitgraphic references

1. Centers for Disease Control and Prevention, *National Health Interview Survey* (Hyattsville, MD: U.S. Department of Health and Human Services, 2013). Available at www.cdc.gov.

2. American College Health Association, *American College Health Association—National College Health Assessment II (ACHA-NCHA II): Undergraduate Reference Group Executive Summary Fall 2012* (Hanover, MD: American College Health Association, 2013)

3. H. Suominen, "Muscle Training for Bone Strength," *Aging Clinical and Experimental Research* 18, no. 2 (2006): 85–93.

4. A. B. Newman et al., "Strength and Muscle Quality in a Well-Functioning Cohort of Older Adults: The Health, Aging and Body Composition Study," *Journal of the American Geriatric Society* 51, no. 3 (2003): 323–30.

LAB 4.1

ASSESSING YOUR MUSCULAR STRENGTH

MasteringHealth™

Name: _____   Date: _____

Instructor: _____   Section: _____

Materials: Calculator, leg press machine, chest press machine

Purpose: To assess your current level of muscular strength

Note: This lab should be performed in the presence of an instructor to ensure proper form and safety.

SCAN TO SEE IT
ONLINE!

SECTION I: MUSCULAR STRENGTH ASSESSMENT

One Repetition Maximum (1 RM) Prediction Assessment

ACSM recommends measuring muscular strength by performing one repetition maximum (1 RM) or multiple RM assessments. This lab estimates 1 RM for the chest press and leg press by finding the amount of weight you can maximally lift 2 to 10 times.

1. **Warm up.** Complete 3 to 10 minutes of light cardiorespiratory activity to warm the muscles. Perform range-of-motion exercises and light stretches for the joints and muscles that you will be using.

2. **Use proper form while executing the chest press and leg press exercises.** For the chest press, position yourself so the bar or handles are across the middle of your chest. Spread your hands slightly wider than shoulder-width. Bring the handles/bar to just above your chest and then press upward/outward until your arms are straight. For the leg press, position yourself so that your knees are at a 90-degree angle. Press the weight away from your body until your legs are straight.

3. **Perform one light warm-up set.** Set the machine at a very light weight and lift this weight about 10 times as a warm-up for your assessment.

4. **Find the appropriate strength-assessment weight and number of repetitions.** Set a weight that you think you can lift at least 2 times but no more than 10 times. Perform the lift as many times as you can (to complete fatigue) up to 10 repetitions. If you can lift more than 10 repetitions, try again using heavier weight. Repeat until you find a weight you cannot lift more than 2 to 10 times. In order to prevent muscle fatigue from affecting your results, attempt this assessment no more than three times to find the proper weight and number of repetitions. If you experience muscle fatigue, rest and perform the test again on another day. Record your results in the Muscular Strength Results section (see step 7).

5. **Find your predicted 1 RM.** Predict your 1 RM based upon the number of repetitions you performed. If the weight you lifted was between 20 and 250 pounds, use the 1 RM Prediction Table to find your predicted 1 RM. If you lifted over 250 pounds, use the Multiplication Factor Table to find your predicted 1 RM. You can find these tables at the end of this lab.

6. **Find your strength-to-body weight ratio.** Divide your predicted 1 RM by your body weight for your strength-to-body-weight ratio (S/BW). Since heavier people often have more muscle, this is a better indicator of muscular strength than just the weight lifted alone. Record your results in the Muscular Strength Results section.

7. **Find your muscle strength rating by using the Strength-to-Body Weight Ratio chart provided on the last page of this lab.** Finding your rating tells you how you compare to others who have completed this test in the past. Record your results on the next page.

Muscular Strength Results

Chest Press: Weight lifted _____ Repetitions _____

_____ × _____ = _____

Weight lifted (lb) Multiplication factor* Predicted 1 RM (lb)

_____ ÷ _____ = _____

Predicted 1 RM (lb) Body weight (lb) S/BW ratio

Rating _____

Leg Press: Weight lifted _____ Repetitions _____

_____ × _____ = _____

Weight lifted (lb) Multiplication factor Predicted 1 RM (lb)

_____ ÷ _____ = _____

Predicted 1 RM (lb) Body weight (lb) S/BW ratio

Rating _____

*Multiplication factor from the Multiplication Factor Table on page 154.

SECTION II: REFLECTION

1. Were your muscular strength results what you expected? Why or why not?

_____

_____

2. Based upon your strength assessment results, what is your basic plan to maintain or improve?

_____

_____

1 RM Prediction Table

Wt (lb)	Repetitions									
	1	2	3	4	5	6	7	8	9	10
20	20	21	21	22	23	23	24	25	26	27
25	25	26	26	27	28	29	30	31	32	33
30	30	31	32	33	34	35	36	37	39	40
35	35	36	37	38	39	41	42	43	45	47
40	40	41	42	44	45	46	48	50	51	53
45	45	46	48	49	51	52	54	56	58	60
50	50	51	53	55	56	58	60	62	64	67
55	55	57	58	60	62	64	66	68	71	73
60	60	62	64	65	68	70	72	74	77	80
65	65	67	69	71	73	75	78	81	84	87
70	70	72	74	76	79	81	84	87	90	93
75	75	77	79	82	84	87	90	93	96	100

(Continued)

1 RM Prediction Table (Continued)

Wt (lb)	Repetitions									
	1	2	3	4	5	6	7	8	9	10
80	80	82	85	87	90	93	96	99	103	107
85	85	87	90	93	96	99	102	106	109	113
90	90	93	95	98	101	105	108	112	116	120
95	95	98	101	104	107	110	114	118	122	127
100	100	103	106	109	113	116	120	124	129	133
105	105	108	111	115	118	122	126	130	135	140
110	110	113	116	120	124	128	132	137	141	147
115	115	118	122	125	129	134	138	143	148	153
120	120	123	127	131	135	139	144	149	154	160
125	125	129	132	136	141	145	150	155	161	167
130	130	134	138	142	146	151	156	161	167	173
135	135	139	143	147	152	157	162	168	174	180
140	140	144	148	153	158	163	168	174	180	187
145	145	149	154	158	163	168	174	180	186	193
150	150	154	159	164	169	174	180	186	193	200
155	155	159	164	169	174	180	186	192	199	207
160	160	165	169	175	180	186	192	199	206	213
165	165	170	175	180	186	192	198	205	212	220
170	170	175	180	185	191	197	204	211	219	227
175	175	180	185	191	197	203	210	217	225	233
180	180	185	191	196	203	209	216	223	231	240
185	185	190	196	202	208	215	222	230	238	247
190	190	195	201	207	214	221	228	236	244	253
195	195	201	206	213	219	226	234	242	251	260
200	200	206	212	218	225	232	240	248	257	267
205	205	211	217	224	231	238	246	255	264	273
210	210	216	222	229	236	244	252	261	270	280
215	215	221	228	235	242	250	258	267	276	287
220	220	226	233	240	248	256	264	273	283	293
225	225	231	238	245	253	261	270	279	289	300
230	230	237	244	251	259	267	276	286	296	307
235	235	242	249	256	264	273	282	292	302	313
240	240	247	254	262	270	279	288	298	309	320
245	245	252	259	267	276	285	294	304	315	327
250	250	257	265	273	281	290	300	310	322	333

Multiplication Factor Table for Predicting 1 RM

Repetitions	1	2	3	4	5	6	7	8	9	10
Multiplication Factor	1.0	1.07	1.11	1.13	1.16	1.20	1.23	1.27	1.32	1.36

Table and multiplication factors generated using the Bryzcki equation:
1 RM = weight (kg)/[1.0278−(0.0278 × repetitions)].

Source: Equation from M. Brzycki, "Strength Testing: Predicting a One-Rep Max from a Reps-to-Fatigue," *Journal of Physical Education, Recreation, and Dance* 64, no. 1 (1993): 88–90.

Strength-to-Body Weight Ratio Ratings

Chest Press						
Men	**Superior**	**Excellent**	**Good**	**Fair**	**Poor**	**Very Poor**
<20 yrs	1.75	1.34–1.75	1.19–1.33	1.06–1.18	0.89–1.05	0.89
20–29 yrs	1.62	1.32–1.62	1.14–1.31	0.99–1.13	0.88–0.98	0.88
30–39 yrs	1.34	1.12–1.34	0.98–1.11	0.88–0.97	0.78–0.87	0.78
40–49 yrs	1.19	1.00–1.19	0.88–0.99	0.80–0.87	0.72–0.79	0.72
50–59 yrs	1.04	0.90–1.04	0.79–0.89	0.71–0.78	0.63–0.70	0.63
>60 yrs	0.93	0.82–0.93	0.72–0.81	0.66–0.71	0.57–0.65	0.57
Women	**Superior**	**Excellent**	**Good**	**Fair**	**Poor**	**Very Poor**
<20 yrs	0.87	0.77–0.87	0.65–0.76	0.58–0.64	0.53–0.57	0.53
20–29 yrs	1.00	0.80–1.00	0.70–0.79	0.59–0.69	0.51–0.58	0.51
30–39 yrs	0.81	0.70–0.81	0.60–0.69	0.53–0.59	0.47–0.52	0.47
40–49 yrs	0.76	0.62–0.76	0.54–0.61	0.50–0.53	0.43–0.49	0.43
50–59 yrs	0.67	0.55–0.67	0.48–0.54	0.44–0.47	0.39–0.43	0.39
>60 yrs	0.71	0.54–0.71	0.47–0.53	0.43–0.46	0.38–0.42	0.38

Leg Press						
Men	**Superior**	**Excellent**	**Good**	**Fair**	**Poor**	**Very Poor**
<20 yrs	2.81	2.28–2.81	2.04–2.27	1.90–2.03	1.70–1.89	1.70
20–29 yrs	2.39	2.13–2.39	1.97–2.12	1.83–1.96	1.63–1.82	1.63
30–39 yrs	2.19	1.93–2.19	1.77–1.92	1.65–1.76	1.52–1.64	1.52
40–49 yrs	2.01	1.82–2.01	1.68–1.81	1.57–1.67	1.44–1.56	1.44
50–59 yrs	1.89	1.71–1.89	1.58–1.70	1.46–1.57	1.32–1.45	1.32
>60 yrs	1.79	1.62–1.79	1.49–1.61	1.38–1.48	1.25–1.37	1.25
Women	**Superior**	**Excellent**	**Good**	**Fair**	**Poor**	**Very Poor**
<20 yrs	1.87	1.71–1.87	1.59–1.70	1.38–1.58	1.22–1.37	1.22
20–29 yrs	1.97	1.68–1.97	1.50–1.67	1.37–1.49	1.22–1.36	1.22
30–39 yrs	1.67	1.47–1.67	1.33–1.46	1.21–1.32	1.09–1.20	1.09
40–49 yrs	1.56	1.37–1.56	1.23–1.36	1.13–1.22	1.02–1.12	1.02
50–59 yrs	1.42	1.25–1.42	1.10–1.24	0.99–1.09	0.88–0.98	0.88
>60 yrs	1.42	1.18–1.42	1.04–1.17	0.93–1.03	0.85–0.92	0.85

Source: Reprinted with permission from The Cooper Institute, Dallas, Texas from *Physical Fitness Assessments and Norms for Adults and Law Enforcement*, available online at www.CooperInstitute.org.

Name: _____   **Date:** _____

Instructor: _____   **Section:** _____

Materials: Leg press machine, bench press machine, exercise mat, yardstick or ruler, tape

Purpose: To assess your current level of muscular endurance

Note: This lab should be performed in the presence of an instructor to ensure proper form and safety.

SECTION I: MUSCULAR ENDURANCE WEIGHT-LIFTING ASSESSMENT
Twenty Repetition Maximum (20 RM) Assessment

The 20 RM assessment is a weight-lifting assessment of your muscular endurance. By performing the assessments before and after completing 8 to 12 weeks of muscular fitness exercises, you can measure your improvement.

1. Prepare for the muscle endurance assessments. If you have just completed the muscular strength assessments in Lab 4.1, you will already be warmed up. If not, follow the position, form, and warm-up instructions for bench press and leg press in Lab 4.1.

2. Find your 20 RM for chest press and leg press. Set a weight that you think you can lift a maximum of 20 times. Perform the lift to see whether you were correct. If not, increase or decrease the weight and try again until you find your 20 RM. In order to be sure that muscle fatigue does not affect your results, try to find your 20 RM within three tries. If it takes longer, rest and perform the test again on another day. Record your results below.

Muscular Endurance Weight Lifting Results

Chest Press: 20 RM weight lifted _____

Leg Press: 20 RM weight lifted _____

SECTION II: MUSCULAR ENDURANCE CALISTHENIC ASSESSMENT
Push-Up Assessment

In this muscular endurance assessment, you will perform as many push-ups as you can. This test will assess the muscular endurance of your pectoralis major, anterior deltoid, and triceps brachii muscles. If you work with a partner, your partner can check your positioning and form and count your repetitions.

SCAN TO SEE IT
ONLINE!

1. Get into the correct push-up position on an exercise mat. Support the body in a push-up position from the knees (women) or from the toes (men). The hands should be just outside the shoulders and the back and legs straight.

2. Start in the "down" position with your elbow joint at a 90-degree angle, your chest just above the floor, and your chin barely touching the mat. Push your body up until your arms are straight and then lower back to the starting position (count one repetition). Complete the push-ups in a slow and controlled manner.

3. Complete as many correct technique push-ups as you can without stopping and record your results in the Muscular Endurance Calisthenic Results section below.

4. Find your muscle endurance rating for push-ups in the chart at the end of this lab and record your results.

Curl-Up Assessment

In this muscular endurance assessment, you will perform as many curl-ups as you can (up to 75). This test will assess the muscular endurance of your abdominal muscles.

1. Lie on a mat with your arms by your sides, palms flat on the mat, elbows straight, and fingers extended. Bend your knees at a 90-degree angle. Mark the start and end positions with tape. Your instructor or partner will mark your starting finger position with a piece of tape under each hand. He or she will then mark the ending position either 12 cm (under 45 years) or 8 cm (45 years or older) away from the first piece of tape, one ending position tape for each hand. Your goal is to rise far enough on the curl-up to achieve a 30-degree trunk elevation. Alternate methods include placing your hands across your chest and having your partner assess your 30-degree trunk elevation with each repetition or moving your hands from your thighs to the tops of your knees with each repetition.

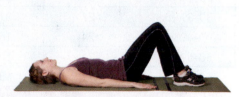

2. Your instructor or partner will set a metronome to 40 beats/min and you will complete the curl-ups at this slow, controlled pace.

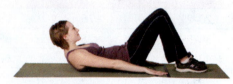

3. To start the test, curl your head and upper back upward, reaching your arms forward along the mat to touch the ending tape. Then curl back down so that your upper back and shoulders touch the floor. During the entire curl-up, your fingers, feet, and buttocks should stay on the mat. Your partner will count the number of correct repetitions you complete. Any curl-ups performed without touching the ending position tape will not be counted in the final results.

4. Perform as many curl-ups as you can without breaking cadence or pausing, to a maximum of 75. Record your score below. Determine your muscular endurance rating for curl-ups using the chart below and record your results.

**Alternative: One-minute timed curl-ups. Your instructor may choose to have you complete as many curl-ups as you can within one minute (without the metronome pacing). Using the same start and end positions, perform controlled repetitions of curl-ups for one minute and record your results below.

Muscular Endurance Calisthenic Results

Push-Ups: Repetitions_____   Rating_____

Curl-Ups: Repetitions_____   Rating_____

**Alternative: One-minute timed curl-ups: Repetitions _____

SECTION III: REFLECTION

1. What was surprising about your muscular endurance results, if anything?

_____

_____

2. How can you use your muscle endurance results to design your muscle fitness program?

_____

_____

Muscular Endurance Rating

Push-ups						
Men	**Superior**	**Excellent**	**Good**	**Fair**	**Poor**	**Very Poor**
20–29 yrs	>36	31–36	24–30	21–23	16–20	<16
30–39 yrs	>30	24–30	19–23	16–18	11–15	<11
40–49 yrs	>25	19–25	15–18	12–14	9–11	<9
50–59 yrs	>21	15–21	12–14	9–11	6–8	<6
60–69 yrs	>18	13–18	10–12	7–9	4–6	<4
Women	**Superior**	**Excellent**	**Good**	**Fair**	**Poor**	**Very Poor**
20–29 yrs	>30	22–30	16–21	14–15	9–13	<9
30–39 yrs	>27	21–27	14–20	12–14	7–11	<7
40–49 yrs	>24	16–24	12–15	10–11	4–9	<4
50–59 yrs	>21	12–21	8–11	6–8	1–5	<1
60–69 yrs	>17	13–17	6–12	4–6	1–3	<1
Curl-ups						
Men	**Superior**	**Excellent**	**Good**	**Fair**	**Poor**	**Very Poor**
20–29 yrs	≥75	56–74	31–55	24–30	13–23	<13
30–39 yrs	≥75	69–74	36–68	26–35	13–25	<13
40–49 yrs	≥75	67–74	51–66	31–50	21–30	<21
50–59 yrs	≥74	60–73	35–59	23–34	13–20	<13
60–69 yrs	≥53	33–52	19–32	9–18	1–8	<1
Women	**Superior**	**Excellent**	**Good**	**Fair**	**Poor**	**Very Poor**
20–29 yrs	≥70	45–69	32–44	21–31	12–20	<12
30–39 yrs	≥55	43–54	28–42	15–27	1–14	<1
40–49 yrs	≥55	42–54	28–41	20–27	5–19	<5
50–59 yrs	≥48	30–47	16–29	3–15	1–2	<1
60–69 yrs	≥50	30–49	19–29	9–18	1–8	<1

Source: Canadian Physical Activity, Fitness & Lifestyle Approach: CSEP - Health & Fitness Program's Appraisal and Counselling Strategy, 3rd edition, ©2003. Reprinted with permission from the Canadian Society for Exercise Physiology.

LAB 4.3

SETTING MUSCULAR FITNESS GOALS

MasteringHealth™

Name: _____   Date: _____

Instructor: _____   Section: _____

Purpose: To learn how to set appropriate muscular fitness goals (short- and long-term).

SECTION I: SHORT- AND LONG-TERM GOALS

Create short- and long-term goals for muscular strength and muscular endurance. Be sure to use SMART (*Specific, Measurable, Action-Oriented, Realistic, Timed*) goal-setting guidelines. Apply information discussed in the chapter and use your results from Labs 4.1 and 4.2. Remember that aiming to improve your assessment scores is a measurable way to set goals. Select appropriate target dates and rewards for completing your goals.

Short-Term Goals (3–6 months)

1. **Muscular Strength Goal:**

_____

Target Date: _____

Reward: _____

2. **Muscular Endurance Goal:**

_____

Target Date: _____

Reward: _____

Long-Term Goals (12+ months)

1. **Muscular Strength Goal:**

_____

Target Date: _____

Reward: _____

2. **Muscular Endurance Goal:**

_____

Target Date: _____

Reward: _____

SECTION II: MUSCULAR FITNESS OBSTACLES AND STRATEGIES

What barriers or obstacles might hinder your plan to improve your muscular fitness? Indicate your top three obstacles below and list strategies for overcoming each obstacle.

a. _____

b. _____

c. _____

SECTION III: GETTING SUPPORT

1. List resources you will use to help change your muscular fitness:

Friend/partner/relative: _____   School-based resource: _____

Community-based resource: _____   Other: _____

SECTION IV: REFLECTION

1. How realistic are the short- and long-term target dates you have set for achieving your muscular fitness goals?

_____

_____

_____

_____

2. Are there any other strategies not listed above that could assist you in reaching your goals?

_____

_____

_____

3. Think about all of the opportunities that present themselves in your daily life to work toward muscular fitness. List as many of these as you can think of:

_____

_____

_____

_____

Name: _____ Date: _____

Instructor: _____ Section: _____

Purpose: To create a basic, personal resistance-training workout plan. Forms for following up and tracking your muscular fitness and your resistance-training program are included.

Directions: Complete the following sections.

SECTION I: MUSCULAR FITNESS PROGRAM QUESTIONS AND MOTIVATIONS

1. How many days per week are you planning to work on your muscular fitness program? _____

2. How experienced are you at resistance training? (select one below)

Novice   **Intermediate (training 1 to 2 years)**   **Advanced (training 3+ years)**

3. Which will you focus on first? (select one)   **Muscular strength**   **Muscular endurance**

4. The best muscular fitness programs are well rounded and work the entire body. However, some people want to focus more heavily on one area than another. Which muscle groups do you want to focus on?

_____

5. Which type of equipment do you plan to use and why? (check all that apply)

☐ **Weight machines**

☐ **Free weights**

☐ **No equipment (calisthenic exercises)**

6. How much time do you plan for your resistance-training program on each workout day?

_____ Does this time estimate include your warm-up and cool-down? _____

7. Do you have a workout partner? Do you plan to work with a partner, trainer, or instructor to help you get started?

_____

*See **Activate, Motivate, & Advance Your Fitness: A Resistance-Training Program** on page 164 for a sample resistance-training program that will match your preferences and goals outlined above.

SECTION II: RESISTANCE-TRAINING PROGRAM DESIGN

In the table on the following page, plan your resistance-training program using resources available to you (facility, instructor, text). Complete one line for each exercise you have chosen to do in your program.

Exercise	Muscle(s) Worked	Frequency (days/week)	Intensity (weight in lb)	Sets (number)	Reps (number per set)	Rest (time between sets)
LOWER BODY						
1.						
2.						
3.						
4.						
5.						
6.						
7.						
8.						
UPPER BODY						
1.						
2.						
3.						
4.						
5.						
6.						
7.						
8.						
9.						
10.						
11.						
12.						
TRUNK						
1.						
2.						
3.						
4.						
5.						

SECTION III: TRACKING YOUR PROGRAM AND FOLLOWING THROUGH

1. **Goal and program tracking:** Use a resistance-training chart (see next page) to monitor your progress. Change the amount of resistance, sets, or repetitions frequently to ensure continuing progress toward your goals.

2. **Goal and program follow-up:** At the end of the course or at your short-term goal target date, reevaluate your muscular fitness and answer the following questions:

    a.   Did you meet your short-term goal or your goal for the course? _____

    b.   If so, what positive behavioral changes contributed to your success? If not, which obstacles blocked your success?

        _____

        _____

    c.   Was your short-term goal realistic? After evaluating your progress during the course, what would you change about your goals or resistance-training plan?

        _____

        _____

DATE																					
EXERCISE	Wt.	Sets	Reps	Wt.	Sets	Reps	Wt.	Sets	Reps	Wt.	Sets	Reps	Wt.	Sets	Reps	Wt.	Sets	Reps	Wt.	Sets	Reps
1.																					
2.																					
3.																					
4.																					
5.																					
6.																					
7.																					
8.																					
9.																					
10.																					
11.																					
12.																					
13.																					
14.																					

Activate, Motivate,
& ADVANCE YOUR FITNESS

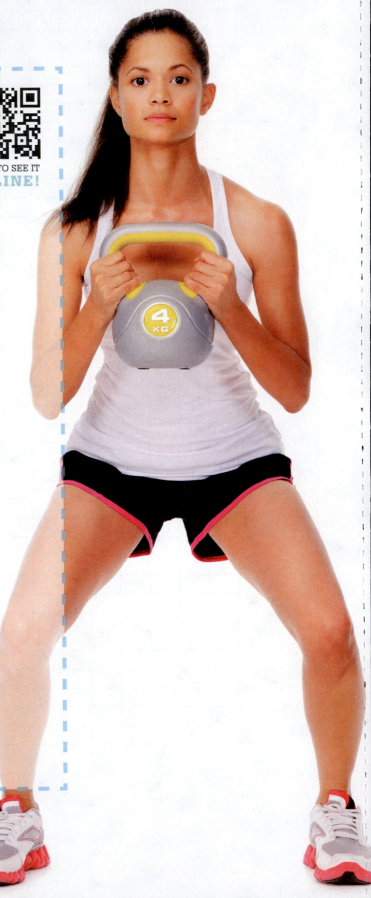

A RESISTANCE-TRAINING PROGRAM

SCAN TO SEE IT ONLINE!

ACTIVATE!

With the long list of health, wellness, and fitness benefits associated with resistance training, there is no doubt you want to get started now and give it all you've got! Just as with your cardiorespiratory program, don't make the mistake of trying to do too much, too soon. Doing too much too soon in a new resistance-training program is a leading cause of injury! Follow these programs to gradually increase the number of times you train each week, the number of exercises you incorporate into your weekly routine and, of course, the load (weight) and the volume (sets/repetitions).

What Do I Need for Resistance Training?

SHOES: For most resistance-training programs, you will want a pair of shoes with good traction and a non-slip sole. This gives you a stable base and prevents slipping when you lift.

CLOTHING: Wear comfortable, supportive clothing that allows for full range-of-motion movements. Choose materials that wick moisture away from your skin to help you regulate your body temperature and stay dry. In addition, you might find a pair of weight lifting gloves helpful for increasing your grip strength and preventing blisters and calluses.

How Do I Start a Resistance-Training Program?

TECHNIQUE: Safe and effective resistance training really depends on proper technique. Be sure to read through each exercise description carefully and learn the proper technique for each exercise to ensure good form. If you need assistance with how to properly use or set up a weight machine or if you need an exercise demonstration, ask your instructor or the fitness specialist at your facility. In addition to maintaining good form, it is important to perform each exercise in a slow and controlled manner through the full range of motion, taking care to avoid "locking out" your joints. If you are unable to maintain good form, decrease the weight or even the number of repetitions. Keep the weight balanced and use collars on weight bars to keep weights stable and secure. When it comes to proper breathing technique, keep it simple. In general, you will want to exhale during the exertion phase (when the exercise is hardest). Finally, when lifting free weights, it is always advisable to have a spotter. This is especially important for heavier weight loads, for maximal efforts, and for exercises that require the weight to pass over your head, face, or chest and even when a weight actually rests on your shoulders.

ETIQUETTE: Most facilities will have posted regulations for all patrons, and there are a few basic guidelines to keep in mind when you are performing resistance training.

Remember, safety first. Place weights, collars, and other equipment back when you finish using them. The next user may not be as strong as you are and may not be able to move the weight plates. The last thing anyone in the gym needs is to be tripping over free weights, so put your weights back on the rack when you finish with them. Be sure to wipe down machines, equipment, and benches after use. Most gyms supply wipes or have spray bottles and rags spread out throughout the weight room, so you shouldn't use your personal sweat towel.

Another common courtesy is to let others use the machines or weights during your rest intervals between sets.

Resistance-Training Tips

AT THE GYM: One of the advantages of resistance training at a gym is access to the wide variety of equipment and the amount of actual weight: weight machines, barbells (long bars with weights attached or slots to add weight plates), dumbbells (smaller, handheld weights), benches (flat, incline, decline), cable stations, the latest the industry has to offer. Utilizing essentials (machines and free weights) and the extras (balls, bands, etc.) provides exercise variety, which reduces boredom and increases exercise adherence. Another advantage to having a wide array of equipment and exercise options available relates to your specific muscular fitness goal and your progression. The exercise options included in the programs below and at the end of the chapter show options and modifications based on the equipment you have available. Feel free to mix up the mode you use for a basic exercise to challenge your body and increase your resistance or effort. Sometimes it is the little changes you make to an exercise that lead to the biggest progress.

AT HOME: You really have everything you need to get started. There are dozens of exercises that use your own bodyweight against gravity to increase your muscular

endurance and strength. That being said, you can always add a few pieces of equipment to your home gym as you progress. Items you might consider include bands or tubing, a stability ball, medicine balls, suspension training systems, kettlebells, and so on. These all store easily and most travel well. Each of these is simply one of many tools available to help you create a resistance to overcome. Training with different exercises and different exercise equipment allows you the opportunity to challenge your body with dynamic or functional exercises that mimic your movements in your activities of daily living (ADL) or your sport by introducing a fresh stimulus for physiological adaptation. For example, training with a medicine ball helps to develop total body power, muscular endurance, and flexibility. Bands can provide exercise options for beginning to advanced exercisers and athletes, an effective yet inexpensive way for your entire family to incorporate resistance training into their weekly routine. Stability balls can be used for improving core stability, static and dynamic balance, strength, and flexibility and can enhance functional and sport performance. You can do an entire workout with a stability ball or use one as part of a well-rounded exercise program for greater variety and effective progression in your resistance-training program.

Resistance-Training Warm-Up and Cool-Down

A resistance-training warm-up and cool-down should include light cardiorespiratory exercises for 5 to 10 minutes. After breaking a light sweat in your warm-up, you will want to add dynamic exercises for increasing your range of motion and maybe a bit of foam rolling. Before you begin your lifts with full weight, you should complete a few repetitions with little or no weight to ensure proper form, posture, and body alignment. After you finish your cool-down, you can hold static stretches longer for improved flexibility.

Resistance-Training Programs

If you are new to resistance training or if you have taken a lay-off of more than three months, start slowly and build gradually. Start with the Beginner Resistance-Training Program. This will help you increase overall muscular fitness (both muscular endurance and strength) and help to keep you injury free! If you are already resistance training two days a week (full body routine), then start with the Intermediate Resistance-Training Program. Adjust intensity, volume, and training days to suit your personal fitness level and schedule; visit the mobile website for more options.

RESISTANCE-TRAINING PROGRAM **GOAL:** Improve overall muscular fitness by performing eight exercises twice a week.

Frequency	Intensity	Time			Number and Type of Exercises
		Reps	*Sets*	*Rest*	
2 nonconsecutive days a week	60% 1RM	12	2	2 minutes between sets	8 multiple-joint exercises

Order of Exercises:

Leg Press

Heel Raises (can be performed through ankle plantar flexion while completing leg press)

Chest Press

Compound Row

Overhead Press

Lat Pull-Down

Abdominal Curl

Back Extension

INTERMEDIATE

RESISTANCE-TRAINING PROGRAM **GOAL:** Continue to improve muscular fitness by performing a split resistance-training program (upper/lower) four days of the week.

Frequency	Intensity	Time			Number and Type of Exercises
		Reps	*Sets*	*Rest*	
4 days a week: Upper body M/W Lower body T/Th	70% 1RM	10	3	2.5 minutes between sets	Upper body: 7 multiple-joint exercises 1 single-joint exercise Lower body: 4 multiple-joint exercises 3 single-joint exercises

M/W Upper Body Order of Exercises:

Chest Press

Row

Chest Fly

Overhead Press

Lat Pull-Down

Upright Row

Biceps Curl

Triceps Extension

T/Th Lower Body Order of Exercises:

Squat

Lunge

Leg Extension

Leg Curl

Heel Raise

Abdominal Curl

Oblique Curl

Back Extension

MOTIVATE!

Create your own exercise log to track your resistance-training program—make note of days, actual exercises, sets, reps, load amounts, and rest intervals—or use the log available through the mobile website. Here are a few other tips to keep your training strong.

ADJUST YOUR TRAINING ROUTINE: Boredom is a motivation killer. Changing your training exercises regularly, incorporating different equipment, and changing your training location from time to time are all ways to keep you engaged and ready for a new challenge.

MOTIVATION THROUGH MEDIA: Listen to music or podcasts during your rest intervals. In your downtime, try reading articles, blogs, or books about fitness, resistance training, healthy lifestyles, or your favorite sport. This helps to keep you interested and engaged to reach your goals.

STAY POSITIVE: Turn around your negative thoughts and self-talk and low energy days by surrounding yourself with positive affirmations and training partners. Stay focused and remember your goals. Take a moment to acknowledge how much you have already accomplished.

JOIN A SOCIAL MEDIA SITE OR FITNESS MESSAGE BOARD: Check out the message boards of fitness websites for inspiration from others who have accomplished their goals or who are working toward exercise goals similar to yours. Most message boards are designed to foster encouragement, discipline, and accountability.

MAKE A HEALTH CONTRACT WITH YOUR FAMILY MEMBERS: Everyone gets one private hour every day to exercise guilt-free. This will help establish your family's goal of a happy, healthy, and active lifestyle.

ADVANCE!

Now that you have established your resistance-training program, challenge yourself. Maybe it is time to try a few new exercises or new equipment. You may want to retake the estimated 1 RM and 20 RM tests and set new goals to take your training to the next level. Remember to follow the "10 percent rule" to safely progress to a new goal: Do not increase frequency, intensity, or time more than 10 percent per week. Below are two more advanced resistance-training programs. You can follow these or log onto the mobile website to find more options or to personalize this program or any of the programs in this book.

MUSCULAR ENDURANCE PROGRAM GOAL: Increase muscular endurance by

performing 12 exercises three days a week.

Frequency	Intensity	Time			Number and Type of Exercises
		Reps	Sets	Rest	
3 nonconsecutive days a week	50% 1RM	15	3	45–60 seconds between sets	10 multiple-joint and 2 single-joint exercise

Order of Exercises:

Push-Up	Upright Row
Assisted Pull-Up	Overhead Press
Squat	Biceps Curl
Lunge	Pullover
Chest Fly	Plank
Row	Side Bridge (each side)

MUSCULAR STRENGTH & MASS PROGRAM GOAL: Build muscular

strength and mass by performing a high-intensity split resistance-training program (upper/lower) four days of the week.

Frequency	Intensity	Time			Number and Type of Exercises
		Reps	Sets	Rest	
4 days a week: Upper body M/W Lower body T/Th	80% 1RM	8	4	3 minutes between sets	Upper body: 7 multiple-joint exercises 1 single-joint exercise Lower body: 4 multiple-joint exercises 3 single-joint exercises

M/W Upper Body Order of Exercises:

Chest Press
Row
Overhead Press
Lat Pull-Down
Lateral Raise
Biceps Curl
Tricep Extension
Back Extension

T/Th Lower Body Order of Exercises:

Leg Press
Leg Extension
Leg Curl
Hip Abduction
Hip Adduction
Heel Raise
Abdominal Curl
Reverse Curl
Oblique Curl

5 Maintaining Flexibility & Back Health

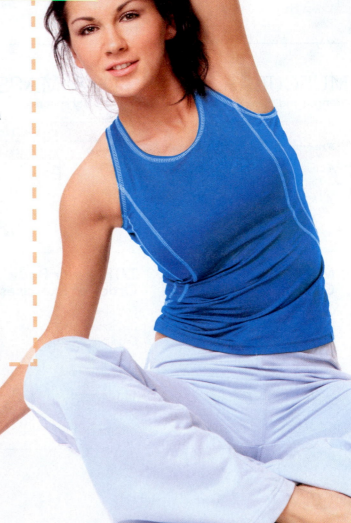

LEARNINGoutcomes

1 Articulate how regular stretching and being flexible can benefit your lifelong fitness and wellness.

2 Identify the body structures, body systems, and individual factors that will determine your joint flexibility and back health over time.

3 Use safe and effective stretching exercises and techniques, reducing stretching-related injuries.

4 Implement a safe and effective stretching program that will maintain or improve your flexibility.

5 Evaluate your personal risk for the primary causes of lower-back pain.

6 Incorporate strategies to reduce your risk for (or manage existing) lower-back pain.

MasteringHealth™

Go online for chapter quizzes, interactive assessments, videos, and more!

case study

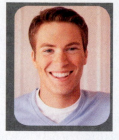

MARK

"Hi, I'm Mark. I live in Colorado Springs, at the foothills of the Rocky Mountains. I love the outdoors. I've been a back-packer, fisherman, and skier my whole life. My girlfriend is a fitness instructor and has been telling me that I should really stretch more, but I'm skeptical. What's so important about stretching? Will it help me be a better hiker or skier? How do I figure out what kind of stretches I should do? And when and how often should I stretch?"

HEAR IT! ONLINE

Flexibility is the ability of joints to move through a full **range of motion**. Flexibility tends to decrease as we get older,[1] so a good time to start a stretching program—if you don't stretch already—is when you are younger. Starting to stretch now will help you feel good and will increase your chances of staying flexible as you get older. A complete fitness program should include **stretching** and range-of-motion exercises to help you maintain flexibility and prevent joint problems.

Flexibility can be classified as static or dynamic. **Static (passive) flexibility** is a measure of the limits of a joint's overall range of motion. **Dynamic (active) flexibility** is a measure of overall joint stiffness during movement (i.e., with muscular contraction). Active movement such as swinging a tennis racket or leaping over a hurdle on a track requires good dynamic flexibility.

In this chapter, we will cover how maintaining your flexibility can improve your mobility, keep your joints healthy, and help you relax. We will discuss the factors that determine how flexible a person is, present strategies for stretching safely and effectively, and provide guidelines for developing a personalized stretching program. We will also discuss the common problem of lower-back pain and offer strategies for incorporating a back-health component into your regular fitness plan.

What Are the Benefits of Stretching and Flexibility?

Like Mark, many people are not in the habit of stretching and are not sure why stretching is important. There are many benefits to stretching, but the most compelling is simple: Being flexible will help you move freely and complete activities you want to do with greater ease.

Improved Mobility, Posture, and Balance

A regular stretching program helps you maintain joint mobility throughout your body. Your joints allow you to move—whether you are bending your knees to tie a shoelace, riding a bicycle around campus, or reaching for a bowl on the top shelf of a cupboard. A reduction in your flexibility can result in a reduction in your ability to move about freely as you perform daily activities. Likewise, an improvement in your flexibility can result in greater freedom of movement. Keeping your body flexible and strong also helps you maintain your balance. Individuals who have better ankle strength and range of motion not only have better balance, but also a greater functional ability—which means fewer falls and injuries.[2]

Regular stretching can also help you maintain a balance of muscle strength and muscle flexibility, which is important for proper joint alignment and posture. For example, if the muscles on the front of your hips get too tight, your pelvis can get pulled forward and cause a larger sway in your lower back. This will alter your posture and could even affect your balance. Good flexibility, developed through stretching, helps you keep your joints and spine aligned and promotes overall body stability.

Healthy Joints and Pain Management

As many as 28 percent of all adults report pain or stiffness in joints. That number increases dramatically with

---

flexibility The ability of a joint (or joints) to move through a full range of motion

range of motion The movement limits of a specific joint or group of joints

stretching Exercises designed to improve or maintain flexibility

static (passive) flexibility A joint's range-of-motion limits with an external force applied

dynamic (active) flexibility A joint's range-of-motion limits with muscular contraction applied

age, and women are more likely to have those joint symptoms. Many adults also have or will develop **arthritis** at some point in their lives; 54 percent of people 75 years and older have been diagnosed with arthritis.[3] Regular exercise, including range-of-motion and flexibility exercises, is essential for people with arthritis to maintain function and manage joint pain.[4] Even in people without arthritis, stretching will increase joint flexibility, improve joint function, and decrease periodic joint pain.[5]

Possible Reduction of Future Lower-Back Pain

Having an adequate level of flexibility may reduce your risk of lower-back pain in the future; however, research on the subject is inconclusive. While poor flexibility has been linked to lower-back pain in adolescents, these relationships are less clear in adults.[6,7,8,9] Despite the mixed evidence, most experts agree that counteracting the natural loss in muscle and connective tissue elasticity that occurs with aging with muscle fitness and stretching exercises can reduce your risk of developing lower-back pain.[10] We will discuss lower-back pain in more detail later in this chapter.

Muscle Relaxation and Stress Relief

After sitting at a computer for hours working on a term paper, doesn't it feel great to stand up and stretch? Staying in one position for too long, repetitive movement, and other stressors can result in stiff and "knotted" muscles. Gentle stretching and relaxation increases blood flow to tight muscles, stimulates the nervous system to decrease stress hormones, and ultimately helps relax areas of tension in your body.

What Determines My Flexibility?

What makes one person a human pretzel, while others can barely touch their toes? Is flexibility genetic, or can it be attributed entirely to the amount of stretching that you do? Many factors can affect your individual level of flexibility. Your joints, muscles, **tendons**, and nervous system—along with other characteristics such as age,

gender, genetics, and activity level—can all influence your flexibility.

Joint Structures, Muscles and Tendons, and the Nervous System

The range of motion possible in a particular **joint** is limited by the structures that comprise that joint, the muscles and tendons that cross over the joint, and the nervous system.

Joint Structures The individual components of a joint all affect the joint's mobility and stability (**Figure 5.1**). *Cartilage* is a strong, smooth tissue that cushions the ends of the bones, preventing them from rubbing directly against one another and providing impact protection. *Ligaments* are fibrous connective tissues that connect bone to bone. Some ligaments form the outer layer of the *joint capsule* to provide a reinforcing structure to the overall joint. Other ligaments, not part of the joint capsule, provide further stability to the joint. The *synovial membrane* forms the inner layer of the joint capsule and secretes *synovial fluid* into the *joint cavity*. Synovial fluid lubricates and protects the joint. *Bursae (singular, bursa)* are small fluid-filled sacs that lubricate the movement of muscles over one another or muscles over bone.

Muscles and Tendons Overall joint structure accounts for 47 percent of the resistance to movement around a

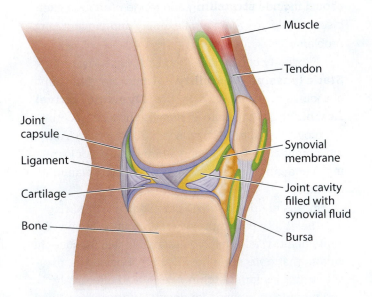

FIGURE **5.1** Joints are surrounded by a supportive joint capsule made of ligaments and synovial membranes. The joint cavity is filled with synovial fluid that (along with cartilage and bursa sacs) cushions and protects bones during movement. The stability of a joint is strengthened by muscle-tendon insertions surrounding the joint.

joint (dynamic flexibility), while individual *soft tissues* (muscles, connective tissue, ligaments, tendons, and skin) account for 53 percent of the resistance to movement.[11] With regular activity and stretching, connective tissues within muscles remain supple and are able to easily lengthen. With disuse and age, connective tissues become stiffer, limiting flexibility. Temperature can also affect the flexibility of soft tissues. When muscle temperature rises, connective tissues become softer and allow muscles to more easily lengthen.

The Nervous System Your nervous system is responsible for stimulating muscle contractions, and it also triggers muscle relaxation. Muscles and tendons contain nervous-system receptors that interpret information about the tension and length of muscles at any given moment. These receptors protect the muscles from damage caused by excessive amounts of tension or by stretching too far. If there is too much tension or force within a muscle, receptors in the tendon (called **golgi tendon organs**) will trigger your muscle to relax.

If your muscle is stretching too far, receptors in the muscle fibers (called **stretch receptors** or **muscle spindles**) will trigger your muscle to contract. This reflexive contraction is called the **stretch reflex**. Have you ever had a doctor tap your knee and watch your leg kick out in response? The doctor was striking your *patellar tendon*. This rapidly stretches your quadriceps muscle, which triggers stretch receptors in the quadriceps to signal your nervous system. Your leg then kicks out because of a reflex contraction of your quadriceps muscle stimulated by the nervous system.

Reducing the stretch reflex and activating the golgi tendon organs allow your muscles to relax, elongate, and gain improvements in flexibility.

Individual Factors

Beyond the anatomical structures and physiological mechanisms that we all share, individual factors such as genetics, gender, age, body type, and activity level also affect flexibility.

Genetics Most people have a moderate level of flexibility. They have flexible and less-flexible areas of their bodies and need to work to maintain their present level of flexibility. However, some people are extremely flexible by nature, while others are exceptionally inflexible. Genetic differences in body structure and the elasticity of soft tissues help account for the wide variety of flexibility levels.

Gender Although it is widely assumed that females are more flexible than males, this may only be true for specific joints, as discussed in the box Men, Women,

and Flexibility on page 172.

Age Flexibility changes throughout the lifespan. Flexible preschool children experience a decrease in joint range of motion until the preteen years, when flexibility increases again to its peak by 18 years of age.[12] In adulthood, flexibility decreases with age due to physical changes in muscles, joints, and connective tissues. These changes are joint specific and are primarily related to inactivity and disuse.

The good news is that with regular exercise, people of all ages can improve their current level of flexibility. In a study of sedentary adult women, researchers observed flexibility improvements when women participated in a 16-week strength training program.[13] The women in the study who also stretched had slightly larger gains in flexibility. These results demonstrate that performing a well-rounded muscle fitness program (with both strength and stretching exercises) may be the key to optimal improvements in flexibility.

Body Type Body type can affect flexibility but typically only at the extremes of body shape and size. For example, body type may affect range of motion if an excessive amount of muscle or fat physically interferes with full joint movement. That said, genetics and training are far more influential factors in determining flexibility than is body type. There are people with long, lean bodies whom you might expect to be flexible

golgi tendon organs Muscle tension receptors located in tendons that are responsible for triggering muscle relaxation to relieve excessive muscle tension

stretch receptors (muscle spindles) Muscle length receptors located within muscle fibers that trigger muscle contractions in response to rapid, excessive muscle lengthening

stretch reflex The reflex contraction of a muscle triggered by stretch receptors (muscle spindles) in response to a rapid overextension of that muscle

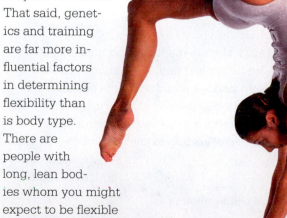

DIVeRSiTY
Men, Women, and Flexibility

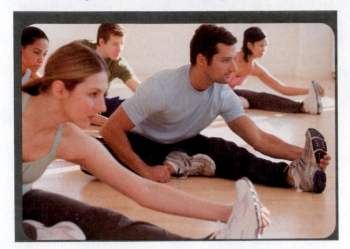

Women are more flexible than men, right? Not necessarily! This commonly held belief is not always true and may lull men into thinking that being inflexible is normal and okay. Women generally are more flexible in the hip joint and hamstrings, which are the most common sites for flexibility testing.[1] Women may have greater flexibility in these areas than males due to their wider hips, hormonal influences, and tendency to partici-

pate in activities that develop greater flexibility. In other joints and areas of the body, however, there is not a large difference between males and females. In fact, males may have greater flexibility in other areas. For example, males may have greater trunk rotation capabilities.[2]

Interestingly, greater joint range of motion and flexibility may increase the chances of injury. Because women tend to have greater hip flexibility and internal rotation of the hip joint, they are more likely to have knee problems.[3] The bottom line is that both men and women can increase flexibility with stretching exercises,[4] and adequate range of motion should be a goal for everyone. Being able to move your body without restriction opens up activity options and makes life easier!

Sources:
1. J. T. Manire et al., "Diurnal Variation of Hamstring and Lumbar Flexibility," *Journal of Strength and Conditioning Research* 24, no. 6 (2010): 1464–71.
2. J. T. Blackburn et al., "Sex Comparison of Hamstring Structural and Material Properties," *Clinical Biomechanics* 24, no. 1 (2009): 65–70.
3. K. M. Sutton and J. M. Bullock, "Anterior Cruciate Ligament Rupture: Differences Between Males and Females," *The Journal of the American Academy of Orthopaedic Surgeons* 21, no. 1 (2013): 41–50.
4. D. J. Cipriani et al., "Effect of Stretch Frequency and Sex on the Rate of Gain and Rate of Loss in Muscle Flexibility During Hamstring-Stretching Program: A Randomized Single-Blind Longitudinal Study," *Journal of Strength & Conditioning Research* 26, no. 8 (2012): 2119–29.

but who actually are not due to genetics or inactivity. Meanwhile, there are people with stocky, muscular builds who are exceptionally flexible, including many gymnasts.

Activity Level Inactivity can result in low levels of flexibility as muscles and connective tissues tighten and shorten with disuse. Overly repetitive physical activity can also result in muscle "stiffness." However, when done properly, stretching and regular physical activity can improve flexibility. We will introduce effective stretches and exercises later in this chapter.

Health Status Certain medical conditions can affect your joint health and range of motion. Diseases that affect your **collagen** and connective tissues can produce overly mobile or exceptionally inflexible joints. For example, arthritis speeds up the destruction of collagen and cartilage, leading to joint inflexibility. In some genetic syndromes, reduced or ineffective collagen causes hypermobility. During pregnancy, many

collagen The primary protein of connective tissues throughout the body

women will experience more flexible joints. Injuries or scar tissue can also affect your ability to move your joints through their full range of motion.

casestudy

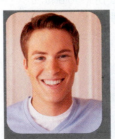

MARK

"I've heard that physical activity is supposed to improve your flexibility. If that's true, why do my muscles feel really stiff after a long day of skiing or hiking? I've noticed that this happens especially when I've gone for my first ski or hike of the season. Are my muscles just out of shape?"

THINK! What might explain Mark's muscle stiffness?

ACT! Create your own flexibility profile chart: In the first column, list out the factors that contribute negatively to your flexibility. In the second column, list out the benefits of stretching that you feel relate most to your life.

HEAR IT! ONLINE

How Can I Assess My Flexibility?

Flexibility levels vary from joint to joint. As a result, most flexibility tests are designed to measure the flexibility of specific muscles and joints, not to measure your body's overall level of flexibility. However, if you take a variety of flexibility tests, you can get a sense of how your body's overall level of mobility is measuring up to recommended target ranges.

Perform the "Sit-and-Reach" Test

One of the most common measures of flexibility is the "sit-and-reach" test. This test measures the flexibility of your lower back, hip, and hamstring muscles. These areas are often tight in individuals who are inactive. This muscular imbalance can negatively influence posture, balance, and risk of back pain. **Lab 5.1** provides instructions for the sit-and-reach test.

DO IT! ONLINE

Perform Range-of-Motion Tests

Having an adequate range of motion in your joints and maintaining that range over time should be the primary goal of a flexibility fitness program. Lab 5.1 provides instructions for performing range-of-motion tests on joints located in your neck, shoulders, trunk, hips, and ankles. By performing these tests, you can evaluate how the range of motion of your joints compares to those of the general population and determine whether your joints are more flexible or less flexible than average. This information will help you design a personalized program for developing flexibility. You can measure your progress over time by retaking the tests after months of training.

How Can I Plan a Good Stretching Program?

Regardless of whether you already stretch regularly, keep in mind the following guidelines to ensure a safe and effective program.

Set Appropriate Flexibility Goals

Decide up front what your goal is. Do you want to *maintain* your current level of flexibility (which is all that many people want to do), or do you want to *improve* your flexibility? Complete the sit-and-reach test and the range-of-motion tests described in Lab 5.1 before making this decision.

Once you've decided on your overall goal, follow the SMART guidelines for setting specific goals. Recall that SMART stands for *specific*, *measurable*, *action-oriented*, *realistic*, and *time-oriented*. An example of a SMART goal designed to *maintain* your flexibility is, "My goal for the next year is to maintain the joint flexibility and range-of-motion levels recorded on my flexibility assessments by incorporating stretching into my workouts at least four times per week." An example of a SMART goal designed to *improve* your flexibility is, "My goal is to regularly stretch so that I can increase my lower-back, hip, and hamstring flexibility from 'poor' to 'good' on the sit-and-reach test by the end of the school semester." For most people, the primary goal should be the ability to move their joints through a normal range of motion. Achieving exceptionally high levels of flexibility may be desirable for some sports and activities but is not necessary for the average person.

Apply the FITT Program Design Principles

Recall that FITT stands for *frequency*, *intensity*, *time*, and *type*. Use the FITT principles to design your own personalized stretching program. **Table 5.1** provides general guidelines from the American College of Sports Medicine (ACSM). Refer to this table as a starting point for designing your own program.

Frequency Notice that the ACSM guidelines in Table 5.1 recommend stretching at least two to three days per week. If you've determined that your current level of flexibility is already within "normal" ranges and you merely want to maintain that level, you should stretch two days per week. If you've determined that your current level of flexibility needs improvement to reach a "normal" range, you should stretch three or more days per week (daily is the most effective). Should you stretch before a workout, after a workout, or both? The box When Should I Stretch? on page 176 explores these questions and others.

Intensity The ACSM guidelines (see Table 5.1) state that you should stretch "to the point of feeling

TABLE **5.1** ACSM's Flexibility Training Guidelines for Healthy Adults	
Frequency	2–3 days/week minimum; daily is most effective
Intensity	Stretch to the point of feeling tightness or slight discomfort
Time	10–30 seconds per static stretch repetition; 2–4 repetitions of each stretching exercise; aim for 60 seconds total time per exercise
Type	Static, dynamic, or PNF stretching of all major muscle groups*

*Ballistic stretching may be appropriate for some individuals in certain sports and recreational activities.

Source: Data from American College of Sports Medicine, *ACSM's Guidelines for Exercise Testing and Prescription*, 9th edition by the American College of Sports Medicine (Baltimore, MD: Lippincott Williams & Wilkins, 2014.)

static stretching Stretching characterized by slow and sustained muscle lengthening

dynamic stretching Stretching characterized by controlled, full-range-of-motion movements that mimic exercise session movements

ballistic stretching Stretching characterized by bouncing, jerky movements, and momentum to increase range of motion

proprioceptive neuromuscular facilitation (PNF) Stretching that is facilitated or enhanced by the voluntary contraction of the targeted muscle group or contraction of opposing muscles

tightness or slight discomfort." If you are feeling pain, you are stretching too far and risking injury. Pay close attention to your body whenever you stretch; your flexibility level may vary slightly from day to day.

Time The ACSM guidelines state that you should perform your stretching program for at least 10 minutes at a time. In that time, stretch all major muscle groups, hold stretches for 10 to 30 seconds each, and repeat stretches two to four times. As soon as you start to stretch, your stretch reflex will activate: You can feel this as a slight increase in muscle tension when you move into a stretch position. By holding your stretches for at least 10 seconds, you are giving the stretch reflex time to lessen. You are also giving your golgi tendon organs time to activate and, thus, allowing your muscles to lengthen farther.

By repeating stretches multiple times, you enable your muscles to relax and lengthen a little bit more each time. If you are beginning a stretching program for the first time and feel uncomfortable with multiple repetitions, you can perform one repetition of each stretch and still obtain benefits. After a few weeks of stretching consistently, gradually increase the number of repetitions to the recommended two to four times per session. Aim to have your total stretching time for each exercise add up to 60 seconds.

Type There are numerous kinds of stretching techniques. The most common are highlighted below.

• **Static stretching** involves moving slowly into a stretch and holding it for a prescribed amount of time. This is the simplest and safest method for individuals who are just starting a stretching program. Static stretching is effective, because the activity of slow stretching and holding reduces the activation of stretch receptors. After a workout, static stretching can help muscles recover and help you to maintain or improve your flexibility.

casestudy

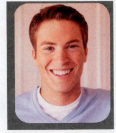

MARK

"The ski season just started. Out of curiosity, I asked a ski instructor for his opinions on stretching. He was surprised that I have been skiing my whole life but wasn't in the habit of stretching! He explained how stretching can help reduce muscle tension, improve my ability to make quick turns, and help prevent strains and stiffness. He recommended quadriceps and hamstrings stretches, for starters. He also suggested some stretching exercises that mimic the motion of skiing, in case I ever wanted to try skiing at a more advanced level."

THINK! Look at the quadriceps and hamstrings stretches in Figure 5.7. Are these static or dynamic stretches? What is the difference?

ACT! Assume that Mark wants to begin a general stretching program in the "off" season when he is not skiing. Write a SMART flexibility goal for him and a basic flexibility program, based on the ACSM guidelines you have learned.

HEAR IT! ONLINE

• **Dynamic stretching** involves stretching through movement. During dynamic stretching, you mimic the motions of your workout or sports activity with slow, fluid movements. Dynamic stretching increases dynamic flexibility and can enhance muscle action during sports and recreational activities.[14] The warm-up phase of an exercise session is a good time to implement dynamic stretching, because it helps prepare the body for the more intense physical activity to come.

• **Ballistic stretching** is a stretching method characterized by bouncing, sometimes jerky, movements and high momentum. Ballistic stretching increases dynamic flexibility and can benefit trained athletes in sports requiring fast, explosive movements such as wrestling, gymnastics, tennis, and basketball. However, the bouncing movements in ballistic stretching rapidly activate the stretch receptors, making this method less effective at increasing static flexibility.

• **Proprioceptive neuromuscular facilitation (PNF)** uses the voluntary contraction of muscle groups to help facilitate relaxation and stretching in target muscles. The most common method of PNF stretching is called *contract-relax PNF*. In contract-relax PNF, the exerciser experiences an isotonic or isometric contraction of the target muscle just prior to slow, passive stretching of that muscle. An example of contract-relax PNF in action is shown in **Figure 5.2**.

Table 5.2 lists some of the pros and cons of each stretching method. For most people starting a

flexibility program on their own, static stretches are the safest option. **Figure 5.7** (starting on page 186) illustrates some common stretching exercises you can select from, and Activate, Motivate, & Advance Your Fitness: A Flexibility Training Program located at the end of the chapter (page 207) offers options for sequencing and combining stretches. **Lab 5.3** walks you through the process of designing your own program. **DO IT! ONLINE**

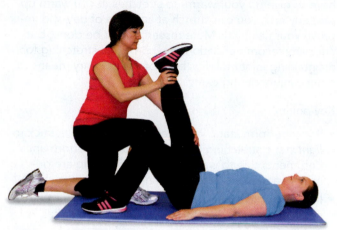

(a) Lie on your back with one leg bent and the other extended toward the ceiling. Have a partner hold your lifted leg as you try to press your leg to the ground for 6 seconds. Your partner can resist enough to allow no movement at all (isometric contraction) or just enough to allow gradual movement toward the ground (isotonic contraction). The contraction stimulates the golgi tendon organs to activate and promote muscle relaxation.

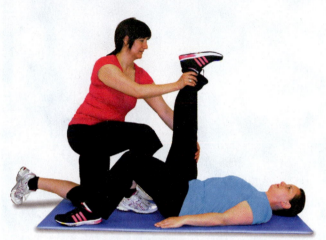

(b) Immediately following the 6-second contraction, relax your muscles and have your partner move your leg up and toward your chest into a passive stretch for the hips, hamstrings, and low back. Hold this stretch for 10–30 seconds and release.

FIGURE **5.2** An example of a contract-relax proprioceptive neuromuscular facilitation (PNF) partner exercise.

TABLE **5.2** Pros and Cons of Common Stretching Methods		
Stretching Method	Pro	Con
Static	Safe, simple to use, effective at increasing static flexibility	Too much can reduce muscle power immediately after stretching, can be time consuming
Dynamic	Increases dynamic flexibility, functional movements, enhances performance	Takes time to learn correct movement patterns
Ballistic	Can be beneficial for ballistic sports, increases dynamic flexibility	Not as effective at increasing overall flexibility, performing ballistic moves quickly can be unsafe
PNF	Effective at increasing static flexibility levels	Need a partner or equipment to perform, complicated method

Q&A When Should I Stretch?

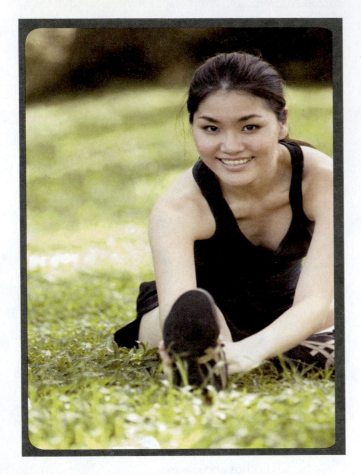

sprint and explosive performance for up to 24 hours. The duration and timing of pre-event stretching is another consideration for competitive and recreational athletes. Even dynamic stretching impairs performance when it lasts too long (inducing fatigue) and is completed too close to the performance time.[2]

It is also now generally accepted that pre-exercise stretching does not reduce overuse injuries.[3] This is a surprise to many people, but it doesn't mean that you have to give up your warm-up stretches. If you warm up properly first, you can stretch at any time of day and improve your flexibility. More research must be done, but flexibility recommendations now promote stretching for maintaining joint mobility, but not as a primary means to reduce injury during exercise.

Key points:

- If you perform static stretches in your warm-up, stick to *light* static stretching (10 to 15 seconds). Performance detriments due to warm-up static stretching are primarily seen with stretches lasting 60 seconds or more.[4]
- If you want to stretch before a workout, be sure to warm up beforehand. Stretching cold muscles can result in injury.
- Emphasize dynamic stretches in your warm-up and make sure the movements are similar to your exercise, sport, or recreational activity.
- Avoid warming-up and stretching to the point of fatigue right before exercise or competition.
- Save most of your static stretching for after the workout—then you can really focus on increasing range of motion in tight areas!

Many people incorrectly think that they *have* to stretch before a workout. In general, it is actually better to perform most of your static stretching *after* a workout, when your muscles are warm and your joint structures are more receptive to stretching.

For *most* individuals, light pre-exercise static stretches will not negatively affect exercise or recreational performance. If you are a power athlete, though, you may want to avoid too much static stretching before a competition or high-intensity workout. Extensive static stretching can result in a reduction in explosive performances for up to 24 hours![1] Conversely, dynamic stretching can improve

Sources:
1. M. Haddad et al., "Static Stretching Can Impair Explosive Performance for at Least 24 Hours," *Journal of Strength & Conditioning Research* (2013): [Epub ahead of print].
2. O. Turki et al., "The Effect of Warm-Ups Incorporating Different Volumes of Dynamic Stretching on 10- and 20-m Sprint Performance in Highly Trained Male Athletes," *Journal of Strength & Conditioning* 26, no. 1 (2012): 63–72.
3. M. P. McHugh and C. H. Cosgrave, "To Stretch or Not to Stretch: The Role of Stretching in Injury Prevention and Performance," *Scandinavian Journal of Medicine & Science in Sports* 20, no. 2 (2010): 169–81.
4. A. D. Kay and A. J. Blazevich, "Effect of Acute Static Stretch on Maximal Muscle Performance: A Systematic Review," *Medicine and Science in Sports and Exercise* 44, no. 1 (2012): 154–64.

Consider Taking a Class

If you would like more structure and instruction in your stretching program, consider enrolling in a class. Yoga, tai chi, Pilates, dance, and martial arts classes can be fun, effective ways to maintain, or improve your flexibility. For more information on these types

of classes, see the box Can I Become Flexible without Stretching? on page 179.

Add Flexibility "Tools"

Alternate methods to achieve increases in joint range-of-motion and functional muscle flexibility have become popular. There are a number of flexibility tools that you can add to your current routine and use in your own home and/or in a gym. These tools can increase the safety and effectiveness of your stretching, plus provide something new for variety and motivation!

Myofascial release therapy is used by physical therapists and other health practitioners to reduce muscle tightness, soft-tissue adhesions, and nervous-system over-activation. In the patient, this results in increased joint and muscle extensibility, muscle balance, and overall function. In recent years, *self*-myofascial release has become popular by competitive and recreational athletes in many sports. Using a foam roller or a massage stick, you can perform these myofascial release techniques on yourself to improve your own muscle range of motion and reduce muscle fatigue.[15] Utilize this self-massage technique to loosen soft tissues before activity, after a workout to assist with muscle relaxation, and/or between workouts for pain relief and muscle balance.

A massage stick is a plastic rod with handles designed to roll over muscles under pressure for myofascial release. Flexibility of the rod varies for more or less intensity, and they are generally sized between 14–30 inches. Massage sticks are a nice alternative to a foam roller for travel. They are available at most sporting goods and running/walking stores for about $20–50.

At some workout facilities you may find a *stretching machine*. This is a machine that facilitates a variety of body stretching positions and provides a deep stretch. It's preferable to use a stretching machine that provides multiple stretching positions. If you see one at your gym, be sure to try it out!

You may have heard of *whole-body vibration* or seen one of these machines in your gym. Developed in the 1960s as a way to help astronauts maintain muscle and bone mass while in space, the whole-body vibration (WBV) platform transmits quick vibrations in one or more directions to the person using the platform, stimulating muscle fiber contractions. The platforms are becoming more common because there is quite a bit of evidence to support the use of these vibration platforms for increased flexibility and muscle action. The evidence seems to be consistent for flexibility gains,[16] even over some of the other benefits such as bone density and muscle strength. Stretching during vibration on a WBV platform appears to be a good adjunct to static stretching and may help you retain the flexibility you gain.[17] If your gym has a WBV platform, talk with a fitness instructor or personal trainer about designing a program for you. Standing or lying muscle fitness exercises can be performed on the platform. Time on the platform should amount to 20 to 30 minutes a day, but work your way up to this. Use the platform a few times per week or every day to increase range of motion, muscle fitness, and bone density.

If a WBV platform is not available for you to use, no worries! There are plenty of other less expensive and widely available flexibility tools that you can use to enhance your stretching program. See **Table 5.3** on the following page for an overview of some of the most popular ones.

> **myofascial release therapy**
> Manual pressure and movement therapy that aims to decrease movement restrictions and pain in muscle tissue and the surrounding fascia

How Can I Avoid Stretching-Related Injuries?

We used to think of stretching as a way to avoid injury, but we now know that stretching can actually *cause* injury if done improperly. To avoid a stretching-related injury, adhere to the following guidelines.

Stretch Only Warm Muscles

An increase in body temperature prepares the joint fluid and structures for stretching and improves muscle elasticity. These changes allow you a greater range of motion while stretching. Increased muscle heat prior to stretching can be achieved via *passive heat* (hot packs or a warm bath) or *active heat* (exercise). Both are effective to prepare you for stretching. However, if you are warming up your muscles prior to your main workout set, use active heat methods. After a workout, you can go right to your static stretching because the muscles have been sufficiently warmed up.

Perform Stretches Safely

One of the keys to safe and effective stretching is to avoid activating stretch receptors when you want a muscle to relax. Stretch receptors are activated when muscles are lengthened rapidly. Muscle injury can occur from quick, bouncing movements, because the muscle is lengthening too far too quickly and the stretch reflex is creating tension at the same time. Avoid the stretch reflex by stretching carefully and slowly. Holding your stretches for at least 10 seconds will allow the stretch receptors and golgi tendon organs to make nervous-system adjustments. These adjustments will allow further relaxation and lengthening of the muscles involved.

TABLE 5.3 Flexibility Tools

Foam Roller	Yoga Tools	Stretching Strap	Whole-Body Vibration
Foam cylinder used for rolling tight body areas	Mat: a thin, long, nonslip mat Blocks: dense foam rectangular blocks Strap: strong cotton strap with a buckle	Long strap with multiple loops or yoga strap that can be used for various static, dynamic, and nonpartner PNF stretches	Platform that vibrates and is used to enhance muscle action while exercising
Sized between 12 and 36 inches; density varies (in general darker rollers are firmer)	Yoga mats are useful for all types of stretching; blocks and straps assist body positioning in poses and stretches	Several feet long, most of these straps have about 10 loops along the length for customizing your stretch position.	Make sure that the platform is large enough for the exercises you want to perform
Choose from a smooth surface or one with ridges for greater massage intensity	Look for a slip-resistant yoga mat that has adequate padding	Some straps come with instructional books or DVDs	Some platforms have a bar or handles for stabilization while working on standing exercises
Cost: $12–50	Cost: Mat $15–40; Blocks $12–20; Strap $6–15	Cost: $12–15	Cost: $200–400

Know Which Exercises Can Cause Injury

Figure 5.3 on page 180 shows common high-risk or **contraindicated** stretches with safer alternatives. Note that this figure is *not* an all-inclusive list. Choosing safe exercises is a highly individual process. Consider your personal limitations and health issues when deciding which exercises are best for your body.

Be Especially Cautious If You Are a Hyperflexible or Inflexible Person

If you are really flexible, you may need to be more careful while stretching than the average exerciser. Excessive hypermobility increases joint laxity or looseness, decreases joint stability, and

contraindicated Not recommended

can lead to permanent changes in connective tissue. Take precautions to avoid overstretching, which may lead to injury or decreases in exercise performance. For example, if you are taking a yoga class, let your instructor know that you are hyperflexible and ask if there are any modified poses that would reduce your risk of overstretching.

Inflexibility is common in many people. If you have limited range of motion in one or more joints, avoid stretching beyond your abilities. Work gradually to improve your range of motion and overall flexibility. People with a very limited range of motion may be more susceptible to sudden acute injuries during sports, to activity-related injuries during daily-living tasks, and to lower-back injuries.

How Can I Prevent or Manage Back Pain?

While you are young, back pain is probably the furthest thing from your mind. However, some 31 percent of all

Q&A Can I Become Flexible without Stretching?

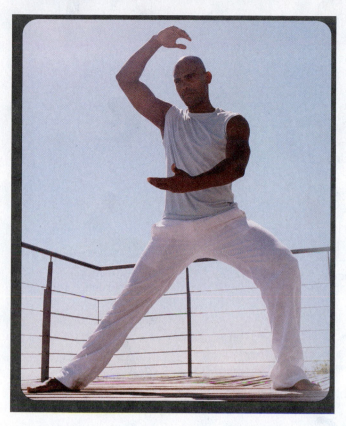

If a regular stretching routine

doesn't appeal to you, try one of these classes to help you reach your flexibility goals:

Yoga originated in India about 5,000 years ago and has become a popular activity in the United States. The forms of yoga most commonly practiced in the United States today require a combination of mental focus and physical effort while performing a variety of postures, or *asanas*. The physical aspect of yoga results in improvements in flexibility, posture, agility, balance, stamina, muscle endurance, and coordination.[1] The mental aspect of yoga promotes attention, controlled breathing, relaxation, a union of mind and body, and an overall psychological sense of well-being.[2]

Tai chi is a martial art that was developed in ancient China by monks wanting to defend themselves. Tai chi practice involves a slow-moving, smooth, and continuous series of positions or forms. These exercises increase balance, muscle endurance, flexibility, and coordination; they also reduce anxiety and stress.[3] Tai chi has become popular with many people, but older individuals in particular are drawn to this safe and effective way to exercise. There are other forms of martial arts that will develop flexibility, as well. You may want to look into classes for one of these popular martial arts: capoeira, karate, jujitsu, or tae kwon do.

Pilates was developed by Joseph Pilates in New York City in the 1920s. Pilates involves performing a sequence of exercises on a mat or specialized equipment designed to stretch and strengthen muscles. Specific breathing patterns are combined with stretching and resistance exercises to increase flexibility and muscle endurance, particularly in the core trunk-supporting muscles.

Dance is a fantastic and fun way to improve your flexibility and your overall fitness level. A group exercise class, such as aerobic dance, will usually give you a chance to work on your flexibility during the cool-down phase.

All of the activities described above require instruction by a trained professional, especially since some exercises can be risky for the untrained or novice participant.

Sources:
1. B. L. Tracy and C. E. Hart, "Bikram Yoga Training and Physical Fitness in Healthy Young Adults," *Journal of Strength and Conditioning Research* 27, no. 3 (2013): 822–30.
2. N. Moliver et al., "Yoga Experience as a Predictor of Psychological Wellness in Women Over 45 Years," *International Journal of Yoga* 6, no. 1 (2013): 11–9.
3. M. Y. Chang et al., "Associations between Tai Chi Chung Program, Anxiety, and Cardiovascular Risk Factors," *American Journal of Health Promotion* (2013): [Epub ahead of print]; H. Liu and A. Frank, "Tai Chi as a Balance Improvement Exercise for Older Adults: a Systematic Review," *Journal of Geriatric Physical Therapy* 33, no. 3 (2010): 103–9.

Americans report limitations due to chronic back conditions.[18] In fact, back and spine problems are the self-reported cause of disability for 7.6 million Americans (16.8 percent), with women affected more often.[19] While Americans spend more than $86 billion each year treating back pain symptoms, the number and symptoms of sufferers continue to rise.[20]

Research has shown that college students are not immune to back-health issues. See the GetFitGraphic on Back Pain and College Students (page 183) for statistics and tips for back pain risk reduction and management. Factors that increase your risk of lower-back pain include obesity, smoking, pregnancy, stress, inactivity, weak and inflexible muscles, and poor posture. In addition, a number of events can trigger back pain or cause a back injury, including accidents, sports injuries, repetitive movements, work trauma, and excessive sitting—especially if you already have other risk factors.

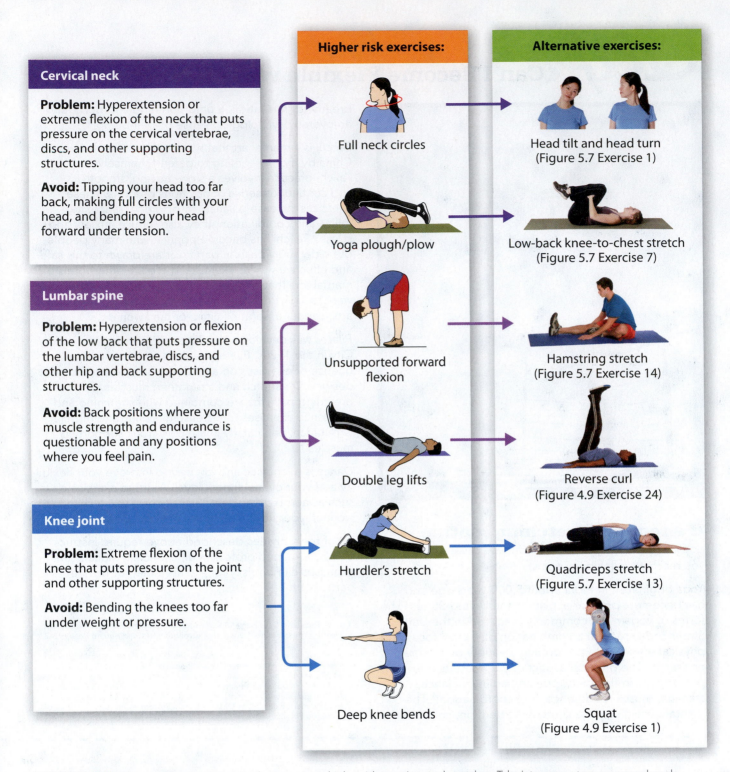

Cervical neck

Problem: Hyperextension or extreme flexion of the neck that puts pressure on the cervical vertebrae, discs, and other supporting structures.

Avoid: Tipping your head too far back, making full circles with your head, and bending your head forward under tension.

Lumbar spine

Problem: Hyperextension or flexion of the low back that puts pressure on the lumbar vertebrae, discs, and other hip and back supporting structures.

Avoid: Back positions where your muscle strength and endurance is questionable and any positions where you feel pain.

Knee joint

Problem: Extreme flexion of the knee that puts pressure on the joint and other supporting structures.

Avoid: Bending the knees too far under weight or pressure.

Higher risk exercises:

Full neck circles

Yoga plough/plow

Unsupported forward flexion

Double leg lifts

Hurdler's stretch

Deep knee bends

Alternative exercises:

Head tilt and head turn
(Figure 5.7 Exercise 1)

Low-back knee-to-chest stretch
(Figure 5.7 Exercise 7)

Hamstring stretch
(Figure 5.7 Exercise 14)

Reverse curl
(Figure 4.9 Exercise 24)

Quadriceps stretch
(Figure 5.7 Exercise 13)

Squat
(Figure 4.9 Exercise 1)

FIGURE **5.3** Choose safer alternatives to these common higher-risk exercises and stretches. Take into account your personal goals, experience, and limitations.

In the next sections, we will cover the causes of back pain, explain how the spine is structured and supported, and present strategies to reduce your risk of back pain. For those who already experience regular episodes of back pain, the next sections will also discuss ways to effectively manage, resolve, and prevent future recurrences of back pain.

Understand the Primary Causes of Back Pain

You experience back pain when your movement causes a sprain, strain, or spasm in one of the muscles, tendons, or ligaments in the back. You may also feel pain when your spine structures become misaligned or injured and the spinal nerves become compressed or irritated. Back pain can also result from age- or disease-related degeneration of the bones and joints of the spine. Ultimately, most back pain is caused by a *sedentary lifestyle,* which results in muscle weakness, inflexibility, and imbalance—all conditions that can lead to poor posture and body mechanics and to a higher risk of back pain and injury.

Muscular Weakness, Inflexibility, and Imbalance

The supporting musculature of the spine is important for maintaining healthy posture, mobility, and spine structures. Weakness and inflexibility in key muscles can lead to muscular imbalances that affect the alignment of your spine. Weak abdominals, for instance, can cause your pelvis to rock forward and create a greater curvature in your lower back. This puts more pressure on spine structures and other spine-supporting muscles, potentially leading to back pain. Inflexible, tight hip flexor muscles can also cause a forward tilt of the pelvis and an increased curvature of the lower back.

Muscles become weak when they are not used on a regular basis. Repetitive movements or long hours of sitting can also cause muscles to shorten and tighten up. Some people have muscles of differing strength and flexibility levels around the spine and other joints. If your spine-supporting musculature does not have a muscle balance that promotes good posture and body mechanics, you may have back pain or injury in the future.

Improper Posture and Body Mechanics
Improper posture can lead to increased forces within the spine structures and eventually to back pain. Altered body mechanics resulting from improper posture puts you at risk for injury during all of your daily activities, but especially during exercise and sports activities.

Acute Trauma, Risky Occupations, and Medical Issues
Acute trauma to the back can happen to anyone at any age. Trauma could be the result of a car accident, a sports-and-recreation injury, or any other accident that affects the spine. Avoiding risky sports and recreational activities will reduce your chance of trauma.

Jobs that involve a lot of bending, twisting, and repeated lifting of heavy objects put workers at especially high risk of developing back pain. Jobs that involve a great deal of sitting every day are also considered high risk. Occupations with a high incidence of back pain include truck driving, nursing, firefighting, construction, and some professional sports (e.g., football, power lifting, golf, and wrestling). Occupations that are highly stressful and require long hours also increase the risk of back pain. Stress is a risk factor for back injury, and long hours at work can reduce the time you have to exercise and relax, further increasing the risk of developing back pain.

Medical issues and individual health factors can also significantly increase your chance of developing lower-back pain. For instance, smokers have an increased risk of low-back pain due to vascular damage, which facilitates disc degeneration.[21] Obesity and weight gain during pregnancy can increase lower-back pain due to greater loads on the spine, misalignment of the pelvis and low back, and muscular weakness. Pain can also result from degenerative conditions such as arthritis or disc disease, osteoporosis or other bone diseases, congenital abnormalities, viral infections, and general conditions that cause irritation to joints or discs.[22]

Understand How the Back Is Supported

The back comprises bones, muscles, and other tissues that form the back side of your trunk. The trunk contains most of your essential organs and bears the weight of your upper body. It is also responsible for transmitting forces and movements from the upper limbs to the lower limbs, and vice versa. If something is amiss with your back or your trunk overall, any upper- or lower-body movement can be difficult. Your back and trunk are supported by the bony structures of the spine and by the core trunk muscles.

The Structure of the Spine

The spine or *spinal column* (also called the *vertebral column*) is the series of bones called *vertebrae* that connect the upper-body and lower-body skeleton and protect the spinal cord. **Figure 5.4** on the following page shows the basic structure of the spine. Note that the spine has four distinct regions and curvatures: *cervical, thoracic, lumbar,* and *sacral.* The curvatures are an essential part of the force-absorbing capabilities of the spine.

Intervertebral discs are round, spongy pads of cartilage that act as shock absorbers. The discs have fibrous outer rings that are filled with gel and water-like substances that will distend slightly when compressed. That distention acts to absorb shock. The discs also

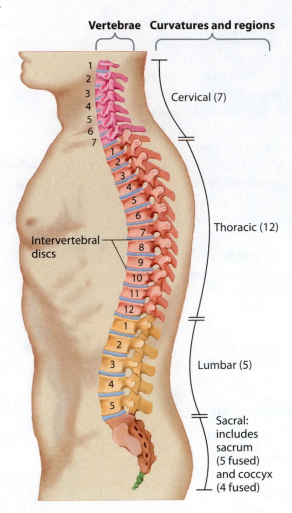

Vertebrae | **Curvatures and regions**

1
2
3
4
5
6
7
— Cervical (7)

1
2
3
4
5
6
7
8
9
10
11
12
— Thoracic (12)

Intervertebral discs

1
2
3
4
5
— Lumbar (5)

— Sacral: includes sacrum (5 fused) and coccyx (4 fused)

FIGURE **5.4** The spine has four distinct regions and curvatures (cervical, thoracic, lumbar, and sacral) made up of individual or fused vertebrae.

ensure that there is adequate space between the vertebrae. When a change in body mechanics or posture occurs—or when an acute injury occurs—the resulting change to spinal alignment can damage the disc structures.

A permanent bulging of a disc out of the normal space is called a **disc herniation**. The disc can bulge toward the spinal column or nerves and cause pain or numbness in the back or other areas of the body. Disc herniations most often occur in the lower lumbar region, where most of the body weight and forces are applied.

Another problem that occurs with trauma or aging is dehydration, hardening, or degeneration of intervertebral

disc herniation A permanent bulging of an intervertebral disc out of its normal space

core muscles Musculature that supports the trunk (back, spine, abdomen, and hips)

discs. Without adequate fluid content and elasticity, discs cannot perform their shock-absorber role very well. The resulting smaller joint space between vertebrae applies pressure to the spinal nerves. This can cause back, hip, or leg pain, and muscle weakness.

The Core Trunk Muscles The bones of the spinal column could not maintain their healthy curvatures and an upright posture without supporting muscles. Core trunk muscles support the trunk while you are standing, sitting, lying down, or moving. These muscles, located all around your body (**Figure 5.5**), are essential for supporting the spine and for performing sports, recreation, and everyday activities. **Core muscles** include back, abdominal, hip, gluteal, pelvis, pelvic floor, and lateral trunk muscles. Core muscles work together to effectively transmit forces between your upper and lower body. While weak core muscles can lead to back pain, strong core muscles can lead to increased performance levels in all of your activities.

Reduce Your Risk of Lower-Back Pain

You can reduce your risk of back pain by improving your body weight, muscle fitness, posture, and movement

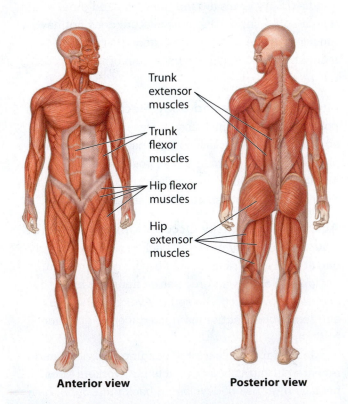

Trunk extensor muscles
Trunk flexor muscles
Hip flexor muscles
Hip extensor muscles

Anterior view　　　**Posterior view**

FIGURE **5.5** Strengthening and stretching of the spine-supporting core muscles is essential for a healthy back. The core muscles include extensors of the trunk and hip and flexors of the trunk and hip.

BACK PAIN
AND COLLEGE STUDENTS

70% of Americans will experience lower-back pain at some point in their lives.

28% of Americans suffer from lower-back pain at any given moment.[1]

43% of college students report regular lower-back pain.[2]

Students who are sad, exhausted, overwhelmed and/or carrying heavy backpacks report the highest amounts of lower-back pain.[3]

WHAT CAN YOU DO TO PREVENT BACK PAIN?

▶ **Strengthen and stretch.** Add core strength and flexibility for back health.

▶ **Lose the backpack.** Carry backpacks no heavier than 10-15% of your weight.[4]

▶ **Study standing.** Try standing at a counter to study or walking around as you review for that midterm.

▶ **Sleep smart.** If you're sleeping on your back, put pillows under your knees to cut down the pressure on your lower lumbar area. Or even better, sleep on your side. Avoid sleeping on your stomach.

▶ **Quit smoking.** Smokers have higher rates of back pain than non-smokers.

▶ **Drop the extra pounds.** Extra weight puts a tremendous strain on your back and can ultimately result in back pain.

▶ **Chill!** Feelings associated with stress increase the risk of back pain among college students.[6] Find ways to relax; your back will thank you!

DO YOU SUFFER FROM AN ACHING BACK?
TRY THESE OPTIONS FOR EASING BACK PAIN![5]

Minimize bed rest (1-2 days max)

Cold treatments (2-3 days)

Heat treatments (as needed after acute pain has lessened)

Light movement therapy (walking, swimming, stretching)

Spine treatments with a chiropractor or physical therapist

Alternative treatments (acupuncture, biofeedback, etc.)

Medical advice/treatment after 3 days if pain persists

Pain medications

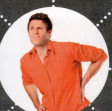

techniques. A review of multiple studies showed that exercise programs prevented back pain episodes in working-age adults, but other strategies, including shoe inserts and back supports, were not effective prevention measures.[23] Incorporating your new fitness knowledge from this course will help you gain strength and stability in your key spine-supporting muscles and reduce your risk of back pain.

Lose Weight The prevalence of lower-back pain rises with increases in body mass index or body weight and body fatness.[24] An increase in body weight puts extra strain and pressure on all the spinal structures. If the additional weight resides in the abdominal region, the pelvis may get pulled forward and result in a greater curvature of the lower back, causing back pain. Lowering your weight and body fat levels to within recommended ranges will reduce your risk of lower-back pain.

Strengthen and Stretch Key Muscles[25] Most people's bodies have "weak" muscle areas, "tight" muscle areas, and areas that are both weak *and* tight.

- *Hip flexor muscles* tend to be tight in most people. This stems from extended sitting, resulting in shortened and inactive muscles. If you have tight hip flexor muscles, add hip flexor stretches (see Figure 5.7) to your weekly workout.

- *Hip extensor muscles* also tend to be tight and weak in many people and can benefit from stretching and strengthening.

- *Trunk flexor muscles* (abdominals) are often weak in individuals who are sedentary or overweight. Having a minimal level of strength in your abdominal muscles will help protect your spine and back and improve your exercise performance.

- *Trunk extensor muscles* are responsible for keeping your spine upright while sitting, standing, and moving. If you do a lot of hunched-over sitting, these muscles are probably weak, and you should add safe back extensor strengthening exercises to your program.

The simplest prescription for back health is to maintain a healthy weight and an active lifestyle. If you are predisposed to back pain due to other reasons (e.g., hyperflexibility, sport history, occupation), try to add some specific back-health exercises to your current exercise routine. **Figure 5.8** (starting on page 192) illustrates back-health exercises that will help you stretch or strengthen the key areas of the trunk and hips; Activate, Motivate, & Advance Your Fitness: A Back-Health Exercise Program at the end of the chapter (page 210) will help you develop a plan to get started.

Maintain Good Posture and Proper Body Mechanics If you have strong and flexible core trunk muscles, maintaining good posture and body mechanics is easier. The problem is that even with good muscular fitness, poor posture can become a habit. You might always hunch over at the computer and feel unnatural sitting up straight. Maybe you slouch back on the couch when you are watching TV. Over time, poor posture can create back problems.

Poor posture and poor muscle fitness can also lead to improper body mechanics while you perform everyday activities. Poor body mechanics put you at risk of muscle strain and back pain. **Lab 5.2** teaches you how to evaluate your posture, and **Figure 5.6** on the following page illustrates proper postures for standing, walking, lifting, sitting, and lying down.

DO IT! ONLINE

- -

THINK! How long each day do you sit hunched over a pile of books, a laptop computer, or looking down at your smart phone?

ACT NOW! Today, notice your posture while sitting and standing. Correct your posture misalignments. Try to self-correct your posture periodically throughout the day. This week, take a break every 20 minutes or so while studying to do shoulder rolls, neck stretches, and dynamic hip and leg movements. In two weeks, write out a plan to keep your back healthy. Include things you can change about your study environment, your exercise plan, and overall lifestyle.

- -

Properly Treat Lower-Back Pain

If you already experience regular back pain, you can do things to help manage your pain and prevent future recurrences. The GetFitGraphic Back Pain and College Students (page 183) lists some strategies for back-pain management.

Standing posture

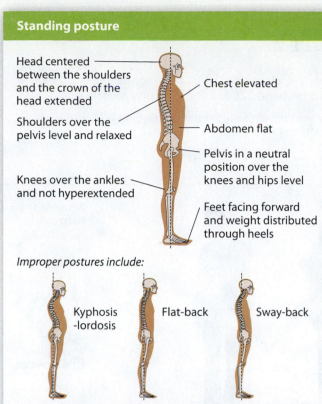

- Head centered between the shoulders and the crown of the head extended
- Shoulders over the pelvis level and relaxed
- Knees over the ankles and not hyperextended
- Chest elevated
- Abdomen flat
- Pelvis in a neutral position over the knees and hips level
- Feet facing forward and weight distributed through heels

Improper postures include:

Kyphosis-lordosis   Flat-back   Sway-back

Walking posture

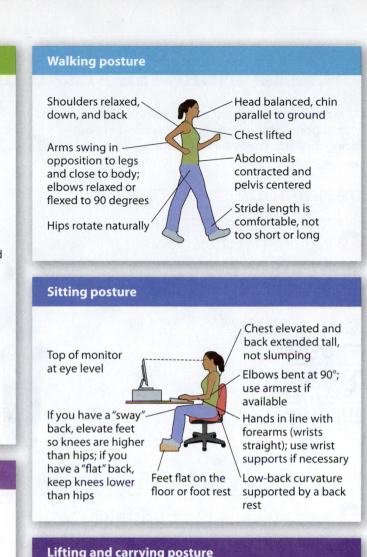

- Shoulders relaxed, down, and back
- Arms swing in opposition to legs and close to body; elbows relaxed or flexed to 90 degrees
- Hips rotate naturally
- Head balanced, chin parallel to ground
- Chest lifted
- Abdominals contracted and pelvis centered
- Stride length is comfortable, not too short or long

Sitting posture

- Top of monitor at eye level
- If you have a "sway" back, elevate feet so knees are higher than hips; if you have a "flat" back, keep knees lower than hips
- Chest elevated and back extended tall, not slumping
- Elbows bent at 90°; use armrest if available
- Hands in line with forearms (wrists straight); use wrist supports if necessary
- Feet flat on the floor or foot rest
- Low-back curvature supported by a back rest

Sleeping posture

Lying on one's back

Medium to firm mattress supports the spine

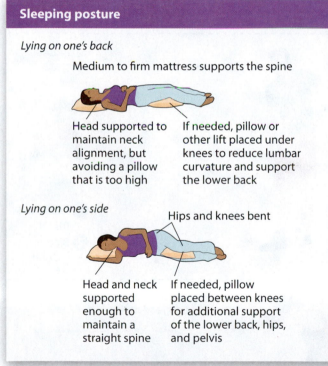

- Head supported to maintain neck alignment, but avoiding a pillow that is too high
- If needed, pillow or other lift placed under knees to reduce lumbar curvature and support the lower back

Lying on one's side

Hips and knees bent

- Head and neck supported enough to maintain a straight spine
- If needed, pillow placed between knees for additional support of the lower back, hips, and pelvis

Lifting and carrying posture

Get help if the weight is too much for you

Bend at the knees and hips; don't bend over at the waist

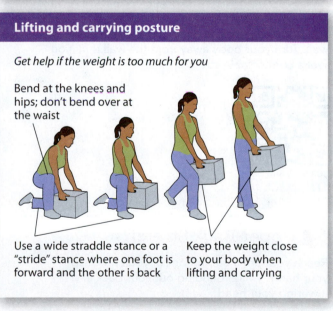

- Use a wide straddle stance or a "stride" stance where one foot is forward and the other is back
- Keep the weight close to your body when lifting and carrying

FIGURE **5.6** Proper posture is important for back health.

FIGURE 5.7

STRETCHES TO MAINTAIN OR INCREASE FLEXIBILITY

All standing stretches should be started or performed from a good posture position (abs pulled in, feet facing forward, knees slightly bent). All one-arm or one-leg stretches should be performed on both sides.

Hold stretches for 10 to 30 seconds. (Refer to Figure 4.8 on page 128 for the full-body muscle diagram.)

Videos for these exercises and more are available online in MasteringHealth.

UPPER-BODY STRETCHES

1 Neck Stretches

(a) **Head turn:** Gently turn your head to look over one shoulder, keeping both of your shoulders down.

(b) **Head tilt:** Keeping your chin level and your shoulders down, tilt your head to one side.

(a)
(b)

SCAN TO SEE IT
ONLINE!

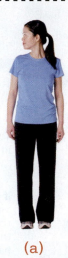

(a)   (b)

Muscles targeted:

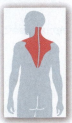

🔟 Trapezius

---

2 Pectoral and Biceps Stretch

Stand arm's length away from a wall. Reach your arm out to the side and place your palm flat on the wall. Turn your body away from the wall until you feel a comfortable stretch.

SCAN TO SEE IT
ONLINE!

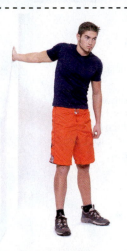

Muscles targeted:

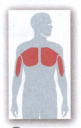

1 Pectoralis major
2 Biceps brachii

---

3 Upper-Back Stretch

Reach your arms out in front of you and clasp your hands while rounding out your back and lowering your head.

SCAN TO SEE IT
ONLINE!

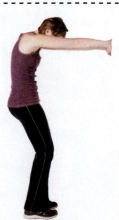

Muscles targeted:

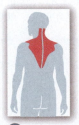

🔟 Trapezius

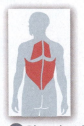

⓫ Rhomboids
⓮ Latissimus dorsi

---

4 Side Stretch

Reach one straight arm over your head and bend sideways at the waist. Focus on reaching up and over with your arm. The opposite hand can reach for the floor or be placed at your hip.

SCAN TO SEE IT
ONLINE!

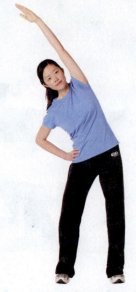

Muscles targeted:

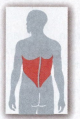 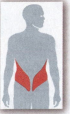

14 Latissimus dorsi   **4** External obliques

5 Shoulder Stretch

Reach one arm across the chest and hold it above or below the elbow with the other hand. Keep both shoulders pressed down.

SCAN TO SEE IT
ONLINE!

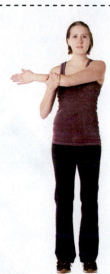

Muscles targeted:

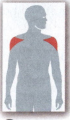

9 Deltoids

6 Triceps Stretch

Lift your arm overhead, reaching the elbow toward the ceiling and the hand down the back. Assist the stretch by using your other hand to either **(a)** press the arm back from the front or **(b)** reach over your head, grasp your arm just below the elbow, and pull back and toward your head.

(a)

SCAN TO SEE IT
ONLINE!

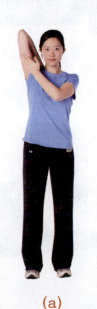

Muscles targeted:

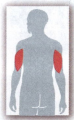

13 Triceps brachii

(a)   (b)

LOWER-BODY STRETCHES

7 Low-Back Knee-to-Chest Stretch

Lie on your back on a mat and lift either **(a)** one knee or **(b)** two knees toward the chest, grasping the leg(s) from behind for support.

(a)

SCAN TO SEE IT
ONLINE!

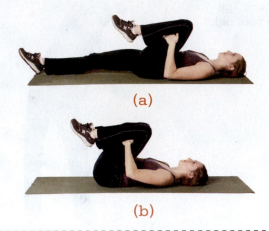

(a)

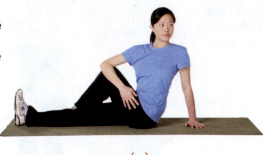

(b)

Muscles targeted:

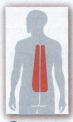

12 Erector spinae

8 Torso Twist and Hip Stretch

(a) Seated twist: Sit on a mat with your legs straight out in front of you. Bend one knee and cross that leg over your other leg. Turn your body toward the bent knee and twist your body to look behind you. Place the opposite arm on the bent leg to gently press into the stretch further.

(b) Lying cross-leg twist: While lying on your back, bend the knee and hip of one leg to 90 degrees. Keep the other leg straight and slowly move the bent leg across your body toward the floor. Keep your arms wide for balance and both shoulders down.

(a)

SCAN TO SEE IT
ONLINE!

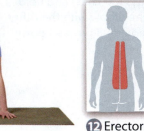

(a)

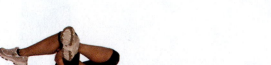

(b)

Muscles targeted:

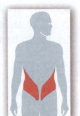

12 Erector spinae

4 External obliques

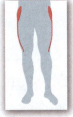

5 Tensor fasciae latae

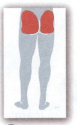

15 Gluteus maximus

9 Gluteal Stretch

Lie on your back with one leg bent and the foot on the floor. Place the ankle of the other leg on your thigh just below the knee. Lift both legs toward the chest and support them with your hands clasped behind your thigh.

SCAN TO SEE IT
ONLINE!

Muscles targeted:

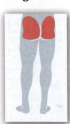

15 Gluteus maximus

10 Hip Flexor Stretch

(a) Standing stretch: Stand tall with one foot forward and one foot back in a lunge position. Lift up the heel of the back leg and press your hips forward.

(b) Low-lunge stretch: Lunge forward and gently place your back knee on a mat and release your foot to point back. Lean forward into the hip and thigh stretch but make sure that your front ankle is directly under your front knee.

(b)

SCAN TO SEE IT
ONLINE!

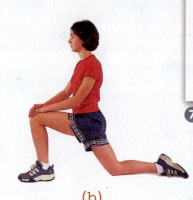

(a)   (b)

Muscles targeted:

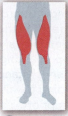

7 Quadriceps

---

11 Inner-Thigh Stretch

(a) Side-lunge stretch: With a wide stance, shift your weight over onto one leg, bending that knee. Press your hips back to ensure that your bent knee does not extend beyond your ankle. Place your hands on your thigh, and keep your chest lifted and back straight.

(b) Butterfly stretch: Sitting on a mat, bring the bottoms of your feet together and pull your feet gently toward you. Actively contract your hip muscles to lower your knees closer to the ground. A slight lean forward will stretch the gluteal and low-back muscles as well.

(b)

SCAN TO SEE IT
ONLINE!

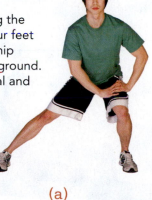

(a)   (b)

Muscles targeted:

6 Adductors

---

12 Outer-Thigh Stretch

Stand at arm's length next to a wall. Place your outside foot on the floor closer to the wall, crossing over the inside leg. Lean your hip closer to the wall while you lean your upper body away from the wall for balance.

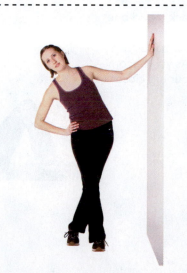

SCAN TO SEE IT
ONLINE!

Muscles targeted:

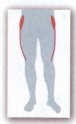

5 Tensor fasciae latae

13 Quadriceps Stretch

Grab your foot from behind and pull it back toward your rear until you feel a stretch in the front of your thighs. Maintain straight body alignment and keep your thighs parallel to one another. When **(a)** standing, assist your balance by holding a wall, a chair, or another form of support. The stretch can also be done from a **(b)** lying down position.

SCAN TO SEE IT
ONLINE!

(a)

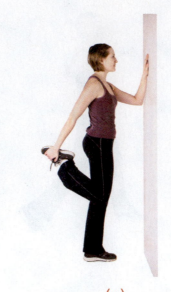

(a)

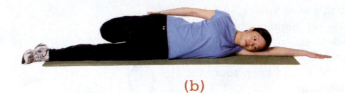

(b)

Muscles targeted:

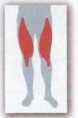

7 Quadriceps

---

14 Hamstrings Stretch

(a) Modified hurdler stretch: Sit with one leg extended and the other leg bent. The bent leg should have the knee facing sideways and the foot placed next to the extended leg near the calf, knee, or thigh. Keeping your back as straight as possible, lean your body forward, moving your chest closer to your extended leg. Your hands can be placed on the floor next to your knee, calf, or ankle for support.

(b) Supine lying: Lying on your back, bend one knee and extend the other toward the ceiling. Support the stretch by placing your hands or a towel above or below the knee. As you become more flexible, work at bringing your leg closer to your chest.

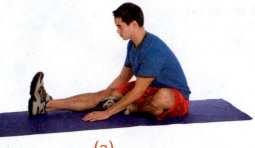

(a)

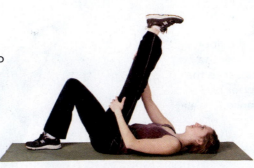

(b)

Muscles targeted:

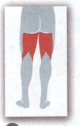

16 Hamstrings

15 Calf Stretches

(a) Gastrocnemius lunge: Lean into a wall in a lunge position, extending one leg straight behind you. Press the heel of your straight leg into the floor as you lean your body and hips into the wall.

(b) Gastrocnemius heel drop: Stand tall and place your toes on a raised surface (mat or step) that will not tip over. Balance by holding on to a wall for support as you lower your heels toward the floor.

(c) Soleus stretch: Starting in a lunge position (a), bend the back knee until you feel a stretch in the soleus muscle.

Muscles targeted:

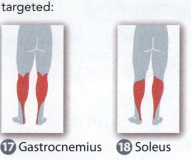

17 Gastrocnemius   18 Soleus

SCAN TO SEE IT
ONLINE!

(a)

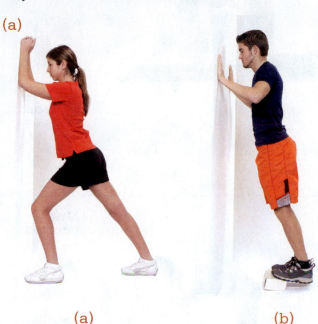

(a)   (b)   (c)

16 Shin Stretch

Reach one leg behind you and place the tips of your toes on the ground. Bend both knees and lower the body slightly as you press the top of your back foot toward the ground. You can use a wall for support if needed.

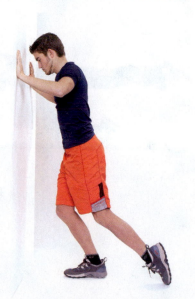

Muscles targeted:

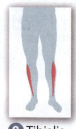

8 Tibialis anterior

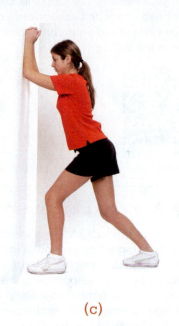

SCAN TO SEE IT
ONLINE!

FIGURE 5.8

EXERCISES FOR A HEALTHY BACK

Perform 3 to 10 repetitions of the back-health exercises, holding where appropriate for 10 to 30 seconds. (See Figure 4.8 on page 128 for a full-body muscle diagram.)

Videos for these exercises and more are available online in MasteringHealth.

1 Cat Stretch

Start on your hands and knees with a flat back. Looking at the ground, align your head with your spine. Drop your head and look back toward your knees while lifting your upper back toward the ceiling.

SCAN TO SEE IT
ONLINE!

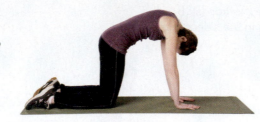

Muscles targeted:

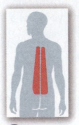 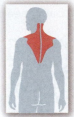

12 Erector spinae   **10** Trapezius; various neck muscles

2 Arm/Leg Extensions

Start on your hands and knees with a flat back. Looking at the ground, align your head with your spine. Extend your arm straight out in front of you while extending the opposite leg straight out behind you. Keep your arm and leg in a straight line with your spine. Do not lift them too high, because this causes too much arch in your lower back.

SCAN TO SEE IT
ONLINE!

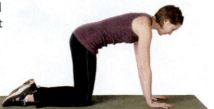

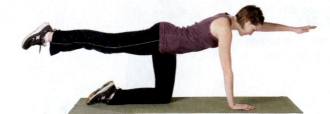

Muscles targeted:

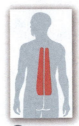 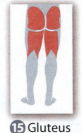

12 Erector spinae   **15** Gluteus maximus
                         16 Hamstrings

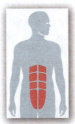

3 Rectus abdominis

③ Pelvic Tilt

Lie on your back with your knees bent and your feet flat on the floor. Relax in a comfortable posture, letting the natural curve of your spine bring your lower back off the mat. Breathe out as you tilt the bottom of your pelvis toward the ceiling, pulling your abdominals in and pressing your lower back flat against the floor.

SCAN TO SEE IT
ONLINE!

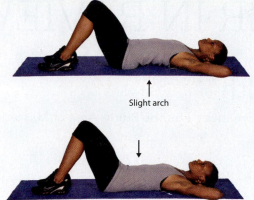
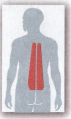

Slight arch

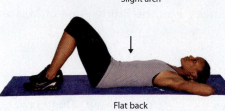

Flat back

Muscles targeted:

⑫ Erector spinae

③ Rectus abdominis; various hip/pelvis stabilizers

---

④ Back Bridge

Lie on your back with your knees bent, your feet flat on the floor, and your arms extended straight along your sides. Lift your hips off the ground and press your pelvis toward the ceiling until your thighs and back are in a straight line. Look at the ceiling and keep your neck extended throughout the exercise (do not tuck your chin to your chest).

SCAN TO SEE IT
ONLINE!

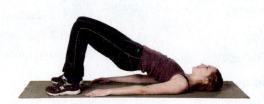

Muscles targeted:

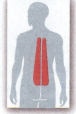
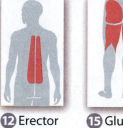

⑫ Erector spinae

⑮ Gluteus maximus
⑯ Hamstrings

Other exercises that can help maintain back health include:

Plank (p. 142)
Side bridge (p. 141)
Knee-to-chest stretch (p. 188)
Hamstring stretch (p. 190)

Torso twist and hip stretch (p. 188)
Hip flexor stretch (p. 189)
Abdominal curl (p. 140)
Oblique curl (p. 141)

CHAPTER IN REVIEW

MasteringHealth™

Build your knowledge—and wellness!—in the Study Area of MasteringHealth with a variety of study tools.

SEE IT! ONLINE

videos
Flexibility Exercises
Core Strength Exercises
Assessments

HEAR IT! ONLINE

audio tools
Audio case study
MP3 chapter review

REVIEW IT! ONLINE

chapter review
Chapter reading quizzes
Glossary flashcards

LIVE IT! ONLINE

programs & behavior change
Customizable four-week flexibility training programs
Customizable four-week back-health exercise programs
Behavior Change Logbook and Wellness Journal

DO IT! ONLINE

labs
Lab 5.1 Assess Your Flexibility
Lab 5.2 Evaluate Your Posture
Lab 5.3 Planning a Flexibility Program
Alternate Labs for Assessing Flexibility

review questions

1. _____ is a measure of your overall joint stiffness during movement.
   a. Dynamic flexibility
   b. Static flexibility
   c. Passive flexibility
   d. Anatomical flexibility

2. Which of the following triggers a muscle to relax when there is too much force or tension in the muscle?
   a. Muscle spindle
   b. Baroreceptor
   c. Golgi tendon organ
   d. Reflex receptor

3. The intensity of each stretch should be stretching until you reach
   a. your toes.
   b. the point of tightness.
   c. moderate burning pain.
   d. your goal.

4. Stretching that involves voluntary muscle contractions to facilitate relaxation describes
   a. static stretching.
   b. dynamic stretching.
   c. ballistic stretching.
   d. PNF stretching.

5. Which of the following exercise styles uses a slow-moving series of forms to increase coordination, balance, and flexibility?
   a. Dance
   b. Pilates
   c. Yoga
   d. Tai chi

6. Which of the following is the primary underlying cause of low-back pain?
   a. Poor posture
   b. Sedentary living
   c. Muscle weakness
   d. Poor flexibility

7. The fluid of an intervertebral disc bulging outward and pressing on the nervous-system structures in the spine is best described as disc
   a. dehydration.
   b. degeneration.
   c. herniation.
   d. hardening.

8. Which of the following sleep postures creates the most tension in your lower back and is not recommended?
   a. Lying on your side
   b. Lying on your stomach
   c. Lying on your back
   d. Sleeping in a chair

9. What approximate percentage of people will experience lower-back pain at some point in their lives?
   a. 25 percent
   b. 50 percent
   c. 70 percent
   d. 100 percent

10. Which of the following acute back pain self-care treatments is not recommended?
    a. Five days of bed rest
    b. Light exercise
    c. Pain relievers
    d. Cold and hot treatments

critical thinking questions

1. Explain how stretching can improve your posture and balance.
2. Describe how reducing the stretch reflex will enhance the effectiveness of your stretches.
3. Have you ever done or been asked to do a contraindicated stretch? What would be an equally effective alternative?
4. List three occupations that present high risk for low-back pain and explain why.

references

1. M. Nolan et al., "Age-related Changes in Musculoskeletal Function, Balance and Mobility Measures in Men aged 30–80 years," *Aging Male* 13, no. 3 (2010): 194–201, doi: 10.3109/13685531003657818.

2. M. J. Spink et al., "Foot and Ankle Strength, Range of Motion, Posture, and Deformity Are Associated with Balance and Functional Ability in Older Adults," *Archives of Physical Medicine and Rehabilitation* 92, no. 1 (2011): 68–75, doi: 10.1016/j.apmr.2010.09.024.

3. J. R. Pleis et al., National Center for Health Statistics, "Summary Health Statistics for U.S. Adults: National Health Interview Survey, 2009," *Vital Health Statistics* 10, no. 249 (2010).

4. H. B. Sun, "Mechanical Loading, Cartilage Degradation, and Arthritis," *Annals of the New York Academy of Science* 1211 (2010): 37–50, doi: 10.1111/j.17496632.2010.05808.x; J. K. Cooney et al., "Benefits of Exercise in Rheumatoid Arthritis," *Journal of Aging Research* (2011): 681640, doi: 10.4061/2011/681640; Y. Escalante, A. García-Hermoso, and J. M. Saavedra, "Effects of Exercise on Functional Aerobic Capacity in Lower Limb Osteoarthritis: A Systematic Review," *Journal of Science and Medicine in Sport* 14, no. 3 (2011): 190–8, doi: 10.1016/j.jsams.2010.10.004.

5. F. R. Moyano et al., "Effectiveness of Different Exercises and Stretching Physiotherapy on Pain and Movement in Patellofemoral Pain Syndrome: A Randomized Controlled Trial," *Clinical Rehabilitation* 27, no. 5 (2013): 409–17, doi: 10.1177/0269215512459277.

6. D. Perich et al., "Low Back Pain in Adolescent Female Rowers: A Multi-Dimensional Intervention Study," *Knee Surgery, Sports Traumatology, Arthroscopy* 19, no. 1 (2011): 20–9, doi: 10.1007/s00167-010-1173-6.

7. I. Calvo-Muñoz, A. Gómez-Conesa, and J. Sánchez-Meca, "Physical Therapy Treatments for Low Back Pain in Children and Adolescents: A Meta-Analysis," *BMC Musculoskeletal Disorders* 14 (2013): 55, doi: 10.1186/1471-2474-14-55.

8. P. W. Marshall, J. Mannion, and B. A. Murphy, "Extensibility of the Hamstrings Is Best Explained by Mechanical Components of Muscle Contraction, Not Behavioral Measures in Individuals with Chronic Low Back Pain," *PM&R: The Journal of Injury, Function, and Rehabilitation* 1, no. 8 (2009): 709–18, doi: 10.1016/j.pmrj.2009.04.009.

9. E. N. Johnson and J. S. Thomas, "Effect of Hamstring Flexibility on Hip and Lumbar Spine Joint Excursions during Forward-Reaching Tasks in Participants with and without Low Back Pain," *Archives of Physical Medicine and Rehabilitation* 91, no. 7 (2010): 1140–2, doi: 10.1016/j.apmr.2010.04.003.

10. National Institute of Neurological Disorders and Stroke, *Low Back Pain Fact Sheet* NIH Publication No. 03-5161 (Bethesda, MD: Office of Communications and Public Liaison, National Institutes of Health, 2003), www.ninds.nih.gov

11. R. J. Johns and V. Wright, "Relative Importance of Various Tissues in Joint Stiffness," *Journal of Applied Physiology* 17, no. 5 (1962): 824–8.

12. H. O. Kendall, F. P. Kendall, and G. E. Bennett, "Normal Flexibility According to Age Groups," *Journal of Bone and Joint Surgery* 30A, no. 3 (1948): 690–4; M. J. Alter, *The Science of Flexibility* (Champaign, IL: Human Kinetics, 2004).

13. R. Simão et al., "The influence of Strength, Flexibility, and Simultaneous Training on Flexibility and Strength Gains," *Journal of Strength & Conditioning Research* 25, no. 5 (2011): 1333–8, doi: 10.1519/JSC.0b013e3181da85bf.

14. M. Amiri-Khorasani, N. A. Abu Osman, and A. Yusof, "Acute Effect of Static and Dynamic Stretching on Hip Dynamic Range of Motion during Instep Kicking in Professional Soccer Players," *Journal of Strength Conditioning Research* 25, no. 6 (2011): 1647–52, doi: 10.1519/JSC.0b013e3181db9f41.

15. G. Z. MacDonald et al., "An Acute Bout of Self-Myofascial Release Increases Range of Motion Without a Subsequent Decrease in Muscle Activation or Force," *Journal of Strength and Conditioning Research* 27, no. 3 (2013): 812–21, doi: 10.1519/JSC.0b013e31825c2bc1; K. C. Healey et al., "The Effects of Myofascial Release with Foam Rolling on Performance," *Journal of Strength and Conditioning Research* (2013): [Epub ahead of print].

16. D. G. Dolny and G. F. Reyes, "Whole Body Vibration Exercise: Training and

Benefits," *Current Sports Medicine Reports* 7, no. 3 (2008): 152–7, doi: 10.1097/01. CSMR.0000319708.18052.a1; R. Di Giminiani et al., "Effects of Individualized Whole-Body Vibration on Muscle Flexibility and Mechanical Power," *Journal of Sports Medicine Physical Fitness* 50, no. 2 (2010): 139–51; S. L. Ferguson et al., "Comparing the Effect of 3 Weeks of Upper Body Vibration Training, Vibration and Stretching, and Stretching Alone on Shoulder Flexibility in College-Aged Males," *Journal of Strength & Conditioning Research* (2013): [Epub ahead of print].

17. J. B. Feland et al., "Whole Body Vibration as an Adjunct to Static Stretching," *International Journal of Sports Medicine* 31, no. 8 (2010): 584–9, doi: 10.1055/s-0030-1254084.

18. National Center for Health Statistics, Health Promotion Statistics Branch, CDC Wonder. *DATA2010… the Healthy People 2010 Database* (Hyattsville, MD: Centers for Disease Control, 2010), http://wonder.cdc.gov

19. Centers for Disease Control and Prevention, "Prevalence and Most Common Causes of Disability among Adults—United States, 2005," *Morbidity and Mortality Weekly Report* 58, no. 16 (2009): 421–6.

20. B. I. Martin et al., "Expenditures and Health Status Among Adults with Back and Neck Problems," *JAMA* 299, no. 6 (2008): 656–64, doi: 10.1001/jama.299.6.656.

21. R. Shiri et al., "The Association Between Smoking and Low Back Pain: A Meta-Analysis," *The American Journal of Medicine* 123, no. 1 (2010): 87.e7–35, doi: 10.1016/j.amjmed.2009.05.028.

22. National Institute of Neurological Disorders and Stroke, *Low Back Pain Fact Sheet,* NIH Publication No. 03-5161 (Bethesda, MD: Office of Communications and Public Liaison, National Institutes of Health, 2003).

23. S. J. Bigos et al., "High-quality Controlled Trials on Preventing Episodes of Back Problems: Systematic Literature Review in Working-Age Adults," *The Spine Journal: Official Journal of the North American Spine Society* 9, no. 2 (2009): 147–68, doi: 10.1016/j.spinee.2008.11.001.

24. D. M. Urquhart et al., "Increased Fat Mass Is Associated with High Levels of Low Back Pain Intensity and Disability," *Spine (Philadelphia, p. 1976)* 36, no. 16 (2011): 1320–5, doi: 10.1097/BRS.0b013e3181f9fb66.

25. K. Ohtsuki, "The Immediate Changes in Patients with Acute Exacerbation of Chronic Lower-Back Pain Elicited by Direct Stretching of the Tensor Fasciae Latae, the Hamstrings and the Adductor Magnus," *Journal of Physical Therapy Science* 24 (2012): 707–9.

getfitgraphic references

1. J. R. Pleis, B. W. Ward, and J. W. Lucas, "Summary Health Statistics for U.S. Adults: National Health Interview Survey, 2009," *Vital and Health Statistics* 10, no. 249 (2010): 1–207.

2. Z. Heuscher et al., "The Association of Self-Reported Backpack Use and Backpack Weight with Low Back Pain among College Students," *Journal of Manipulative Physiological Therapy* 33, no. 6 (2011): 432–7, doi: 10.1016/j.jmpt.2010.06.003; C. Kennedy et al., "Psychosocial Factors and Low Back Pain among College Students," *Journal of American College Health* 57, no. 2 (2008): 191–5, doi: 10.3200/JACH.57.2.191-196.

3. Ibid.

4. North American Spine Society, Back Pack Safety, www.knowyourback.org

5. C. Kennedy et al., "Psychosocial Factors and Low Back Pain Among College Students," 2008.

6. National Institute of Arthritis and Musculoskeletal and Skin Diseases, Back Pain NIH Publication No. 09-5282 (Information Clearinghouse, National Institutes of Health: Bethesda, MD, 2010).

LAB 5.1

ASSESS YOUR FLEXIBILITY

MasteringHealth™

Name: _____   Date: _____

Instructor: _____   Section: _____

Materials: Exercise mat, sit-and-reach box, a partner

Purpose: To assess your current level of lower-back, hip, and hamstring flexibility and your current level of joint mobility or range of motion.

SECTION I: THE SIT-AND-REACH TEST

This test measures the general flexibility of your lower back, hips, and hamstrings. The results are specific to those regions of your body and do not reflect your flexibility in other body areas.

1. Warm up. Complete 3 to 10 minutes of light cardiorespiratory activity to warm up your body and then perform light range-of-motion exercises and stretches for the joints and muscles that you will be using.

2. Prepare for the box sit-and-reach test.

SCAN TO SEE IT
ONLINE!

Place the sit-and-reach box against a wall to prevent it from moving during the test. Sit without shoes behind the box, place your feet flat against the box at the 26-cm mark (the "zero" or foot mark for this test), and put your hands on top of the box.

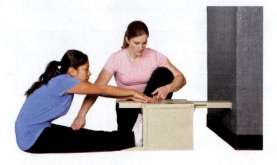

3. Properly perform the test. Keep one hand on top of the other. It is important that fingertips remain together and that your hands remain in contact with the box ruler at all times. Reach forward as far as you can by slowly bending forward, reaching with your arms, and sliding your fingertips out along the box. Keep your legs straight, drop your head between your arms, and breathe out as you perform the test. Hold your ending position for at least two seconds. Your partner will watch to ensure that you have proper hand position and straight legs during the test.

4. Find your reach distance. Your *reach distance* is the most distant point reached with both fingertips. If you cannot keep your hands from separating, the most distant point reached by the fingertips of the *hand that is farthest back* should be considered the reach distance. Record the reach distance in centimeters. Perform the test twice. Have your partner point to your reach distance for each trial. Record your best reach distance of the two trials in the RESULTS section on the next page.

FLEXIBILITY RESULTS

Box Sit-and-Reach Test: Reach Distance (cm): _____   Rating: _____

5. **Find your flexibility rating by using the charts provided below.** Your rating tells you how you compare to others who have completed this test in the past. Record your rating in the RESULTS section above.

BOX Sit-and-Reach Test (centimeters)					
Men (age in years)	**Excellent**	**Very Good**	**Good**	**Fair**	**Needs Improvement**
15–19	≥39	34–38	29–33	24–28	≤23
20–29	≥40	34–39	30–33	25–29	≤24
30–39	≥38	33–37	28–32	23–27	≤22
40–49	≥35	29–34	24–28	18–23	≤17
50–59	≥35	28–34	24–27	16–23	≤15
60–69	≥33	25–32	20–24	15–19	≤14
Women (age in years)	**Excellent**	**Very Good**	**Good**	**Fair**	**Needs Improvement**
15–19	≥43	38–42	34–37	29–33	≤28
20–29	≥41	37–40	33–36	28–32	≤27
30–39	≥41	36–40	32–35	27–31	≤26
40–49	≥38	34–37	30–33	25–29	≤24
50–59	≥39	33–38	30–32	25–29	≤24
60–69	≥35	31–34	27–30	23–26	≤22

Source: *Canadian Physical Activity, Fitness & Lifestyle Approach: CSEP-Health & Fitness Program's Health-Related Appraisal & Counseling Strategy*, 3rd edition © 2003. Reprinted with permission from the Canadian Society for Exercise Physiology.

SECTION II: JOINT MOBILITY—RANGE-OF-MOTION TESTS

Range-of-motion tests assess your joints' ability to move through a normal range of motion. Follow the instructions for each of the tests shown below. Perform each test on both your right and left sides. Stop each movement when you feel resistance. To avoid injury, do not try to push past your normal range. Have a partner observe your movements, "eyeball" your estimated joint angle, and record your range-of-motion results on page 200.

SCAN TO SEE IT
ONLINE!

1. **Neck Lateral Flexion—** Sit or stand with your head neutral and looking forward. Tilt your head to the side and drop your ear toward your shoulder.

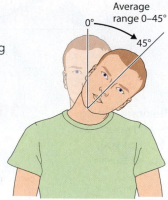

Average range 0–45°

0°
45°

2. **Shoulder Flexion—** Starting with your arms at your sides, reach a straight arm forward and up toward your head.

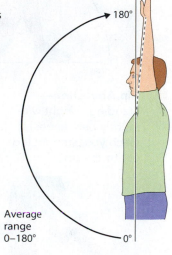

180°

0°

Average range 0–180°

3. **Shoulder Extension—** With your arms at your sides, reach a straight arm behind you and up.

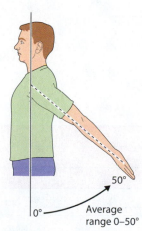

50°

0°

Average range 0–50°

4. **Shoulder Abduction—** Reach your straight arm out to the side and up to your head.

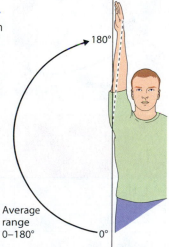

180°

0°

Average range 0–180°

5. **Shoulder Adduction—**Reach your straight arm down and across your body in front.

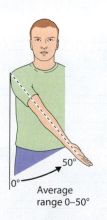

50°

0°

Average range 0–50°

6. **Trunk Lateral Flexion—** Standing upright with slightly bent knees and your arms at your sides, bend your torso sideways and reach your arm down your leg for support.

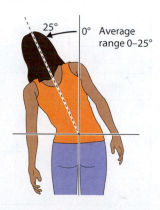

25°
0° Average range 0–25°

7. Hip Flexion—Lying on your back, lift a straight leg up into the air while keeping the other leg bent with the foot flat on the ground.

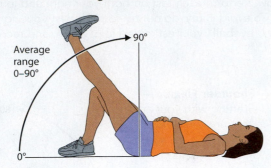

8. Hip Extension—Lying on your stomach with your head on the mat, reach your straight leg up behind you, keeping the other leg flat on the ground.

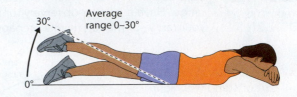

9. Hip Abduction—Standing upright with slightly bent knees, reach your straight leg out to the side.

10. Ankle Dorsiflexion—Sitting without shoes and your legs extended in front of you, flex your foot back toward your knee.

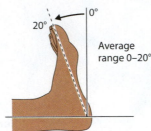

11. Ankle Plantar Flexion—Sitting without shoes and your legs extended in front of you, point your foot toward the floor.

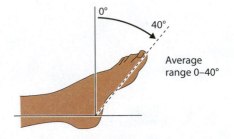

Joint Mobility RESULTS				
	Movement and Average Range (degrees)	**Full Average Joint Range?**		
Joint		*Right Side*		*Left Side*
1. Neck	Lateral Flexion 0–45	_____ Yes _____ No		_____ Yes _____ No
2. Shoulder	Flexion 0–180	_____ Yes _____ No		_____ Yes _____ No
3. Shoulder	Extension 0–50	_____ Yes _____ No		_____ Yes _____ No
4. Shoulder	Abduction 0–180	_____ Yes _____ No		_____ Yes _____ No
5. Shoulder	Adduction 0–50	_____ Yes _____ No		_____ Yes _____ No
6. Trunk	Lateral Flexion 0–25	_____ Yes _____ No		_____ Yes _____ No
7. Hip	Flexion 0–90	_____ Yes _____ No		_____ Yes _____ No
8. Hip	Extension 0–30	_____ Yes _____ No		_____ Yes _____ No
9. Hip	Abduction 0–40	_____ Yes _____ No		_____ Yes _____ No
10. Ankle	Dorsiflexion 0–20	_____ Yes _____ No		_____ Yes _____ No
11. Ankle	Plantar Flexion 0–40	_____ Yes _____ No		_____ Yes _____ No

Sources: Adapted from American College of Sports Medicine, *ACSM's Health-Related Physical Fitness Assessment Manual*, 3rd edition (Baltimore, MD: Lippincott Williams & Wilkins, 2009); American College of Sports Medicine, *ACSM's Resource Manual for Guidelines for Exercise Testing and Prescription*, 6th edition (Baltimore, MD: Lippincott Williams & Wilkins, 2009).

SECTION III: REFLECTION

1. Were your flexibility and range-of-motion results what you expected? Why or why not?

_____

_____

_____

_____

_____

2. Based upon your flexibility assessment results, is your basic plan to maintain or improve flexibility?

_____

_____

_____

_____

_____

Name: _____   Date: _____

Instructor: _____   Section: _____

Purpose: To evaluate your posture.

SECTION I: POSTURE EVALUATION

Before you begin: Wear clothing that will not interfere with the assessment of your posture. If it is comfortable, men should wear shorts only, and women should wear shorts and a tank top. Remove your shoes. If you have long hair, pull it back into a ponytail for the assessment.

Stand against a wall and have a partner evaluate your posture using the chart on page 203. Your partner should assign you a score of between 1 and 5 for each of the 10 areas of your body shown on the next page.

SCAN TO SEE IT
ONLINE!

Posture Results	
Posture Score	*Posture Rating*
45 or higher	Excellent
40–44	Good
30–39	Average
20–29	Fair
19 or less	Poor

Source: Based on the *New York State Physical Fitness Test for Boys and Girls Grades 4–12. A Manual for Teachers of Physical Education*, Division of Physical Education and Research, State University of New York (Albany, NY: New York State Education Dept., 1972).

SECTION II: REFLECTION

1. Did your partner find anything surprising to you about your posture? If so, why do you think you were not aware of it?

_____

_____

2. Based upon your posture evaluation results, is your basic plan to maintain or improve your posture?

_____

_____

	Good—5	Fair—3	Poor—1	Score
Head	Head erect, gravity passes directly through center	Head twisted or turned to one side slightly	Head twisted or turned to one side markedly	
Shoulders	Shoulders level horizontally	One shoulder slightly higher	One shoulder markedly higher	
Spine	Spine straight	Spine slightly curved	Spine markedly curved laterally	
Hips	Hips level horizontally	One hip slightly higher	One hip markedly higher	
Knees and **Ankles**	Feet pointed straight ahead, legs vertical	Feet pointed out, legs deviating outward at the knee	Feet pointed out markedly, legs deviated markedly	
Neck and **Upper back**	Neck erect, head in line with shoulders, rounded upper back	Neck slightly foward, chin out, slightly more rounded upper back	Neck markedly forward, chin markedly out, markedly rounded upper back	
Trunk	Trunk erect	Trunk inclined to rear slightly	Trunk inclined to rear markedly	
Abdomen	Abdomen flat	Abdomen protruding	Abdomen protruding and sagging	
Lower back	Lower back normally curved	Lower back slightly hollow	Lower back markedly hollow	
Legs	Legs straight	Knees slightly hyperextended	Knees markedly hyperextended	
			Total score	

LAB 5.3

PLANNING A FLEXIBILITY PROGRAM

MasteringHealth™

Name: _____ **Date:** _____

Instructor: _____ **Section:** _____

Materials: Results from Lab 5.1

Purpose: To learn how to set appropriate flexibility goals and create a personal flexibility program.

SECTION I: SHORT- AND LONG-TERM GOALS

Create short- and long-term goals for flexibility and back health. Be sure to use SMART goal-setting guidelines. Select appropriate target dates and rewards for completing your goals.

Short-Term Goal for Flexibility (3 to 6 months)

_____

_____

Target Date: _____

Reward: _____

Optional: Short-Term Goal for Back Health (3 to 6 months)

_____

_____

Target Date: _____

Reward: _____

Long-Term Goal for Flexibility (12+ months)

_____

_____

Target Date: _____

Reward: _____

Optional: Long-Term Goal for Back Health (12+ months)

_____

_____

Target Date: _____

Reward: _____

SECTION II: FLEXIBILITY PROGRAM DESIGN

Complete one line for each exercise you have chosen to do in your program.

Stretching Exercises	Frequency (days/week)	Time (sec)	Reps (number)	Total Time (sec)
LOWER BODY				
1.				
2.				
3.				
4.				
5.				
6.				
7.				
8.				
UPPER BODY				
1.				
2.				
3.				
4.				
5.				
6.				
7.				
8.				

SECTION III: TRACKING YOUR PROGRAM AND FOLLOWING THROUGH

1. **Goal and Program Tracking:** Use the following chart to monitor your progress. Change the frequency, time, sets, and reps frequently to ensure continuing progress toward your goals.

2. **Goal and Program Follow-up:** At the end of the course or at your short-term goal target date, reevaluate your flexibility and answer the following questions:

a. Did you meet your short-term goal or your goal for the course? _____

b. If so, what positive behavioral changes contributed to your success? If not, which obstacles blocked your success?

_____

_____

c. Was your short-term goal realistic? After evaluating your progress during the course, what would you change about your goals or training plan?

_____

_____

Flexibility Training Log		
Date	Stretches Completed (with time/reps)	Comments (e.g., stretches modified, stretches held longer, how you felt)

Activate, Motivate,
& ADVANCE YOUR FITNESS

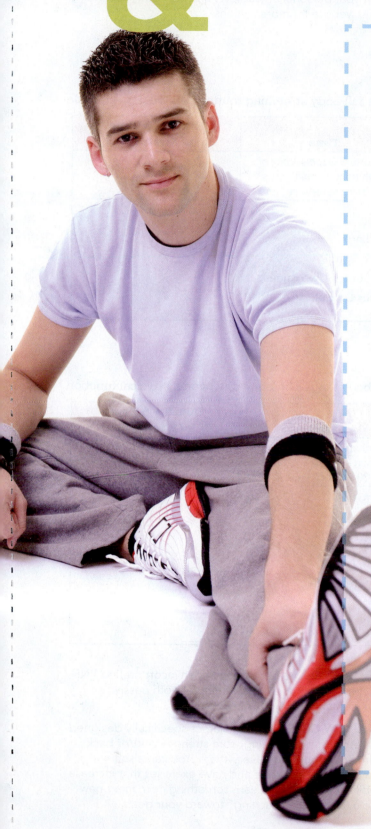

A FLEXIBILITY TRAINING PROGRAM

SCAN TO SEE IT **ONLINE!**

ACTIVATE!

Looking to improve your posture, circulation, and joint mobility? Follow these programs to gradually incorporate regular stretching into your weekly exercise routines.

What Do I Need for Flexibility Training?

GEAR: For flexibility training programs, you'll want a mat, towel, and something stable to hold onto for standing stretches. While you really don't need any other equipment for stretching, you may want to use a strap, foam roller, yoga block, or even a training partner.

CLOTHING: Wear comfortable clothing that allows for full range-of-motion movements.

How Do I Start a Flexibility Training Program?

TECHNIQUE: Safe and effective flexibility training depends on good body alignment and awareness. Read through each exercise description and take time to learn the proper form. If you need assistance, ask your instructor or a fitness specialist at your facility. Perform static stretches in a slow and controlled manner. Hold at the point of tightness but not pain. Exhale with the stretching exercise to help you relax and increase your flexibility.

ETIQUETTE: Most facilities will have mats, equipment, and a designated stretching area for you to use. Wipe down your mat or any other equipment after use.

STRETCHING BEFORE A WORKOUT: Dynamic stretching (stretching through movement) performed during your warm-up can prepare your body for the upcoming more intense activity. Incorporate slow and controlled movements that mimic the motions of your workout.

STRETCHING AFTER A WORKOUT: After your workout program, your muscles are warm and ready to be stretched. Static or PNF stretching performed at this time will result in the biggest gains in flexibility, particularly after a cardiorespiratory workout.

Flexibility Training Warm-Up & Cool-Down

Warming-up prior to stretching is crucial and should include gentle cardiorespiratory exercises for 5 to 10 minutes. After breaking a light sweat, add dynamic movements that increase your range of motion. Ease into the first repetition of each static or PNF stretching exercise. Ensure proper form, posture, and body alignment as you move into your full range of motion.

Flexibility Training Programs

If you are new to flexibility training or if you have not stretched for more than three months, start slowly and build gradually with the Beginner program. If you already stretch two days a week, then start with the Intermediate program. Adjust intensity, volume, and training days to suit your personal fitness level and schedule; visit the mobile website for more options.

BEGINNER

FLEXIBILITY PROGRAM GOAL: Incorporate a full-body stretching routine into weekly schedule

Frequency	Intensity	Time	Number & Type of Stretches
2 nonconsecutive days a week	Stretch to a point of mild tightness, not pain	Perform 2–3 repetitions of each stretch, holding for 10–20 seconds each time	8 static stretches

Order of Stretches

Side Stretch

Upper-Back Stretch

Pectoral and Biceps Stretch

Inner-Thigh Side Lunge

Quadriceps Stretch (Standing)

Hamstrings Stretch (Supine Lying)

Low-Back Knee-to-Chest Stretch (Two Knees)

Calf Stretch (Gastrocnemius Lunge)

INTERMEDIATE

FLEXIBILITY PROGRAM GOAL: Improve full body range of motion and overall physical function

Frequency	Intensity	Time	Number & Type of Stretches
3 nonconsecutive days a week	Stretch to a point of mild tightness, not pain	Perform 2–4 repetitions of each stretch, holding for 20–30 seconds each time	12 static stretches

Order of Stretches

Neck Stretches (Head Turn)

Side Stretch

Upper-Back Stretch

Shoulder Stretch

Pectoral and Biceps Stretch

Inner-Thigh Side Lunge

Outer-Thigh Stretch

Quadriceps Stretch (Lying)

Hamstrings Stretch (Supine Lying)

Low-Back Knee-to-Chest Stretch (Two Knees)

Gluteal Stretch

Calf Stretch (Heel Drop)

MOTIVATE!

Create your own exercise log to track your flexibility training program—make note of days, actual stretches, type of stretch, repetitions, time—or use the log available through the mobile website. Here are a few tips to keep you stretching.

FIND A PARTNER: With a stretching partner, you can keep each other accountable, help each other reach goals, and have greater options when incorporating PNF stretches, as well as a wider variety of both passive and active stretches. Bye-bye boredom!

TRY A NEW CLASS: Shorter classes specifically designed for stretching, foam rolling, core strength, and/or back health are popping up everywhere. You can also try a yoga or martial arts class and have exercises that increase flexibility built right in! Learn something new, meet new people, and keep "reaching" toward your goals.

STRESS? WHAT STRESS? Take a deep breath. Exhale. Slowly move into your stretch. Hold for at least 10 seconds. Repeat three more times. Before you know it you will feel refreshed and relaxed from head to toe. The simple act of performing your flexibility program can increase your circulation, decrease your blood pressure, and keep you calm and focused. Stretch more, stress less!

ADVANCE!

Now that you have established your flexibility program, you might find that you want more stretches that are specific to your sport or activity. Below are three more advanced flexibility programs specific for walkers/runners, cyclists, and swimmers. You can follow these or log onto the mobile website to find more options or simply to personalize this program or any of the programs in this book.

WALKING/RUNNING

FLEXIBILITY PROGRAM GOAL: Add stretches of specific use for walkers and runners

Frequency	Intensity	Time	Number & Type of Stretches
3 nonconsecutive days a week	Stretch to a point of mild tightness, not pain	Perform 2–4 repetitions of each stretch, holding for 20–30 seconds each time	5 additional static stretches*

*Perform following a walking/running cardiorespiratory workout, and in addition to the Intermediate Flexibility Program.

Stretches to Add

Hip Flexor Stretch (Standing for walkers and Low Lunge for runners)

Torso Twist and Hip Stretch (Seated Twist)

Hamstrings Stretch (Modified Hurdler)

Calf Stretch (Soleus Stretch)

Shin Stretch

CYCLING

FLEXIBILITY PROGRAM GOAL: Add stretches of specific use for cyclists

Frequency	Intensity	Time	Number & Type of Stretches
3 nonconsecutive days a week	Stretch to a point of mild tightness, not pain	Perform 2–4 repetitions of each stretch, holding for 20–30 seconds each time	5 additional static stretches*

*Perform following a cycling cardiorespiratory workout, and in addition to the Intermediate Flexibility Program.

Stretches to Add

Neck Stretches (Head Tilt)

Hip Flexor Stretch (Standing or Low Lunge)

Torso Twist and Hip Stretch (Seated Twist)

Calf Stretch (Soleus Stretch)

Shin Stretch

SWIMMING

FLEXIBILITY PROGRAM GOAL: Add stretches of specific use for swimmers

Frequency	Intensity	Time	Number & Type of Stretches
3 nonconsecutive days a week	Stretch to a point of mild tightness, not pain	Perform 2–4 repetitions of each stretch, holding for 20–30 seconds each time	5 additional static stretches

*Perform following a swimming cardiorespiratory workout, and in addition to the Intermediate Flexibility Program.

Stretches to Add

Neck Stretches (Head Tilt)

Triceps Stretch

Hip Flexor Stretch (Standing)

Torso Twist and Hip Stretch (Seated Twist)

Shin Stretch

Activate, Motivate,
& ADVANCE YOUR FITNESS

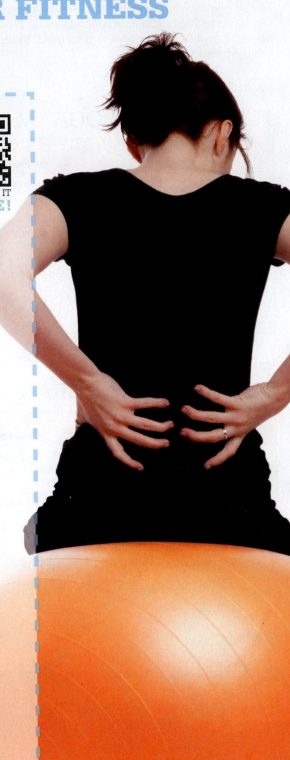

A BACK-HEALTH EXERCISE PROGRAM

SCAN TO SEE IT
ONLINE!

Want to avoid back pain or manage pain you may already have? Try the core stretching and strengthening exercise programs outlined on the next page. They are specifically designed to help you increase the strength of your core trunk muscles and decrease tightness. Combine the Core Muscular Endurance and the Core Flexibility programs for a full-core back-health program. Together, these programs can stand alone; however, the exercises are designed to be incorporated into your current muscular fitness and flexibility programs. Visit the mobile website to find more options or to personalize this or any of the programs in this book.

CORE MUSCULAR ENDURANCE PROGRAM FOR BACK HEALTH

GOAL: Increase core muscle endurance and strength

Frequency	Intensity	Time			Number & Type of Exercises
		Reps	*Sets*	*Rest*	
2 nonconsecutive days a week	60% 1RM	12	2	2 minutes between sets	8 core muscle exercises

Core Strength Exercises

Arm/Leg Extensions

Plank (hold each plank for 15 to 30 seconds and complete 2 to 4 repetitions)

Back Extension

Abdominal Curl

Reverse Curl

Oblique Curl

Pelvic Tilt

Side Bridge (hold each side bridge for 15 seconds and complete 4 repetitions)

CORE FLEXIBILITY PROGRAM FOR BACK HEALTH

GOAL: Decrease core muscle tightness

Frequency	Intensity	Time	Number & Type of Exercises
2 nonconsecutive days a week	Stretch to a point of mild tightness, not pain	Perform 2–4 repetitions of each stretch, holding for 10–30 seconds each time	8 core stretch exercises

Core Stretches

Back Bridge

Low-Back Knee-to-Chest Stretch (Two Knees)

Gluteal Stretch

Hamstrings Stretch (Supine Lying)

Quadriceps Stretch (Lying)

Torso Twist and Hip Stretch (Seated Twist)

Cat Stretch

Hip Flexor Stretch (Low Lunge)

6 Understanding Body Composition

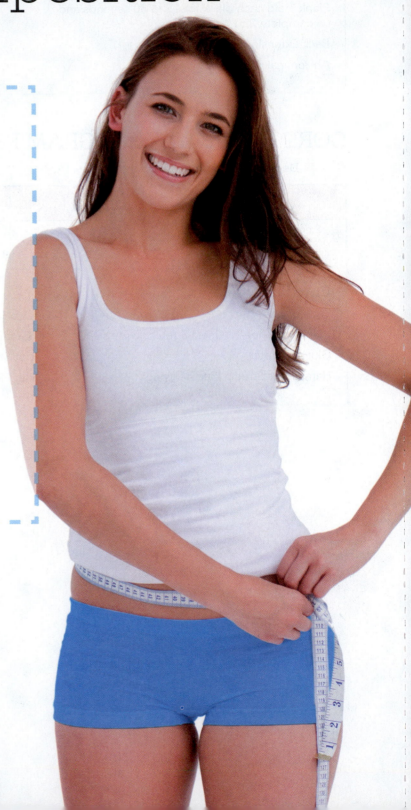

LEARNINGoutcomes

1 Discuss how body composition is related to life-long fitness and wellness.

2 Describe how the assessment of body size and shape differs from the assessment of body composition.

3 Evaluate your BMI and body circumferences and relate your scores to your overall health status.

4 Set and continually reevaluate goals to reach your healthy body fat percentage.

MasteringHealth™

Go online for chapter quizzes, interactive assessments, videos, and more!

casestudy

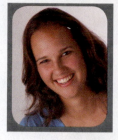

JESSIE

"Hi, I'm Jessie. I started running and resistance training two months ago and feel great! I like the new muscle tone in my legs, and I've made a lot of friends from the running group I joined. The ironic thing is, I started working out mainly because I wanted to lose weight, but I actually weigh a little bit more right now than I did when I first started. It doesn't make any sense to me, because my clothes fit better and I look more 'toned.' I've heard that muscle weighs more than fat, but that doesn't make any sense, either—doesn't a pound of muscle weigh the same as a pound of fat?"

HEAR IT! ONLINE

How much of your body is composed of fat? It's impossible to get an exact answer to that question, but you can estimate it. Body fat is a component of your total **body composition**, along with the amount of lean tissue in your body. Although this health-related component of physical fitness is not measured by your physical performance on a task like the others, body composition is an important determinant of overall health. Estimating body composition involves determining your lean body mass, fat mass, and percent body fat. Your **lean body mass** is your body's total amount of lean or fat-free tissue (muscles, bones, skin, other organs, and body fluids). Your **fat mass** is body mass made up of fat (adipose) tissue. **Percent body fat** is the percentage of your total weight that is fat tissue— that is, the weight of fat divided by total body weight.

All fat tissue can be labeled as either essential fat or storage fat. **Essential fat** is necessary for normal body functioning; it includes fats in the brain, muscles, nerves, bones, lungs, heart, and digestive and reproductive systems. Men need a minimum of 3 to 5 percent essential body fat. Women need significantly more (12% essential body fat) because of reproductive system-related fat deposits in their breasts, uterus, and elsewhere (**Figure 6.1**, page 214). **Storage fat** is nonessential fat stored in tissue near the body's surface and around major body organs. Storage fat provides energy, insulation, and padding. Men and women have similar amounts of storage fat but may differ in the location of larger fat stores. Your individual amount of storage fat depends upon many factors, including your lifestyle and genetics.

In this chapter, you will learn why body size, shape, and composition are useful measurements of fitness and wellness. You'll also learn how each of these measurements is determined and how you can change or maintain your body composition. (In Chapter 8, you will combine your knowledge of physical activity, body composition, and diet to create your own weight-management plan.)

Why Do My Body Size, Shape, and Composition Matter?

You might think of body size, shape, and composition mainly in terms of your physical appearance, but they encompass more than how you look. They are important components (as well as measurements) of your overall fitness and wellness.

Knowing Your Body Composition Can Help You Assess Your Health Risks

From the mid-1970s to 2010, the number of overweight children and adolescents increased from a mere 5 to 18 percent of the U.S. population![1] This is a problem because

body composition The relative amounts of fat and lean tissue in the body

lean body mass Body mass that is fat-free (muscle, skin, bone, organs, and body fluids)

fat mass Body mass that is fat tissue (adipose tissue)

percent body fat Percentage of total weight that is fat tissue

essential fat Body fat that is essential for normal physiological functioning

storage fat Body fat that is not essential but does provide energy, insulation, and padding

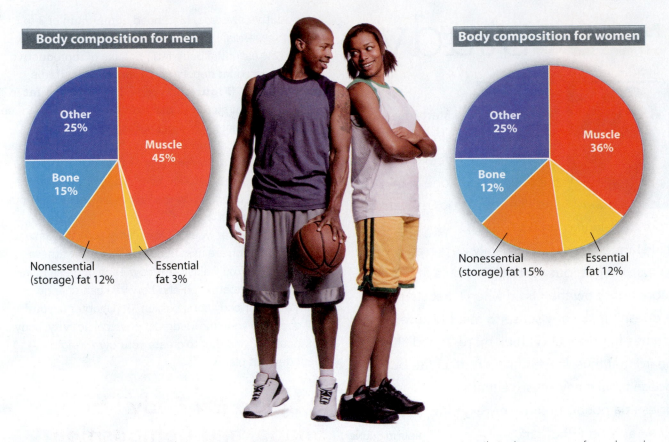

Body composition for men

- Other 25%
- Muscle 45%
- Bone 15%
- Nonessential (storage) fat 12%
- Essential fat 3%

Body composition for women

- Other 25%
- Muscle 36%
- Bone 12%
- Nonessential (storage) fat 15%
- Essential fat 12%

FIGURE **6.1** The body compositions of typical 20- to 24-year-old men and women vary primarily in the amounts of muscle and essential fat.

Data from: McArdle et al., *Exercise Physiology: Energy, Nutrition, and Human Performance*, 7th edition (Baltimore, MD: Lippincott Williams & Wilkins, 2010).

childhood obesity significantly increases your risk for heart disease and premature death and disability in adulthood.[2] Although research indicates that the rate of increase in obesity appeared to slow between 1999 and early 2012 for many populations, current rates of obese adults are extremely high, with more than 68 percent of U.S. adults being overweight or obese. Of those, approximately 35 percent are classified as obese![3]

Studies of obesity, however, often rely on measurements of total body weight rather than measurements of body composition. While measurements of total body weight can be useful in studying large populations, they are less useful in assessing an individual's health risks and body changes. For individuals, estimates of body composition—specifically, of lean and fat mass—provide additional important information. By knowing your percent body fat, you can more effectively determine your risks for chronic disease and decide just how much weight you should try to lose (or gain).

Evaluating Your Body Size and Shape Can Help Motivate Healthy Behavior Change

If you are just beginning an exercise program for fitness, it is often more useful to assess changes in body size and shape as a measurement of your progress, rather than weighing yourself daily on a bathroom scale. The reason: Healthy increases in muscle tissue (achieved by exercise) may cause you to temporarily gain weight, until the process of body fat loss catches up with muscle tissue gains. This is a *good* thing, but you would not know it if you relied solely on the scale to determine your progress. The box What Is Muscle Tone and How Is It Related to Body Composition? on page 219 discusses muscle mass, body fat, and the term "muscle tone."

By monitoring improvements in your body size and shape instead, you can get a more realistic sense of your achievement and stay motivated to stick with an exercise program.

How Can I Evaluate My Body Size and Shape?

How do you determine whether your body size and shape are "healthy"? This is a much-debated topic, but there are three common methods of doing so: calculating your body mass index, measuring your body circumferences, and identifying the patterns of fat distribution on your body. (Evaluating your body composition is a somewhat more complicated process, which we discuss later in this chapter.)

Calculate Your Body Mass Index (BMI) but Understand Its Limitations

Body mass index (BMI) is one of the most common measurements that doctors and researchers use to assess risk of weight-related disease, death, and disability. BMI is a measurement based on your weight and height. You can calculate your BMI now, using the chart in **Figure 6.2**.

BMI scores place individuals in categories as follows[4]:

Underweight (BMI of <18.5)

Normal weight (BMI of 18.5 to 24.9)

Overweight (BMI of 25.0 to 29.9)

Obese—Class I (BMI of 30.0 to 34.9)

Class II (BMI of 35.0 to 39.9)

Class III (BMI of >40.0)

Figure 6.3 on page 216 illustrates that very low and very high BMI scores are correlated with greater risk of death and disability.

> **body mass index (BMI)**
> A number calculated from a person's weight and height that is used to assess risk for health problems

The limitation with using BMI scores to assess "fitness" or "fatness" is that they do not differentiate between fat mass and lean mass. BMI is solely determined by height and weight. While BMI measurements can be helpful for individuals of average muscle and bone density, they can be misleading for athletes, bodybuilders, and short or petite individuals. For instance, someone who has an exceptionally heavy skeleton and larger-than-average muscle mass may have a BMI score that classifies him or her as "overweight," even if his or her percent body fat is in the "healthy" range. Because of BMI's limitations, it helps to also consider other factors, such as percent body fat, when assessing the overall picture of a person's fitness. **Lab 6.1** walks you through how to calculate your own BMI.

DO IT! ONLINE

Weight (pounds)

Height (feet and inches)	100	110	120	130	140	150	160	170	180	190	200	210	220	230	240	250	260
4'6"	24	27	29	31	34	36	39	41	43	46	48	51	53	55	58	60	63
4'8"	22	25	27	29	31	34	36	38	40	43	45	47	49	52	54	56	58
4'10"	21	23	25	27	29	31	33	36	38	40	42	44	46	48	50	52	54
5'0"	20	22	23	25	27	29	31	33	35	37	39	41	43	45	47	49	51
5'2"	18	20	22	24	26	27	29	31	33	35	37	38	40	42	44	46	48
5'4"	17	19	21	22	24	26	28	29	31	33	34	36	38	40	41	43	45
5'6"	16	18	19	21	23	24	26	27	29	31	32	34	36	37	39	40	42
5'8"	15	17	18	20	21	23	24	26	27	29	30	32	33	35	37	38	40
5'10"	14	16	17	19	20	22	23	24	26	27	29	30	32	33	34	36	37
6'0"	14	15	16	18	19	20	22	23	24	26	27	29	30	31	33	34	35
6'2"	13	14	15	17	18	19	21	22	23	24	26	27	28	30	31	32	33
6'4"	12	13	15	16	17	18	20	21	22	23	24	26	27	28	29	30	32
6'6"	12	13	14	15	16	17	19	20	21	22	23	24	25	27	28	29	30
6'8"	11	12	13	14	15	17	18	19	20	21	22	23	24	25	26	28	29
6'10"	11	12	13	14	15	16	17	18	19	20	21	22	23	24	25	26	27
7'0"	10	11	12	13	14	15	16	17	18	19	20	21	22	23	24	25	26

Key:
- Underweight
- Normal weight
- Overweight
- Obese

FIGURE **6.2** Estimate your BMI by finding where your weight and height intersect.

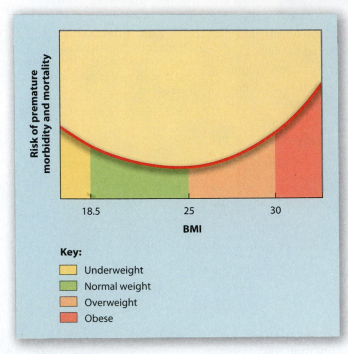

FIGURE **6.3** Extremely low or extremely high BMIs are associated with a greater risk of premature death and disability.

Data from: Katherine Flegal et al., "Excess Deaths Associated with Underweight, Overweight, and Obesity," *Journal of the American Medical Association* 293, no. 15 (2005): 1861–67.

Key:
- Underweight
- Normal weight
- Overweight
- Obese

Measure Your Body Circumferences

You can measure circumferences of various parts of your body to monitor your body's changes over time and to further assess your risk of disease. If you want to gain or lose weight, you can measure the circumference of your waist, hips, neck, upper arm, chest, thigh, and calf and then monitor changes in your body over time. You can also use waist and hip circumferences to assess disease risk. As shown in **Table 6.1** on the following page, waist circumference (a marker of abdominal fat) can indicate greater risk of diabetes, high blood pressure, and heart disease if it is greater than 102 cm in males or 88 cm in females.[5] As the table also shows,

waist-to-hip ratio (WHR) Waist circumference divided by hip circumference

android Body shape described as "apple-shaped," with excess body fat distributed primarily on the upper body and trunk

gynoid Body shape described as "pear-shaped," where excess body fat is distributed primarily on the lower body (hips and thighs)

subcutaneous fat Adipose tissue that is located just below the surface of the skin

visceral fat Adipose tissue that surrounds organs in the abdomen

the people at greatest risk are those with high waist circumferences *and* high BMIs.

You can also use waist and hip circumferences to determine your waist-to-hip ratio (WHR). **Waist-to-hip ratio** is your waist circumference divided by your hip circumference. A higher WHR is associated with more health risks. Young men with a WHR of 0.94 or more and young women with a WHR of 0.82 or more fall into a high-risk category.[6] **Lab 6.2** will walk you through the process of measuring your body circumferences and determining your WHR. Although waist circumference and WHR are both measures of disease risk, waist circumference is generally preferred because it is simpler, because of its relationship with abdominal fat, and because of its strong association to disease risk factors.[7]

DO IT! ONLINE

Identify Your Body's Patterns of Fat Distribution

Body fat distribution patterns are mostly genetically determined. You have probably noticed that people take after one parent in the way they "wear their fat." Some individuals tend to accumulate fat around their midsections; others collect it in the lower body or hips. These distributions contribute to an overall body shape that can be correlated to a higher or lower risk of disease.

The two most common body shapes are **android** ("apple-shaped") and **gynoid** ("pear-shaped") (**Figure 6.4**, see the following page). A person with *android pattern obesity* has excess body fat on the upper body and trunk and has a greater risk of developing chronic disease than a person with *gynoid pattern obesity*, who carries excess body fat in the lower body. Higher waist circumferences due to excess abdominal fat are associated with higher levels of **subcutaneous fat** and **visceral fat**.[8] Although both are associated with metabolic diseases, fat in the abdominal cavity (visceral fat) has a stronger relationship to disease risk.[9] The good news is that a reduction in total body fat will result in reductions in subcutaneous fat, visceral fat, and disease risk.[10,11] While men tend to store fat in the abdomen and women tend to store it in

TABLE 6.1 Waist Circumference, BMI, and Disease Risk

Weight Classification	BMI (kg/m²)	Waist Circumference and Disease Risk*	
		Smaller Waist Men ≤102 cm (40 in) Women ≤88 cm (35 in)	Larger Waist Men >102 cm (40 in) Women >88 cm (35 in)
Underweight	<18.5	—	—
Normal weight	18.5–24.9	—	—
Overweight	25.0–29.9	Increased	High
Obese—I	30.0–34.9	High	Very high
Obese—II	35.0–39.9	Very high	Very high
Obese—III	>40.0	Extremely high	Extremely high

*Risk for type 2 diabetes, hypertension, and cardiovascular disease, relative to normal weight and waist circumference.

Source: Adapted from National Heart, Lung, and Blood Institute—Expert Panel on the Identification, Evaluation, and Treatment of Overweight in Adults, "Clinical Guidelines on the Identification, Evaluation, and Treatment of Overweight and Obesity in Adults: Executive Summary," *American Journal of Clinical Nutrition* 68 (1998): 899–917. Reprinted with permission.

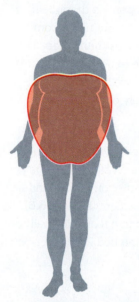 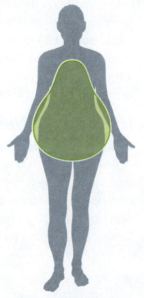

(a) Android ("apple-shaped") fat patterning

(b) Gynoid ("pear-shaped") fat patterning

FIGURE **6.4** (a) Android ("apple-shaped") fat distribution, associated with greater risk of heart disease and diabetes, is more common in men of all ages and postmenopausal women; (b) gynoid ("pear-shaped") fat distribution is more common in premenopausal women.

the lower body, there are exceptions, and fat distribution is strongly influenced by genetics. If you have an "apple-shaped" body, understanding the health risks can help motivate you to keep your "apple" from getting too large and round!

casestudy

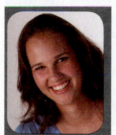

JESSIE

"My friend Emily explained to me that I probably gained weight after starting my exercise program because I was building muscle faster than I was losing fat and that I shouldn't worry about it. She suggested that I check my body measurements instead of getting on the scale. I like that idea, and she offered to help, but now I am not sure which ones to do. My problem areas have always been my hips and thighs. Should I measure those areas and call it good?"

THINK! Why would body measurements/circumferences be a better way for Jessie to measure her progress than body weight? What body shape, gynoid or android, does Jessie most likely have? Does her shape increase or decrease her risk for disease?

ACT NOW! Today, write three specific short-term process-oriented goals incorporating the SMART guidelines to help improve or maintain your current level of body fatness or body shape (i.e., I will go to the gym three times next week). This week, assess how you did and reevaluate your goals if necessary. In two weeks, add three longer-term goals.

HEAR IT! ONLINE

What Methods Are Used to Assess Body Composition?

Unlike BMI and body circumference measurements, body composition (lean mass vs. fat mass) can only be estimated indirectly. A true, direct assessment of body composition requires dissection after death; in fact, researchers judge the accuracy of the indirect measures by comparing them with dissection results from cadavers.

Methods of estimating body composition range from assessments that trained fitness instructors can easily administer, such as skinfold measurements and bioelectrical impedance analysis, to sophisticated tests that must be conducted by clinicians in a lab or hospital setting. The most accurate estimates of body composition are body scans such as an MRI (magnetic resonance imaging) or a CT (computed tomography) scan. These are used in medical settings to diagnose injury and illness but are not often used for body composition analysis alone. In the next section, we discuss methods that are commonly used to assess body composition.

Skinfold Measurements

Skinfold measurements are an easy, inexpensive way to estimate your percent body fat. **Calipers** (shown in Lab 6.3) are used to measure the thickness of a fold of skin and subcutaneous adipose tissue. Skinfold measurements at specific sites around the body are recorded and entered into an equation that predicts percent body fat. This prediction of percent body fat has an error range of 3 to 4 percent[12]; for example, if your body fat measurement is 16 percent, the true value could be anywhere from about 12 to 20 percent. More recent research has shown that current equations to predict body fat from skinfolds will underestimate percent body fat levels by about 1.3 percent in men and 3.0 percent in women (compared to DXA measured body fat levels), and may result in additional over- or underestimates for ethnically and racially diverse populations.[13] If you use this method to estimate your body fat, remember it is just that—an estimate! **Lab 6.3** provides instructions for skinfold measurements. Performing an accurate skinfold assessment takes education and practice, so be sure to ask a qualified fitness instructor to help you. Also, the difference between technicians can be a major source of error. Make sure the same technician performs the measurements if you are tracking body fat change over time.

DO IT! ONLINE

Dual-Energy X-Ray Absorptiometry

Dual-energy X-ray absorptiometry (DXA) is the practical "gold-standard" reference method for body composition assessment in clinical and research settings (**Figure 6.5**). In a DXA scan, low-radiation X rays are used to distinguish fat, bone mineral, and bone-free lean components of the body. Measuring bone mineral (in addition to fat and lean mass) increases the accuracy of body fat estimates. In the medical setting, DXA scans are most often used to determine bone density for osteoporosis diagnosis. Body composition estimates can be obtained from whole body DXA scans that take less than three minutes. However, DXA tests are expensive, require a trained technician, and are not well designed to examine people who are extremely obese.

Hydrostatic Weighing

Hydrostatic weighing (also called *underwater weighing*) was widely used in research and college settings and prior to DXA was considered the criterion (gold-standard) method of body composition assessment (**Figure 6.6**). Recently, it has been replaced by more technologically advanced techniques like DXA and the Bod Pod (described

skinfold A fold of skin and subcutaneous fat that is measured with calipers to determine the fatness of a specific body area

calipers A handheld and spring-loaded instrument with calibrated jaws and a meter that reads skinfold thickness in millimeters

dual-energy X-ray absorptiometry (DXA) A technique using two low-radiation X rays to scan bone and soft tissue (muscle, fat) to determine bone density and to estimate percent body fat

hydrostatic weighing A technique that uses water to determine total body volume, total body density, and percent body fat

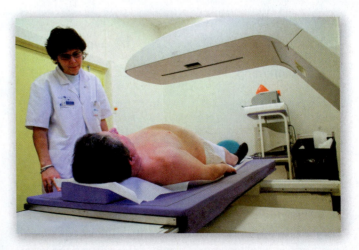

FIGURE **6.5** A DXA machine uses low-radiation X rays to determine body composition.

Q&A What Is Muscle Tone and How Is It Related to Body Composition?

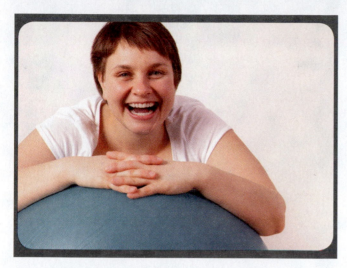

Muscle tone is an overused and technically misused term. The scientific definition of muscle tone is the residual tension or contraction of muscle. In other words, it is the unconscious low level of contraction of your muscles at rest. This definition is vastly different from how most people think about the term "tone." Generally, muscle tone is considered having muscles that appear defined and feel firm and tight.

Firmness and definition is best accomplished through resistance training.

Will high repetitions and light weight result in toned muscles? For years, women (and men) wanting long, lean muscles have been told they can get "toned" and avoid bulky muscles by lifting very light weights and performing lots of repetitions. This is a major exercise misconception. There is no evidence that using light weights and doing high repetitions (15–25) results in more muscle tone over lifting heavier weights. In fact, using heavier weights with lower repetitions (8–12) is best for maximizing strength and muscle changes.

However, a strength-trained muscle that is covered with layers of fat will not appear tone. Thus, you may need to decrease your body fat percentage to help showcase your muscles. This is best accomplished through dietary modifications and increasing your energy expenditure through physical activity. So it is the *combination* of an exercised, trained muscle and a low overall body fat that result in what most people consider good muscle tone. A word of caution: Be wary of exercise infomercials that guarantee increased muscle tone. Since there is no way to measure muscle tone (combination of definition and firmness) companies don't have to prove their products really work!

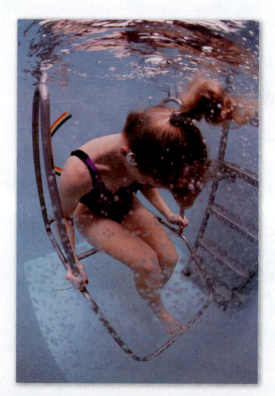

FIGURE **6.6** Hydrostatic (underwater) weighing uses total body water displacement to calculate estimated percent body fat.

in the next section). In hydrostatic weighing, a person is first weighed outside a water tank and then weighed while completely submerged in the tank. Since fat is less dense than water it will float, while lean body mass will sink as it is more dense than water. Therefore, a person with a high percent of body fat will weigh less in water compared to a leaner person of the same body weight. From this technique body density can be calculated and used to estimate percent body fat. The method is valid and reliable, but access to an equipped facility may be limited and not everyone is comfortable with being submerged. It is also time consuming and requires special equipment for the measurement of residual lung volume (the air you cannot expire).

> **Bod Pod** An egg-shaped chamber that uses air displacement to determine total body volume, total body density, and percent body fat

Air Displacement (Bod Pod)

Air displacement plethysmography, commercially known as the **Bod Pod**, measures total body *air* displacement (**Figure 6.7**). The person being assessed puts on a

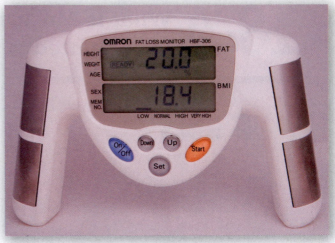

FIGURE **6.8** Bioelectrical impedance analysis (BIA) machines measure the resistance of different body tissues to electrical currents. These measurements are then used to estimate percent body fat. A handheld BIA machine is shown here.

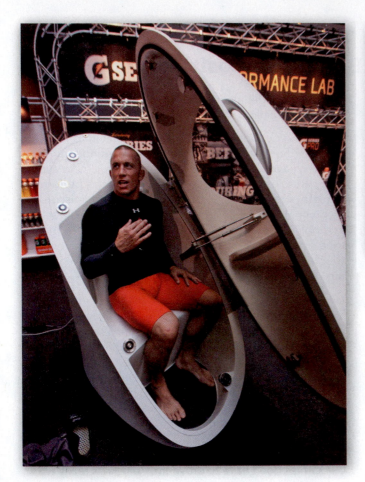

FIGURE **6.7** The Bod Pod uses total body air displacement to calculate estimated percent body fat.

swimsuit and then sits in the egg-shaped Bod Pod chamber while the air displacement is measured. The volume of air displaced (moved) is equal to the subject's body volume as he or she sits in the chamber. Body density is easily calculated (Density = Mass/Volume) and converted to a body fat percentage. Bod Pod percent body fat measurements are generally within 1 to 2 percent of hydrostatic weighing and DXA-measured levels of percent body fat.[14] Bod Pod measurements are available in many clinical and college settings, but availability in fitness settings is still somewhat limited.

Bioelectrical Impedance Analysis

In **bioelectrical impedance analysis (BIA)**, a machine measures the resistance of various body tissues to electrical currents. BIA machines send small electrical currents through the body via the hands, feet, or both (**Figure 6.8**). Fat does not conduct electricity

bioelectrical impedance analysis (BIA) A technique that distinguishes lean and fat mass by measuring the resistance of various body tissues to electrical currents

very well, so fat tissues will demonstrate a resistance to the currents. Fat-free tissues, namely muscle, have more body water and conduct electricity well; thus, fat-free tissues do not offer as much resistance to the currents. These resistance differences are used to estimate percent body fat. Higher resistance indicates higher levels of overall body fat. The error range of BIA is 3 to 4 percent but accuracy depends upon the quality of the machine and upon the subject's preparation, especially concerning his or her water intake.[15] Higher or lower levels of body water will significantly alter a BIA machine's results, so it is important to hydrate normally. BIA is an acceptable method of tracking body fat change if conditions are consistent (Lab 6.3).

How Can I Change My Body Composition?

After you assess your body size, shape, and composition, the next steps are evaluation, goal setting, and (if your results are not within healthy ranges) planning for change.

Determine Whether Your Percent Body Fat Is within a Healthy Range

Because people accumulate fat very differently and not all fat is the same, it is difficult to specify the exact level of body fat that is "healthy" or "unhealthy" for an individual. For instance, abdominal fat increases your risk for disease much more than fat on your calves does. Because of these differences, researchers do not agree upon desired body fat percentages for people of all ages, and you will find that research articles, books, and websites differ in their recommendations. **Table 6.2** provides percent body fat norms.

TABLE 6.2 Percent Body Fat Norms for Men and Women*

Body Fat Rating	Women (%)	Men (%)
Athletic/Low	14–20	6–13
Fitness	21–24	14–17
Acceptable	25–31	18–25
Obese	>32	>26

*Please note that there are no agreed-upon standards for recommended percent body fat; however, a range of 10–22% for men and 20–32% for women is considered healthy.

Source: From "Percent Body Fat Norms for Men and Women" in *ACE Lifestyle and Weight Management Coach Manual*, © 2013 American Council on Exercise. Reprinted with permission from the American Council on Exercise® (ACE®), www.acefitness.org.

Set Reasonable Body Composition Goals

You have many choices in setting body composition goals. If you are already in the healthy ranges, you can set additional goals for increasing lean mass or decreasing fat mass (within the low limits). Keep in mind that real body composition changes take time. Quick

SEE IT! ONLINE
A Real Look at Real Women

weight loss is easier for those with more weight to lose, but most weight that is lost quickly consists of water and muscle—the very things you *don't* want to lose. To lose fat only, you have to be committed to exercise and slow, consistent weight loss. Aim for a body composition goal and a target weight that is healthy and that you can maintain for a lifetime. See the GetFitGraphic on page 223 for more on spot training and the need for a whole-body approach to body composition.

Follow a Well-Designed Exercise and Nutrition Plan

True body changes come from sticking with a carefully planned and executed nutrition and exercise program. This book will help you get started. For additional assistance, seek out qualified medical, nutrition, and fitness experts.

Monitor Your Body Size, Shape, and Composition Regularly

Stay motivated in your body change program by monitoring your progress regularly. Since body fat changes may take time, allow two to four months between body composition (percent body fat) assessments. Other types of assessments can be done more frequently. Here is a suggested schedule:

- Body size/shape (mirror and fit of clothes)—assess daily or weekly
- Weight—assess weekly
- Circumferences—measure monthly (or less frequently)
- BMI—measure monthly (or less frequently)
- Percent body fat—measure every other month (or less frequently)

casestudy

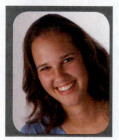

JESSIE

"A trainer at my gym gave me a skinfold test. I was amazed how much of my body is fat—50 lbs, wow! The trainer said that 50 lbs sounds like a lot, but my body fat percentage is actually 31 percent. Since this number is marginally high for my age, she said she would help me with a program to lower it. We are planning to retest my skinfolds in three months to see how all of my exercise is paying off!

THINK! What advice would you give Jessie if her body fatness doesn't change much despite all of her exercise? What other methods could Jessie use to determine her body composition? What methods of assessing body composition are readily available to you?

ACT! Use one body composition measurement method to determine your body fat. Make a note in your calendar to get retested in three months to check your progress.

HEAR IT! ONLINE

DIVeRSiTY

Self-Esteem and Unhealthy Body Composition Behaviors

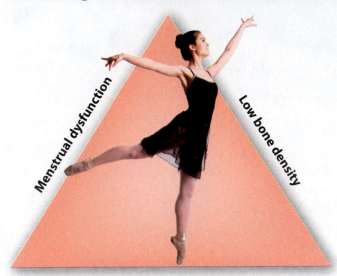

Menstrual dysfunction

Low bone density

Low energy availability

Body composition can become a major problem for athletes in certain sports—not because they are too fat, but because they are too thin. This is true for both sexes, though the problem is more common in females, who are at risk of developing the female athlete triad. Men may also develop disordered eating habits, as well as a body composition disorder known as muscle dysmorphia, in which men who are of normal weight and even unusually muscular think that they are "puny." (Muscle dysmorphia is discussed further in Chapter 8.) Some sports—gymnastics, figure skating, wrestling, ballet dancing, body-building—place a huge emphasis on appearance and having a lean body. The pressure to look lean and to weigh less can push athletes to cut back on what they eat and increase their workouts to the point where they lose too much weight.

An athlete's self-esteem can make a big difference. Lower self-esteem can lead to believing that life events are out of your control (external locus of control) and vice versa. One study has shown that if a female athlete has an internal locus of control (or belief that she has power or control over her body and training), she will be more immune to coach and social pressures that can lead to disordered eating.[1] This can help her avoid the female athlete triad (see figure), a triangle of three interrelated problems: menstrual dysfunction, low bone density, and low energy availability as a result of disordered eating or eating disorders. In the triad, too little caloric intake coupled with too much exercise can lead to hormonal changes and the stopping of menstruation.[2] Improper nutrition, including too little calcium and vitamin D intake, can lead to altered hormones and to bone loss and a risk of fractures. Such changes taking place in adolescence or early adulthood can permanently reduce the size of a woman's skeleton and increase her lifelong risk for osteoporosis. In dancers, one study has shown that the triad negatively affects cardiovascular health.[3]

Athletes with low self-esteem and at high risk for the female athlete triad should carefully monitor their body composition, menstrual health, eating habits, and perhaps bone density. If the triad is suspected, the athlete should eat more nutritious food and/or exercise less, and may need to seek treatment for an eating disorder.

SEE IT! ONLINE

Young Boys Exercising to Extremes

Sources:
1. S. Scoffier, Y. Paquet, and F. d'Arripe-Longueville, "Effect of Locus of Control on Disordered Eating in Athletes: The Mediational Role of Self-regulation of Eating Attitudes," *Eating Behaviors* 11, no. 3 (2010): 164–9.
2. A. M. McManus and N. Armstrong, "Physiology of Elite Young Female Athletes," *Medicine and Sport Science* 56 (2011): 23–46.
3. A. Z. Hoch et al., "Association between the Female Athlete Triad and Endothelial Dysfunction in Dancers," *Clinical Journal of Sport Medicine* 21, no. 2 (2011): 119–25.

In addition to tracking these measurements, log how you're feeling. Remember, improving your body composition should help you feel good about yourself! The box Self-Esteem and Unhealthy Body Composition Behaviors talks about some problems to be watchful for.

Keep a separate log, journal, or notebook of your progress, but do not feel burdened by it. Some people are more motivated by journaling than others—find the monitoring system that works best for you, and use it consistently.

CAN I GET RID OF **FAT** AND **CELLULITE** IN ONE AREA OF MY BODY?

Have you ever thought, "I don't need to work on my whole body. I just need to lose some fat off my hips (or thighs or abdomen)!" Well unfortunately, spot reducing fat and cellulite just doesn't work!

WHAT ARE SOME COMMON METHODS PEOPLE USE TO TARGET FAT AND CELLULITE IN SPECIFIC AREAS?

1 Ab-crunchers, thigh-slimmers, or arm-toners

DO THEY WORK? These machines increase the strength, endurance, and firmness of the underlying muscles, but there's no change in fat in the target area without changes in overall caloric expenditure and consumption.

2 Laser therapy or liposuction

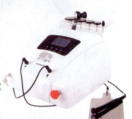

DO THEY WORK? These procedures will take out and/or change fat cells, but in order to maintain such changes, you must adjust your diet and exercise.[1]

3 Skin creams

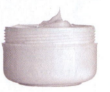

DO THEY WORK? Skin creams may decrease the appearance of cellulite by causing the skin to swell, but the effect is minimal and non-lasting.

IS CELLULITE A SPECIAL TYPE OF FAT?

NO! Cellulite is **enlarged fat cells** that bulge out of their connective tissue compartments and **push into the skin, causing a bumpy appearance.**[2] More women than men have it due to greater irregularity in patterns of connective tissue.

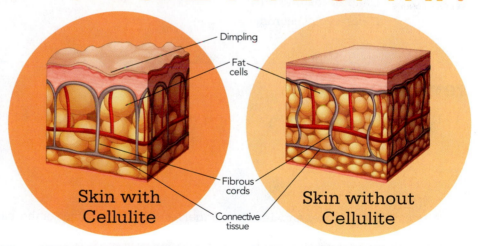

Dimpling

Fat cells

Skin with Cellulite

Fibrous cords

Connective tissue

Skin without Cellulite

WHAT CAN I DO TO REDUCE CELLULITE?[3]

EAT A HEALTHY DIET rich in fruits, vegetables, and fiber

STAY HYDRATED with plenty of fluids

EXERCISE REGULARLY to keep muscles firm and bones strong

MAINTAIN a healthy weight

DON'T smoke

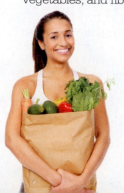
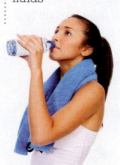
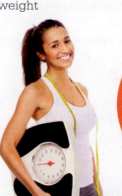
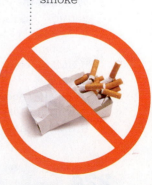

CHAPTER IN REVIEW

MasteringHealth™

Build your knowledge—and wellness!—in the Study Area of MasteringHealth with a variety of study tools.

SEE IT! ONLINE

videos

Measuring Hip-to-Waist Ratio

Skinfold Measurement

A Real Look at Real Women

Young Boys Exercising to Extremes

HEAR IT! ONLINE

audio tools

Audio case study

MP3 chapter review

REVIEW IT! ONLINE

chapter review

Chapter reading quizzes

Glossary flashcards

LIVE IT! ONLINE

programs & behavior change

Take Charge of Your Health! Worksheets

Behavior Change Log Book and Wellness Journal

DO IT! ONLINE

labs

Lab 6.1 How to Calculate Your BMI

Lab 6.2 Measure and Evaluate Your Body Circumferences

Lab 6.3 Estimate Your Percent Body Fat (Skinfold Test and BIA Test)

---

reviewquestions

1. The proportion of your total weight that is fat is called
   a. body composition.
   b. lean mass.
   c. percent body fat.
   d. BMI.

2. Women have a greater amount of *essential fat* due to
   a. larger calves and thighs.
   b. their eating habits.
   c. less physical activity.
   d. reproduction-related fat deposits.

3. Which of the following statements about BMI is true?
   a. Your BMI is an estimate of your body fat percentage.
   b. BMI differentiates between lean mass and fat mass.
   c. Very low and very high BMI scores are associated with greater risk of mortality.
   d. BMI stands for "Basic Measure Indices."

4. Which of the following BMI ratings is considered "overweight"?
   a. 20
   b. 25
   c. 30
   d. 35

5. Which of the following circumference measures indicates an increased risk of disease?
   a. A waist circumference over 100 cm for men and over 80 cm for women
   b. A waist circumference over 102 cm for men and over 88 cm for women
   c. A waist-to-hip ratio of 0.50 or higher
   d. A waist-to-hip ratio of 0.75 or higher

6. Which of the following body shapes or body fat distribution patterns is associated with an increased risk of heart disease and diabetes?
   a. Bell-shaped
   b. Android pattern obesity
   c. Pear-shaped
   d. Gynoid pattern obesity

7. Skinfold measurements are used to assess the amount of
   a. subcutaneous fat.
   b. visceral fat.
   c. essential fat.
   d. intramuscular fat.

8. Which of the following body composition measurement methods uses air displacement to estimate total body volume, density, and percent body fat?
   a. Bioelectrical impedance analysis
   b. Hydrostatic weighing
   c. The Bod Pod
   d. Skinfold measurement

9. Which body composition measurement method relies heavily on body water or hydration levels being normal (not too low or too high)?
   a. Bioelectrical impedance analysis
   b. Hydrostatic weighing
   c. The Bod Pod
   d. Skinfold measurement

10. The female athlete triad consists of the following interrelated issues:
   a. disordered eating, low bone density, and menstrual dysfunction.
   b. weak eyesight, poor nutrition, and brittle bones.
   c. low body weight, poor nutrition, and diabetes.
   d. excessive exercise, high blood pressure, and menstrual issues.

---

critical thinkingquestions

1. Explain the usefulness and limitations of using BMI to determine fitness goals.

2. What factors should you consider when determining a healthy percent body fat range for yourself?

---

references

1. C. D. Fryar, M. D. Carroll, and C. L. Ogden, "Prevalence of Obesity Among Children and Adolescents: United States, Trends 1963–1965 Through 2009–2010," *National Center for Health Statistics, Health E-Stats* (2012), www.cdc.gov

2. J. J. Reilly and J. Kelly, "Long-term Impact of Overweight and Obesity in Childhood and Adolescence on Morbidity and Premature Mortality in Adulthood: Systematic Review," *International Journal of Obesity (London)* 35, no. 7 (2011): 891–8, doi: 10.1038/ijo.2010.222; J. L. Baker, L. W. Olsen, and T. I. Sorensen, "Childhood Body-Mass Index and the Risk of Coronary Heart Disease in Adulthood," *New England Journal of Medicine* 357, no. 23 (2007): 2329–37, doi: 10.1056/NEJMoa072515.

3. K. M. Flegal et al., "Prevalence of Obesity and Trends in the Distribution of Body Mass Index among U.S. Adults, 1999–2010," *Journal of the American Medical Association* 307, no. 5 (2012), doi: 10.1001/jama.2012.39.

4. National Heart, Lung, and Blood Institute—Expert Panel on the Identification, Evaluation, and Treatment of Overweight in Adults, "Clinical Guidelines on the Identification, Evaluation, and Treatment of Overweight and Obesity in Adults: Executive Summary," *American Journal of Clinical Nutrition* 68, no. 4 (1998): 899–917.

5. Ibid.

6. V. H. Heyward, *Advanced Fitness Assessment and Exercise Prescription*, 6th edition (Champaign, IL: Human Kinetics, 2010).

7. J. P. Reis et al., "The Relation of Leptin and Insulin with Obesity-Related Cardiovascular Risk Factors in U.S. Adults," *Atherosclerosis* 200, no. 1 (2008): 150–60.

8. A. Bosy-Westphal et al., "Measurement Site for Waist Circumference Affects Its Accuracy as an Index of Visceral and Abdominal Subcutaneous Fat in a Caucasian Population," *The Journal of Nutrition* 140, no. 5 (2010): 954–61, doi: 10.3945/jn.109.118737.

9. C. S. Fox et al., "Abdominal Visceral and Subcutaneous Adipose Tissue Compartments: Association with Metabolic Risk Factors in the Framingham Heart Study," *Circulation* 116, no. 1 (2007): 39–48.

10. G. Fisher et al., "Effect of Diet with and without Exercise Training on Markers of Inflammation and Fat Distribution in Overweight Women," *Obesity (Silver Spring)* 19, no. 6 (2011): 1131–6, doi: 10.1038/oby.2010.310.

11. B. H. Goodpaster et al., "Effects of Diet and Physical Activity Interventions on Weight Loss and Cardiometabolic Risk Factors in Severely Obese Adults: A Randomized Trial," *JAMA* 304, no. 16 (2010): 1795–802, doi: 10.1001/jama.2010.1505.

12. V. H. Heyward, *Advanced Fitness Assessment and Exercise Prescription*, 2010.

13. A. S. Jackson et al., "Cross-validation of Generalised Body Composition Equations with Diverse Young Men and Women: The Training Intervention and Genetics of Exercise Response (TIGER) Study," *British Journal of Nutrition* 101, no. 6 (2009): 871–8.

14. D. A. Fields, M. I. Goran, and M. A. McCrory, "Body-composition Assessment via Air-displacement Plethysmography in Adults and Children: A Review," *American Journal of Clinical Nutrition* 75, no. 3 (2002): 453–67.

15. V. H. Heyward, *Advanced Fitness Assessment and Exercise Prescription*, 2010.

getfitgraphic references

1. M. K. Caruso-Davis et al., "Efficacy of Low-Level Laser Therapy for Body Contouring and Spot Fat Reduction," *Obesity Surgery* 21, no. 6 (2010): 722–9, doi: 10.1007/s11695-010-0126-y.

2. National Library of Medicine, National Institutes of Health, Medline Plus, "Cellulite," Updated August 2011, www.nlm.nih.gov

3. R. B. Kreider et al., "A Structured Diet and Exercise Program Promotes Favorable Changes in Weight Loss, Body Composition, and Weight Maintenance," *Journal of the American Dietetic Association* 111, no. 6 (2011): 828–43, doi: 10.1016/j.jada.2011.03.013.

LAB 6.1

HOW TO CALCULATE YOUR BMI

MasteringHealth™

Name: _____ Date: _____

Instructor: _____ Section: _____

Purpose: To learn how to calculate your BMI.

Materials: Weight scale, measuring tape, calculator

SECTION I: CALCULATE YOUR BMI

1. Record your weight and height below:

Weight _____ lb   Height _____ inches

2. Convert your weight and height to metric units:

Weight _____ lb ÷ 2.2 = _____ kg

Height _____ inches × 2.54 = _____ cm ÷ 100 = _____ meters (m)

3. Calculate your BMI:

BMI = _____ ÷ [_____ × _____]
      (weight in kg)   (height in m)   (height in m)

BMI = _____ kg/m^2

Note: Square the height (multiply by itself) before dividing into weight.

4. Indicate your BMI rating in the table below:

Weight Classification	BMI (kg/m^2)
Underweight	_____ <18.5
Normal Weight	_____ 18.5–24.9
Overweight	_____ 25.0–29.9
Obese—I	_____ 30.0–34.9
Obese—II	_____ 35.0–39.9
Obese—III	_____ >40.0

SECTION II: REFLECTION

1. Is your BMI category what you thought it would be?

_____

2. Remember that BMI categories can be misleading for individuals with above-average muscle mass. Do you fall into this category? _____

3. Monitoring changes to your BMI over time is one way to assess your progress with a fitness program. Within this course or on your own, recalculate your BMI two months after you begin a new exercise program. How has your BMI changed?

_____

LAB 6.2

ASSESS YOURSELF
MEASURE AND EVALUATE YOUR BODY CIRCUMFERENCES

MasteringHealth™

Name: _____ **Date:** _____

Instructor: _____ **Section:** _____

Purpose: To learn how to measure your body circumferences.

Materials: Measuring tape, partner

SCAN TO SEE IT
ONLINE!

SECTION I: MEASURING CIRCUMFERENCES

Using a cloth or plastic tape measure, have a partner assist you with the following circumference measures. Be sure to mark your measurements (centimeters or inches) and record them to the nearest 0.5 cm or 0.25 inch. You can perform these measurements again to track how your body shape changes over time.

Site	Description	Measurement
Waist	For those with a visible waist, measure at the narrowest part of the torso; for those with a larger torso, measure at the navel.	
Hip	Measure with the legs slightly apart. Measure where the hip/buttock circumference is the greatest.	
Upper Arm	Measure midway between the shoulder and elbow.	Right: Left:
Forearm	Measure at the greatest circumference between the wrist and elbow.	Right: Left:
Thigh	Measure with your leg on a bench or chair (knee at 90 degrees). Measure half way between the crease in your hip and your knee.	Right: Left:
Calf	Measure at the greatest circumference between the knee and ankle.	Right: Left:
Neck	Measure midway between the head and shoulders.	

Source: Based on American College of Sports Medicine, *ACSM's Guidelines for Exercise Testing and Prescription*, 8th edition (Baltimore, MD: Lippincott Williams & Wilkins, 2010).

SECTION II: EVALUATING CIRCUMFERENCES AND DISEASE RISK

1. Calculate your waist-to-hip ratio (WHR):

WHR = _____ + _____

　　　　　(waist circumference)　　(hip circumference)

WHR = _____

2. Evaluate your WHR using the table below:

Disease Risk and WHR				
Age (years)	Low	Moderate	High	Very High
Men: 20–29	<0.83	0.83–0.88	0.89–0.94	>0.94
30–39	<0.84	0.84–0.91	0.92–0.96	>0.96
40–49	<0.88	0.88–0.95	0.96–1.00	>1.00
50–59	<0.90	0.90–0.96	0.97–1.02	>1.02
60–69	<0.91	0.91–0.98	0.99–1.03	>1.03
Women: 20–29	<0.71	0.71–0.77	0.78–0.82	>0.82
30–39	<0.72	0.72–0.78	0.79–0.84	>0.84
40–49	<0.73	0.73–0.79	0.80–0.87	>0.87
50–59	<0.74	0.74–0.81	0.82–0.88	>0.88
60–69	<0.76	0.76–0.83	0.84–0.90	>0.90

Source: Reprinted, with permission, from W.H. Heyward, 2010. *Advanced Fitness Assessment and Exercise Prescription*, 6th ed. (Champaign, IL: Human Kinetics), 222.

Evaluate your waist circumference using the table below:

Waist Circumference (WC)		
Disease Risk Category	Women	Men
Very Low	<70 cm (<28.5 in)	<80 cm (<31.5 in)
Low	70–89 cm (28.5–35.0 in)	80–99 cm (31.5–39.0 in)
High	90–109 cm (35.5–43.0 in)	100–120 cm (39.5–47.0 in)
Very High	>110 cm (>43.5 in)	>120 cm (>47.0 in)

Source: From G. A. Bray, "Don't Throw the Baby Out with the Bath Water," *American Journal of Clinical Nutrition* 70, no. 3 (2004): 347–9, by permission of the American Society for Nutrition.

3. Record your disease risk from WHR and waist circumference below:

Disease rating for WHR: _____

Disease rating for WC: _____

SECTION III: REFLECTION

1. Do your ratings for disease risk based upon circumferences surprise you? _____

2. Which of your circumference measures are you most interested in changing and why?

_____

Name: _____ **Date:** _____

Instructor: _____ **Section:** _____

Materials: Skinfold calipers, BIA machine, appropriate clothing (shorts, tank top, sports bra for women)

Purpose: To assess your current percent body fat using either the skinfold procedure or a BIA machine or both.

Directions: Complete the sections below with a trained instructor.

SCAN TO SEE IT
ONLINE!

SECTION I: SKINFOLD MEASUREMENT

You will need an experienced, trained instructor to complete your measurements. Note the time of day of your measurements and perform any follow-up measurements at the same time of day.

1. Identify the correct skinfold locations. If you are male, locate the chest, abdomen, and thigh locations (see photos). If you are female, locate the triceps, suprailiac, and thigh locations (see photos). Your instructor should mark these locations on the right side of the body with a pen before using the caliper.

| Chest | A diagonal fold measured midway between the shoulder/armpit crease and the nipple. | |
| Abdomen | A vertical fold measured one inch to the right of the navel. | |

Thigh	A vertical fold measured midway between the crease in your hip and the top of your knee.	
Triceps	A vertical fold on the back of the upper arm midway between the shoulder and elbow.	
Suprailiac	A diagonal fold just above the hip bone, on the side of the body at the front edge of your relaxed arm.	

Source: Based on American College of Sports Medicine, *ACSM's Guidelines for Exercise Testing and Prescription*, 8th edition (Baltimore, MD: Lippincott Williams & Wilkins, 2010).

2. Your instructor will measure each skinfold location using the technique below. Record the results below and then add up the numbers for the three skinfold sites to obtain your overall skinfold sum.

Skinfold measurement technique: After locating the correct sites, grab a double fold of skin on both sides of the skinfold location. Open your fingers about three inches when lifting the fold (> than three inches is required for larger individuals). Holding the fold in place, pick up the calipers with your other hand. While still holding the fold, place the caliper jaws on the skinfold location, measuring halfway between the crest and the base of the fold. You should measure perpendicular to the fold and about one cm away from your fingers. Read the measurement two to three seconds after placing the calipers and record the skinfold numbers to the nearest 0.5 mm. For accuracy, measure each site three times and average the two closest numbers.

Men			Women		
Chest	_____	mm	Triceps	_____	mm
Abdomen	_____	mm	Suprailiac	_____	mm
Thigh	_____	mm	Thigh	_____	mm
Sum of 3 =	_____	mm	Sum of 3 =	_____	mm

3. Using the sum of three skinfolds, find your estimated percent body fat in the tables for women and men.

Sum of Skinfolds (mm)	Percent Body Fat Estimates for WOMEN (from triceps, suprailiac, and thigh skinfolds)								
	AGE (years)								
	Under 22	23–27	28–32	33–37	38–42	43–47	48–52	53–57	Over 57
23–25	9.7	9.9	10.2	10.4	10.7	10.9	11.2	11.4	11.7
26–28	11.0	11.2	11.5	11.7	12.0	12.3	12.5	12.7	13.0
29–31	12.3	12.5	12.8	13.0	13.3	13.5	13.8	14.0	14.3
32–34	13.6	13.8	14.0	14.3	14.5	14.8	15.0	15.3	15.5
35–37	14.8	15.0	15.3	15.5	15.8	16.0	16.3	16.5	16.8
38–40	16.0	16.3	16.5	16.7	17.0	17.2	17.5	17.7	18.0
41–43	17.2	17.4	17.7	17.9	18.2	18.4	18.7	18.9	19.2
44–46	18.3	18.6	18.8	19.1	19.3	19.6	19.8	20.1	20.3
47–49	19.5	19.7	20.0	20.2	20.5	20.7	21.0	21.2	21.5
50–52	20.6	20.8	21.1	21.3	21.6	21.8	22.1	22.3	22.6
53–55	21.7	21.9	22.1	22.4	22.6	22.9	23.1	23.4	23.6
56–58	22.7	23.0	23.2	23.4	23.7	23.9	24.2	24.4	24.7
59–61	23.7	24.0	24.2	24.5	24.7	25.0	25.2	25.5	25.7
62–64	24.7	25.0	25.2	25.5	25.7	26.0	26.2	26.4	26.7
65–67	25.7	25.9	26.2	26.4	26.7	26.9	27.2	27.4	27.7
68–70	26.6	26.9	27.1	27.4	27.6	27.9	28.1	28.4	28.6
71–73	27.5	27.8	28.0	28.3	28.5	28.8	29.0	29.3	29.5
74–76	28.4	28.7	28.9	29.2	29.4	29.7	29.9	30.2	30.4
77–79	29.3	29.5	29.8	30.0	30.3	30.5	30.8	31.0	31.3
80–82	30.1	30.4	30.6	30.9	31.1	31.4	31.6	31.9	32.1
83–85	30.9	31.2	31.4	31.7	31.9	32.2	32.4	32.7	32.9
86–88	31.7	32.0	32.2	32.5	32.7	32.9	33.2	33.4	33.7
89–91	32.5	32.7	33.0	33.2	33.5	33.7	33.9	34.2	34.4
92–94	33.2	33.4	33.7	33.9	34.2	34.4	34.7	34.9	35.2
95–97	33.9	34.1	34.4	34.6	34.9	35.1	35.4	35.6	35.9
98–100	34.6	34.8	35.1	35.3	35.5	35.8	36.0	36.3	36.5
101–103	35.3	35.4	35.7	35.9	36.2	36.4	36.7	36.9	37.2
104–106	35.8	36.1	36.3	36.6	36.8	37.1	37.3	37.5	37.8
107–109	36.4	36.7	36.9	37.1	37.4	37.6	37.9	38.1	38.4
110–112	37.0	37.2	37.5	37.7	38.0	38.2	38.5	38.7	38.9
113–115	37.5	37.8	38.0	38.2	38.5	38.7	39.0	39.2	39.5
116–118	38.0	38.3	38.5	38.8	39.0	39.3	39.5	39.7	40.0
119–121	38.5	38.7	39.0	39.2	39.5	39.7	40.0	40.2	40.5
122–124	39.0	39.2	39.4	39.7	39.9	40.2	40.4	40.7	40.9
125–127	39.4	39.6	39.9	40.1	40.4	40.6	40.9	41.1	41.4
128–130	39.8	40.0	40.3	40.5	40.8	41.0	41.3	41.5	41.8

Source: A. S. Jackson and M. L. Pollock, "Practical Assessment of Body Composition," *The Physician and Sportsmedicine* 13, no. 5 (1985): 76–90. Copyright © 1985 JTE Multimedia, LLC. Used with permission.

Sum of Skinfolds (mm)	Percent Body Fat Estimates for MEN (from chest, abdomen, and thigh skinfolds)								
	AGE (years)								
	Under 22	23–27	28–32	33–37	38–42	43–47	48–52	53–57	Over 57
8–10	1.3	1.8	2.3	2.9	3.4	3.9	4.5	5.0	5.5
11–13	2.2	2.8	3.3	3.9	4.4	4.9	5.5	6.0	6.5
14–16	3.2	3.8	4.3	4.8	5.4	5.9	6.4	7.0	7.5
17–19	4.2	4.7	5.3	5.8	6.3	6.9	7.4	8.0	8.5
20–22	5.1	5.7	6.2	6.8	7.3	7.9	8.4	8.9	9.5
23–25	6.1	6.6	7.2	7.7	8.3	8.8	9.4	9.9	10.5
26–28	7.0	7.6	8.1	8.7	9.2	9.8	10.3	10.9	11.4
29–31	8.0	8.5	9.1	9.6	10.2	10.7	11.3	11.8	12.4
32–34	8.9	9.4	10.0	10.5	11.1	11.6	12.2	12.8	13.3
35–37	9.8	10.4	10.9	11.5	12.0	12.6	13.1	13.7	14.3
38–40	10.7	11.3	11.8	12.4	12.9	13.5	14.1	14.6	15.2
41–43	11.6	12.2	12.7	13.3	13.8	14.4	15.0	15.5	16.1
44–46	12.5	13.1	13.6	14.2	14.7	15.3	15.9	16.4	17.0
47–49	13.4	13.9	14.5	15.1	15.6	16.2	16.8	17.3	17.9
50–52	14.3	14.8	15.4	15.9	16.5	17.1	17.6	18.2	18.8
53–55	15.1	15.7	16.2	16.8	17.4	17.9	18.5	19.1	19.7
56–58	16.0	16.5	17.1	17.7	18.2	18.8	19.4	20.0	20.5
59–61	16.9	17.4	17.9	18.5	19.1	19.7	20.2	20.8	21.4
62–64	17.6	18.2	18.8	19.4	19.9	20.5	21.1	21.7	22.2
65–67	18.5	19.0	19.6	20.2	20.8	21.3	21.9	22.5	23.1
68–70	19.3	19.9	20.4	21.0	21.6	22.2	22.7	23.3	23.9
71–73	20.1	20.7	21.2	21.8	22.4	23.0	23.6	24.1	24.7
74–76	20.9	21.5	22.0	22.6	23.2	23.8	24.4	25.0	25.5
77–79	21.7	22.2	22.8	23.4	24.0	24.6	25.2	25.8	26.3
80–82	22.4	23.0	23.6	24.2	24.8	25.4	25.9	26.5	27.1
83–85	23.2	23.8	24.4	25.0	25.5	26.1	26.7	27.3	27.9
86–88	24.0	24.5	25.1	25.7	26.3	26.9	27.5	28.1	28.7
89–91	24.7	25.3	25.9	26.5	27.1	27.6	28.2	28.8	29.4
92–94	25.4	26.0	26.6	27.2	27.8	28.4	29.0	29.6	30.2
95–97	26.1	26.7	27.3	27.9	28.5	29.1	29.7	30.3	30.9
98–100	26.9	27.4	28.0	28.6	29.2	29.8	30.4	31.0	31.6
101–103	27.5	28.1	28.7	29.3	29.9	30.5	31.1	31.7	32.3
104–106	28.2	28.8	29.4	30.0	30.6	31.2	31.8	32.4	33.0
107–109	28.9	29.5	30.1	30.7	31.3	31.9	32.5	33.1	33.7
110–112	29.6	30.2	30.8	31.4	32.0	32.6	33.2	33.8	34.4
113–115	30.2	30.8	31.4	32.0	32.6	33.2	33.8	34.5	35.1
116–118	30.9	31.5	32.1	32.7	33.3	33.9	34.5	35.1	35.7
119–121	31.5	32.1	32.7	33.3	33.9	34.5	35.1	35.7	36.4
122–124	32.1	32.7	33.3	33.9	34.5	35.1	35.8	36.4	37.0
125–127	32.7	33.3	33.9	34.5	35.1	35.8	36.4	37.0	37.6

Source: A. S. Jackson and M. L. Pollock, "Practical Assessment of Body Composition," *The Physician and Sportsmedicine* 13, no. 5 (1985): 76–90. Copyright © 1985 JTE Multimedia, LLC. Used with permission.

4. Record your estimated percent body fat.

% body fat = _____

SECTION II: BIA MEASUREMENT

1. Use a BIA machine to estimate your percent body fat. Remember to hydrate normally, as especially high or low levels of body water can skew results.

2. Record your estimated percent body fat.

% body fat = _____

SECTION III: BODY FAT RATING

Based on your estimated percent body fat from the skinfold test and/or BIA test, indicate your body fat rating below:

Body Fat Rating	Women	Men
Athletic/Low	14–20%	6–13%
Fitness	21–24%	14–17%
Acceptable	25–31%	18–25%
Obese	>32%	>26%

Source: From "Percent Body Fat Norms for Men and Women" in *ACE Lifestyle and Weight Management Coach Manual*, © 2013 American Council on Exercise. Reprinted with permission from the American Council on Exercise® (ACE®), www.acefitness.org.

Body fat rating: Skinfold test = _____

Body fat rating: BIA test = _____

SECTION IV: REFLECTION

1. Did your estimated percent body fat or rating surprise you? _____

2. If you performed both tests, how does your percent body fat rating for the skinfold test compare to the BIA test? If the results differ greatly, can you identify possible sources of error (such as technique, hydration, type of machine, etc.)?

_____

_____

3. How does your percent body fat rating compare with your other disease risk ratings from Lab 6.2?

_____

_____

7 Improving Your Nutrition

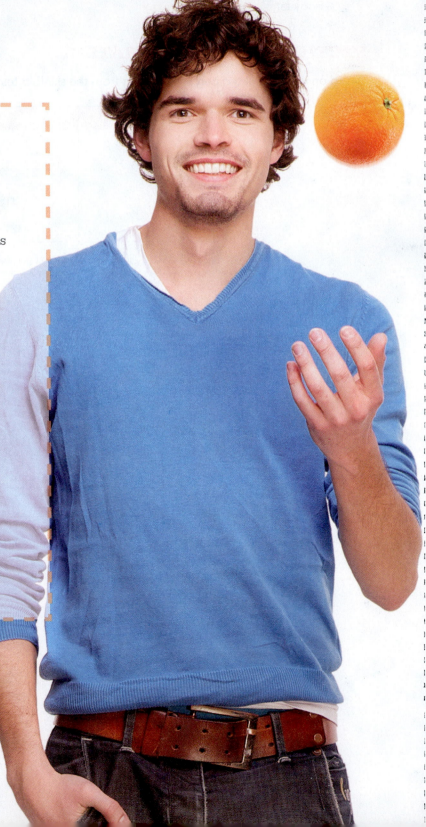

LEARNING outcomes

1. Describe obstacles to a healthy diet during the college years and a few ways to overcome them.

2. Identify the main nutrients in food and their roles in the body.

3. Discuss the role of portion size, food labels, food groups, and whole foods in maintaining a balanced diet.

4. Describe the special dietary needs of elite athletes versus everyday exercisers.

5. List some special nutritional needs of women, children, adults over 50, and vegetarians, and examine your own specific nutritional needs.

6. Assess your current diet and create a behavior change plan for improved nutrition.

MasteringHealth™

Go online for chapter quizzes, interactive assessments, videos, and more!

casestudy

CHAU

"Hi, I'm Chau. I'm a freshman and I live on campus in a dorm with my roommate, Tom. I moved here to Connecticut from Chicago. Living away from home for the first time has been quite an experience! I've been studying hard, taking a full load of classes, and trying to figure out if I want to major in history or political science. Plus, I'm in a few clubs and I'm playing a lot of soccer. I'm not on the team, but I like to play for fun. I'll jump into just about any pick-up game if I have time. I'm always rushing, though, and then I realize I'm starving! When I lived at home, there was always food around. My meal plan at the cafeteria covers 60 meals a month. For the others, I'm often scrambling at the last minute to find something to eat."

HEAR IT! ONLINE

Hunger is one of our basic motivators. Eating—seeing, smelling, and tasting food—is one of life's great pleasures. Hunger compels us to seek and consume the food that will supply our bodies with energy and raw materials. The pleasure of eating compels us to find the foods we enjoy or even crave. Our challenge is to eat a healthy balance of the food our bodies need and the foods we want to eat.

Food contains **nutrients**, chemical compounds that supply the energy and raw materials for survival. Our cells break down food molecules and, in the process, change their shapes and release energy stored in their chemical bonds. The energy becomes available to drive the activities within our cells, tissues, and organs. The breakdown of nutrients also liberates raw materials that cells can take in, modify, and use in repair and growth.

Nutrition is the study of how people consume and use the nutrients in food. Nutrition researchers explore some of the basic questions about what we should be eating and how food affects our long-term health and disease. Is it better to eat butter or margarine? Should you drink tea, coffee, both, or neither? Should you take a daily vitamin pill? Is red meat okay? How much salt is too much?

Nutritional findings are sometimes contradictory. Since the 1970s, consumers have been advised to throw away butter and use margarine instead; then to do just the reverse; then to avoid almost all fats; then to avoid almost all carbohydrates, and so on. Understandably, some people have grown skeptical about nutritional information. As in every area of science, new studies in nutrition occasionally contain data that appear to invalidate older studies. Nevertheless, the field has made tremendous advances toward understanding our daily **diets**—the foods and drinks we select—as well as what we *should* be eating, what we should be *avoiding*, and why. The kinds of healthy diets we discuss in this chapter can help you stay fit and well. Keep in mind:

- A balanced diet helps sustain desirable body mass and weight and helps keep your fat-to-lean ratios within a recommended range. This, in turn, can improve appearance, make you more comfortable in your body, and reduce the risk of chronic illnesses related to excess weight and obesity.

- A good diet can help alleviate feelings of stress and depression, while a poor diet can contribute to them.

- A good diet can help prevent chronic diseases, frequent colds and infections, and the effects of vitamin deficiency. Conversely, poor diet is one of the biggest contributors to cardiovascular disease, diabetes, obesity, arthritis, osteoporosis, and several types of cancers.

If you are young and currently healthy, chronic diseases may seem improbable and remote. However, establishing good dietary habits now can both improve your current wellness and diminish your later risk of chronic illness. Optimal fitness and wellness—both now and in your future—require good nutrition and good **eating habits**. This chapter helps you analyze and improve both.

nutrients Chemical compounds in food that are crucial to growth and function; including proteins, carbohydrates (starches and sugars), lipids (fats and oils), vitamins, and minerals

nutrition The study of how people consume and use the nutrients in food

diets The foods and drinks we select to consume

eating habits When, where, and how we eat; with whom we eat; what we choose to consume; and our reasons for choosing it

Why Are My College Years a Nutritional Challenge?

If you are like most college students, you often reach for cheap snacks and fast food to save time and money. You grab something tasty. You eat it quickly, maybe even while you walk or drive to the next class, job, study session, or social event. You may worry about calories and weight. But most students don't think much about vitamins, minerals, and other nutrients or worry much about the challenge of eating well during the college years.

The typical student's diet resembles the typical American diet: Nearly one-third of Americans' total calories come from chips, cookies, donuts, desserts, french fries, candy bars, sugary drinks, beer, wine, and other alcoholic beverages.[1] The number-one takeout food is pizza, followed by Chinese food and fast food (burgers, fries, and so on). Other favorite "staples" of the American diet are coffee drinks, tacos, burritos, sandwiches, and salads. The most frequently eaten vegetables in America are iceberg lettuce and potatoes.[2]

Most Students Have Less-Than-Optimal Eating Habits

Eating habits describe when, where, and how we eat; with whom we eat; what we choose to consume; and why we choose it. Like most Americans, college students, in general, have poor eating habits. Examples of poor eating habits are eating fast food and eating while driving or watching television. Good eating habits include sitting down to a relaxed meal and consuming fresh fruits and vegetables every day. How are your eating habits? **Figure 7.1** can help you find out.

The GetFitGraphic Do Students Make the Grade When It Comes to Healthy Eating? on the next page

Less healthy eating habits	More healthy eating habits
Consuming sugary soft drinks with and between meals	Drinking water with and between meals
Skipping meals then gorging once or twice per day	Eating three meals plus one or two small, nutritious snacks at regular times
Eating large amounts of red meats, fatty meats, or fried meats	Choosing fish, lean poultry, tofu, or other proteins that are low in saturated fats
Choosing processed foods	Choosing whole foods such as fruits, vegetables, whole grains, nuts, seeds, and lean sources of protein
Hurriedly bolting down food on the run, in a car, or on a bike	Sitting down to eat a relaxed meal with friends or family
Finishing the large portions served at restaurants	Eating half of a large restaurant portion and taking the rest home
Snacking before bed	Eating earlier in the evening
Eating heartily to be social, regardless of appetite	If you're not very hungry, drinking a low-cal beverage or eating a piece of fruit to be social
Eating out of habit or boredom, for example, while watching TV	Sitting down at a table to eat only when hungry, finding another outlet for boredom
Reaching for food when feeling stressed or angry	Learning stress reduction techniques

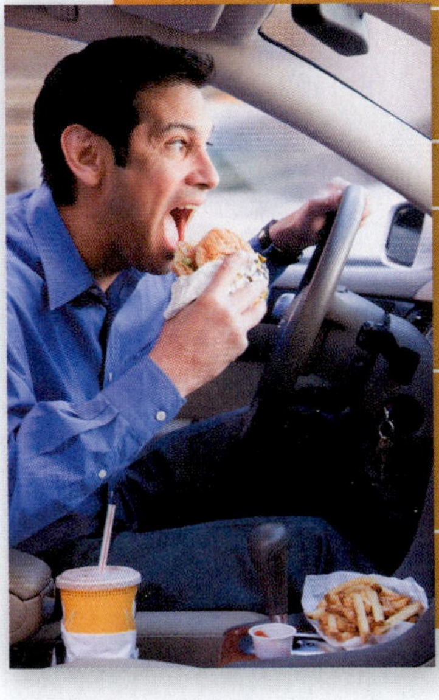

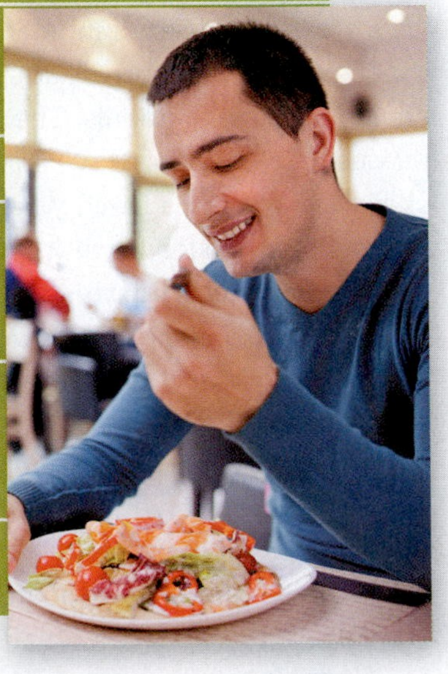

FIGURE **7.1** You can examine your own eating and snacking habits by comparing what, when, where, and how much you eat and drink to the sliding scale for each habit. You can also get ideas here for improving your daily diet.

Adapted from U.S. Department of Agriculture and U.S. Department of Health and Human Services, "Dietary Guidelines for Americans, 2010, 7th ed," 2013, www.health.gov

DO STUDENTS MAKE THE GRADE WHEN IT COMES TO HEALTHY EATING?

The college student nutrition report card is in!

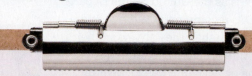

HOW DO STUDENTS' DIETS COMPARE TO THE USDA RECOMMENDATIONS?[1]

✓ Good ✗ Bad

Nutrient	USDA Recommended Daily Consumption	Students' Average Daily Consumption	Grade
TOTAL PROTEIN	10–35% of calories	~16% of calories	✓
TOTAL CARBOHYDRATES	45–65% of calories	~53% of calories	✓
TOTAL FAT	25–35% of calories	~30% of calories	✓
SATURATED FAT & SUGARS	<10% of calories	~30% of calories	✗
CHOLESTEROL	<300 mg	~295 mg	✓
FIBER	~31 g	~19 g	✗
VITAMIN E	15 mg	~6.5 mg	✗✗
POTASSIUM	4,700 mg	~2695 mg	✗✗
SODIUM	1500–2300 mg	~3300 mg	✗
FOLATE	400 mcg	~390 mcg	✓
CALCIUM	1000 mg	~975 mg	✓
VITAMIN D	15 mcg	~4 mcg	✗
FRUITS & VEGETABLES	5–9 servings	~2.5 servings	✗

LET'S LOOK AT THREE NUTRIENT AREAS WHERE STUDENTS AREN'T MAKING THE GRADE: SODIUM, FATS, AND FRUITS & VEGETABLES.

SODIUM

Stop shaking the salt! Students consume an average of **1000 mg sodium** over the USDA recommendations. Where does all that salt come from?[2]

65% Foods from grocery stores

25% Foods eaten in restaurants

10% Foods cooked at home

FATS

75% of college freshman eat fried or high-fat fast foods at least three times a week

25% of college freshman eat fried or high-fat fast foods fewer than three times a week[4]

10 TROUBLEMAKERS

These ten foods supply 44% of the sodium in a typical American diet:[3]

1 Breads and rolls **2** Cold cuts and cured meats **3** Pizza **4** Poultry **5** Soups
6 Sandwiches **7** Cheese **8** Pasta dishes **9** Meat dishes **10** Snacks

FRUITS & VEGETABLES

Fill half your plate with fruits and veggies at every meal! The majority of students are getting less than half of the USDA recommendations for fruits and vegetables, with only 1-2 servings per day.[5]

0 servings = **6.6%**

1-2 servings = **61.6%**

3-4 servings = **27.1%**

5+ servings (USDA recommendation) = **5.3%**

provides data on the typical student diet and how it stacks up. Most students, for example, eat half as many fruit and vegetable servings as the United States Department of Agriculture (USDA) recommends; get one and a half to two times more sodium than they should in their salted foods; and take in three times more refined sugar and saturated fat than the government deems healthy.[3] Understanding the information throughout this chapter and in our discussion of weight management can make a measurable difference in your nutritional wellness, including the energy you need for studying, exercising, and other daily activities.

College Life Presents Obstacles to Good Nutrition

Food is easy to find in the many vending machines, cafeterias, bars, restaurants, and markets on campus and off. But nutritious foods—low in saturated fat, salt, and sugars, for instance, and high in fiber and vitamin content—are much harder to find on and near campus. Food choice is an important obstacle to student nutrition in addition to other obstacles: time and money pressures, lack of home-cooking facilities, personal habits and attitudes, and the emotional stresses college can present.

Fast food and takeout solve both time and money issues, but the food at these restaurants often provides poor nutrition. Even when students cook for themselves, however, nutritional misconceptions and a tight budget can still impede a healthy diet. If you do shop and cook, a few simple steps can help you achieve a balanced, affordable diet: Buy seasonal fruits and vegetables. Watch for sales, use coupons, and shop at discount stores. Make a shopping list and stick to it. Buy more plant proteins (e.g., beans and tofu) and less meat, fish, or poultry. And if possible, double your recipes and freeze portions for later.

Another obstacle to good nutrition is our natural human craving for sweet, fatty, salty, and high-protein foods. We love those treats! Students sometimes come to college with preexisting preferences and eating habits and then, away from parental influence for the first time, tip over into unhealthy dietary routines such as regularly eating junk food, skipping breakfast, snacking frequently, and limiting fruit and vegetable consumption.

Meal skipping or protein loading can also be an offshoot of body dissatisfaction at a time when social interaction and physical attractiveness are emphasized. Three-fifths of female college students and half of males are dissatisfied with their body size and shape.[4] Most students want to lose weight, while a few want to gain weight or add muscle. Body

casestudy

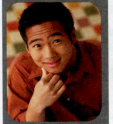

CHAU

"I like eating in the dorm cafeteria but I have to take care of about 30 meals on my own each month. The idea was that I'd eat two meals a day in the dorm—probably breakfast and dinner—and grab lunch somewhere between classes. So far, though, it's not quite working out that way. On days when I don't have an early class, I tend to sleep through breakfast. Then, I've got to rush to my 11:00, which means grabbing donuts and coffee in the campus store. Sometimes I manage to get back to the dorm for lunch, but if I don't, I usually eat something on the run at the food court. The good thing is that my dorm has a late night café that accepts my meal plan. So if I'm up late studying, I can grab a pizza or bowl of cereal. I don't pay much attention to my diet or how many calories I'm eating. I figure at my age, it's more about getting enough calories than eating a 'balanced meal.' Doesn't it all kind of balance out naturally?"

THINK! What aspects of college life are influencing Chau's dietary choices? How does your own living situation and schedule affect your efforts to eat right?

ACT! Make a list of small lifestyle changes you could make to improve your diet and try to incorporate at least one in the coming week, another the following week.

HEAR IT! ONLINE

- - - - - - - - - - - - - - - - - - - -

dissatisfaction leads some students to skip meals; avoid particular classes of foods such as fats or carbohydrates; go on drastic very-low-calorie diets; or take other measures that can cause an imbalance of nutrients, vitamins, and minerals.

Stress and social eating contribute to poor diet, as well. Stress itself can cause people to eat more, especially high-calorie "comfort" foods. Stress can also reduce sleep, which can lead to using food, caffeine, sugar, and alcohol to alter mood and energy levels. People under stress also tend to seek out the relief of socializing for relaxation, and when people get together, they eat and drink. The box Tips for Ordering at Restaurants on pages 239–240 helps you learn to recognize and choose healthy items from a variety of menus.

TOOLS FOR CHANGE

Tips for Ordering at Restaurants

No matter what type of cuisine you enjoy, there will always be healthier and less healthy options on the menu. To help you order wisely, here are lighter options and high-fat pitfalls. "Lighter" choices contain fewer than 30 grams of fat, a generous meal's worth for an active, medium-sized woman. They also have a higher ratio of nutrients to calories. "Heavier" choices have up to 100 grams of fat; often have hefty sodium levels; and have a lower ratio of nutrients to calories.

Cuisine	Lighter	Heavier	Tips
Italian	Pasta with red or white clam sauce Spaghetti with marinara or tomato and meat sauce	Eggplant parmigiana Fettuccine Alfredo Fried calamari Lasagna	Stick with plain bread instead of garlic bread made with butter or oil. Avoid cream- or egg-based sauces. Try vegetarian pizza. Don't ask for extra parmesan.
Mexican	Bean burrito (no cheese) Chicken fajitas with lots of vegetables	Beef chimichanga, deep fried Chile relleno, battered and fried	Choose soft tortillas with fresh salsa. Order grilled shrimp, fish, or chicken, or an entrée salad. Ask for black or pinto beans made without lard or fat. Avoid cheeses and sour cream or ask for a small portion on the side.
Chinese	Hot-and-sour soup Stir-fried vegetables Shrimp with garlic sauce Szechuan shrimp Wonton soup	Crispy chicken Kung pao chicken Moo shu pork Sweet-and-sour pork	Request brown rice instead of white. Ask for vegetables steamed or stir-fried with less oil. Avoid fried rice, breaded dishes, egg rolls and spring rolls, and items loaded with peanuts or cashews. Avoid high-sodium sauces (those containing soy sauce).
Japanese	Steamed rice and vegetables Tofu as a meat substitute Broiled or steamed chicken and fish	Fried rice dishes Miso Tempura	Avoid soy sauces. Avoid deep-fried dishes such as tempura. Ask for extra vegetables and half as much rice. Eat sashimi and sushi (raw fish) only where the food is freshly made to avoid possible bacteria or parasites.
Thai	Clear broth soups Stir-fried chicken and vegetables Grilled meats	Coconut milk soup with chicken Peanut sauces for satay Deep-fried or batter-fried meats and vegetables	Avoid coconut-based soups and curries. Ask for steamed brown rice, not fried or white rice. Avoid Thai iced tea, which is filled with sugar and high-fat evaporated milk.
American Breakfast	Hot or cold cereal with nonfat or 1 percent milk Pancakes or French toast with a small amount of syrup Scrambled eggs with hash browns and plain toast	Belgian waffle with sausage Sausage and eggs with biscuits and gravy Ham-and-cheese omelet with hash browns and toast	Ask for whole-grain cereal or shredded wheat with nonfat milk. Ask for whole wheat toast without butter or margarine. Order omelets without cheese. Order fried eggs without bacon or sausage.
Sandwiches	Veggies and tofu spread Roast beef Turkey	Tuna salad Reuben Submarine	Ask for mustard. Hold the mayonnaise and high-fat cheese. Load on dark green lettuce and sliced vegetables.
Seafood	Broiled bass, halibut, or snapper Grilled scallops Steamed crab or lobster	Fried seafood platter Blackened catfish	Order fish broiled, baked, grilled, or steamed—not pan fried or sautéed. Ask for lemon instead of tartar sauce. Avoid creamy and buttery sauces.

Cuisine	Lighter	Heavier	Tips
Fast Food	Grilled chicken sandwich Lean roast beef sandwich Entrée salad, dressing on the side Water, nonfat milk, unsweetened iced tea Fresh fruit and yogurt	Double-patty sandwiches Added cheese French fries and onion rings Fried chicken Fish fillets Chicken nuggets Apple pie Colas	Order sandwiches without mayo or special sauce. Avoid deep-fried items. Go for oil and vinegar instead of creamy salad dressings. Choose a fruit salad rather than a fruit pastry.
Coffee-house	Latte or brewed coffee with nonfat milk and no or low-cal sweetener Chai with nonfat milk and no or low-cal sweetener Hot black, green, or herbal tea with no or low-cal sweetener	Carmel or vanilla latte with whipped cream Chai with whole or evaporated milk and sugar Hot chocolate or mocha with whipped cream	Avoid whipped cream. Request fat-free milk in blended drinks. Avoid extra sugar; try flavoring drinks with a dash of cinnamon or nutmeg.

There are several keys to overcoming the food obstacles in college life:

- Learn about nutrition and what your body needs to maintain maximum wellness.

- Learn to distinguish good food choices from poor ones and good eating habits from bad ones.

- As often as possible, frequent those restaurants, stores, and cafeterias that offer a wide selection of healthy foods.

- Improve your eating habits and hang out with other students who care about nutritious eating.

What Are the Main Nutrients in Food?

Humans share the need to "refuel" with every other kind of animal, from soaring eagles to drifting sea cucumbers. Our bodies can't originate energy-containing raw materials for activity, growth, and repair. Like all animals, we must consume enough of these compounds in foods and liquids to supply our daily needs. Our required nutrients are water, proteins, carbohydrates (starches and sugars), lipids (fats and oils), vitamins, and minerals (**Figure 7.2**, page 241). Within each class of nutrients, the three-dimensional molecular shapes of the individual kinds of sugars, fats, and so on determine the nutrients' unique chemical properties and, in turn, their roles in the body.

Nutritionists use the term **essential nutrients** for those compounds we must get from foods to maintain normal body functioning. Consuming nutrients keeps our internal "production line" efficiently manufacturing cell parts and usable energy compounds.

Nutritionists can measure the nutrients in individual foods—the natural sugars and starches in an apple, for example. They can measure the energy stored within those carbohydrates. And they can study the way our bodies release that stored energy during the digestion process. They measure the released energy in **calories**. One calorie (with a lowercase c) is the amount of energy required to raise the temperature of 1 gram of water 1 degree Celsius. When they refer to specific foods, nutritionists usually apply the larger measure **kilocalories (kcal) or Calories (C)**. One kilocalorie or Calorie (spelled with a capital C) equals 1,000 calories. A small-sized apple, for example, about the size of a tennis ball might have about 50 or 60 C.

To avoid confusion, this book will use "calories" when referring to food energy in general as well as when designating the energy in a specific food. Active adults need about 2,000 to 2,500 calories of food energy per day. The more you exercise, the higher your need for calories.

Proteins Are Building Blocks of Structure and Function

About 50 to 60 percent of your body weight is water; of the remainder, about half is protein. At 150 pounds, your

essential nutrients Nutrients necessary for normal body functioning that must be obtained from food

calories A measure of the amount of chemical energy that foods provide. One calorie (lowercase c) can raise 1 gram of water 1 degree Celsius.

kilocalories (kcal) or Calories (C) A measure of energy equal to one thousand calories; also designated kilocalorie (kcal); nutritionists use kcal or C when they refer to specific foods.

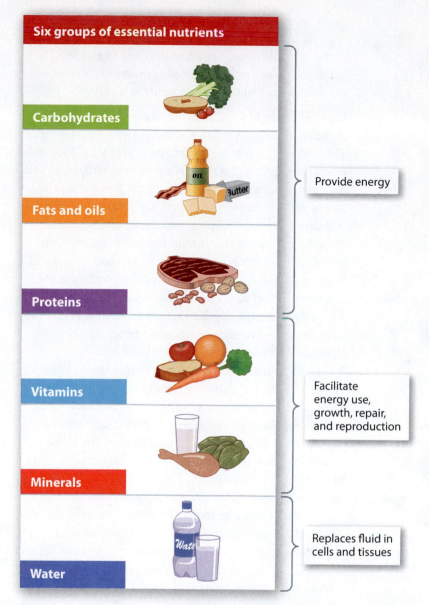

Six groups of essential nutrients	
Carbohydrates	
Fats and oils	Provide energy
Proteins	
Vitamins	
Minerals	Facilitate energy use, growth, repair, and reproduction
Water	Replaces fluid in cells and tissues

FIGURE **7.2** The six groups of essential nutrients in our foods provide energy, facilitate vital activities, and supply needed fluid for cells and tissues.

body would contain about 75 pounds of water and about 37.5 pounds of protein, depending on your muscle mass. **Proteins** are major structural components of nearly every cell and are especially important to the building and repairing of bone, muscle, skin, and blood cells. Proteins also make up the antibodies that protect us from disease, the enzymes that control all chemical reactions in the body, and the many types of hormones that regulate body activities. And proteins help transport oxygen, carbon dioxide, and various nutrients to body cells. When the body runs low on fats and carbohydrates as sources of ready energy, it can break down its own proteins and convert them to energy compounds. Protein supplies four calories of energy per gram.

Protein molecules are chains of subunits called *amino acids*. Sometimes called the "building blocks

of life," amino acids contain carbon, hydrogen, oxygen, and nitrogen arrayed in particular ways. There are 20 different kinds of amino acids, each with a different three-dimensional shape. Your body uses the 20 types of amino acids to build tens of thousands of kinds of proteins. Many of these are *structural proteins* that make up parts of cells, tissues, and organs. Many kinds of structural proteins enable cells to move, to divide, and to transport materials around internally. Other structural proteins make up your hair strands, your fingernails and toenails, and the lenses of your eyes. A steady supply of amino acids in the diet allows your body to continuously build, repair, and replace its own structural proteins.

Proteins that perform crucial functions (rather than make up physical structures) are called *functional proteins* and include **enzymes**, which enable thousands of kinds of chemical reactions to occur simultaneously within each body cell every second, including the enzyme reactions that break down food, absorb nutrients, and build new cell parts.

Proteins in the Diet Our bodies can manufacture only 11 of the 20 kinds of amino acids. Nutritionists call the other nine, which we must consume in food, the **essential amino acids**. Dietary protein that supplies all the essential amino acids is called *complete protein*, or *high-quality protein*. Typically, protein from animal products is complete. *Incomplete proteins* lack some of the essential amino acids and therefore some of the building blocks we need to produce the full spectrum of proteins for growth, repair, and activity. Proteins from plant sources are often incomplete, lacking one or two of the essential amino acids. Nevertheless, a vegetarian can

proteins Biological molecules composed of amino acids. Proteins serve as crucial structural and functional compounds in living organisms.

enzymes Proteins that facilitate chemical reactions but are not permanently altered in the process; biological catalysts

essential amino acids Collectively, the 9 of the 20 types of amino acids, or building blocks, that our bodies cannot manufacture and that we must consume in our foods

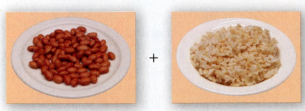

Legumes and grains

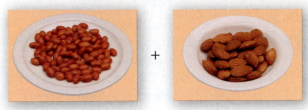

Legumes and nuts and seeds

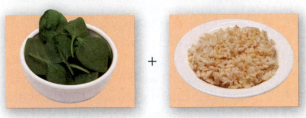

Green leafy vegetables and grains

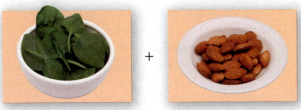

Green leafy vegetables and nuts and seeds

FIGURE **7.3** Combining plant foods from different groups (e.g., grains and legumes) on the same day can provide complementary proteins and all the necessary amino acids, even without eating meat or other animal foods.

easily combine plant foods to obtain *complementary proteins* from plant sources (**Figure 7.3**). Eating peanut butter on whole grain bread is one good example of combining plant foods to get all the essential amino acids. Eating corn and beans together is another.

Daily Protein Needs Nutritionists typically recommend that you get about 10 percent of your calories (or about 200 calories or more) from protein in a 2,000-calorie diet. Over a billion of the world's people face daily protein deficiency, but few Americans suffer it. The average American consumes between 60 and 100 grams (250 to 400 calories or more) of protein daily, with as much as 70 percent of it coming from animal parts and products and dairy products high in saturated fats and cholesterol. Consuming too much protein, particularly animal protein, can place added stress on the liver and kidneys and can cause a painful disease called *gout.* An overload of protein may also increase calcium excretion in urine, which can increase your risk of bone loss and bone fractures.[5]

Use **Figure 7.4** to calculate your daily protein needs. Here's an example: A healthy young woman weighing 132 pounds (60 kg) would need about 48 grams (60 × 0.8). One gram is equal to 0.035 ounce; therefore, she would need about 1.68 ounces of protein (0.035 × 48 = 1.68), which she could get, for example, by consuming one cup of skim milk, one-half cup of tofu, and one cup of cooked beans or 3 ounces of salmon during the course of a day.

In recent years, millions of people have tried the Atkins diet and similar diets that nearly eliminate carbohydrates and prescribe large quantities of protein. While these diets *can* lead to weight loss, the dieter is losing weight due to total calorie reduction, not due to some magical property of dietary protein itself. Diets that are

Group	Daily protein requirement (g/kg body weight)
Most adults	0.8 g/kg
Recreational athletes	1.0–1.1 g/kg
Elite athletes in training	1.2 –1.6 g/kg

Calculating your daily protein requirement	Example (for average adult)
❶ Determine your body weight	❶ Weight = 132 lb
❷ Convert pounds to kilograms: lb ÷ 2.21 lb/kg = kg	❷ 132 lb ÷ 2.21 lb/kg = about 60 kg
❸ Multiply by 0.8 g/kg for average adult to get requirement in grams per day	❸ 60 kg × 0.8 g/kg = 48 g Result: A 132 lb adult would need 48 g of protein a day

FIGURE **7.4** Use these formulas to determine your daily protein requirements, depending on your activity level.

not nutritionally balanced are almost always flawed. People with fluid imbalances, kidney or liver problems, or cardiovascular disease should avoid these diets altogether, as they usually contain higher levels of saturated fat and sodium, have lower levels of important vitamins, and raise risk factors for various chronic diseases. Others who choose to try such unbalanced diets should limit the length of time they follow them.

Protein and Fitness It is fairly common for athletes and fitness buffs to load up on animal protein under the misguided notion that eating more protein will cause them to build bigger muscles. But muscles grow in response to being worked: You must use them to grow them! The many vegetarian Olympic athletes are proof that training and effort—not mountains of animal protein—are the crucial ingredients. Research has also shown that 0.8 to 0.9 grams per kilogram of protein is enough for all but the top athletes, most of whom can get all they need for heavy endurance and strength training in 1.2 to 1.6 grams per kilogram per day.[6]

It's true that under some circumstances, you may need extra protein for cellular repair and replacement, such as when you are fighting off a serious infection, or if you are a pregnant woman. Most of us, though, need to be much more concerned with getting proteins low in saturated fat than with meeting our daily protein needs.

Carbohydrates Are Major Energy Suppliers

Carbohydrates, including the sugars and starches, have ring- and chain-like three-dimensional structures that allow them to store and supply much of the energy we need to sustain normal daily activity. The **simple carbohydrates** or **sugars** are common in whole, unprocessed foods such as beets, sugarcane, carrots, other vegetables, and fruits such as grapes (**Figure 7.5a**). The **complex carbohydrates** include the starches found abundantly in grains (such as rice and wheat), cereals (such as oats), some fruits and vegetables (such as bananas and squash), and many root vegetables (such as potatoes, yams, and turnips) (**Figure 7.5b**).

Our cells can rapidly break down sugar molecules and release energy stored in their chemical bonds. For this reason, simple sugars such as glucose, sucrose (table sugar), and lactose (milk sugar) are a source of immediate energy for the body. Your muscle cells and your brain and nerve cells are particularly dependent on a steady supply of glucose, whether from fruits and vegetables or from the starches in grains. This dependence is the reason low blood sugar, or *hypoglycemia,* can leave you feeling foggy-headed, weak, and shaky. According to research outlined in the USDA's *2010 Dietary Guidelines for Americans,* most of us consume a diet that is too heavy in added sugars and other sweeteners. The box What Sweeteners Should I Use? (page 244) explains how to recognize the many kinds of sweeteners listed on food labels and why we should limit our consumption of sweetened food.

carbohydrates A class of nutrients containing sugars and starches; supply most energy for daily activity

simple carbohydrates or sugars Carbohydrates made up of one or two sugar subunits that deliver energy in a quickly usable form

complex carbohydrates Energy-storing and structural compounds made up of long chains of sugar molecules; most deliver energy slowly

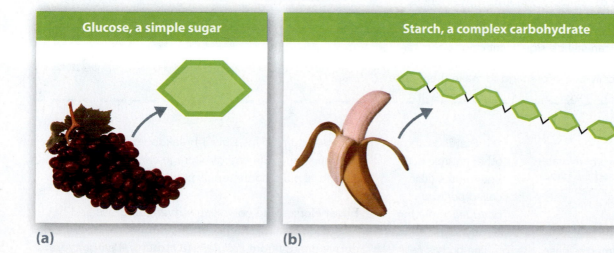

Glucose, a simple sugar

Starch, a complex carbohydrate

(a)

(b)

FIGURE **7.5** (a) Grapes are rich in glucose, a simple sugar. (b) Bananas contain starch, a complex carbohydrate.

Q&A What Sweeteners Should I Use?

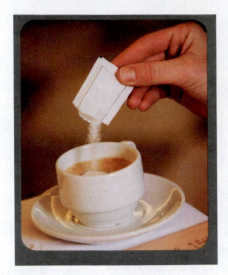

Full-Calorie Sweeteners

The average American consumes more than 355 calories (more than 22 teaspoons per day) of sugars, such as honey, corn syrup, or sucrose (table sugar) added to their foods and beverages. Most of this is in processed foods. Sweeteners can boost flavor, texture, and bulk. However, added sugars have health consequences: They add calories but virtually no other nutrients. They promote tooth decay. They tend to replace more nutritious foods in the diet such as fruits, vegetables, seeds, nuts, and whole grains. And they raise triglyceride levels in the blood; this, in turn, can contribute to cardiovascular disease.[1] The American Heart Association recommends a maximum daily limit of 100 calories of added sugars (the equivalent of six teaspoons of sugar) for most women, and 150 calories (equivalent to nine teaspoons) for most men.[2]

Reduced-Calorie Sweeteners

Many products that claim to be "low in sugar" or "sugar free" include sugar alcohols: carbohydrates with a sweet flavor and a particular type of chemical structure. Examples of these ingredients include mannitol, sorbitol, xylitol, and hydrogenated starch hydrolysates. The products sometimes contain nonnutritive sweeteners, as well (see below). These "dietetic" foods do provide fewer calories—only about half of the calories in regular sweeteners—but can still be significant calorie and carbohydrate sources, depending on how much you consume.[3] They typically cost more, and to make them taste good, the manufacturers often add fat. Be sure to scan such food labels for these sweeteners as well as for *trans* fats and saturated fats.

Nonnutritive Sweeteners

Artificial sweeteners contain synthetic compounds or chemicals derived from naturally occurring herbs or sugars. The products in this class are intensely sweet and provide essentially no calories. Most "sugar free" gums and beverages, for example, contain an artificial sweetener such as aspartame (Equal, NutraSweet); sucralose (Splenda); neotame; acesulfame potassium (Sunett, Sweet One), or saccharin (Sugar Twin, Sweet'N Low). A recently released product, Truvia, contains the sweet-tasting nonnutritive compound rebiana derived from the leaves of the stevia plant. In addition to rebiana, Truvia contains a sugar-alcohol. Despite some concerns about the safety of nonnutritive sweeteners based on experiments feeding animals with saccharin, health agencies, including the National Cancer Institute, find no sound scientific evidence that artificial sweeteners raise cancer risk or promote other serious health problems. Some researchers, however, have suggested an association between weight gain and artificial sweetener use, for unknown reasons.[4] A recent study of frequent diet soda drinkers found changes in the way their brains' reward circuitry responds to the sweet taste of saccharin and sugar compared to nondiet soda drinkers. The researchers speculate that while these brain changes need to be studied in greater depth, they may help explain why people can over-consume carbohydrates and other nutrients and gain weight despite drinking zero-calorie beverages.[5]

SEE IT! ONLINE
Ditching Sugar

Sources:
1. Mayo Clinic Staff, "Added Sugar: Don't Get Sabotaged by Sweeteners," MayoClinic Online, October 2012, www.mayoclinic.com
2. American Heart Association, "Sugars and Carbohydrates," June 2012, www.heart.org
3. American Diabetes Association, "Sugar Alcohols," February 2013, www.diabetes.org
4. Mayo Clinic Staff, "Artificial Sweeteners: Understanding These and Other Sugar Substitutes," Mayo Clinic Online, October 2012, www.mayoclinic.com
5. E. Green and C. Murphy, "Altered Processing of Sweet Taste in the Brain of Diet Soda Drinkers," *Physiology and Behavior* 107, no. 4 (2012): 560–567.

---

fiber Indigestible carbohydrates in the diet that speed the passage of partially digested food through the digestive tract

Starches and other complex carbohydrates (also called *polysaccharides*, meaning "many sugars") can be a source of "timed release" energy. The body's cells must break starch molecules down into sugar subunits before releasing the chemical bond energy contained in those sugars. This slower breakdown makes most starches important energy-storage compounds and structural building materials in plants and animals.

Fiber Horses and cows can survive on grass and hay alone because their digestive systems break down and derive energy from *cellulose* (a structural carbohydrate that makes up the cell walls of plants). In humans, cellulose acts as indigestible **fiber** in one of two forms.

Insoluble fiber, found in bran, whole grain breads and cereals, and in most fruits and vegetables, speeds the passage of foods and reduces bile acids and certain bacterial enzymes. *Soluble fiber,* which is in oat bran, dried beans, and some fruits and vegetables, attaches to water molecules. Soluble fiber appears to help lower blood cholesterol levels and the risk of cardiovascular disease. Both kinds of fiber assist the passage of partially digested food through the digestive tract. They also help control appetite and body weight by creating a feeling of fullness without adding extra calories.

Fiber-rich foods contain nutrients that may help reduce cancer risk and have other health benefits.[7] Fiber also helps prevent constipation by absorbing moisture like a sponge and producing softer, bulkier stools that are easily passed. Fiber-induced gas may also initiate bowel movements. Reducing constipation helps protect against diverticulosis—the formation of tiny pouches in the colon that bulge out through the intestinal wall the way an inner tube protrudes through holes in a tire. These pouches tend to get inflamed and can cause intestinal pain, bloating, bleeding, blockages, and other symptoms.

The USDA's *2010 Dietary Guidelines for Americans* recommends that we increase our daily consumption of whole, ground, cracked, or flaked grains (including whole oats, whole wheat, and brown rice), and decrease our consumption of refined carbohydrates such as white rice or white flour (made into white bread, sandwich buns, pastries, and so on). **Table 7.1** lists many whole and refined grains. For tips on how to increase the fiber in your diet, see the box Tips for Eating More Fiber on page 246.

TABLE **7.1** Whole Grains and Refined Grains

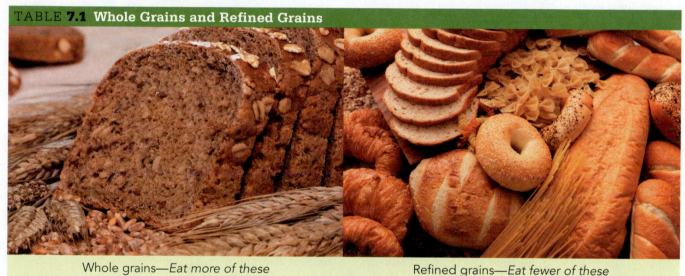

Whole grains—*Eat more of these*		Refined grains—*Eat fewer of these*	
brown rice	whole wheat bread	cornbread*	pitas*
buckwheat	whole wheat crackers	corn tortillas*	pretzels
bulgur (cracked wheat)	whole wheat pasta	couscous*	white bread
oatmeal	whole wheat sandwich buns	crackers*	white sandwich buns
popcorn	and rolls	flour tortillas*	and rolls
whole grain barley	whole wheat tortillas	grits	white rice
whole grain cornmeal	wild rice	noodles*	
whole rye		pasta*	*Ready-to-eat breakfast cereals*
	Less common whole grains:		corn flakes
Ready-to-eat breakfast cereals:	amaranth		
whole wheat cereal flakes	millet		
muesli	quinoa		
	sorghum		
	triticale		

*Most of these products are made from refined grains. Some are made from whole grains. Check the ingredient list for the words *whole grain* or *whole wheat* to decide whether they are made from a whole grain. Some foods are made from a mixture of whole and refined grains.

Source: United States Department of Agriculture ChooseMyPlate, "Food Groups: Grains," May 2012, www.ChooseMyPlate.gov

Tips for Eating More Fiber

Most Americans should double their daily fiber intake. To increase the fiber in your diet, think "whole" and "traditional" foods instead of refined foods and choose more of these:

SEE IT! ONLINE
High Fiber Diet

- Whole grains, including stone-ground wheat, bulgur wheat, wheat bran, wheat berries, whole barley, whole millet, whole quinoa, oatmeal, oat bran, popcorn, barley, cornmeal, whole rye, brown rice, and rice bran
- Peas, beans, nuts, and seeds
- Leafy greens such as baby spinach, endive, radicchio, arugula, mizuna, watercress, or dandelion greens
- Bran or flaxseed
- Fresh fruits and vegetables including, when edible, their cleanly scrubbed skins
- Plenty of liquids each day

At the same time, choose fewer of these:

- White bread, buns, or flour tortillas
- Cereals that list "enriched" flour as the main ingredient
- Cookies, pastries, desserts, or candies

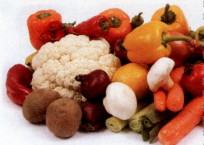

THINK! What is your average daily intake of fiber?

ACT NOW! <mark>Today,</mark> keep a food diary (or look at one you are already keeping) and, using food labels and other available information, calculate the total grams of fiber in your foods. <mark>This week,</mark> make a list of the fiber-containing foods you have eaten in the past week and next to each, write a food that you could swap for even more fiber. For example: "white rice–brown rice," or "white bread bun–whole wheat pita." <mark>In two weeks,</mark> keep a food diary for an entire day and again calculate the total number of fiber grams you consumed. Did you improve your fiber consumption? How does your new level compare with the USDA recommendation of 28 grams (females ages 19–30) and 34 grams (males ages 19–30)?

The daily recommended amount of fiber for an adult is 25 to 30 grams, but most Americans—including most college students—get less than that amount.[8] Some professional groups believe the requirements should be higher, perhaps even double the recommended amount. Food labels must list the fiber contents of foods and often break that number down into insoluble and soluble fiber.

The Glycemic Index of Foods Nutritionists use a tool called the **glycemic index** to measure the rate at which foods raise levels of glucose in the blood. If you eat food with a high glycemic index, especially in large portions, your bloodstream becomes flooded with glucose, and this, in turn, leads to an upsurge of the hormone insulin. The combination of glycemic index plus portion size is called *glycemic load*. Over time, this flooding and surging can contribute to certain cancers; to overweight, obesity, and type 2 diabetes; and perhaps to heart disease.[9]

Using the glycemic index of foods to control the amount of sugar in your bloodstream requires some practice. A glycemic index chart can help you predict the effect a given food will have on your blood sugar levels. (See this book's website for links to these charts.) Note that not all sweet foods have a high index and many starchy or fatty foods do. The glycemic index of foods can help you plan a healthy diet, but it is just one factor to consider because some low–glycemic index foods are poor nutritional choices overall (e.g., premium ice cream, sausages), whereas some high–glycemic index foods are good choices overall (e.g., bran flakes, watermelon). The best approach to control your sugar intake is to develop a habit of reading food labels before you buy or eat something to discover the amount of dietary sugars contained in foods. Then, use glycemic index and glycemic load charts to help you get a feel for which foods raise your blood sugar levels quickly and which do not.

glycemic index A measurement of the rate at which foods raise levels of glucose in the blood and, in turn, trigger the release of insulin and other blood-sugar regulators

"Low-Carb" Foods In recent years, food manufacturers have introduced thousands of "low-carb" foods, influenced, in part, by the popularity of high-protein weight loss diets. As we've seen, however, whole grain foods are packed with healthful nutrients and fiber. The culprit is not the "carbs" themselves but the quantity most people eat and the refining of the carbohydrates. Whole fruits and vegetables, and foods made with whole grains, seeds, and nuts, are nutrient-dense and retain the fibrous cellulose in their skins and husks. Most "low-carb" foods are highly processed and contain substitute sugars such as mannitol, sorbitol, and dextrose. There is no solid evidence that "low-carb" products made with sweeteners protect you from diseases, and they cost much more than simple fruits, vegetables, whole grains, nuts, seeds, and beans.

Fats Are Concentrated Energy Storage

The "low-carb" diet craze was preceded by a "low-fat" craze that labeled all fats and oils as harmful. In fact, fats play vital roles in maintaining healthy skin and hair, padding the body organs against shock, insulating us against temperature extremes, storing energy to fuel muscle activity, and promoting healthy cell function. Although they are widely misunderstood nutrients, fats make foods taste better; carry the fat-soluble vitamins A, D, E, and K to cells; and provide certain essential compounds we can't get from other foods or manufacture in our own cells. They also provide a concentrated form of energy and raw materials that can stand in whenever carbohydrates are in short supply.

Types of Fats *Fat* is a common term for **lipids**, a class of molecules that includes fats and oils. **Fats**, such as butter, lard, and bacon grease, are solid at room temperature. **Oils** are usually liquid at room temperature; examples are corn and olive oils. Lipids also include *waxes,* such as beeswax, and *steroids,* such as steroid hormones, cholesterol, and certain vitamins.

Structurally, fats and oils are made up of long chains of carbon atoms called **fatty acids**. The fatty acids in most foods and in the body occur in the form of **triglycerides**, molecules that have a "head," which contains the compound glycerol, and three tails (**Figure 7.6a**, page 248). The "tails" are made up of fatty acid chains of various lengths.

In lipid molecules of all types, the chemical bonding of carbon atoms is the key to whether the chains remain straight and form solid fats, or kink and form liquid oils (**Figure 7.6b**).

In a fatty acid chain where every available carbon bond is *saturated* or filled with hydrogen atoms, the fat itself is called a **saturated fat**. Saturated chains remain straight and can pack solidly against each other. This explains why butter, beef fat, and lard—all saturated fats—occur as solids at room temperature (**Figure 7.6c**).

In an oil, there are also chains of carbon atoms, but double bonds between certain carbons leave fewer bonds to be saturated (filled with hydrogen molecules). The chains are said to be **unsaturated**. These double-bonded spots also cause the chains to kink and bend. Because the chains can't pack tightly together, they create a liquid oil rather than a solid fat. Fatty acid chains containing just one kinked (unsaturated) region are called **monounsaturated fatty acids** (**MUFAs**; *mono* means "one"). Olive oil, canola oil, and cashew oil are all rich in monounsaturated fatty acids. Chains containing two or more linked regions are called **polyunsaturated fatty acids** (**PUFAs**; *poly* means "many"). Corn oil, safflower oil, and cottonseed oil are all rich in polyunsaturated fatty acids (**Figure 7.6d**).

Food manufacturers sometimes alter the properties of oils by adding hydrogen atoms to liquid oils, a process called hydrogenation. This results in partially hydrogenated oils that contain some *trans* fatty acids or **trans fats**. These have cooking properties of solid fats as well as their potentially negative effects on health.

lipids A category of compounds, including fats, oils, and waxes, that do not dissolve in water

fats Lipids, such as butter, lard, and bacon grease, which are usually solids at room temperature

oils Lipids, such as corn and olive oil, which are usually liquids at room temperature

fatty acids The most basic units of triglycerides

triglycerides Lipid molecules made up of three fatty acid chains or "tails" attached to one glycerol "head" containing a three-carbon backbone; common form of fats in foods and in organisms

saturated fat A lipid, usually a solid fat such as butter, in which most of the chains of carbon atoms are loaded (or "saturated") with as many hydrogen atoms as the chain can carry

unsaturated fat A lipid, usually a liquid oil, in which most carbon chains lack the maximum load of hydrogen atoms

monounsaturated fatty acids (MUFAs) Lipids whose fatty acid chains have just one kinked (unsaturated) region

polyunsaturated fatty acids (PUFAs) Lipids whose fatty acid chains have two or more kinked (unsaturated) regions

trans fats Unsaturated lipids or oils with hydrogen atoms added to cause more complete saturation and make the oil function as a solid

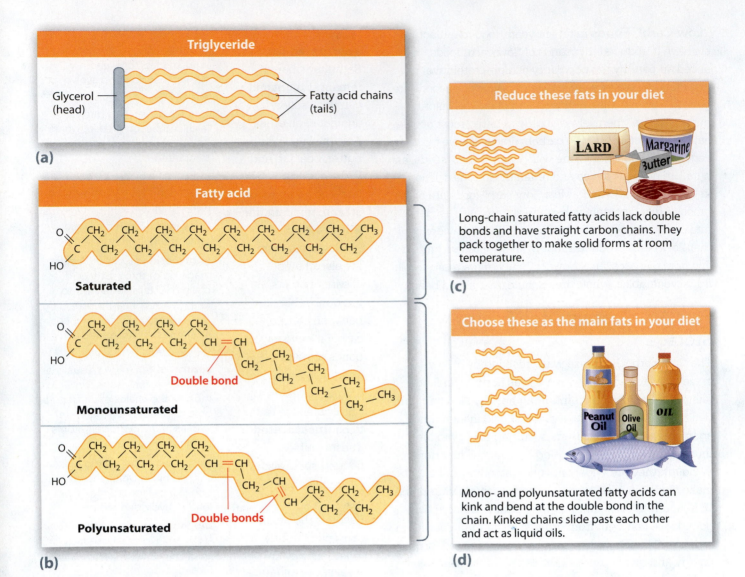

FIGURE **7.6** (a) Structure of triglyceride. (b) The chemical makeup of fatty acid chains in fats and oils helps explain why saturated fats (c) such as lard or butter are usually solid, and why mono- and polyunsaturated fats (d) such as olive and corn oil are usually liquids.

Figure from *Nutrition: An Applied Approach*, 3rd Edition, by Janice Thompson and Melinda Manore. Copyright ©2012 Pearson Education. Reprinted and Electronically reproduced by permission of Pearson Education, Inc., Upper Saddle River, New Jersey.

Margarines, shortenings, and many processed foods contain *trans* fats. Dairy products and meat naturally contain small amounts of *trans* fats, as well, created when certain bacteria act upon unsaturated fats. Nutritionists often recommend that we avoid or greatly decrease the intake of foods containing *trans* fats. The *trans* fat content of foods is now indicated on food labels. We will discuss the health consequences of eating *trans* fats later.

All of our food sources of fats and oils contain both saturated and unsaturated fats, in different ratios (**Figure 7.7**, page 249). For example, a tablespoon of safflower oil contains 0.8 gram of saturated fat, 10.2 grams of monounsaturated fat, and 2 grams of polyunsaturated fat. A tablespoon of butter typically contains 7.2 grams of saturated fat, 3.3 of grams monounsaturated fat, and

a trace of polyunsaturated fat. In general, lipids high in saturated fats are unhealthy for you, especially if you eat them frequently. Animals tend to make saturated fats, and plants tend to make unsaturated fats. Some plants, however, generate oils that are very high in saturated fats. Cocoa butter, palm kernel oil, and coconut oil contain more saturated fat per tablespoon than butter, beef fat, or lard! Since lipids high in mono- and polyunsaturated fats are much healthier for you than those high in saturated fat, it pays to learn about the types of oils so you can choose wisely. Figure 7.7 shows the oils containing the widest purple and red bands (which designate mono- and polyunsaturated fatty acids) are the healthiest. The fats and oils with the widest blue bands (which designate saturated fatty acids) are the least healthy.

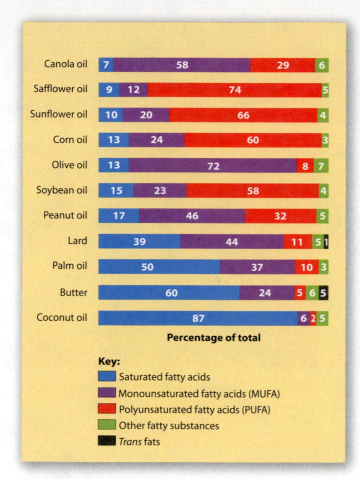

Canola oil, Safflower oil, Sunflower oil, Corn oil, Olive oil, Soybean oil, Peanut oil, Lard, Palm oil, Butter, Coconut oil

Percentage of total

Key:
- ■ Saturated fatty acids
- ■ Monounsaturated fatty acids (MUFA)
- ■ Polyunsaturated fatty acids (PUFA)
- ■ Other fatty substances
- ■ *Trans* fats

FIGURE **7.7** Common fats and oils have varying percentages of saturated and unsaturated fats, making them more or less healthful in the diet.

Omega-3 and Omega-6 Fatty Acids

Our cells cannot synthesize certain types of fatty acids and therefore we must consume each of them in our diet. These fatty acids are called **essential fatty acids**. They include *linoleic acid,* an omega-6 fatty acid, and *linolenic acid,* an omega-3 fatty acid. An **omega-6 fatty acid** is polyunsaturated and has double-bonded carbons at two sites, including one at the sixth carbon along the carbon chain. An **omega-3 fatty acid** has double-bonded carbons at three sites, including one at the third carbon along the chain. Other omega-3 fatty acids include EPA and DHA, which the human body can modify into linolenic acid. Polyunsaturated oils such as canola oil, corn oil, soybean oil, and sunflower oil all contain high levels of omega-6 fatty acids. Polyunsaturated oils such as flaxseed oil, walnut oil, and, to a lesser degree, certain fish oils, canola oil, and soybean oil contain relatively high percentages of omega-3 fatty acids. The body can modify both types of essential fatty acids into various fats we need for blood clotting, building cell membranes in the brain, contributing to healthy blood vessel walls, and counteracting inflammation.

As a result, they lower the risks for heart disease and Alzheimer's disease, and help prevent inflammatory and autoimmune diseases, such as ulcerative colitis and rheumatoid arthritis.[10] Recent studies have shown that eating foods rich in omega-3s such as flaxseed, walnuts, and the flesh of oily fish (sardines, mackerel, salmon) is more protective than simply taking supplements (pills) containing the oil.[11]

Dietary Fats and Your Health

As your body breaks down the fats and oils in a food, it packages the lipids into particles called **lipoproteins** that can move along easily in the bloodstream. Lipoproteins contain lipid and protein portions, and carry both triglycerides and **cholesterol**, the most common steroid in the body (recall that steroids are one structural class of fats). Our cells need and make cholesterol to keep membranes pliable and use it as a building block for making steroid hormones and other substances. In common usage, lipoproteins carrying cholesterol are simply called *cholesterol.* When we consume more calories than we need, the body makes extra triglycerides and stores them as body fat.

Eating saturated fat and *trans* fat raises the level of both triglycerides and so-called bad cholesterol or **low-density lipoproteins (LDLs)** in your bloodstream. Over time, elevated levels of LDLs can lead to plaque deposits inside the blood vessels. These plaques can constrict blood flow, raise blood pressure, and lead to heart disease, heart attacks, and strokes. Eating saturated fat also raises the level of so-called good cholesterol or

essential fatty acids Lipid components, including linolenic acid, EPA, DHA, and linoleic acid, which the body cannot manufacture and which we must obtain in polyunsaturated oils

omega-6 fatty acid A polyunsaturated fatty acid that has double-bonded carbons at two sites, including one at the sixth carbon along the chain

omega-3 fatty acid A polyunsaturated fatty acid that has double-bonded carbons at three sites, including one at the third carbon along the chain

lipoproteins Lipid-plus-protein transport particles that can move along easily in the bloodstream; carry triglycerides or cholesterol

cholesterol A waxy lipid in the steroid class that is an important component of cell membranes and is transported in the blood by carriers called *LDL* and *HDL*

low-density lipoproteins (LDLs) A form of lipoprotein sometimes called "bad cholesterol"; LDL levels rise in response to saturated fats in the diet and can contribute to plaque deposits inside blood vessels

high-density lipoproteins (HDLs) in the blood, but to a lesser degree. Eating polyunsaturated oils raises HDL levels to a much greater degree. HDLs prevent and reduce plaque deposits in the blood vessels and therefore help protect against cardiovascular disease, strokes, and heart attacks. That's the main reason nutritionists urge us to choose oils over saturated fats.

You may be wondering how something the human body makes and needs for its own cell membranes and hormones can be harmful in the diet. When some people consume cholesterol, their body cells make less cholesterol and their overall level stays constant. In other people, however, that "leveling mechanism" works inefficiently, and they tend to accumulate the extra dietary cholesterol in blood-vessel-narrowing plaques.[12] Researchers are still trying to untangle the interconnections between cholesterol, triglycerides, HDLs, LDLs, body fat, and disease. The USDA recommends that you consume *less* cholesterol in your diet by cutting back on fatty meats, egg yolks, high-fat dairy products, and all other sources of saturated fats, cholesterol, and *trans* fats.

Research shows that *trans* fatty acids can be even more damaging than saturated fats. *Trans* fats increase LDLs and simultaneously lower HDLs, a doubly negative effect. A person who gets just 2 percent of his or her calories from *trans* fats would be raising his or her risk for heart disease by 23 percent and for sudden cardiac death by 47 percent.[13] The USDA recommends choosing products with little or no *trans* fats.[14] In fact, the USDA's ChooseMyPlate.gov website—which provides specific daily food recommendations based on your sex, size, age, and activity level—now classifies *trans* fats along with saturated fats and sugars as "empty calories." The site suggests you restrict your overall daily consumption of such empty calories to 260 per day (if you are a woman aged between 19 and 30) and to 330 per day (if you are a man in that same age group).

Trans fats also raise triglyceride levels. After a meal, the liver takes cholesterol and triglycerides that we don't use immediately in our tissues, packages them into HDLs and LDLs, and sends them through the blood for storage in fat cells.[15] Coincidentally, consuming large quantities of refined starches, sugars, and/or alcohol also raises blood triglycerides. This helps explain why eating big helpings of such starches and sugars, as so many Americans do, can lead to obesity, diabetes, and heart disease.

Eating mono- and polyunsaturated fats lowers LDLs and raises HDLs, a doubly positive effect. As Figure 7.7 shows, most kinds of cooking oil are high in mono- and polyunsaturated fats and low in saturated fats, but there are exceptions, such as palm kernel oil and coconut oil. That's one reason it is important to read food labels rather than make assumptions about the fats in particular foods.

Some nutritionists encourage people to consume more oils. A popular plan called the Mediterranean diet encourages people to use olive oil liberally in cooking and at the table. Spanish researchers studying nearly 7,500 middle-aged men and women with identified risk factors for suffering a heart attack or stroke recently drew an important conclusion about the menus so common in Mediterranean countries such as Italy, Greece, and Spain: A diet that is rich in nuts, olive oil, fish, fruits, vegetables, and wine with meals, but that contains very little red meat, processed meats, dairy products, or sweets *can cut the incidence of stroke or heart attack by 30 percent.*[16] Nutritionists from Harvard Medical School also encourage people to eat healthful plant oils, including but not limited to olive oil, at most meals.[17] The USDA ChooseMyPlate.gov website recommends a daily consumption of six teaspoons of mono- and polyunsaturated oils per day for women aged 19 to 30 and seven teaspoons for men of the same age.

A Healthy Plan for Fats in Your Diet

LIVE IT! ONLINE
Worksheet 24
Cutting Out the Fat

Most of us need to cut down on saturated fats while getting more heart-healthy fats into our diet. Here are some ideas:

- Always read food labels, looking at both the amount of saturated fat and the percentage it represents of your daily recommended maximum for saturated fat and total fat.

- Don't be fooled into thinking that cookies, crackers, or chips are healthy foods because they are labeled "low-fat." Watch out for high levels of added sugars, refined flour, salt, and *trans* fats (the label may read "vegetable shortening" or "partially hydrogenated vegetable oil").

- For salad dressings, sautéing, and other cooking needs, choose oils such as canola, soy, olive, and safflower that contain high levels of mono- and polyunsaturated fats.

- Whenever possible, instead of butter or margarine, use soft, buttery spreads that list "0 *trans* fats" on the label. For topping bread and crackers, alternatives to butter include all-fruit jams (no sugar added), fat-free cream cheese, salsa, hummus, olive oil, or low-fat salad dressing.

- For protein, choose beans, nuts, seeds, tofu, lean meats, fish, or poultry instead of fatty meats such as bacon, sausages, hot dogs, bologna, pepperoni, or organ meats. Remove skin. Avoid frying. Drain off fat after cooking.

- Choose dairy products that have 0 or 1 percent fat, such as skim milk, nonfat yogurt, and fat-free cottage cheese. Avoid reduced-fat dairy products (2 percent fat) and whole-milk dairy products (4 percent fat) whenever possible. Choose nonfat or low-fat frozen yogurt or sorbet rather than ice cream. Cut back on cheese: Cheese is a major source of saturated fat and cholesterol (as well as sodium) in the American diet.

- Cook with chicken broth, wine, vinegar, low-calorie salad dressings, or unsaturated oils (mono- and polyunsaturated) rather than butter, margarine, sour cream, mayonnaise, and creamy salad dressings.

- To increase omega-3s, eat walnuts, flaxseed, tofu, beans, winter squash, and fatty fish (i.e., salmon, tuna, bluefish, herring, or sardines). Be aware, however, that salmon, canned tuna, North Atlantic mackerel, and catfish can contain high levels of mercury, so you must limit yourself to no more than 12 ounces (two servings) of them per week. Other fish such as King mackerel, tilefish, swordfish, and shark can have higher levels of mercury—so high, in fact, that reproductive-age women and children should avoid them completely and others should eat them with caution.[18]

- Add green leafy vegetables, walnuts, walnut oil, and milled flaxseed to your diet.

- Limit processed and convenience foods. These often contain refined carbohydrates and high levels of sodium in addition to *trans* fats.

Don't demand daily nutritional perfection from yourself. Try to balance your intake of different foods over a few meals and a couple of days at a time. If you have a high-fat breakfast or lunch, balance it with a low-fat dinner. If you forget to eat at least five servings of fruits and vegetables today, eat extra servings tomorrow. And closely monitor your diet to avoid consuming more than the small daily allotment the USDA recommends for empty calories such as sugars and saturated fats (no more than about 10 percent of daily calories).

Vitamins Are Vital Micronutrients

Vitamins are organic compounds that we need in tiny amounts to promote growth and help maintain life and health. Vitamins take part in the minute-by-minute cellular reactions that help maintain our nerves and skin, contribute to the production of blood cells, help us build bones and teeth, assist in wound healing, and help convert food energy to accessible fuel for cellular activities. Some vitamins are toxic in high doses, and for many vitamins, time spent on the shelf, the heat from cooking, and certain other environmental conditions can diminish their potency in foods.

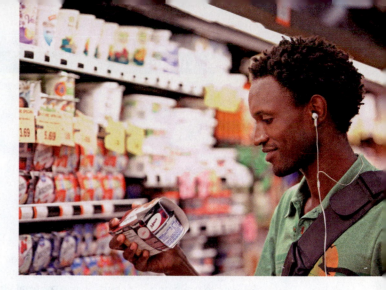

Some vitamins can dissolve only in water and some only in fat. *Water-soluble vitamins,* including vitamin C and the B vitamins, dissolve easily in water and can be absorbed directly into the bloodstream.[19] Excess water-soluble vitamins are usually excreted in the urine and cause few toxicity problems. Because they are not stored in the liver, body fat, or other tissues, we must consume water-soluble vitamins on a regular basis in our foods. *Fat-soluble vitamins,* including vitamins A, D, E, and K, must associate with fat molecules in order to be absorbed through the intestinal tract. Excess, unused quantities of the fat-soluble vitamins tend to be stored in the body. High levels can accumulate in the liver and cause damage. **Table 7.2** on pages 252–253 lists 13 vitamins, their food sources, their chief functions in the body, and the symptoms caused by consuming too little or too much of each.

Vitamin vendors often make various claims about the benefits of taking vitamin supplements to augment what we consume in foods. For the most part, a carefully chosen diet will provide your vitamin needs, but because many people eat too few fruits and vegetables, they don't get optimal levels. In addition, certain groups of people, and all of us at certain life stages, do have special vitamin needs. People over 50, for example, must be careful to get enough vitamin B_{12} since absorption of certain nutrients, including B_{12}, declines naturally with age. The box Do I Have Special Vitamin and Mineral Needs? on page 254 discusses both the vitamin needs of specific groups and the issue of taking vitamin supplements versus getting vitamins from food alone. Few Americans suffer from true vitamin deficiencies if they eat a fairly balanced diet. Taking very high levels of certain vitamins can even lead to a toxic condition known as *hypervitaminosis.*

vitamins Organic compounds in foods that we need in tiny amounts to promote growth and help maintain life and health

TABLE 7.2 Guide to Vitamins

Vitamin RDI	Best Food Sources	Main Functions in Body	Deficiency Symptoms	Toxicity Symptoms
Water-Soluble Vitamins				
B_1 (Thiamin) 1.5 *milligrams (mg)*	Meat, pork, liver, fish, poultry, whole grain and enriched breads and cereals, pasta, nuts, legumes	Energy harvest and use from nutrients; normal appetite; nervous system function	Poor appetite, heart irregularities, mental confusion, muscle weakness, poor growth	None known
B_2 (Riboflavin) 1.7 *mg*	Dairy products, dark green vegetables, liver, meat, whole grain and enriched breads and cereals	Energy harvest and use from nutrients; healthy skin, normal vision, normal growth	Eye problems, skin cracking around nose and mouth	None known
Niacin 20 *mg*	Meat, eggs, poultry, fish, milk, whole grain and enriched breads and cereals, nuts, legumes, yeast, all protein foods	Energy harvest and use from nutrients; healthy skin, nervous system function, digestion	Skin rash, loss of appetite, dizziness, weakness, irritability, fatigue, mental confusion, indigestion	Flushing, blurred vision, glucose intolerance, abnormal liver function
B_6 (Pyridoxine) 2.0 *mg*	Meat, poultry, fish, shellfish, legumes, whole grain foods, leafy greens, bananas	Breakdown of proteins and fats, formation of red blood cells and antibodies, conversion of niacin	Nervous disorders, skin rash, muscle weakness, anemia, convulsions, kidney stones	Sensory nerve damage, skin lesions
Folate 0.4 *mg*	Leafy greens, liver, legumes, seeds	Forming red blood cells, breakdown of proteins, cell division, proper formation of neural tube in embryo	Anemia, heartburn, diarrhea, smooth tongue, poor growth and development	Nerve damage; high levels may mask a vitamin B_{12} deficiency
B_{12} 6 *micrograms (mcg)*	Meat, fish, poultry, shellfish, milk, cheese, eggs, yeast	Nerve cell maintenance, red blood cell formation, building of new genetic material	Anemia, smooth tongue, fatigue, nerve degeneration progressing to paralysis	None known
Pantothenic acid 10 *mg*	Widespread in foods	Crucial factor in energy harvest and use	Rare; sleep disturbances, nausea, fatigue	None known
Biotin 0.3 *mg*	Widespread in foods	Crucial factor in energy harvest and use, building fat molecules, energy storage in muscles	Loss of appetite, nausea, depression, muscle pain, weakness, fatigue, rash	None known
C (Ascorbic acid) 60 *mg*	Citrus fruits, cabbage-type vegetables, tomatoes, potatoes, dark green vegetables, peppers, cantaloupe, strawberries, mangos, papayas	Helps heal wounds; maintains connective tissue, bones, and teeth; strengthens blood vessels; antioxidant; boosts immunity; aids absorption of iron	Scurvy, anemia, blood vessel damage, depression, frequent infections, loose teeth, bleeding gums, bleeding, muscle wasting, rough skin, weak bones, poor wound healing	Nausea, abdominal cramps, diarrhea, red blood cell breakdown in some people, kidney stones in people with kidney disease. Upon withdrawing from high doses, deficiency symptoms may appear

TABLE **7.2** *(Continued)*

Vitamin RDI	Best Food Sources	Main Functions in Body	Deficiency Symptoms	Toxicity Symptoms
Fat-Soluble Vitamins				
A 5000 *international units (IU)*	Milk, cream, cheese, butter, eggs, liver, dark leafy greens, broccoli, deep orange fruits and vegetables	Healthy vision, growth and repair of tissues, formation of bones and teeth, immunity, building hormones, cancer protection	Night blindness; rough skin; frequent infections; impaired growth, especially of bones and teeth; eye problems leading to blindness	Miscarriage, birth defects, red blood cell breakage, nosebleeds, abdominal cramps, nausea, blurred vision, bone pain, dry skin, rashes, hair loss
D 200 IU	Sunlight on skin; fortified milk and margarine, eggs, liver, fish	Healthy bones and teeth; aids absorption of calcium and phosphorus	Rickets in children, weakened bones and bone problems in adults, abnormal growth, joint pain, soft bones	Raised blood calcium, constipation, weight loss, irritability, weakness, nausea, kidney stones, mental and physical retardation, calcium deposits
E 30 IU	Vegetable oils, leafy greens, wheat germ, whole grains, butter, liver, egg yolk, milk, nuts, seeds, fortified cereals, soybeans, avocado	Healthy red and white blood cells, healthy cell membranes in lungs and elsewhere, antioxidant activity	Muscle wasting, weakness, damage to red blood cells, anemia, bleeding, fibrocystic breast disease	Interference with anticlotting medication, intestinal discomfort, increased risk of stroke
K	Liver, milk, leafy greens, cabbage-type vegetables, vegetable oils	Aids digestion, blood clotting, regulation of calcium in blood, builds bone tissue	Bleeding	None known

Minerals Are Elemental Micronutrients

The micronutrients called **minerals** allow our nerves to transmit impulses, our hearts to beat, oxygen to reach our tissue cells, and our digestive tracts to absorb vitamins from food. They are usually not toxic, and we excrete excess quantities of most minerals from the body. The **major minerals** (also called *macrominerals*) are elements that the body needs in relatively large amounts. We need smaller amounts of the **trace minerals** (also called *microminerals*). **Table 7.3** on pages 255–256 lists most of the major and trace minerals, their functions, food sources, and symptoms of deficiency and/or toxicity. We discuss three minerals—sodium, calcium, and iron—in more detail because of their crucial roles in the body and their excesses or deficiencies in diets.

Sodium We need sodium, the Na in sodium chloride (NaCl), or table salt, for regulating the water contents of blood and body fluids; for the transmission of nerve impulses; for muscle contraction, including the heartbeat; and for several metabolic functions inside cells. However, most of us consume much more than we need.[20] Nutritionists estimate that the average American consumes around 3,400 milligrams per day, mostly from salted snacks and processed foods.[21] The average adult at rest and not sweating profusely needs only 180 to 500 milligrams of sodium (about one-quarter teaspoon) per day for

minerals Elements such as calcium or sodium that allow vital physiological processes, including nerve transmission, heartbeat, oxygen delivery, and absorption of vitamins

major minerals Elements needed in relatively large amounts, including sodium, calcium, phosphorus, magnesium, potassium, and chloride

trace minerals Elements the body needs in very tiny amounts; includes iron, zinc, copper, iodine, selenium, fluoride, and chromium

DIVeRSiTY

Do I Have Special Vitamin and Mineral Needs?

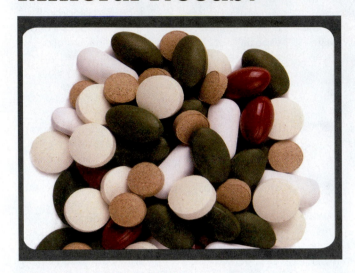

Most nutritionists agree that you should try to get your daily vitamins and minerals from a healthful diet rather than eating carelessly and relying on supplements. People in a number of population groups, however, are at risk for vitamin deficiencies. If you belong to one of these groups, you should pay extra attention to your diet and perhaps consider taking a multivitamin.[1]

- Women of reproductive age who could become pregnant need 400 micrograms of folate per day to prevent potential neurological defects in a developing fetus. Pregnant women need 600 micrograms per day.

- Premenopausal women, especially those with heavy menstrual bleeding, need 18 milligrams of iron per day in foods or in total from foods and a multivitamin. They must also get enough vitamin C to help them absorb iron from foods. Men and postmenopausal women need 10 milligrams per day and should be careful not to get too much.

- Everyone needs a good supply of calcium each day from low-fat dairy products, fortified juices, and other sources. The daily value for people under 50 is 1,000 milligrams. Pregnant women, nursing mothers, teens, and older adults need extra calcium (1,200 to 1,500 mg/day) for the development and maintenance of bones and to lower the risk of osteoporosis.

- Older adults need sufficient potassium for normal muscle contraction and nerve transmission and sodium within a healthy range to supply cellular needs but lower the risk of high blood pressure.

- Older adults, dark-skinned individuals, and people who do not get regular exposure to sunlight have a special need for vitamin D. The government currently recommends that people under 50 consume 200 IU (International Units) of vitamin D per day, people between 50 and 70 consume 400 IU per day, and people over 70 consume 600 IU per day.

- People over 50 naturally produce less stomach acid and absorb less vitamin B_{12} from foods. Older adults should be careful to get at least 2.4 micrograms of B_{12} per day or more, especially if they take stomach acid blockers.

- Cigarette smoking decreases bone density and interferes with the body's normal use of vitamin C. Smokers therefore need to consume higher levels of calcium (1,200 mg/day) and of vitamin C (110 mg in women, 125 mg/day in men) compared to 90 milligrams for nonsmoking adults.

- People with diseases that disrupt normal metabolism or nutrient absorption (e.g., diabetes and certain cancers) can develop vitamin or mineral deficiencies. Physicians often recommend special diets or multivitamins as part of their treatment.[2]

- The USDA dietary guidelines provide specific pointers for parents and guardians to help kids and teens get the balance of nutrients they need to support their growth and development.

- Details about the special nutritional needs of vegetarians and diabetics are covered on page 270.

If you plan to take a multivitamin, apply common sense. There is no need to get more than the RDI for vitamins and minerals. Doses exceeding 100 percent can lead to serious side effects. Since fat-soluble vitamins and certain minerals can build up in the body, be sure a multivitamin has less than the RDI for vitamins A, D, E, and K and for magnesium, chromium, selenium, and zinc.[3] To be safe, people in high-risk groups should consult a doctor before taking supplements regularly.

Sources:
1. Center for Science in the Public Interest, "The Multivitamin Maze" and "How to Read a Multi Label," *Nutrition Action Healthletter* (March 2006): 6–7.
2. U.S. Department of Agriculture and U.S. Department of Health and Human Services, *Dietary Guidelines for Americans, 2010*, 7th Edition (Washington, DC: U.S. Government Printing Office, 2010).
3. National Institutes of Health, "NIH State of the Science Panel Urges More Informed Approach to Multivitamin/Mineral Use for Chronic Disease Prevention," May 2006, www.nih.gov

TABLE **7.3** Guide to Selected Minerals

Mineral RDI	Best Food Sources	Main Functions in Body	Deficiency Symptoms	Toxicity Symptoms
Calcium 1.0 g	Milk and dairy products, small fish with bones, tofu, leafy greens, legumes	Building bones and teeth, muscle contraction and relaxation, nerve function, blood clotting, blood pressure	Stunted growth in children, bone weakness and thinning in adults	Mineral imbalances, shock, kidney failure, fatigue, mental confusion
Phosphorus 1.0 g	All animal tissues	Component of every cell, helps regulate pH balance	Unknown	Can unbalance calcium; can lead to calcium deficiency, spasms, convulsions
Magnesium 400 mg	Nuts, legumes, whole grains, deep leafy greens, seafood, chocolate	Bone hardening, protein synthesis, enzyme activity, normal function of muscles and nerves	Weakness, confusion, poor growth, impaired hormone production, muscle spasms, disturbed behavior	Mega-doses can lead to nausea, cramps, dehydration, death
Sodium 2400 mg	Salt, soy sauce, processed foods, cured, canned, pickled foods	Helps maintain normal fluid balance and pH within body	Muscle cramps, mental apathy, loss of appetite	Hypertension, water retention, increased calcium loss
Chloride 2300 mg	Salt, soy sauce, processed foods, cured, canned, pickled foods	Component of stomach acid and needed for digestion, helps maintain normal fluid balance	Dangerous changes in pH, irregular heartbeat	Vomiting
Potassium 3500 mg	Meats, fruits, milk, vegetables, grains, legumes	Involved in biochemical reactions that help build protein, maintain fluid balance, transmit nerve impulses, contract muscles	Muscle weakness, paralysis, confusion; accompanies dehydration; can cause death	Muscular weakness, vomiting, irregular heartbeat; can stop heart
Iodine 150 mcg	Iodized salt, seafood	Component of thyroid hormone, helps regulate metabolism	Goiter; mental and physical retardation due to thyroid deficiency	Goiter or enlargement of thyroid gland
Iron 18 mg	Beef, fish, poultry, shellfish, eggs, legumes, dried fruits	Crucial component of hemoglobin in red blood cells, myoglobin in muscles; takes part in oxygen transfer, energy use	Anemia, weakness, pallor, headaches, frequent infections, difficulty concentrating	Nausea, vomiting, dizziness, rapid heartbeat, damage to organs, death
Zinc 15 mg	Meats, fish, poultry, grains, vegetables	Component of insulin and many enzymes; takes part in DNA, protein synthesis, immune response, taste, wound healing, normal development, sperm production, vitamin A transport	Growth failure in children, delayed sexual development, loss of taste, poor wound healing	Fever, nausea, vomiting, diarrhea, headaches, depressed immune function

TABLE **7.3** *(Continued)*

Mineral *RDI*	Best Food Sources	Main Functions in Body	Deficiency Symptoms	Toxicity Symptoms
Copper 2 mg	Meats, drinking water	Absorption of iron, component of several enzymes	Anemia, bone changes (rare)	Liver damage if toxicity is due to certain diseases; nausea, diarrhea, vomiting
Fluoride 10 mg	Drinking water (natural or fluoridated), tea, seafood	Formation and maintenance of bones and teeth	Susceptibility to tooth decay and bone loss	Discoloration of teeth, joint pain, stiffness
Selenium 400 mcg	Seafood, meats, grains	Helps protect body compounds from oxidation	Muscle pain and possible deterioration, possible damage to nails and hair	Vomiting, nausea, rash, brittle hair and nails, cirrhosis of liver
Chromium 30 mcg	Meats, whole foods, fats, vegetable oils	Associated with insulin, needed for breakdown and use of glucose	Diabetes-like condition with poor glucose utilization	Unknown. Occupational overexposure damages skin and kidneys

normal body functioning.[22] The *2010 Dietary Guidelines for Americans* recommends that everyone restrict sodium to less than 2,300 milligrams (less than 1 teaspoon) per day, and that certain groups (those over 51 years old, African Americans, and people with hypertension, diabetes, or chronic kidney disease) reduce their sodium consumption to under 1,500 milligrams per day. Pickles, salty snack foods, processed cheeses, many breads and bakery products, and smoked meats and sausages often contain several hundred milligrams of sodium per serving. Many fast-food entrées and convenience entrées pack 500 to 1,000 milligrams of sodium per serving.

Many experts believe that there is a link between excessive sodium intake and hypertension (high blood pressure).[23] Researchers began recommending, several years ago, that people with hypertension cut back on sodium to reduce their risk of cardiovascular disorders.[24]

You can shake your own salt habit by choosing low-sodium or salt-free food products. For example, order popcorn without salt. Switch to kosher salt—an equivalent measure has less sodium than regular table salt. Instead of adding salt to food you prepare, try using fresh or prepackaged herb blends to season foods. These small changes can add up to a significant reduction in unneeded sodium.

osteoporosis A disease of thinning, weakened, porous bones during which too little calcium is deposited or retained in the bones

Calcium High sodium intake may also increase calcium loss in urine, which increases your risk for debilitating fractures as you age.[25] The element calcium (Ca) is crucial for the development and maintenance of bones and teeth, blood clotting, muscle contraction, nerve transmission, and fluid balance between the cell's interior and its environment. Nevertheless, most Americans consume less than the 1,000 to 1,300 milligrams of calcium per day recommended by government guidelines.[26]

Osteoporosis is a disease of thinning, weakened, porous bones that affects more than 44 million Americans (women and men) over age 50. The risk for it climbs if you consume too little calcium during childhood and adolescence when bones are developing, if you have a small skeleton (or "frame"), and/or if you consume too little calcium during adulthood. Bone weakness can lead to pain, stooped posture, and fractures, and can diminish mobility and independence. Forty to 50 percent of women and 13 to 22 percent of men will break a bone as a result of osteoporosis.[27]

Dairy products are among the richest dietary sources of calcium, but calcium-fortified orange juice, almond milk, or soy milk are also good sources, as are leafy green vegetables and many other foods (see Table 7.3). Be aware that the added phosphoric acid (phosphate) in carbonated colas and certain other soft drinks can cause you to excrete calcium and thus deplete needed calcium from your bones.[28] Calcium/phosphorus imbalance may lead to kidney stones and bone spurs and to the deposits or plaques inside blood vessels that contribute to cardiovascular diseases.

Vitamin D improves absorption of calcium; that's why dairies are required by law to add it to milk. In some studies, deficiencies of Vitamin D also appear linked to the risks for heart disease, cancer, and arthritis.[29]

Sunlight shining on your skin also increases your body's own manufacture of vitamin D, so a moderate amount of sunlight helps improve calcium absorption. The best way to obtain calcium with vitamin D is to consume them as part of a balanced diet. Fat-free dairy products are a good source, as are fortified soy and almond milk, salmon, tuna, eggs, and fortified cereals. Additionally, certain people do need calcium supplements (see the Diversity box on page 254).

Iron Each of us needs the element iron (Fe) for producing healthy blood, for muscle function, and for normal cell division. Women aged 19 to 50 need about 18 milligrams per day; men aged 19 to 50 need about 8 milligrams per day. Worldwide, iron deficiency is the most common nutrient deficiency, affecting more than 1 billion people. In developing countries, more than one-third of the children and women of childbearing age suffer from **iron-deficiency anemia**, in which the body fails to produce enough of the red hemoglobin pigment in the blood, leading to unusually low oxygen levels and unusually high carbon dioxide levels and resulting in mental and physical fatigue. About 5 percent of all Americans get too little iron in their food.[30] Among toddlers, adolescent girls, and women of childbearing age, about 10 percent show iron-deficiency anemia. Table 7.3 on pages 255–256 lists good dietary sources of iron.

Getting the right amount of iron is important. Researchers have linked iron deficiency to a host of problems, including poor immune system functioning and a propensity toward certain cancers. Some research has also suggested a link between too much iron in the diet and/or stored in the body and a higher risk for cardiovascular disease, cancer, and Alzheimer's and other brain diseases.[31]

Acute iron toxicity due to ingesting too many iron-containing supplements remains the leading cause of accidental poisoning in small children in the United States. Dozens of children have died from overdoses of as few as five iron tablets.[32]

Water Is Our Most Fundamental Nutrient

Imagine you are stranded on a desert island for a reality TV show and you can take along just one provision.

Would you choose food, water, or a cell phone? We hope you said water!

Humans are mostly water—close to 60 percent. Watery fluids bathe each of our internal cells. They help maintain a proper balance of salts within our blood and tissues, help maintain pH balance, and help facilitate the transport of substances throughout the body. Human blood plasma (the fluid portion of blood exclusive of red and white blood cells and other solid components) is approximately 91.5 percent water.[33] This proportion must remain fairly constant for blood to efficiently carry oxygen and nutrients to the cells and carry away carbon dioxide and other wastes.

Even under the most severe conditions, the average person can live for weeks on the energy stored in body fat. You can also get along without certain vitamins and minerals from foods for an equal amount of time before experiencing serious deficiency symptoms. Without water, however, you would become **dehydrated**, or depleted of normal levels of body fluids, within hours. Within one day without drinking water, you would probably begin to feel sluggish, dizzy, and nauseated, and would experience headaches, muscle cramps, or weakness. After a few days without water, your tongue would be parched and swollen, your heart would be racing, and you'd very likely go into shock and die.

A person's need for water varies dramatically based on age, size, diet, exercise, overall health, and environmental temperature and humidity levels. Most of us get enough water through foods and beverages just by satisfying our thirst.[34] People with certain diseases such as diabetes or cystic fibrosis, however, excrete extra fluid and must generally take in a higher volume. On a hot day, especially if exercising, you need to consciously replace fluids lost to sweat and exhalation. It is possible, though, to take in too much water and become nauseated, confused, or weak or even to lose consciousness from excess hydration leading to *hyponatremia* (sometimes called water intoxication). This condition results from too much water in the blood and therefore a salt concentration that is too low due to dilution. It often occurs in conjunction with heavy perspiration. If you are forcing

iron-deficiency anemia A disease in which the body takes in too little iron and makes too little oxygen-carrying hemoglobin

dehydrated Depleted of normal, necessary levels of body fluids

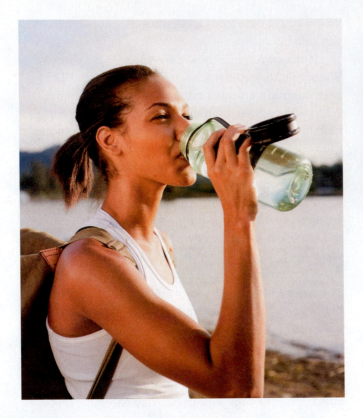

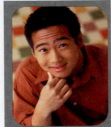

CHAU

"I kind of understand that your body uses different nutrients for different things. But I've never had a weight problem, so I've been more concerned with quantity than quality. I realize I'm eating a lot more carbs than I used to, mostly cereal and white bread. And Tom's girlfriend is always baking him cookies, so I load up on those. I also eat cheese and pepperoni pizzas in the cafeteria. Still, I don't worry about eating fat or being fat. Everyone in my family is thin!"

THINK! Chau often eats meals prepared on campus, where he has no access to nutrition labels. How could Chau estimate the amount of protein, carbohydrate, and fat in his diet? Given what you know about Chau's diet, which nutrients might he be deficient in? Which nutrients might he be consuming too much of?

ACT NOW! Today, analyze your own diet. What nutrients, if any, are you deficient in? This week, begin to calculate specific nutrients such as protein. How much should you be consuming each day? Are you taking in more protein than you really need? In two weeks, do the same for total carbohydrates and for fats.

HEAR IT! ONLINE

yourself to drink extra water even when you don't feel thirsty, or if your intake is so high that you gain water weight during an active exercise session, you may be imbibing more than you need. Thirst is a good indicator for most people during regular activity and all but the most extreme exercise. Thirst can be less reliable in children and the elderly, however, and some may need to consume water on a schedule while exercising.[35]

Commercial energy drinks can help exercisers replenish water lost through sweat and to restore salt and sugar. Many people dilute them with water, however, to prevent taking in more salt and sugar than they actually lose during exercise. One recent study found that drinking water and eating part of a banana every 15 minutes during a 2- to 3-hour bicycle race has a benefit equal to consuming a sports drink but provides more vitamins and fiber.[36] Some energy drinks include ingredients that are ineffectual or that can be harmful in large quantities. For example, researchers have failed to confirm any health benefit for ingredients such as taurine, bee pollen, and ginkgo biloba.[37] High concentrations of added sugars can boost energy in the short term but can create sluggishness later. Added vitamins C and B are unnecessary in a balanced diet. If overused, energy drinks containing the stimulants caffeine

and/or ginseng can speed bone loss, raise blood pressure, and increase the risk of cardiovascular diseases.

How Can I Achieve a Balanced Diet?

The average American adult consumes about 1,000 calories more per day than the average citizen worldwide and yet still gets unbalanced nutrition. To counter these trends toward overeating and substandard nutrition, the U.S. government:

- Sets guidelines for minimum and recommended levels of nutrients, vitamins, and minerals
- Requires standardized nutrition labels on most packaged and processed foods
- Determines appropriate portion sizes

- Publishes an interactive website, ChooseMyPlate.gov, to help individuals manage their daily nutrition, including calorie counting and energy expenditure through exercise, and
- Regulates the safety of our food supply

This massive effort is designed to improve our national wellness, and the many tools the USDA, FDA, National Academy of Sciences, and other governmental agencies provide can help you achieve a better diet, maintain a healthy weight, and help prevent several chronic diseases.

Follow Guidelines for Good Nutrition

There are so many parts to the government's nutritional advice to the public that they publish an overview— think of it as a cheat sheet for nutrition—called the *Dietary Guidelines for Americans*. A version came out in 2010 from the USDA and U.S. Department of Health and Human Services; the next version appears in 2015. We discuss the government's nutritional guidelines for specific sex, age, and ethnic groups later in this chapter. Here, we summarize the major recommendations in the 2010 version:

- *Balance calories to maintain weight.*
  - Balance the calories you take in from food with the calories your burn through activity and exercise. For most people, this means eating less and exercising more.
  - Learn about standard portion sizes so you can avoid oversized portions.
- *Increase certain foods and nutrients in your diet.*
  - Make at least half of your plate fruits and vegetables and eat a variety of produce types.
  - Consume at least half of your daily grains as whole grains and reduce refined grains.
  - Switch to fat-free or low-fat (1 percent) dairy products.
  - Eat proteins low in solid (saturated) fats such as eggs, beans, seeds, nuts, soy, fish, poultry, and lean meats.
  - Eat more vegetables, whole grains, and fat-free or low-fat dairy products to increase potassium, dietary fiber, calcium, and vitamin D.
- *Decrease consumption of certain foods and components.*
  - Compare sodium in foods such as soup, bread, and frozen meals—and choose the foods with the lower numbers.
  - Drink water instead of sugary drinks.

- Avoid *trans* fats and reduce saturated fat. Increase mono- and polyun- saturated oils to recommended levels for your sex, age, size, and activity level.
- Reduce cholesterol.
- Reduce added sugars and count the calo- ries as "empty."
- Reduce refined grains to less than half of your daily grains.
- Limit alcohol consumption.

- *Build healthy eating patterns.*
  - Eat so that you can balance your nutrient and caloric needs over time.
  - Keep track of what you eat and drink and make sure they fit your long-term pattern.
  - Follow safety rules for food preparation and eating to avoid foodborne illnesses.

Several government scientific advisory boards serve up an "alphabet soup" of specific recommended daily minimum and maximum intakes for each type of nutrient (fat, carbohydrates, proteins), and for the various types of vitamins and minerals:

- **DRI (Dietary Reference Intake)** is a listing of 26 nutrients essential to maintaining health. The DRI listing identifies recommended and maximum safe intake levels of the nutrients for healthy people, and identifies minimum levels needed to prevent deficiencies and diseases. DRIs are an umbrella category for several older classifications. The National Academy of Sciences Food and Nutrition Board publishes DRIs.

- **RDAs (Recommended Dietary Allowances)** are a listing of the average daily nutrient intake levels of vitamins and minerals that meet most people's daily needs.

- **RDIs (Reference Daily Intakes)** are a listing of needed daily nutrients based on the RDAs. Tables 7.2 (pages 252–253) and 7.3 (pages 255–256) list the current RDIs for various vitamins and minerals.

DRIs (Dietary References Intakes) A listing of 26 nutrients essential to maintaining health, including recommended and maximum safe intake levels of the nutrients for healthy people and minimum levels needed to prevent deficiencies and diseases

RDAs (Recommended Dietary Allowances) A listing of the average daily nutrient intake level for a list of vitamins and minerals that meets most people's daily needs

RDIs (Reference Daily Intakes) A listing of needed daily nutrients based on the RDAs. The National Academy of Sciences introduced RDAs in 1941 and updates the list periodically

DRVs (Daily Reference Values) Set of general intake guidelines of total fat, saturated fat, cholesterol, carbohydrates, protein, fiber, sodium, and potassium

DVs (Daily Values) A listing of all the important nutrients from two less-inclusive government lists—the RDIs (Reference Daily Intakes) and the DRVs (Daily Reference Values); DVs are printed on all nutrition labels

- *DRVs (Daily Reference Values)* cover some nutrients the RDIs left out that proved to be important for daily dietary monitoring. They cover fat (including saturated fat and cholesterol), carbohydrates (including fiber), protein, sodium, and potassium. **Table 7.4** on page 261 lists the current DRVs for these nutrients.

- *DVs (Daily Values)* are the RDIs and the DRVs as printed on food labels. American consumers need to know what's in their food and what they should be eating without sorting through a bunch of confusing acronyms. Therefore, the U.S. Food and Drug Administration (FDA) invented a simpler term, DV, for all the important nutrients from the RDI and DRV lists to include on food labels. If you look on any food label, you will see a column labeled "% Daily Value."

Reading Food Labels The U.S. government requires nutrition labels on the packages of most food products, including the familiar panel entitled "Nutrition Facts" (**Figure 7.8**). Reading and understanding these labels can help you judge both appropriate portion sizes and the nutritional merits of the foods you eat. By law, every food package must

- prominently identify the product, such as "multigrain cereal" or "fat-free milk";

- state the quantity of food product in the package by weight, volume, or number of pieces so you can judge the value of what you are buying;

- list all the ingredients by common name in order of amount from most to least by weight;

- give contact information for the food company in case you want more information; and

- supply nutritional information in a standardized panel so you can compare and judge the dietary merits of the product before you buy it.

The Nutrition Facts panel provides the greatest concentration of information; it identifies a serving size

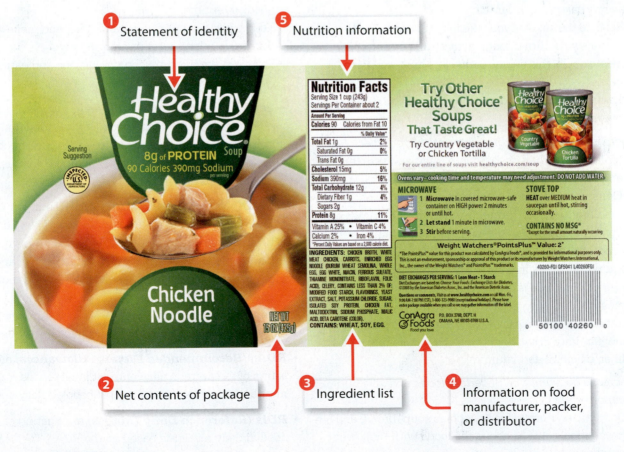

① Statement of identity

⑤ Nutrition information

② Net contents of package

③ Ingredient list

④ Information on food manufacturer, packer, or distributor

FIGURE **7.8** An important part of improving personal nutrition is reading food labels and understanding the information they provide.

Image © ConAgra Foods, Inc. Used with permission.

and how many servings you'll get in a package. For example, the serving size of the soup in Figure 7.8 is 1 cup. The panel tells you how many calories each serving provides and how many of those calories come from fat. It lists daily recommended values (DVs) for nutrients that people should limit in their diets, including total fat, saturated fat, cholesterol, carbohydrates, and sodium. It also lists nutrients that many people should increase in their diets, such as vitamins A and C, calcium, and iron, giving the % Daily Value for each nutrient.

In 2010, First Lady Michelle Obama launched the "Nutrition Keys" front-of-package nutrition labeling initiative. She requested that the U.S. food industry create a new system of simplified front-of-package food labels that would act as a kind of "CliffsNotes" for quickly scanning and judging a food's nutrient content. In early 2011, some manufacturers responded by using streamlined front labels that highlight calories-per-serving information and the values per serving for three nutrients of interest for that type of food (**Figure 7.9**). A package of cookies, for example, might include calories, grams of saturated fat and sugar, and milligrams of sodium per serving. Other foods might highlight calories per serving and three other types of nutrients such as vitamins A, C, or D; calcium; fiber; or protein content.

The 2010 initiative also required chain restaurants (with more than 20 sites) to label the calorie content on all menus and menu boards (including drive-throughs) and have printed information available to hand out on request for nutrient content: sodium, total fat, saturated fat, cholesterol, *trans* fat, total carbohydrates, sugars, fiber, and protein. In 2012, the USDA added a requirement for vending machines to provide calorie counts.[38]

Without simplified front "keys" and more detailed side label panels, it would be easy for a consumer to eat half of a large bag of potato chips and think of that as one serving. Or to pick out a box of sweetened granola with 250 calories in one-half cup and mistakenly

consider that food to be the nutritional equivalent of high-fiber, low-sugar multigrain flakes with only 100 calories in three-quarters of a cup. Individual consumers are responsible for reading those labels, understanding the issues behind the various values, and making intelligent choices.

Determining Your Calorie Needs If you read the fine print near the bottom of any nutrition label, you will see that the listings of nutrients are based on diets of either 2,000 or 2,500 calories per day. The U.S. government chose a 2,000 calorie-per-day diet as the basis for recommending the daily values of 65 grams of fat, 300 grams of carbohydrates, and 50 grams of protein (see Table 7.4 below). Does that mean you should be eating 2,000 calories per day regardless of whether you are 4' 9" tall and weigh 90 pounds, or 6' 9" and weigh 230 pounds? And does it mean that you should adhere to those daily values regardless of your activity level? No, on both counts.

A round number like 2,000 calories makes it easy to extrapolate your actual calorie needs and serving sizes. It is also a maintenance level of energy input for a medium-sized person—about 150 pounds—who expends a medium amount of energy such as 30 minutes of moderate activity a few times per week. Food labels usually also provide a second level, 2,500 calories, as a calculation base for larger or more active people. Your actual calorie needs are determined by your size, age, gender, activity level, and medical conditions and your basal metabolic rate (BMR), which is partly inborn and partly activity-based.

TABLE **7.4** Daily Reference Values (DRVs)	
Food Component	DRV
Fat	65 grams (g)
Saturated Fatty Acids	20 g
Cholesterol	300 milligrams (mg)
Total Carbohydrate	300 g
Dietary Fiber	25 g
Protein*	50 g

(Based on 2,000 calories a day for adults and children over 4 only)
*DRV for protein does not apply to certain populations; Reference Daily Intake (RDI) for protein has been established for these groups: children 1 to 4 years: 16 g; infants under 1 year: 14 g; pregnant women: 60 g; nursing mothers: 65 g.

Adapted from U.S. Food and Drug Administration, "FDA Food Labeling Guide," October 2009, www.fda.gov

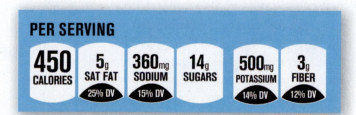

FIGURE **7.9** One serving of this imaginary product has a whopping 450 calories, contains one-quarter of a day's saturated fat, one-sixth of a day's sodium, and the gram equivalent of three teaspoons of sugar. It does, however, also provide some potassium and fiber.

Your BMR, the amount of energy your body uses in a given time period while resting or sleeping, accounts for 50 to 70 percent of your calorie consumption each day and allows you to maintain a steady heartbeat, a temperature of about 98.6°F, and so on. You use another 20 percent of your calories moving around and doing physical work such as walking, talking, carrying things, running, or sweeping the floor. Finally, eating and digesting food itself uses up about 5 to 10 percent of the calories you burn each day.

In determining calorie needs, the big variables are body size, BMR, and energy expenditure through physical activity. Larger people, more muscular people, and those who do hard physical work or exercise burn extra calories. You can get a specific calorie estimate based on your own height, weight, and activity level by using diet analysis tools such as www.ChooseMyPlate.gov. Use your own personal calorie estimate to calculate appropriate serving sizes and numbers when reading food labels and planning your diet.

Understanding Portion Sizes
One reason that Americans eat an average of nearly 3,500 calories per day rather than the world average of 2,400 to 2,600 is that our typical food portions are too big. The U.S. government recommends that each of us eat a certain number of servings each day from each food group based on standard serving sizes. Most Americans, however, don't know how to recognize standard portions. It helps to have some visual aids for estimating proper serving sizes and recognizing the right amount of food. **Figure 7.10** illustrates various foods, healthy serving sizes in cups and ounces, and visual devices for remembering proper portions. For example, one serving of cooked whole-wheat pasta or brown rice is half a cup, about the size of half a baseball. This figure puts into startling perspective the servings we receive at most restaurants: the mountains of pasta, the big wedges of pie, the stacks of plate-sized pancakes, the bucket-sized soft drinks, and the other servings we accept and expect as normal.

Using Food Guides
The USDA has issued Food Guides since the 1940s to help Americans select healthy diets as defined by contemporary nutritionists. They have used wheels, rectangles, pyramids, and most recently a divided plate to summarize and illustrate their recommendations simply for the public.[39] The plate icon introduced in 2011 uses segments of certain colors and sizes to symbolize the kinds and relative amounts of foods and nutrients consumers should select each day (half the plate are fruits and vegetables;

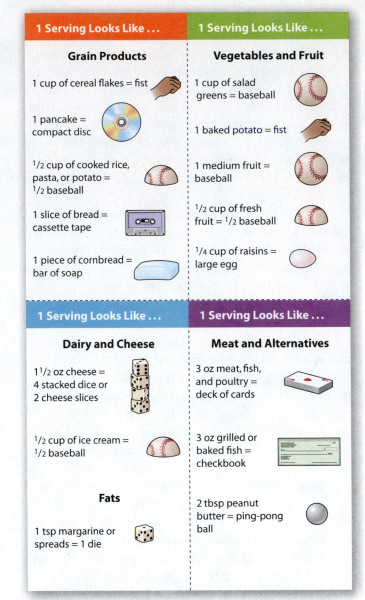

FIGURE **7.10** One of the challenges of following a healthy diet is judging how big a portion size should be and how many servings you are really eating. The comparisons on this card can help you recall what a standard food serving looks like. For easy reference, photocopy or cut out this card, fold on the dotted line, and keep it in your wallet. You can even laminate it for long-term use.

Source: National Heart, Lung, and Blood Institute, "Serving Size Card," 2010, http://hp2010.nhlbihin.net

a little more than one-quarter of the plate are grains; less than one-quarter is protein; and a small amount is dairy) (see **Figure 7.11** on page 263). The supporting website (www.ChooseMyPlate.gov) provides specific personalized diet, nutrition, and exercise recommendations based on your sex, age, size, and activity level.

Nongovernment nutritionists have published several alternative food plans. A pyramid published by Harvard Medical School's Department of Nutrition recommends that you minimize all sugars and refined or low-fiber carbohydrates such as white flour, white rice, pasta, and peeled

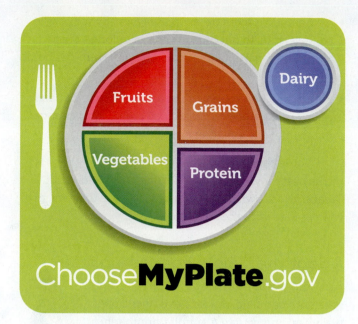

FIGURE 7.11 The ChooseMyPlate.gov icon shows the proper proportion of each food group in a healthy diet. The supporting website provides each visitor with an individualized recommendation for daily servings and portion sizes of each food type.

Source: USDA Choose MyPlate, 2013, www.ChooseMyPlate.gov

potatoes. It also discourages the consumption of red meat, butter, cheese, and other sources of saturated fat. At the same time, it encourages consumption of vegetables, whole grains, nuts, beans, and unsaturated fats from plant oils. On the Internet, you can find alternative pyramids for Mediterranean, Asian, Latin American, and vegetarian eating patterns.

Acquire Skills to Improve Your Nutrition

Do you know the nutritional value of your own diet? Do you know how to find out? A few simple skills will help you analyze and improve your diet. Developing a habit of quickly checking eight items from the typical food label can greatly improve your daily nutrition. **Lab 7.1** will walk you through this process. Here are the eight items you should look for regularly:

DO IT! ONLINE

- *How many calories are in a normal serving*? Most of us need to consider the calorie contents of the foods in our diets to keep from ingesting more calories than we expend in routine activities and exercise.

- *What is the normal serving size?* Let's say you bought a bag of corn chips and were planning to eat the whole thing. The label, however, says it contains 8.5 servings. That provides a valuable hint about the calorie density of that food, not to mention the amount of fat and sodium in the whole bag. If you decide to eat

just one serving, you can count out your seven or eight chips and enjoy them—slowly!

- *What is the main ingredient?* If it is water, corn syrup, or enriched (translation, "white") flour, are you getting your money's worth—and good nutrition?

- *How do the total fats and saturated fats compare to the listed daily values?* Just one tablespoon of butter, for example, will provide one-third of your DV for saturated fat. Do you really want to consume that much fat in one pat?

- *What is the* trans *fat content?* Reduce or eliminate *trans* fats because of their potentially negative health consequences.

- *How does the sodium compare to the % Daily Value?* People diagnosed with high blood pressure, diabetes, kidney disease, and certain other conditions must limit sodium levels. Others should limit sodium to within recommended levels.

- *Does the food provide any fiber?* If not, could you substitute something that does—for example, baby spinach leaves instead of iceberg lettuce in a salad, or a fresh apple instead of canned pineapple, or brown rice instead of white?

- *Finally, how does the sugar content compare to the % Daily Value of sugars?* Technically, there is no DV for sugars or other sweeteners, but you can see the content in grams listed on food labels. Sugars are common in cereals, sauces, and other processed foods and add empty calories that you could devote to more filling and nutritious foods. For example, instead of eating a cup of raisin bran with 19 grams of sugar and 188 calories of food energy, try choosing one cup of bran flakes with only 5 grams of sugar and 122 calories, and then adding a cup of sliced, fresh strawberries (high in volume, flavor, vitamin C, and fiber and containing only 55 calories).

Keeping a Food Diary Did you have three servings of fruit yesterday or two? 200 calories of fats and sugars or 600? If you are like most people, you can only remember a highlight or two from yesterday's meals, and not much of what you ate the other days of the week. To get an accurate idea of whether your diet is nutrient rich or poor and whether it provides enough fiber, try to record snacks and meals for a few days. This is best done immediately after eating, not hours later when you have discarded wrappers with nutrient labels or lost count of serving sizes. For dieters or those working to manage their weight, keeping track of food, calorie, and nutrient intake doubles the amount of weight lost.[40]

LIVE IT! ONLINE
Worksheet 19
Food Log

One way to track your diet is to fill in a food diary. Keeping a food diary helps you learn to judge serving sizes. It requires you to read and apply the information on nutrition labels, learn the value of your typical foods, and substitute healthier items for the foods you usually choose. Many free food diary apps are now available for downloading to smart phones and tablets.

Using Diet Analysis Software An online program such as www.ChooseMyPlate.gov is a powerful tool for keeping track of what you eat, analyzing its nutrient content, and making needed changes to your diet. It is just one of several such programs that can streamline your efforts to achieve better nutrition.

To use this USDA website and its personalized features, visit www.ChooseMyPlate.gov. Find the box "I want to…," and select "Get a Personalized Plan." Enter your age, sex, weight, height, and general activity level. The next screen will present you with the number of daily calories you should consume; the number of servings you should eat from each of the five food groups (grains, vegetables, fruits, dairy, and protein foods); pointers for eating enough whole grains and for varying your vegetables each week so you include some dark green ones, some orange ones, some legumes, some starchy vegetables, and others; a reminder to consume enough healthful oils; and advice on limiting the calories in fats and sugars.

You can then print out a personalized food plan based on your individual information. Beyond the personalized plan, the site also provides these features:

- You can use a meal tracking worksheet to keep tabs on each food you ate on a given day and save this for comparison with additional days.

- You can use the ChooseMyPlate Tracker to assess the nutrients—calories, fats, carbohydrates, vitamins, and so on—in specific foods such as a tuna fish sandwich or a slice of pizza (see **Lab 7.2**).

DO IT! ONLINE

- You can make a data bank of nutritional information for foods or meals you eat routinely— say, your typical breakfast of cereal, juice, and toast—so you don't have to enter them individually each time.

- You can do a more detailed analysis of your physical activities to get an estimate of calories burned as you do a particular exercise for a certain period of time.

- Finally, you can keep track of trends in your diet and physical activity over time if you are making changes to benefit your fitness and wellness.

Choose the method—online or on paper—that works best for you, as that's the one you'll stick with. Creating your own nutrition plan (see page 273) will give you practice with the new tools.

Adopt the Whole Foods Habit

Analyzing your daily foods for calories and nutrients can help you achieve nutritional wellness, and so can a simpler approach: making each bite you take more nutritious by choosing primarily **whole foods**, or dietary items produced with the minimum of refining, preservatives, or processing for quick preparation.

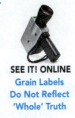

SEE IT! ONLINE
Grain Labels Do Not Reflect 'Whole' Truth

LIVE IT! ONLINE
Worksheet 18 Grocery Shopping List

Decades ago, virtually all food was "whole," or real and unchanged. Many packaged foods today, however, have long lists of ingredients and additives that reduce the cost of ingredients, extend shelf life, intensify flavor, and make food preparation easier. People have learned to like the taste and convenience of processed foods, but these products tend to contain hidden fats and sugars, relatively large amounts of sodium, and various additives and preservatives. They also tend to have less naturally occurring fiber and fewer vitamins. Let's compare a medium-sized fresh apple, for example, with one cup of processed, preserved, and dried apple slices. The fresh apple contains about 95 calories, 17 grams of carbohydrates, 3 grams of fiber, and 13 grams of sugars. The cup of dried apple slices (derived from two or more whole apples) contains 209 calories, 51 grams of carbohydrates, 7 grams of fiber, and 49 grams of sugars, and may contain added sucrose or corn syrup and preservatives such as sulfur.

Shifting from a diet heavy in processed foods to one rich in whole foods doesn't mean you have to sacrifice good taste or feel hungry or dissatisfied. In fact, you will probably find snacks and meals very filling and delicious if you choose as many foods as possible that are nutrient-dense, high in volume but low in calories, high in fiber, and rich in antioxidants.

Nutrient-Dense Foods You may have heard people talk about foods—sugar, for example—that provide only "empty calories." What they mean is that such foods provide calories for energy without supplying other healthful nutrients. By contrast, **nutrient-dense foods** provide rich sources of vitamins, minerals, antioxidants, and fiber and minimize saturated fat, added sugars, sodium, and refined carbohydrates. Choosing nutrient-dense foods means striving to maximize the food value of each and every meal and snack you consume.

To see what this means in a practical way, compare two small meals—a glass of cola and a hot dog versus a glass of low-fat milk and a small serving of salmon. The cola provides 105 calories, all from refined carbohydrates. In about the same number of calories, the milk provides 8 grams of protein along with vitamin D and calcium. The cola is nutrient-poor; the milk is nutrient-dense.

Now compare the hot dog and salmon. A hot dog on a white-bread bun supplies 420 calories. It contains more than a whole day's recommended amount of saturated fat, 9 grams of protein, most of a day's allotted sodium, and refined white flour lacking much fiber. In contrast, a serving of salmon provides fewer than 200 calories, 10 grams of heart-healthy omega-3 fatty acids, twice as much protein, and a small fraction of the sodium. The hot dog has fewer healthful nutrients, while the salmon is nutrient-dense.

Learning to reach for nutrient-dense foods every time you get hungry will greatly benefit your lifelong fitness and wellness. If your diet consists primarily of processed foods such as pastries, coffee drinks, pizza, hamburgers, and cola, you may not even know what wellness feels like! Why should you care about eating too many calories, too much saturated fat, too many refined carbohydrates, and too much sodium? Because dietary excesses can affect your appearance, energy level, athletic performance, social life, ability to fight off infections, and overall sense of well-being. Try shifting toward nutrient-dense foods and away from empty calories, and watch for positive changes in those short-term measures. Focus on establishing habits, including the whole foods habit, that keep you looking and feeling vibrantly well today and your lifelong wellness will improve, too.

> **nutrient-dense foods** Foods or beverages that provide a high level of nutrients and thus maximize the nutritional value of each meal and snack consumed

High-Volume, Low-Calorie Foods We eat for many reasons, but the primary one is *satiety*: a feeling of fullness and the physical and emotional pleasure it brings. Nutrition researchers have discovered that each of us has a characteristic weight of food that we eat in a day. You can eat that weight of food in candy bars, potato chips, steak, and ice cream, but you will be getting too few nutrients and too many calories and you probably wouldn't feel full for very long between meals. You could eat that same weight of food in celery, iceberg lettuce, and bran and still get too few nutrients, but the volume would help keep you full. The proper goal is a filling, calorie-appropriate diet that also emphasizes nutrient density. Relatively recent nutritional research has shown that eating nutritious foods with more volume due to higher air or water content can help people feel full and satisfied longer.[41] This is especially helpful for dieters or for people who want to maintain their weight and not gain more.

Foods with high contents of water, fiber, or protein tend to keep you full and satisfied longer, while those with high contents of fat, sugar, or refined carbohydrates leave you feeling hungry sooner. However, the water must be in the food (as in soups, fruits, and vegetables) and not just in a glass accompanying your meal. Apparently, your brain's satiety center knows the difference and isn't fooled by drinking water coupled with

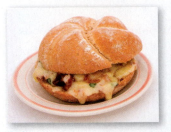

(a)

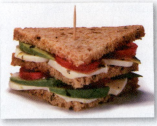

(b)

FIGURE **7.12** These two sandwiches have approximately the same number of calories (300), but one (a) is small and filled with saturated fat. It contains mayonnaise, butter, cheese, and bacon on a white roll. The other sandwich (b) is large, high-volume, and rich in fiber and vitamins. It contains whole wheat bread, tomato, lettuce, green and red peppers, and cheese.

a candy bar. **Figure 7.12** compares two sandwiches with approximately the same number of calories, but very different ingredients. **Table 7.5** lists familiar foods by calorie density.

High-Fiber Foods Fiber adds bulk and, often, a chewy quality to food. Both help satisfy hunger better and for longer periods. Soluble fiber such as that in oats, barley, and apples, for example, lowers LDL

antioxidants Compounds in foods that help protect the body against the damaging effects of oxygen derivatives called *free radicals*

cholesterol. Grains that are intact (such as brown rice or bulgur wheat) instead of finely ground (as in whole wheat flour) have a lower glycemic index. High-fiber foods also improve the passage of digested material through the digestive tract.

Antioxidant-Rich Foods *Free radicals* are molecules with unpaired electrons that the body produces in excess when it is overly stressed. Free radicals can damage or kill healthy cells, cell proteins, or genetic material in cells. **Antioxidants** produce enzymes that scavenge free radicals, slow their formation, and actually repair oxidative stress damage. Thus, the theory goes that if you consume lots of antioxidants, you will nullify or greatly reduce the negative effects of oxidative stress. Among the more commonly cited nutrients touted as providing a protective effect are vitamin C, vitamin E, beta-carotene and other carotenoids, and the mineral selenium.

How valid is the theory? To date, many claims about the benefits of antioxidants in reducing the risk of heart disease, improving vision, and slowing down the aging process have not been fully investigated; conclusive statements about their true benefits are difficult to make. Large, longitudinal epidemiological studies support the hypothesis that antioxidants in foods, mostly fruits and vegetables

TABLE **7.5** Comparing Calorie Density in Common Foods

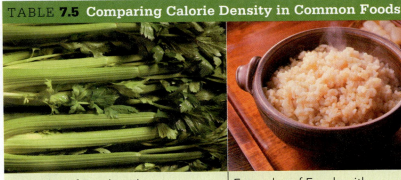

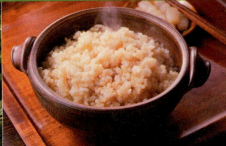

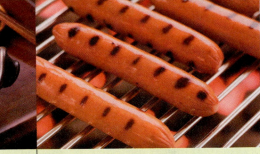

Examples of Foods with Low Calorie Density— *Consume a variety of these daily*	Examples of Foods with Medium Calorie Density— *Consume a few of these daily*	Examples of Foods with High Calorie Density— *Reduce consumption of these daily*
Raw celery (1250 g = 200 calories)	Brown rice, cooked (179 g = 200 calories)	Hot dog, Oscar Meyer beef (61 g = 200 calories)
Watermelon (666 g = 200 calories)	Enriched spaghetti, cooked (126 g = 200 calories)	French fries, McDonald's (59 g = 200 calories)
Raw broccoli (588 g = 200 calories)	Chicken breast, roasted (121 g = 200 calories)	Potato chips, plain salted (37 g = 200 calories)
Red or green grapes (290 g = 200 calories)	Salmon, cooked, Alaskan wild (110 g = 200 calories)	Peanut butter, smooth salted (34 g = 200 calories)

Data from Nutrient Data Laboratory Home Page U.S. Department of Agriculture, "USDA National Nutrient Database for Standard Reference Release 25," Agricultural Research Service, 2012.

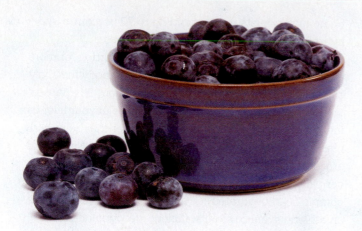

FIGURE **7.13** Fruits and vegetables such as blueberries and kale are high in antioxidants.

(**Figure 7.13**), help protect against cognitive decline and risk of Parkinson's disease. However, because of problems with study design and difficulties in isolating dietary effects from supplement effects, it is difficult to assess overall benefits of antioxidants.[42]

Some studies indicate that when people's diets include foods rich in vitamin C, they seem to develop fewer cancers, but other studies detect no effect from dietary vitamin C.[43] Early studies seemed to show that vitamin E had antioxidant effects that could help prevent heart disease and cancer. Large trials involving hundreds of people taking vitamin E and/or selenium supplements, however, have shown very mixed results, with some indicating no benefit and others showing actual harm.[44] The vitamin E in foods does seem to help protect the cell membranes of red blood cells and the delicate surface lining our lungs.

Many people take a daily multivitamin pill as "insurance" against deficiencies in their diets. Is this a good plan? The body's cells can absorb and use the vitamins in food more easily and fully than it can the compounds in supplements, so a vitamin-rich diet is always a better choice. In addition, research results are mixed on whether to take multivitamins to reduce diseases: One recent study of 14,000 men showed that those who took a multivitamin daily for 10 years had 8 percent fewer cancers than those taking placebos.[45] Yet an equally large and long trial found that multivitamins had very little preventative effect for cardiovascular disease risk.[46]

Phytochemicals Plants make thousands of compounds collectively called *phytochemicals* (meaning literally "plant chemicals"), many of which have antioxidant properties. Fruit, flowers, and plant leaves form a bright palette of colors, in part because plants can generate pigments with antioxidant properties such as *beta-carotene* (yellow and orange pigments), *lycopene* (red pigments), and *lutein*, found in various green, red, yellow, and orange foods.[47]

One phytochemical called sulphorophane, found in broccoli and other cruciferous vegetables (including kale, brussels sprouts, cauliflower, cabbage, collard greens, and bok choy), actually targets and kills cancer cells.[48] However, while people love the idea of "magic bullets"—pills that will quickly solve their health problems with no other effort—most nutrition researchers recommend getting antioxidants and phytochemicals in nutrient-dense foods rather than in supplements.[49]

Foods Containing Folate **Folate** (also called *folic acid* or sometimes vitamin B$_9$) is a form of vitamin B that plays a role in the development of the spinal cord. Folate also helps break down the compound homocysteine, which is produced as the body digests meat and other high-protein foods. By helping break down homocysteine, folate may also protect against cardiovascular disease, heart attacks, and strokes.[50] Foods rich in folate include sunflower seeds, dark leafy greens, bean sprouts, cooked beans, asparagus, and peanuts. Many people, including reproductive-age women, consume low levels of folate in their diet. For this reason and to help prevent developmental defects such as spina bifida, the FDA in 1998 started requiring food manufacturers to fortify with folate all bread, cereal, rice, and macaroni products sold in the United States.

Do I Need Special Nutrition for Exercise?

Fitness requires physical activity, but does it also require a special diet? Active people may need some extra nutrients—a little more protein, perhaps, and some extra carbohydrates for fast energy and endurance. But big imbalances in the major nutrients, such as those caused by a high-protein diet or a low-carbohydrate regimen, cannot support improved fitness.

Most Exercisers Can Follow General Nutritional Guidelines

Exercisers often look for an "edge" and wonder what they can eat, drink, or swallow in pill form that will help them get into shape faster or better. Significantly, sports physiologists and nutritionists have conducted hundreds of studies of recreational, collegiate, and professional athletes, trying to determine optimal energy and nutrient levels for peak performance. Their findings may surprise and disappoint many fitness enthusiasts:

folate A form of vitamin B that is vital for spinal cord development and helps break down homocysteine as the body digests proteins

They closely follow general nutritional guidelines with only a few minor adjustments, and they emphasize the same "food first" philosophy (rather than supplements) that athletic trainers are adopting in greater and greater numbers.[51]

Carbohydrates The best source of energy before and during exercise is carbohydrates; they should provide up to about 55 to 65 percent of daily calories.[52] Restricting carbohydrates can impede your fitness efforts by leaving you energy-deprived. Sugars can give a little energy boost but can also cause a rise in insulin and a drop in blood sugar that produces fatigue.

Proteins For moderate strengthening and endurance exercise, most of us need about 0.75 to 0.8 gram of protein per kilogram of body weight per day. Protein does not in itself help build muscle. Only activity, including weight training, adds new muscle.

Elite Athletes Have Extra Nutritional Needs

While most exercisers can get complete nutrition from a balanced diet of nutrient-dense foods, some elite athletes—those with the potential for intercollegiate, Olympic, or professional sports—do need to modify their eating patterns for better training and performance.

Calories People in regular training for competitive sports need extra calories. Athletes often have greater muscle mass than the average person, and muscle tissue consumes more calories than fat tissue, even at rest. A tall young man training with a football or basketball team, for example, could require 5,000 calories or more daily. High activity levels sustained for long periods—the running during a soccer match, for example—also require extra fuel. About 55 to 65 percent of that extra athletic fuel should come from complex carbohydrates—bread, pasta, cereals, grains, vegetables, and fruits.[53]

Some nutritionists recommend up to 70 percent carbohydrates for sustained high-level activities.

Endurance events requiring heavy exertion for more than 90 minutes use two types of internal body fuels, glycogen and fat. Your muscles can store about 90 minutes' worth of glycogen, and additional storage in your liver can fuel a few more minutes of exercise. After that, your body uses its own fat to fuel activity (**Figure 7.14**). Endurance athletes such as marathon runners, swimmers, and soccer players often consume 60 or 70 percent of their diet in complex carbohydrates starting two to three days before an athletic event to store sufficient glycogen and fat. Consuming 5 to 7 grams of carbohydrates per kilogram of body weight per day is usually enough for general training, while 7 to 10 grams per kilogram per day will fuel endurance training and strenuous one-time events.

Pre- and Post-Event Meals Trainers usually instruct athletes to drink plenty of water; to eat complex carbohydrates three or four hours before an event; and to avoid proteins, fats, refined sugars, caffeine, and gas-producing foods in the pregame meal. They recommend avoiding protein, because protein takes more time to digest and can lead to increased urination and dehydration. Likewise, fats and oils are slow to digest. Sugar is on the list because it induces a surge of insulin in the blood and later, during the event, can cause an energy dip. A small amount of caffeine can boost your energy during the event, but a large amount can lead to increased urination and dehydration and to an accelerated heartbeat. Gas-producing foods can upset digestion.

Most athletes need water and additional carbohydrates during the event, and many choose sports drinks diluted with water to sustain energy and provide sufficient hydration. You can learn more about this by visiting the American College of Sports Medicine's website (www.acsm.org) to view its guidelines on exercise and fluid replacement.[54]

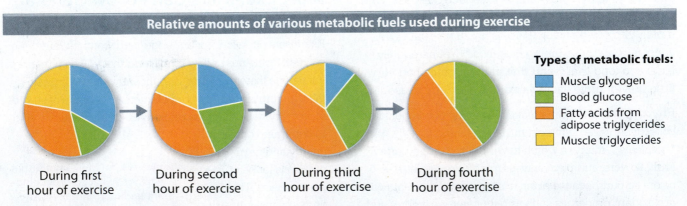

Relative amounts of various metabolic fuels used during exercise

During first hour of exercise

During second hour of exercise

During third hour of exercise

During fourth hour of exercise

Types of metabolic fuels:
- Muscle glycogen
- Blood glucose
- Fatty acids from adipose triglycerides
- Muscle triglycerides

FIGURE **7.14** If you exercise for less than one hour, your body uses mostly glycogen and fatty acids (triglycerides) stored in your muscles. If you exercise for four hours, the fuel ratios shift dramatically and your activity is mainly powered by blood sugar and the breakdown of fat (adipose) tissue.

Selecting foods for post-performance meals is also important to help restore the muscles' energy supply. Soon after a training or performance session you should eat some protein as well as some simple and complex carbohydrates. Good suggestions include cereal with fat-free dairy, soy, or almond milk; whole-wheat crackers or pretzels and hummus; or part of a turkey sandwich with lots of veggies.[55]

Is the popular practice of carbo-loading necessary? If you define *carbo-loading* as eating one huge starch meal the night before an athletic event, then no, it is not necessary or desirable. This kind of consumption can cause the body to retain water, the muscles to feel stiff the next day, and the athlete to feel slow and sluggish when the event starts.

If you define *carbo-loading* as eating 55 to 65 percent of your calories as complex carbohydrates at every meal for one or two days before an event, then it is desirable because it can load the muscles with glycogen for sustained activity if previous carbohydrate intake was low. A recent study suggests that marathon runners who carbo-load for 24 to 36 hours before an event perceived more energy and less fatigue half way through the race.[56] Manipulating the pre-exercise diet with more or less sugar, fat, or protein seems to have little effect on most people's performance.[57]

Vitamins and Minerals The body's energy production and use requires B vitamins; bone- and blood-building require iron and calcium; sweating causes the loss of sodium and potassium that must be replenished during or after events. A balanced diet provides most athletes with enough vitamins and minerals to meet recommended intakes.

Supplements Optimal muscle growth and strength gain do not require nutritional supplements. Most competitive athletes in high school and college do take various kinds of supplements, including megadoses of certain vitamins and minerals as well as purported muscle builders.[58] Where there is no deficiency to start with, these megadoses provide little or no benefit to performance.[59] The popular creatine monohydrate is chemically related to a natural substance called *creatine phosphate*, which helps fuel muscle contraction. Vendors claim creatine monohydrate helps build muscle, increases energy to improve performance, and delays muscle fatigue. Objective scientific studies suggest that taking creatine orally may cause muscles to temporarily retain more water, and this may boost short-term performance under anaerobic conditions. Thus, it may pump up the muscles a bit so they feel bigger, but it is not

helpful for endurance events. And it does not do what many athletes are hoping for: build permanently bigger muscles. This requires regular physical strength training.

Also popular are individual, concentrated amino acid supplements such as taurine, arginine, glutamine, and leucine. Eating protein-rich foods provides these very same building blocks but in safe concentrations and in naturally occurring mixtures of multiple amino acids. In contrast, supplements provide artificially high concentrations of individual amino acids that may block your body's absorption of the full amino acid spectrum. What's more, amino acid supplements can become contaminated and are far more expensive than eating protein-rich foods. Most importantly, vendors claim that amino acid supplements will help build muscle and sustain muscle contraction, but there is no good evidence of these benefits.

Meal Timing People use the term *meal timing* in various ways, and some trainers claim that *when* you eat fats, proteins, and carbohydrates will determine

casestudy

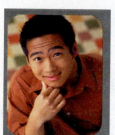

CHAU

"I'm not an 'athlete,' but I do like sports. I've never worried too much about supplementing my diet with extras. I figure as long as I eat enough to feel satisfied, my body's getting what it needs. Some of my friends—like Tom, who's a cross-country runner—are always drinking sports drinks and eating energy bars. I've also noticed Tom often has a pasta dinner two days before a big run, and then he will eat a lighter meal the night before the race. He's also pretty strict about taking a multivitamin every day. It makes me wonder if I should start taking vitamins too."

THINK! How do Chau's and Tom's nutritional needs differ? Should Chau begin taking vitamin supplements? Why would Tom eat pasta two nights before a big run, instead of the night before the race?

ACT NOW! Today, analyze your own physical activity. Could you benefit from consuming more or fewer calories? This week, calculate your calorie expenditures during physical activity each day for three days in a row. In two weeks, add or subtract some calories depending on what you discover.

HEAR IT! ONLINE

how quickly you can build muscles in the gym or how well you can sustain activity during a long bike ride. Carbo-loading and pre- and post-event meals are all forms of meal timing. So are regimens that instruct you to eat proteins early in the day, carbohydrates at lunch, and so on.

Research shows that the most significant thing about meal timing is the effect on your appetite. Skipping meals, getting ravenously hungry, then "gorging" most of your day's calories at dinner is far more likely to cause fat accumulation than "grazing" on five or six small meals throughout the day. Sumo wrestlers deliberately apply this principle to put on hundreds of pounds of fat. If they spread their daily 6,000 calories into five or six meals instead of two, they would weigh up to 25 percent less![60]

Do I Have Special Nutritional Needs?

In its *Dietary Guidelines for Americans*, the USDA highlights several groups with special nutritional needs and concerns, including children, teens, adults over 50, vegetarians, and diabetics. We review the needs of vegetarians and diabetics here.

Vegetarians Must Monitor Their Nutrient Intake

More and more people today are choosing partial or strict vegetarian diets. Between 5 and 15 percent of all Americans claim to be one of the following, arranged in order from the strictest and most exclusive of animal products to the least: Strict *vegetarians* (also called *vegans*) avoid all foods of animal origin, including dairy products and eggs; *lacto-vegetarians* avoid animal flesh but eat dairy products; *ovo-vegetarians* avoid animal flesh and dairy products but eat eggs; *lacto-ovo-vegetarians* consume both dairy products and eggs; and *semi-vegetarians* consume fish and/or poultry but no red meat.

Vegetarian diets have certain benefits.[61] Most people who follow a balanced vegetarian diet weigh less than nonvegetarians of similar height. Most also have healthier cholesterol levels, less constipation and diarrhea, and a lower risk of dying from heart disease or cancer than those who eat red meat.[62] Vegetarians consume less saturated fat, and this, in addition to lifestyle factors such as avoiding tobacco and exercising more, helps lower their morality risk. Based on these benefits of vegetarian diets as well as the environmental concerns of additional greenhouse gases released during the production of meat and other animal foods, many universities are initiating "Meatless Monday Dinners" in campus dining halls.[63]

Despite their benefits, vegetarian diets can have deficiencies; with careful food choices, however, vegetarians can avoid deficiencies. Semi-vegetarians who eat dairy products and small amounts of chicken or fish are seldom nutrient-deficient. Vegans can get enough essential amino acids through complementary combinations of plant products (review Figure 7.3 on page 242). Lacto-vegetarians usually get enough vitamins D and B_{12} from dairy products, while strict vegans can develop deficiencies. Fortified products such as soy or almond milk can usually provide enough of these vitamins. Vegans are sometimes deficient in vitamin B_2 (riboflavin) since it is found mainly in meat, eggs, and dairy products. They can get enough B_2, however, by eating generous amounts of broccoli, asparagus, almonds, and fortified cereals. Because meat is rich in iron and dairy products are rich in calcium, vegans who avoid both can develop deficiencies of these minerals. Solutions include choosing mineral-rich plant foods (see Table 7.3) and/or taking multivitamin/mineral supplements.

In general, vegetarians can stay in excellent health by eating a wide variety of grains, legumes, fruits, vegetables, and seeds each day. **Figure 7.15** on page 271 shows some meal planning ideas (based on www.ChooseMyPlate.gov).

Those with Diabetes Must Reduce Carbohydrates

Anyone diagnosed with type 1 or type 2 diabetes will receive specific information from medical providers about both necessary drug treatments and dietary changes. Because diabetes is a disorder of blood-sugar regulation, patients usually must cut back on sweets and desserts, both to reduce surges of sugar in the blood and to control obesity, which can lead to and intensify diabetes. Choosing foods with a lower rather than higher glycemic index (see page 246) is also beneficial, and this usually means less-processed foods and reduced fat content. The American Diabetes Association advises diabetics to eats lots of nonstarchy vegetables and fruits, to choose whole grains over processed grain products, to include beans and lentils in the diet, to eat fish two to three times per week, to choose lean meats and nonfat dairy products, to drink water and diet drinks instead of sugary drinks, to avoid saturated fats and *trans* fats during cooking, and to watch portion sizes.[64]

Good Food Safety Practices Are for Everyone

Sometimes people think they have the flu when it is actually "food poisoning." Foodborne illnesses usually cause diarrhea, nausea, cramping, and vomiting. They usually occur five to eight hours after eating and last only a day or two. For the healthy people, food poisoning is unpleasant and inconvenient. For the very young, the elderly, or people with cancer, diabetes, AIDS, or other severe illnesses, it can be fatal.

Every year, millions of Americans become sick from unclean or poorly handled foods, sometimes with life-threatening consequences. The Centers for Disease Control and Prevention estimates that every year 48 million Americans are sickened, 128,000 are hospitalized, and 3,000 die from foodborne illnesses.[65]

A rise in imports of fresh fruits and vegetables from developing countries, as well as increased urbanization, industrialization, travel, and restaurant dining, raises the risk of unsafe food handling and results in illness. Here are some tips for avoiding foodborne illness:

- Be aware of cleanliness in stores and restaurants. When purchasing food, be aware of the expiration dates on perishable foods.

- Use proper at-home techniques for storing and handling food.
  - Keep hands and cooking surfaces clean.
  - Separate raw foods from cooked foods during storage and cooking.
  - Scrub and thoroughly rinse produce before eating it.
  - Heat foods to high enough temperatures to kill germs.
  - Refrigerate perishable foods.
  - Safely handle the most common sources of foodborne illness: raw eggs, meat, poultry, and fish; unwashed or outdated bean or alfalfa sprouts; and unpasteurized milk and juices.

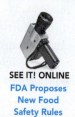

<ol start="1">
<li>SEE IT! ONLINE</li>
</ol>

FDA Proposes New Food Safety Rules

Some people have concerns about the safety of foods produced with the use of genetically modified organisms or their products, or foods that are irradiated to kill microorganisms and prolong shelf life. You can learn more about these issues by visiting the Web links listed on this book's website.

Breakfast

1 cup cooked oatmeal with 1 cup of mixed berries
½ banana
1 cup nonfat soy, rice, almond, or cow's milk

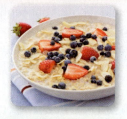

Lunch

1 whole wheat wrap, filled with:
  1 tablespoon nonfat cream cheese, hummus, and/or salsa
  ½ cup chopped vegetables (such as red peppers, green onions, avocado)
  1 cup mixed leafy greens
  ½ to 1 cup black or kidney beans
  2 tablespoons grated soy cheese or nonfat cow's milk cheese
Sliced apple sprinkled with cinnamon
Iced tea or club soda with a lemon slice

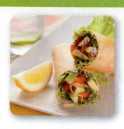

Snack

1 ounce roasted unsalted almonds or ½ cup baby carrots with 2 tablespoons hummus
An orange or grapefruit

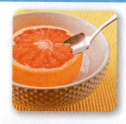

Dinner

Grilled veggie burger on whole wheat bun with condiments (lettuce, ketchup, mustard, salsa, pickles)
Side salad with oil and vinegar dressing and chopped veggies (such as tomatoes, cucumbers, celery, carrots)
1 cup steamed broccoli with 1 teaspoon whipped butter or butter-like spread
½ cup lemon sorbet with sliced strawberries and two small cookies
Water or tea

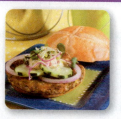

FIGURE 7.15 Vegetarians can plan healthy meals by making careful food choices. Here's one example of a daily vegetarian diet that includes protein, calcium, B vitamins, and other nutrients.

Based on: United States Department of Agriculture, *Health Eating Tips, Sample Menus, and Healthy Lunchtime Challenge,* www.ChooseMyPlate.gov

How Can I Create a Behavior Change Plan for Nutrition?

You've no doubt heard the famous phrase, "You are what you eat." But did you know that its origin was a book written in 1825 by Anthelme Brillat-Savain—a French lawyer who loved the pleasures of the table above all else? What he actually wrote was, "Tell me what you eat and I shall tell you what you are." We could modify that slightly to make it perfectly relevant to this book and to you, the reader: Tell us what you eat and we'll tell you how fit and well you're likely to be now and in the future!

Assess Your Current Diet

Would you benefit from changes to your current diet? The most successful way to change long-ingrained eating habits is to break the task into steps and keep track of your progress.

Recording What You Eat If you filled in Lab 7.2 using either a manual food diary or the food tracker at www.ChooseMyPlate.gov, then you are on your way to a better diet. Self-awareness is the necessary starting point for change, followed by your own actions for self-improvement.[66]

LIVE IT! ONLINE
Worksheet 20
Your Eating Habits

You should get a pretty clear idea of how many calories your daily diet provides and whether your diet meets, exceeds, or falls short of the daily values for carbohydrates, fats, proteins, fiber, vitamins, and minerals. If there are gaps in your food diary, keep track of your hour-by-hour food consumption for another day or two so you have a clear picture of your typical nutritional profile.

Identifying Your Patterns Go through your food diary and analyze your reasons for eating each meal and snack. Was it primarily hunger? Primarily socializing? Primarily boredom? If it is hunger, are you satisfying that need with nutrient-dense foods? If it is primarily socializing, are you even hungry at the time? Does peer pressure persuade you to eat an after-dinner snack of pizza and frozen yogurt when you could be happy with a salad, an apple, or a low-cal beverage? If you are eating out of boredom or stress—snacking on chips and cola while studying, for example—could

you find a more nutritious alternative such as carrot sticks, whole wheat crackers, unsalted peanuts, popcorn, or grapes?

By reflecting on and identifying your own reasons for food preferences and eating habits, you can start to understand your patterns and perhaps change them for the better. It is seldom easy or automatic to improve your diet because it means breaking long-standing habits. But new behaviors become somewhat simpler if you realize when and why you reach for certain foods and that the resistance to change may come from within yourself or your family and friends.

Review Your Behavior Change Skills

Examining your current eating patterns is just one part of applying behavior change skills to improve your nutrition. Here are some other ways you can incorporate the behavior change model:

- *Look at your motivation.* Do you really want a different and better diet? What do you see as the immediate benefits of improved nutrition? What do you expect over the long term? Solidifying your motivation can help you get ready for change.

- *Identify barriers to a better diet.* What are some of the difficulties you foresee in achieving better nutrition? Time? Money? Eating in less-than-optimal ways with friends and family? Naming some of those barriers and coming up with alternatives can help you on the path to change. If you have trouble brainstorming solutions, the student health service or counseling center may be able to help you.

- *Make a commitment to learning about better nutrition.* Based on what you learn, list ways in which an improved diet will benefit your life. What could eating more whole grain fiber do for you? How about consuming more fruits and vegetables? Listing these will help you stick with your plan for change.

- *Choose a target behavior by identifying your biggest nutritional concern.* What is the most pressing issue with your current diet? Review your food diary. If you see that you're getting too much saturated fat every day, outline an approach for getting less saturated fat in your meals and snacks. If you discover that fried meats and cheese (on hamburgers, nachos, pizzas, etc.) are pushing up your daily total, think of lower-fat alternatives for those items.

- *Note where you stand in the typical stages of change.* Are you contemplating change? If so, gathering more information or talking more with friends and family might help. Are you planning for change and getting ready to take action?

- *Have you noticed any helpful role models?* Do you know people with good eating habits and a nutritious diet? Observing their food choices and talking to them about your nutritional issues may help you learn to counter your current habits with others based on better food choices, more successful eating patterns, and solid nutritional information.

Get Set to Apply Nutritional Skills

With this chapter, you've already begun to learn and apply nutritional skills. Review your use of them and look for ways to improve those skills and call upon them daily.

Examine food guides to compare your daily servings of various food groups with the amounts that nutritionists recommend from governmental agencies or from academic institutions. Read food labels more often and watch for those nutrients you've identified as problematic in your own diet. For example, watch for hidden fats and sugars and look for opportunities to increase fiber.

Recognize proper portion sizes and note when the helping you are served in a restaurant or cafeteria is way too big (e.g., three cups of pasta instead of half a cup) or way too small (e.g., a side salad the size of a golf ball instead of a softball). Use www.ChooseMyPlate.gov or other kinds of diet software to get an individual analysis of the daily calories and nutrients you consume and how they compare with the recommended daily intakes of each and to keep track of what you eat.

Both behavior-change skills and nutritional tools can help you plan your own program for improved nutrition. Working on this plan can give you practice

at recognizing nutrient-dense foods. You can start to choose high-volume, low-density alternatives to high-density, high-calorie foods. You may find that you now prefer whole grains to refined ones. And you may start to savor the colors, flavors, and textures of fruits and/or vegetables with every snack and meal.

Your plan may be your first deliberate application of nutritional tools and behavioral-change skills for nutrition. In time, however, it should become a continual and automatic part of each day. The goal is to balance nutrients and control calories naturally as part of your long-term efforts for fitness and wellness and your ongoing management of body mass and weight.

Create a Nutrition Plan

Begin planning your own program using **Lab 7.3**. As you work through the lab, write down your own notes and observations and swap them with others in your class, perhaps during a class discussion or in a small discussion group.

DO IT! ONLINE

Keep track of calories for your new plan. Are you on track? Where could you cut or add without increasing saturated fats or sugars?

After two weeks, discuss the plan and your results with your fitness/health instructor, and revise if necessary. Again, if possible, discuss your experiences with others in your class to exchange successful ideas and get support for your efforts.

For several weeks, continue tracking your daily diet, either manually or using www.ChooseMyPlate .gov—at least for the number of servings of the main food groups. This helps you eat sufficient amounts of the foods you needed to increase (e.g., whole grains, fruits, vegetables, beans, nuts) and helps you cut back on those that are already overrepresented (e.g., saturated fat or refined carbohydrates). Be sure to continue applying nutritional skills such as reading labels and comparing serving sizes to the portions in Figure 7.10 (on page 262).

Don't try for perfection! Approach your diet in sets of two or three days at a time. When you have a day with too few fruits and vegetables, increase them the next day. When you have a day with too little protein, have more the next day. If you get too much protein one day, eat less the next or eat less-concentrated protein foods such as tofu, beans, or skim milk. See the Activate, Motivate, & Advance Your Well-being: A Program to Eat More Fruits and Vegetables (on pages 281–284) for further guidance in planning your diet.

CHAPTER IN REVIEW

MasteringHealth™

Build your knowledge—and wellness!—in the Study Area of MasteringHealth with a variety
of study tools.

SEE IT! ONLINE

videos

Ditching Sugar

High Fiber Diet

Grain Labels Do Not Reflect
  'Whole' Truth

FDA Proposes New Food
  Safety Rules

HEAR IT! ONLINE

audio tools

Audio case study

MP3 chapter review

REVIEW IT! ONLINE

chapter review

Chapter reading quizzes

Glossary flashcards

LIVE IT! ONLINE

programs & behavior change

Take Charge of Your Health! Worksheets:

  Worksheet 18 Grocery Shopping List

  Worksheet 19 Food Log

  Worksheet 20 Your Eating Habits and Extra Calories

  Worksheet 24 Cutting Out the Fat

Behavior Change Log Book and Wellness Journal

DO IT! ONLINE

labs

Lab 7.1 Reading a Food Label

Lab 7.2 Keeping a Food Diary and Analyzing Your
  Daily Nutrition

Lab 7.3 Improving Your Nutrition

reviewquestions

1. Which of the following would be considered a
   healthy, nutrient-dense food?
   a. Cheddar cheese
   b. Soft drink
   c. Potato chips
   d. Fat-free milk

2. Essential amino acids are
   a. found only in animal proteins.
   b. found only in plant proteins.
   c. best taken as supplements.
   d. protein building blocks your body can't produce.

3. Simple carbohydrates
   a. are important amino acid compounds.
   b. act as structural compounds in plants.
   c. provide fiber in the diet.
   d. deliver energy in a quickly usable form.

4. Using the glycemic index, one can determine
   a. the percentage of glucose in a food.
   b. the percentage of glycine in a food.
   c. how quickly a food will boost your blood sugar levels.
   d. the caloric content of a food.

5. What do nutritionists sometimes call "bad cholesterol"?
   a. Saturated fat
   b. Butter
   c. HDLs
   d. LDLs

6. Which of these is a poor source of essential fatty acids?
   a. Omega-3 fatty acids
   b. Omega-6 fatty acids
   c. Polyunsaturated oils
   d. Saturated oils such as palm kernel or coconut

7. Vitamins can
   a. act as structural components of bones and teeth.
   b. act as hormones that help regulate the body's use of
      glucose.
   c. help us convert food molecules into cellular fuel.
   d. delay wound healing.

8. Calcium can
   a. cause osteoporosis (brittle bones).
   b. delay blood clotting.
   c. prevent proper nerve impulse transmission.
   d. play an important role in muscle contraction.

9. An example of an antioxidant would be
   a. vitamin C.
   b. vitamin B_{12}.
   c. selenium.
   d. iron.
10. For proper food handling and safety
    a. use all produce straight from the garden or market without washing.
    b. avoid pasteurized milk and juices.
    c. observe expiration dates on food packaging.
    d. store raw and cooked foods together in airtight containers.
11. By law, a food label must
    a. tell the exact number of items in the package.
    b. give the manufacturer's business address.
    c. calculate the percentage of calories from fat.
    d. provide a recommended serving size.

critical thinkingquestions

1. Write out a healthy menu for yourself for one breakfast, one lunch, and one dinner, including portion sizes for each type of food you select.
2. Excluding water, what are the major types of nutrients in food? What are the main roles of each?
3. Name several protective functions of dietary fiber.
4. Differentiate *trans* fat and saturated fat. Name two dietary sources of each. Which is worse, and why?
5. How do antioxidants protect the body against the damaging effects of free radicals?
6. Describe the requirements for calcium and vitamin D in children, women of childbearing age, and people over 50.

references

1. U.S. Department of Agriculture, Agriculture Research Service, "What We Eat in America, NHANES 2007–2008," August 2010, www.ars.usda.gov
2. U.S. Department of Agriculture, Agricultural Marketing Service, *How to Buy Fresh Vegetables*, Home and Garden Bulletin No. 258, 1994.
3. USDA Dietary Guidelines for Americans, 2010, www.dietaryguidelines.gov; J. S. Morrell et al., "Metabolic Syndrome, Obesity, and Related Risk Factors Among College Men and Women," *Journal of American College Health* 60, no. 1 (2012) 82–89.
4. W. D. Hoyt, S. B. Hamilton, and K. M. Rickard, "The Effects of Dietary Fat and Caloric Content on the Body-Size Estimates of Anorexic Profile and Normal College Students," *Journal of Clinical Psychology* 59, no. 1 (2003): 85–91.
5. P. W. Lemon, "Is Increased Dietary Protein Necessary or Beneficial for Individuals with a Physically Active Lifestyle?" *Nutrition Review* 54, no. 4 pt. 2 (1996): S169–S175.
6. S. M. Phillips, D. R. Moore, and E. J. Tang, "A Critical Examination of Dietary Protein Requirements, Benefits, and Excesses Athletes," *International Journal of Sports Nutrition and Exercise Metabolism* 17 (2007): S58–S76.
7. American Cancer Society, "ACS Guidelines on Nutrition and Physical Activity for Cancer Prevention: Common Questions About Diet and Cancer," January 2012, www.cancer.org
8. U.S. Food and Drug Administration, "How to Understand and Use the Nutrition Facts Label," February 2012, www.fda.gov; USDA Dietary Guidelines for Americans, 2010, www.dietaryguidelines.gov; J. S. Morrell et al., "Metabolic Syndrome, Obesity, and Related Risk Factors Among College Men and Women," 2012.
9. J. Hu et al., "Glycemic Index, Glycemic Load, and Cancer Risk," *Annals of Oncology* 24, no. 1 (2013): 245–51; F. Jingyao et al., "Dietary Glycemic Index, Glycemic Load, and Risk of Coronary Heart Disease, Stroke, and Stroke Mortality A Systematic Review with Meta-Analysis," *PLoS ONE* 7, no. 12 (2012): 1–12.
10. F. Sacks, "Ask the Expert: Omega-3 Fatty Acids," The Nutrition Source, Harvard School of Public Health, February 2011, www.hsph.harvard.edu; N. D. Riediger et al., "A Systemic Review of the Roles of n-3 Fatty Acids in Health and Disease," *Journal of the American Dietetic Association* 109, no. 4 (2009): 668–79.
11. E. C. Rizos et al., "Association Between Omega-3 Fatty Acid Supplementation and Risk of Major Cardiovascular Disease Events: A Systematic Review and Meta-Analysis," *Journal of the American Medical Association* 308, no. 10 (2012): 1024–33.
12. J. Thompson and M. Manore, *Nutrition: An Applied Approach*, 3rd Edition (San Francisco: Pearson, 2012).
13. W. Willett and D. Mozaffarian, "*Trans* Fats in Cardiac and Diabetes Risk: An Overview," *Current Cardiovascular Risk Reports* 1, no. 1 (2007): 16–23.
14. United States Department of Agriculture, "Empty Calories: What Are 'Solid Fats'?" June 2011, www.choosemyplate.gov
15. American Heart Association, "What Are Triglycerides?," American Heart Association internet publication, www.americanheart.org
16. R. Estruch et al., "Primary Prevention of Cardiovascular Disease with a Mediterranean Diet," *New England Journal of Medicine*, February 2013, doi: 10.1056/NEJMoa1200303.
17. F. B. Hu and W. C. Willett, "Optimal Diets for Prevention of Coronary Heart Disease," *Journal of the American Medical Association* 288, no. 20 (2002): 2569–78.
18. U.S. Food and Drug Administration, "Mercury Levels in Commercial Fish and Shellfish, 1990–2010," January 2013, www.fda.gov
19. J. May, "Ascorbic Acid Transporters in Health and Disease," Paper given at Linus Pauling Diet and Optimum Health Annual Conference, Portland, OR, May 2007.
20. L. J. Appel and C. A. M. Anderson, "Compelling Evidence for Public Health Action to Reduce Salt Intake," *New England Journal of Medicine* 362, no. 7 (2010): 650–2.
21. U.S. Department of Agriculture, "Table 1," *What We Eat in America, NHANES 2007–2008*, (2010); C. Ayala et al., "Application of Lower Sodium Intake Recommendations to Adults—United States, 1999–2006," *Morbidity and Mortality Weekly* (MMWR) 58, no. 11 (2009): 281–83.
22. Centers for Disease Control and Prevention, "Americans Consume Too Much Sodium (Salt)," February 2013, www.cdc.gov
23. H. W. Cohen et al., "Sodium Intake and Mortality in the NHANES II Follow-Up Study," *American Journal of Medicine* 119, no. 3 (2006): 275.e7–14; J. Feng et al., "Salt Intake and Cardiovascular Mortality," *American Journal of Medicine* 120, no. 1 (2007): e5–c7; H. Karppanen and E. Mervaala, "Sodium Intake and Hypertension," *Progress in Cardiovascular Diseases* 49, no. 2 (2006): 59–75.
24. J. Midgley et al., "Effects of Reduced Dietary Sodium on Blood Pressure: A Meta-Analysis of Randomized Controlled Trials," *The Journal of the American Medical Association* 275, no. 20 (1996): 1590–1597.
25. R. P. Heaney, "Role of Dietary Sodium in Osteoporosis," *Journal of the American*

College of Nutrition 25, no. 3 suppl (2006): 271S–276S.

26. J. Ma, R. Johns, and R. Stafford, "Americans Are Not Meeting Current Calcium Recommendations," *American Journal of Clinical Nutrition* 85, no. 5 (2007): 1361–6.

27. I. A. Dontas and C. K. Yiannakopoulos, "Risk Factors and Prevention of Osteoporosis-Related Fractures," *Journal of Musculoskeletal and Neuronal Interactions* 7, no. 3 (2007): 268–72.

28. K. Tucker et al., "Colas, but Not Other Carbonated Beverages, Are Associated with Low Bone Mineral Density in Older Women: The Framingham Osteoporosis Study," *American Journal of Clinical Nutrition* 84, no. 4 (2006): 936–42.

29. Mayo Clinic.com, "Vitamin D: Evidence," September 2012, www.mayoclinic.com

30. World Health Organization, "Micronutrient Deficiencies: Iron Deficiency Anaemia," 2013, www.who.int

31. Office of Dietary Supplements; National Institutes of Health, "Dietary Supplement Fact Sheet: Iron," February 2013, http://ods.od.nih.gov; M. Loef and H. Walach, "Copper and Iron in Alzheimer's Disease: A Systematic Review and Its Dietary Implications," *British Journal of Nutrition* 107, no. 1 (2012): 7–19, doi: 10.1017/S000711451100376X.3233

32. Office of Dietary Supplements, National Institutes of Health, "Dietary Supplement Fact Sheet: Iron," 2013.

33. J. Postlethwait and J. Hopson, *Explore Life* (Pacific Grove, CA: Brooks/Cole, 2003): 400–1.

34. Institute of Medicine of the National Academies, Food and Nutrition Board, *Dietary Reference Intakes for Water, Potassium, Sodium, Chloride, and Sulfate* (Washington, DC: The National Academies Press, 2004).

35. B. M. Popkin et al., "Water, Hydration, and Health," *Nutrition Review* 68, no. 8 (2010): 439–58.

36. D. C. Nieman et al., "Bananas as an Energy Source During Exercise: A Metabolomics Approach" *PLoS One* 7, no. 5 (2012): e37479, doi: 10.1371/journal.pone.0037479.

37. Consumers Union, "A Guide to the Best and Worst Drinks," *Consumer Reports on Health* (July 2006): 8–9.

38. USDA, "New Menu and Vending Machines Labeling Requirements," *Food Labeling and Nutrition*, June 2012, www.fda.gov

39. USDA, Center for Nutrition Policy and Promotion, "A Brief History of USDA Food Guides," June 2011, www.choosemyplate.gov

40. J. F. Hollis et al., "Weight Loss During the Intensive Intervention Phase of the Weight-Loss Maintenance Trial," *American Journal of Preventative Medicine* 35, no. 2 (2008): 118–26.

41. B. J. Rolls, E. A. Bell, and B. A. Waugh, "Increasing the Volume of a Food by Incorporating Air Affects Satiety in Men," *American Journal of Clinical Nutrition* 72, no. 2 (2000): 361–8.

42. A. Asherio, "Dietary Antioxidant Intakes and Neurological Disease Risks," Paper Presented at the Linus Pauling Diet and Optimum Health Annual Conference (Portland, OR: May 2007).

43. J. Thompson and M. Manore, *Nutrition: An Applied Approach,* 3rd Edition (San Francisco: Pearson Education, 2012).

44. E. R. Miller III and others, "Meta-Analysis: High-Dosage Vitamin E Supplementation May Increase All-Cause Mortality," *Annals of Internal Medicine* 142, no. 1 (2005): 37–46; E. A. Klein et al., "Vitamin E and the Risk of Prostate Cancer: The Selenium and Vitamin E Cancer Prevention Trial (SELECT)," *Journal of the American Medical Association* 306, no. 14 (2011): 1549–56.

45. W. Willett, *Eat, Drink, and Be Healthy: The Harvard Medical School Guide to Healthy Eating* (New York: Free Press, 2003).

46. J. D. Clarke et al., "Differential Effects of Sulforophane on Histone Deacteylases, Cell Cycle Arrest, and Apoptosis in Normal Prostate Cells Versus Hyperplastic and Cancerous Prostate Cells," *Molecular Nutrition and Food Research* 55, no. 7 (2011): 999–1009.

47. B. Frei, "Closing Remarks Summary, 2001," Paper presented at the Linus Pauling Institute International Conference on Diet and Optimum Health (Portland, OR: May 2001).

48. Ibid.

49. J. L. Buell et al., "National Athletic Trainers' Association Position Statement: Evaluation of Dietary Supplements for Performance Nutrition," *Journal of Athletic Training* 48, no. 1 (2013): 124–36.

50. M. Gonzalez-Gross et al., "Nutrition in the Sport Practice: Adaptation of the Food Guide Pyramid to the Characteristics of Athletes Diet," *Archives of Latino American Nutrition* 51, no. 4 (2001): 321–331.

51. L. M. Burke et al., "Carbohydrates and Fat for Training and Recovery," *Journal of Sports Science* 22, no. 1 (2004): 15–30.

52. M. N. Sawka, "American College of Sports Medicine Position Stand: Exercise and Fluid Replacement," *Medicine and Science in Sports and Exercise* 39, no. 2 (2007): 377–90.

53. L. M. Burke et al., "Carbohydrates and Fat for Training and Recovery," *Journal of Sports Science* 22, no. 1 (2004): 15–30.

54. M. N. Sawka, "American College of Sports Medicine Position Stand: Exercise and Fluid Replacement," *Medicine and Science in Sports and Exercise* 39, no. 2 (2007): 377–90.

55. N. Clark, "Recovering from Hard Exercise," *American Fitness* 30, no. 5 (2012): 64–65.

56. P. B. Wilson et al., "Dietary Tendencies as Predictors of Marathon Time in Novice Marathoners," *International Journal of Sport Nutrition and Exercise Metabolism*, (2012) [Epub ahead of print] www.ncbi.nlm.nih.gov

57. W. H. Saris and L. J. van Loon, "Nutrition and Health: Nutrition and Performance in Sports," [article in Dutch] *Nederlands Tijdschrift voor Geneeskunde* 148, no. 15 (2004): 708–12.

58. J. J. Crowley and C. Wall, "The Use of Dietary Supplements in a Group of Potentially Elite Secondary School Athletes," *Asia-Pacific Journal of Clinical Nutrition* 13, suppl. (2004): S39.

59. R. Maughan, "The Athlete's Diet: Nutritional Goals and Dietary Strategies," *Proceedings of the Nutritional Society* 61, no. 1 (2002): 87–96.

60. J. B. Anderson et al., *Eat Right! Healthy Eating in College and Beyond* (San Francisco: Benjamin Cummings, 2007).

61. American Dietetic Association, "Position of the American Dietetic Association: Vegetarian Diets," *Journal of the American Dietetic Association* 109, no. 7 (2009): 1266–82.

62. A. Pan et al., "Red Meat Consumption and Mortality," *Archives of Internal Medicine* 172, no. 7 (2012): 555–63.

63. D. White, "Where's the Beef? Dining Makes Moves Toward Meatless Meals," *University of California at Santa Cruz News*, June 2012, http://news.uscs.edu

64. American Diabetes Association, "Making Healthy Food Choices," September 2011, www.diabetes.org

65. Centers for Disease Control and Prevention, "CDC Estimates of Foodborne Illness in the United States: CDC 2011 Estimates: Findings," October 2012, www.cdc.gov

66. J. Kurman, "Self-Enhancement, Self-Regulation, and Self-Improvement Following Failures," *British Journal of Social Psychology* 45, p. 2. (2006): 339–56.

getfitgraphic references

1. USDA Dietary Guidelines for Americans, 2010, www.dietaryguidelines.gov; J. S. Morrell et al., "Metabolic Syndrome, Obesity, and Related Risk Factors Among College Men and Women," *Journal of American College Health* 60, no. 1 (2012): 82–9.

2. Tufts University Health and Nutrition Letter Special Report, "Where is Your Sodium Coming From," May 2012, 4–5.

3. Centers for Disease Control and Prevention, Vital Signs, "Where's the Sodium? There's too much in many common foods," February 2012, www.cdc.gov

4. S. B. Racette et al., "Weight Changes, Exercise, and Dietary Patterns During Freshman and Sophomore Years of College," *Journal of American College Health* 53, no. 6 (2005): 245–51.

5. American College Health Association, American College Health Association-*National College Health Assessment II: Reference Group Data Report Fall 2012* (Hanover, MD: American College Health Association, 2013), www.acha-ncha.org

Name: _____ Date: _____

Instructor: _____ Section: _____

Purpose: To learn how to read food labels and analyze the nutritional content of a packaged food.

Directions: Select any packaged food item from your kitchen or from a grocery store. Find the "Nutrition Facts" panel on the package and answer the following questions.

1. What is the name of the packaged food you are examining?

_____

2. What is the "serving size" stated on the Nutrition Facts panel?

_____

Does this "serving size" match the portion you typically consume of this food in one sitting? Is it bigger or smaller than the amount that you typically consume?

_____

3. Examine the ingredients. What are the main ingredients (i.e., which items are listed first)?

_____

Does this list of main ingredients surprise you? How nutritious are the main ingredients?

_____

4. Complete the following table for your chosen food, listing amounts and % Daily Value (% DV) for various nutrients:

Calories (per serving)	Total Fat	Saturated Fat	Trans Fat	Sodium	Dietary Fiber	Sugars	Vitamins/ Minerals
	Amount:	Amount:	Amount:	Amount:	Amount:	Amount:	Amount:
	% DV:	% DV:	% DV:	% DV:	% DV:		% DV:

Examine your data. Is this food excessively high in fat, saturated fat, *trans* fat, or sodium? Does it provide any dietary fiber? How much sugar is in this food? Does this food supply any vitamins and minerals?

_____

_____

5. What is your overall assessment of the nutritional value of the packaged food you have examined? How does the particular food you examined compare to other typical foods in your daily diet?

_____

_____

6. Healthy eaters make regular label reading a part of every shopping trip. What can you add to your behavior-change contract for nutrition that will help you develop a life-long food-label-reading habit?

_____

_____

Name: _____ Date: _____

Instructor: _____ Section: _____

Purpose: To get an initial assessment of your current nutrition and identify areas to be improved.

Directions: Follow the instructions below. You will need Internet access to complete this lab.

1. Log on to https://www.supertracker.usda.gov/foodtracker.aspx

2. Click "CREATE PROFILE" in the upper right-hand corner of the page if you are accessing this site for the first time. Click "LOG IN" if you are returning.

3. Click on "Track Food & Activity" at the top of the page and select "Food Tracker." Enter all of the food items you have eaten today. (It's best to complete this at the end of the day when you have finished all of your meals.) Enter each food individually by entering the name of the food in the search field and clicking "Go." If you cannot find the exact food you are looking for, select the food that is the most similar. After you have located a food, it should show up on the left side of the screen. Select a serving size from the drop-down menu and enter the number of servings you consumed. Choose a meal time and click "Add" to save the food in your tracker. Repeat until you have entered all of the foods you consumed today. (Don't forget to include any snacks and beverages!)

4. Click on the "My Reports" tab, and select "Food Groups & Calories." Select a date range and click "Create Report." How does your food intake compare to the recommendations for food groups and calories?

_____

_____

_____

_____

5. Click on "Nutrients Reports" at the top of the screen. Select a date range and click "Create Report." This report will illustrate how your intake of specific nutrients compares to the recommendations.

   a. Does your intake of any nutrient fall short of the recommendations? If so, which nutrient(s)?

_____

_____

   b. Does your intake of any nutrient exceed the recommendations? If so, which nutrient(s)?

_____

_____

   Note: For more accurate results, record your intake for at least three consecutive days, and then analyze your data again.

PLAN FOR CHANGE
IMPROVING YOUR NUTRITION

MasteringHealth™

Name: _____ Date: _____

Instructor: _____ Section: _____

Purpose: To create a detailed plan for improving your personal nutrition.

Materials: Results from Lab 7.2.

SECTION I: PLANNING CHANGES TO YOUR DIET

1. Look back at your results for Lab 7.2. Which nutrients do you consume too little of?

_____

_____

List at least three foods you could add to your diet in order to increase your consumption of these nutrients:

Food: _____ Rich in: _____

Food: _____ Rich in: _____

Food: _____ Rich in: _____

(**Hint:** To get ideas for new foods to try, go to the Food Groups section of www.ChooseMyPlate.gov and choose the food groups one by one. You will see a listing of fruits, vegetables, grains, protein rich foods, and dairy foods.)

2. Do you consume too much protein, fat, saturated fat, cholesterol, or sodium? If so, what foods high in these substances could you reduce or eliminate from your diet? List at least 3:

Food: _____ High in: _____

Food: _____ High in: _____

Food: _____ High in: _____

3. How closely did your diet match up with the USDA recommendations? Fill in the blanks below.

Current dairy intake: _____ cups   Recommended dairy intake: _____ cups

Current intake of protein rich foods: _____ oz.   Recommended intake of protein rich foods: _____ oz.

Current vegetables intake: _____ cups   Recommended vegetables intake: _____ cups

Current fruits intake: _____ cups   Recommended fruits intake: _____ cups

Current grains intake: _____ oz.   Recommended grains intake: _____ oz.

How can you adjust your diet to more closely meet recommended intake levels for each food group?

- I would like to increase/decrease my milk intake by _____ cups.

- I would like to increase/decrease my meat and beans intake by _____ oz.

- I would like to increase/decrease my vegetables intake by _____ oz.

- I would like to increase/decrease my fruits intake by _____ cups.

- I would like to increase/decrease my grains intake by _____ oz.

SECTION II: SHORT- AND LONG-TERM GOALS

Create short- and long-term goals for your healthy eating plan. Be sure to use SMART (specific, measurable, action-oriented, realistic, time-limited) goal-setting guidelines and the information obtained from Section I of this lab and all of your Lab 7.2 materials. Choose appropriate target dates and rewards for completing your goals.

1. Short-Term Goal (3–6 Months)

   a. Goal: _____

   _____

   b. Target Date: _____

   c. Reward: _____

2. Long-Term Goal (12+ Months)

   a. Goal: _____

   _____

   b. Target Date: _____

   c. Reward: _____

SECTION III: BARRIERS TO GOOD NUTRITION; STRATEGIES FOR OVERCOMING THEM

1. What barriers or obstacles might hinder your plan for nutrition changes? Indicate your top three nutritional barriers here:

   a. _____

   b. _____

   c. _____

2. Overcoming these barriers to change will be an important step in reaching your goals. List three strategies for overcoming the obstacles listed:

   a. _____

   b. _____

   c. _____

SECTION IV: GETTING SUPPORT

List resources you will use to help you change your nutritional behavior and how each of these resources will support your goals:

Friend/partner/relative: _____

School-based resource: _____

Community-based resource: _____

Other: _____

Activate, Motivate,
&ADVANCE YOUR WELL-BEING

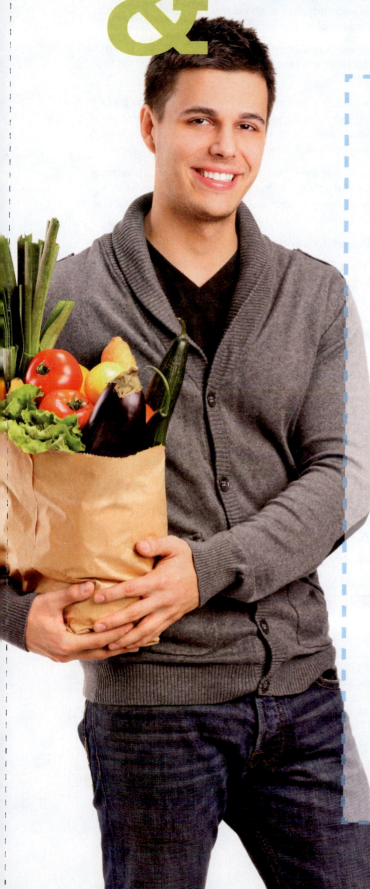

A PROGRAM TO EAT MORE FRUITS AND VEGETABLES

SCAN TO SEE IT
ONLINE!

ACTIVATE!

Fruits and vegetables are important components of a nutritious diet, and eating them is also helpful for managing your weight. Fruits and vegetables are low in calories and high in the nutrients Americans under-consume such as folate, magnesium, potassium, dietary fiber, and vitamins A, C and K. Fruits and vegetables also help prevent diseases such as heart attacks, stroke, and certain cancers. The following programs can help you successfully increase your vegetable and fruit consumption and variety!

What Do I Need to Do to Eat More Fruits?

KNOW WHAT COUNTS: All fresh, frozen, canned, and dried fruits and 100% fruit juices count as fruit.

MORE ABOUT JUICE: 100% fruit juice can be part of a healthy diet, but it lacks dietary fiber and it can add extra calories to your diet. Most of the fruit you eat should come from whole fruits rather than juice. When choosing juice, aim for 100% juice and look for notation on the package saying "100% juice." Fruit drinks that have little juice are considered sugar-sweetened beverages rather than fruit juice. This recommendation also goes for juice in canned fruit; look for fruit canned in 100% fruit juice.

CHOOSE OLD FAVORITES AND NEW: Create a list of fruits you like or want to try for the first time. Remember that fruit may come in different forms (such as peaches which you may enjoy fresh, canned, or frozen). Having a list of fruits you are interested in should help you plan ahead to get more into your day.

What Do I Need to Do to Eat More Vegetables?

KNOW WHAT COUNTS: All fresh, frozen, canned, and dried vegetables and 100% vegetable juices count.

VARIETY IS KEY: Eat a variety of vegetables, especially dark-green and red and orange vegetables and beans and peas.

CHOOSE OLD FAVORITES AND NEW: Create a list of vegetables you like, types that are available to you, and ones you'd like to try for the first time. Remember that vegetables come in different forms (such as spinach which you may enjoy fresh, frozen, or canned). A list can help you plan ahead to eat more helpings each day.

Tips to Eating More Fruits and Vegetables

KEEP PRODUCE HANDY: Keep a bowl of whole fruit on the table, on the counter, or in the refrigerator. You can also keep a piece of fruit in your bag for an easy to grab snack. Individual containers of fruits like peaches or applesauce are also easy and convenient.

Keep vegetables on-hand ready for snacking. Carrots, broccoli, cauliflower, bell peppers, and baby tomatoes are all great with dips like hummus, low-fat ranch, or cottage cheese.

CHOOSE MEALS WISELY: Try a salad as a main dish for lunch (go light on the salad dressing). Include a green salad with your dinner every night. Add beans and peas to salads or get creative and try topping them with dried fruit, oranges, apples, or berries.

When eating out (or in the dining hall) look for options that include the most vegetables, such as a pizza topped with mushrooms and green peppers or a veggie burrito or omelet. Add vegetables such as tomatoes, lettuce, and avocado to your sandwiches and subs. Choose split pea or lentil soups or add beans into other soup choices.

Replace large portions of high-calorie foods such as chips or cookies with lower-calorie fruit- based choices such as smoothies with low-fat yogurt or milk blended with frozen fruit; 100% juice frozen fruit bars; yogurt topped with fresh fruit; sliced fruit dipped in flavored yogurt; or even a "baked" apple cooked in the microwave with cinnamon and raisins.

Choose fresh fruits in season, as they will likely taste best and cost less.

Always top your cereal (hot or cold), pancakes, and waffles with fruit. Some ideas include sliced bananas, dried fruit, frozen or fresh berries, and chopped apples or peaches.

COOKING AND SHOPPING: If you are cooking, add shredded carrots or canned pumpkin to muffins and breads and chopped or shredded vegetables to soups, stews, casseroles, stir-fries, and tomato sauces.

Buy baked beans or refried beans in cans to use them for side dishes or snacks, such as adding refried beans to a quesadilla.

Buy vegetables that are easy to prepare, such as bags of baby carrots, bagged salad mixes, or lower-sodium canned vegetables or soup. Frozen vegetables are quick and easy to cook in the microwave.

Buy fruits that are dried, frozen, and canned (in water or 100% juice) as well as fresh, so that you always have a supply on hand. Choose packaged fruits that do not have added sugars.

Keep vegetables and fruits visible when storing them.

4 Week Program to Boost Fruit and Vegetable Intake

Very few adults in the United States eat the recommended 5 to 9 cups of fruits or vegetables per day, so this is a program from which most everyone can benefit. You could start by focusing on fruits, vegetables, or more specifically on the choices within those food groups. Adjust the program to suit your personal meal schedule.

What Counts As a Cup?

In general, what counts as a cup is: 1 cup of fruit, 1 cup of raw or cooked vegetables, 1 cup of 100% juice, 2 cups of raw leafy greens, or ½ cup of dried fruit. Visit www.choosemyplate.gov for more information on portion sizes.

EATING MORE FRUITS AND VEGETABLES PROGRAM **GOAL:** Increase fruit and vegetable intake to 5 cups of fruits and vegetables per day by progressively including them in meals and snacks over four weeks.

	Mon	Tue	Wed	Thurs	Fri	Sat	Sun
Week 1	2 cups of fruits and vegetables	2 cups of fruits and vegetables	2 cups of fruits and vegetables	2 cups of fruits and vegetables	2 cups of fruits and vegetables	2 cups of fruits and vegetables	2 cups of fruits and vegetables
Week 2	3 cups of fruits and vegetables	3 cups of fruits and vegetables	3 cups of fruits and vegetables	3 cups of fruits and vegetables	3 cups of fruits and vegetables	3 cups of fruits and vegetables	3 cups of fruits and vegetables
Week 3	4 cups of fruits and vegetables	4 cups of fruits and vegetables	4 cups of fruits and vegetables	4 cups of fruits and vegetables	4 cups of fruits and vegetables	4 cups of fruits and vegetables	4 cups of fruits and vegetables
Week 4	5 cups of fruits and vegetables	5 cups of fruits and vegetables	5 cups of fruits and vegetables	5 cups of fruits and vegetables	5 cups of fruits and vegetables	5 cups of fruits and vegetables	5 cups of fruits and vegetables

Note: This program assumes you are already eating 1-2 cups of fruits and vegetables per day. If you are eating <1-2 cups of fruits and vegetables per day, increase your intake before beginning the program to 2 cups per day. If you are already eating >2 cups of fruits and vegetables per day, start by adding one more cup of fruit and vegetables each week until you reach 5 cups per day.

MOTIVATE!

Track your fruit and vegetable intake on your personal planner, on an online food planner site (such as www.supertracker.usda.gov), or on the mobile website. Make note of the meal or snack, types of produce, and amounts. Here are some tips for boosting the nutrition of your choices:

FRUIT: For the benefits of dietary fiber, choose whole or cut-up fruit rather than fruit juice.

Select fruits with more potassium often, such as bananas, prunes and prune juice, dried peaches and apricots, and orange juice.

When choosing canned fruits, select fruit canned in 100% fruit juice or water rather than syrup.

Vary your fruit choices. Fruits differ in nutrient content.

Try to eat different colors of fruits to make consuming a good variety easier.

VEGETABLES: Select often vegetables that contain higher levels of potassium, such as sweet potatoes, white potatoes, white beans, tomato products (paste, sauce, and juice), beet greens, soybeans, lima beans, spinach, lentils, and kidney beans.

Keep in mind that sauces and seasonings can add calories, saturated fat, and sodium to vegetables. Use the Nutrition Facts label to compare the calories and % Daily Value for saturated fat and sodium in plain and seasoned vegetables.

Prepare more foods from fresh ingredients to lower sodium intake. Most of the sodium we eat comes from packaged or processed foods.

Buy canned vegetables labeled "reduced sodium," "low sodium," or "no salt added." If you want to add a little salt it will likely be less than the amount in the regular canned product.

ADVANCE!

Now that you have boosted your fruit and vegetable intake, challenge yourself to explore and consume even more produce, or try cooking an old favorite in a new way. Below is a program to help you increase your variety of produce. Choose new varieties from the lists following the program. On days without a new fruit or vegetable in your program, continue incorporating the new varieties from the previous day(s).

INCREASING YOUR FRUIT AND VEGETABLE VARIETY PROGRAM

GOAL: To eat a variety of fruits and vegetables, especially including vegetables from the following sub-groups: dark-green vegetables, red and orange vegetables, and beans and peas, progressively over a four week period.

	Mon	Tue	Wed	Thurs	Fri	Sat	Sun
Week 1	Try 1 new fruit or vegetable		Try 1 new fruit or vegetable				
Week 2	Try 1 new fruit and 1 new vegetable		Try 1 new fruit and 1 new vegetable				
Week 3	Try 1 new fruit and 1 new vegetable		Try 1 new fruit and 1 new vegetable		Try 1 new fruit and 1 new vegetable		
Week 4	Try 2 new fruits and 2 new vegetables		Try 1 new fruit and 1 new vegetable		Try 2 new fruits and 2 new vegetables		

Common Fruit Choices to Add for Variety

Apples	Kiwi fruit	Pineapple
Apricots	Lemons	Plums
Bananas	Limes	Prunes
Blueberries	Mangoes	Raisins
Cantaloupe	Nectarines	Raspberries
Cherries	Oranges	Strawberries
Grapefruit	Peaches	Tangerines
Grapes	Pears	Watermelon
Honeydew	Papaya	

Common Vegetable Choices to Add for Variety

Dark Green
Bok choy
Broccoli
Collard greens
Dark green leafy lettuce
Kale
Mesclun
Mustard greens
Romaine lettuce
Spinach
Turnip greens
Watercress

Red and Orange
Acorn, butternut or
    hubbard squash
Carrots
Pumpkin
Red peppers
Sweet potatoes
Tomatoes or tomato juice

Beans and Peas
Black beans
Black-eyed peas

Garbanzo beans (chickpeas)
Kidney beans
Lentils
Navy beans
Pinto beans
Soy beans
Split peas
White beans

Starchy
Cassava
Corn
Green peas
Green lima beans
Plantains
Potatoes
Taro
Water chestnuts

Other
Artichokes
Asparagus
Avocado
Bean sprouts
Beets

Brussels sprouts
Cabbage
Cauliflower
Celery
Cucumbers
Eggplant
Green beans
Green peppers
Iceberg (head) lettuce
Mushrooms
Okra
Onions
Turnips
Wax beans
Zucchini

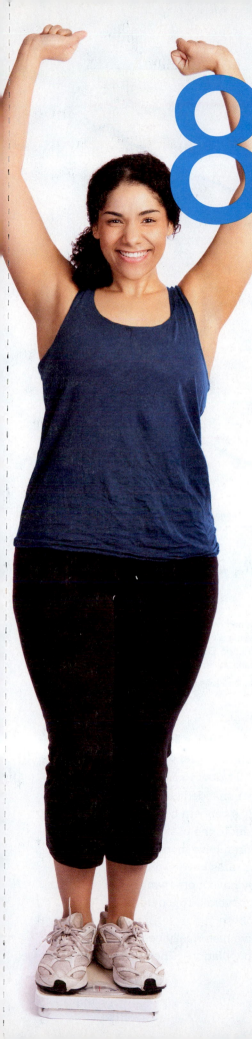

8 Managing Your Weight

MasteringHealth™

Go online for chapter quizzes, interactive assessments, videos, and more!

casestudy

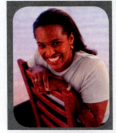

MARIA

"My name is Maria. I'm 25 and a full-time student in southern Florida, finishing a BA in child development. I was halfway through college when my daughter, Anna, was born. Now that she's in pre-school, I'm back to taking a full load of classes and hope to finish college in two more years. I love being a mom. The only thing I'd like to change is my weight! Ever since Anna was born, I've been trying to get back into my prepregnancy clothes. I've tried lots of ways to lose the extra pounds—diet pills, liquid diets, Atkins, Paleo—you name it, I've tried it! Sometimes it works for a while, but eventually the weight always comes back. I'm willing to try again, but how do I find a plan that will stick?"

HEAR IT! ONLINE

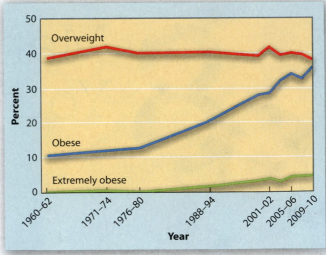

(a) Men

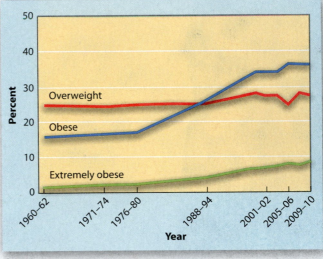

(b) Women

FIGURE **8.1** For the past half century, one-third of Americans have been overweight despite massive government campaigns and personal efforts at weight reduction. During that same period, the percentages of obese Americans have more than doubled.

Source: NCHS E-Stat: Prevalence of Overweight, Obesity and Extreme Obesity among Adults: United States, Trends 1960–1962 through 2009–2010, National Health and Nutrition Examination Survey.

Weight is a serious and growing health issue in America. While introducing a new campaign to combat obesity, First Lady Michelle Obama warned that the rising rate of obesity in America is a "public health crisis" threatening our nation and our future.[1] Over two-thirds of Americans over age 20 have a body mass index, or BMI, of at least 25 or above, categorizing them as **overweight** or **obese**.[2] About half of these adults (33.3 percent of the total adult population) are overweight (see **Figure 8.1**), meaning that their body weight is more than 10 percent over the recommended range and their BMI is between 25 and 29.9.[3] The other half (35.7 percent of the total adult

overweight In an adult, a BMI of 25 to 29 or a body weight more than 10 percent above recommended levels

obese In an adult, a BMI of 30 or more or a body weight more than 20 percent above recommended levels

underweight In an adult, a BMI below 18.5 or a body weight more than 10 percent below recommended levels

population) are obese, with a BMI of 30 or above.[4] Only about 1.7 percent of Americans older than age 20 are **underweight**, with a BMI below 18.5 or a weight 10 percent below the recommended range.[5]

Part of the First Lady's concern comes from the alarming trend in children: In the past 25 years, obesity rates for young children have more than doubled; for kids aged 6 to 11, the rates have nearly tripled; and for adolescents, they have more than tripled (**Figure 8.2,** page 287).[6] Overall, 16.9 percent of American children are obese.[7]

College students have historically been in better shape than other adult populations. There is evidence,

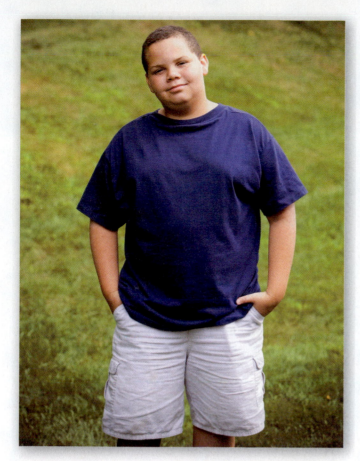

FIGURE **8.2** In the past 30 years, obesity rates for children aged 2 to 5 years have more than doubled, going from 5% to 12.1%, while rates for those aged 6 to 11 years went from 6.5% to 18.0%. The biggest increase was in adolescents aged 12 to 19 years, whose obesity rates more than tripled from 5% to 18.4%!

Source: Data from NCHS E-Stat: Prevalence of Obesity among Children and Adolescents: United States, Trends 1960–1962 through 2009–2010, National Health and Nutrition Examination Survey.

however, that overweight is increasing in college populations. A recent study of nearly 3,000 college students indicated that between one-quarter to one-half of students are overweight or obese.[8] Of even greater concern, three-quarters of all the male college students they surveyed had at least one criterion for *metabolic syndrome*: a set of interrelated physical and physiological symptoms that increase the risk for stroke, heart disease, and diabetes.[9]

Regardless of your age and stage of life, you should keep several key points in mind as you assess your own diet, exercise, and **weight management** strategies:

- The changes you make in your diet and exercise habits cannot be short-term fixes; they must become a new way of life—and your payoff will be increased energy, greater self-acceptance, and a trimmer appearance. No diet program, product, or service will magically make weight melt away. Successful weight loss takes time, effort, motivation, and a commitment to permanently adopting positive habits.

- Recognize that your overall percentage of body fat is more important than your weight or the amount of weight you lose.

- Understand that fast weight loss usually involves a temporary decrease in tissue fluids and often a loss in lean muscle mass, as well. "Healthy weight loss" means the slow, sustained loss of fat, coupled with increases in muscle mass and the preservation and maintenance of lean body mass.

- Learn how long-term weight management balances calories consumed in foods with calories expended through metabolism, activity, and exercise—an equation called **energy balance**.

This chapter presents the tools and techniques you need to determine a healthy target weight and create a sound plan for reaching and maintaining it. Incorporating weight management into your ongoing wellness program will allow you to realize the significant benefits—physiological, social, and emotional—of sustaining your body mass and body composition within recommended ranges throughout adult life.

Why Is Obesity on the Rise?

In 2013, the World Health Organization (WHO) estimated that 46 percent of the world's adults (over 1.4 billion people) were overweight or obese and that the number could increase substantially by 2025.[10] Obese adults represent 11 percent of the world's adult population and number over 500 million worldwide.[11] The WHO coined the new term *globesity* to describe this trend. Surprisingly, obesity is a problem in high-income industrialized countries as well as in low- and middle-income developing countries.[12] Diets high in processed fats, meats, sugars, and refined starches provide excess calories, while labor-saving devices and sedentary lifestyles reduce energy expenditure. In developing countries, entire cultures are moving away from traditional diets—rich in fruits, vegetables, grains, and low-fat proteins—as well as from manual labor. As a result, they are experiencing the same gain in body fat percentages and weight that Americans did three decades ago. Only the poorest countries of sub-Saharan Africa do not reflect this worldwide trend.[13]

weight management A lifelong balancing of calories consumed and calories expended through exercise and activity to control body fat and weight

energy balance The relationship between the amount of calories consumed in food and the amount of calories expended through metabolism and physical activity

Several Factors Contribute to Overweight and Obesity in America

In the last quarter century, the number of obese adults has more than doubled.[14] The maps in **Figure 8.3** reveal that the rapid increase is distributed unevenly: The southern and upper Midwestern states show the highest rates of obesity in the United States. Several factors contribute to the rapid increase.

Overconsumption and Eating Calorie-Dense Foods Americans consume an average of 523 calories more per day now than they did in 1970, according to the U.S. Department of Agriculture.[15] Without additional exercise, the extra calories lead to weight gain. Eating certain calorie-dense foods also contributes to weight gain: A 20-year study of over 120,000 Americans revealed that weight gain was closely associated with consuming foods such as potato chips, potatoes, sugary beverages, and red and processed meats.[16]

LIVE IT! ONLINE
Worksheet 23
Why Do
You Eat?

Many societal factors encourage overeating, such as "portion distortion," the constant availability of food, advertising, and price. Food portions in restaurants and supermarkets have grown steadily over the past half-century (**Figure 8.4**). Researchers have also found that people don't read their own "fullness signals," or feelings of *satiety,* very well. So, the bigger the portions, the more they will eat overall.[17]

Easy access to unhealthy food also encourages overeating.[18] Today, most drugstores, gas stations, schools, and public buildings sell packaged junk food. People eat more treats if they are available in plain sight than if the same food is less accessible.[19] Fast-food franchises also offer highly visible and easily accessible foods loaded with saturated fat, salt, and/or sugar. On average, Americans aged 20 to 39 eat 15 percent of their daily calories from fast food.[20]

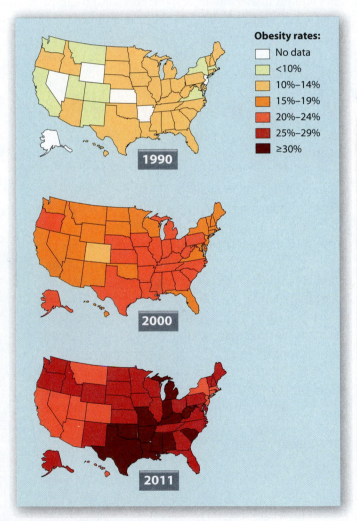

Obesity rates:
- No data
- <10%
- 10%–14%
- 15%–19%
- 20%–24%
- 25%–29%
- ≥30%

1990

2000

2011

FIGURE **8.3** Obesity rates have risen dramatically over recent decades. Rates are highest in the upper Midwest and in the South.

Note: Historical maps are provided for a reference only, as differences in the analysis of prevalence rates for 2011 make direct comparisons to previous years incompatible.

Source: Centers for Disease Control, "U.S. Obesity Trends," 2012, www.cdc.gov

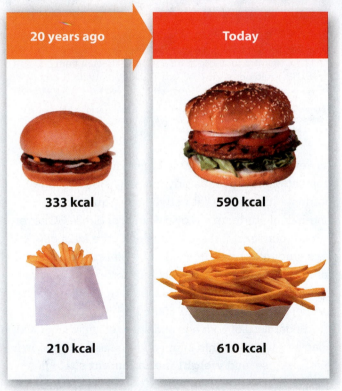

20 years ago → **Today**

333 kcal   590 kcal

210 kcal   610 kcal

FIGURE **8.4** Today's serving portions are significantly larger than those of past decades. A 25-ounce prime-rib dinner served at one local steak chain contains nearly 3,000 calories and 150 grams of fat. That's twice as many calories and more than three times the fat than many adults need in a whole day, and it's just the meat part of the meal!

Source: Data are from National Heart, Lung, and Blood Institute, "Portion Distortion," September 2011, http://hp2010.nhlbihin.net

Advertising contributes to overeating of nutritionally poor sweets, sodas and fruit drinks, alcoholic beverages, and salty snacks. Amazingly, one-third of our daily calories come from just a few categories of these highly advertised junk foods.[21] Food price also influences consumption, as junk foods tend to be inexpensive.[22]

Too Little Exercise The ease of our modern life is an improvement over the hard physical labor of past generations. Yet the exertion we are spared amounts to hundreds of calories per day that we *don't* burn off as we sit at our desks, drive our vehicles, or change channels with a remote control.[23] Even the layout of modern towns and cities contributes to reduced energy expenditure. Walkable neighborhoods with open space for recreation and grocery stores that sell fresh produce have child obesity rates *half* as high as neighborhoods without these amenities.[24] And in neighborhoods with fewer exercise opportunities and poorer food choices, adults are more likely to weigh more and have high blood pressure, heart disease, cancer, diabetes, and other diseases.[25]

Hereditary Factors With all these overconsumption factors in play, why isn't *everyone* overweight or obese? Part of the answer lies in heredity. If most of your relatives are overweight or obese, you are more likely to gain weight during adulthood. If most of your relatives are thin, you are more likely to be thin as well. Researchers have learned that dozens—perhaps hundreds—of genes help determine your weight.[26] Genes control whether our metabolism is fast, burning off most of our excess calories, or "thrifty," tending to conserve food energy.[27]

> **non-exercise activity** Routine daily activities such as standing up and walking around that use energy but are not part of deliberate exercise

Non-Exercise Activity Uses Energy In recent years, researchers have studied the human "fidget factor": the tendency of some people to conserve energy by sitting quietly for long stretches and being generally less active all day, while others use energy by being fidgety, jiggling their head, hands, and feet, and getting up to walk around every few minutes. James Levine and colleagues at the Mayo Clinic have demonstrated that lean people burn 279 to 477 more calories per day than obese people through this type of **non-exercise activity**—an expenditure that can significantly affect fat storage and body weight.[28] The box Get Up from Your Chair! explores how even small, deliberate breaks from sitting can assist in weight management.

TOOLS FOR CHANGE

Get Up from Your Chair!

Researchers have discovered that sitting for long periods day after day can negatively impact your health—even if you exercise on those same days. Several studies have shown that people who spend the most time sitting also have the highest mortality rates from cardiovascular disease and other illnesses.[1]

Conversely, recent research shows that people who interrupt sedentary time with movement "breaks" have narrower waistlines and lower risk of cardiovascular disease and diabetes.[2] Scientists in Australia interpreted data from a large American study sponsored by the Centers for Disease Control and Prevention. They found correlations with a trimmer waistline and less risk for cardiovascular diseases in 4,750 participants who wore devices that monitored movement and recorded breaks in sedentary time.[3]

The team recommends that people take a "whole day approach" to increasing physical activity, adding physical exercise but also breaking up sedentary time with "lifestyle exercise" to benefit wellness. Consider this: Expending one minute of sit-ups or jumping jacks instead of sitting during TV commercials, two minutes of stair climbing a few times per day, five minutes of leaf raking, ten minutes of walking around while you talk on your cell phone, or shopping with two small hand grocery baskets instead of pushing one larger cart on wheels can add up to the benefits of a 30-minute trip to the gym![4]

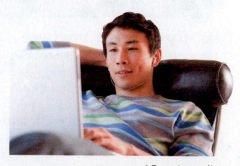

(Continued)

THINK! How much time do you spend sitting each day as you study, attend class, drive your car, and so on?

ACT NOW! Today, keep a log of your "lifestyle exercise." As you move throughout your day, accurately jot down the number of minutes you spend walking, doing chores around your room or house, and so on. This week, make a list of new ways to increase your lifestyle activity, and add one. Do the same each day for a few days. In two weeks, retrack your lifestyle activity to see how many additional minutes you have added to getting up out of your chair!

Sources:
1. N. Owen, A. Bauman, and W. Brown, "Too Much Sitting: A Novel and Important Predictor of Chronic Disease Risk?" *British Journal of Sports Medicine* 43, no. 2 (2009): 81–83.
2. J. Henson et al., "Associations of Objectively Measured Sedentary Behavior and Physical Activity with Markers of Cardiometabolic Health," *Diabetologia* (2013), doi: 10.1007/s00125-013-2845-9.
3. G. Healy, et al. "Sedentary Time and Cardio-Metabolic Biomarkers in U.S. Adults; NHANES 2003–06," *European Heart Journal* (2011), doi: 10.1093/eurheartj/ehq451.
4. P. D. Loprinzi et al., "Association between Biologic Outcomes and Objectively Measured Physical Activity Accumulated in ≥10-Minute Bouts and <10 Minute Bouts," *American Journal of Health Promotion* 27, no. 3 (2013): 143, doi: 10.4278/ajhp.110916-QUAN-348.

Demographic and Lifestyle Factors A mix of demographic factors both biological and nonbiological—including sex, race/ethnicity, culture, education, and economic level—all influence weight. As the Diversity box Race/Ethnicity, Gender, and Weight explains, your body weight and likelihood of overweight or obesity vary by race/ethnic group as well as by sex. Biological and cultural factors interact, of course: Our family and ethnic group influences what, when, and how much we eat, as well as how much we exercise and participate in other activities. The choice of high-fat, high-calorie foods, for instance, is partly based on family upbringing, habit, and preference. The same is true for leisure time activity: 40 percent of Americans engage in no exercise, sports, or other physical activity at all during their leisure time.[29] Education and income influence these choices; the higher a person's education level, and the more money he or she makes, the more likely the individual is to be physically active.[30] About 24 percent of adults with college graduate degrees are sedentary, compared to 70 percent of those with less than a ninth-grade education.[31]

DIVeRSiTY
Race/Ethnicity, Gender, and Weight

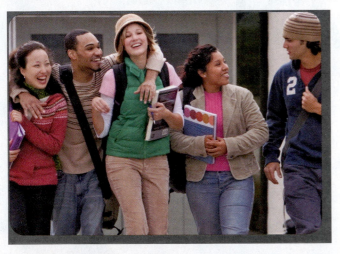

Body weight varies by racial/ethnic groups to some degree, based on genes as well as on cultural preferences for food and exercise. The highest percentages of overweight adults in the United States are: Native American males (78 percent) and females (65 percent), Hispanic males (76 percent) and females (66 percent), African American males (69 percent) and females (72 percent), Pacific Islander males (87 percent) and females (70 percent), and white males (70 percent). White females have somewhat lower percentages of overweight (54 percent), and Asian American men and women have the lowest percentages of overweight (52 percent and 32 percent, respectively).[1]

Some ethnic groups appear to have "thrifty genes" that helped their ancestors survive during extended periods of famine by slowing down metabolism to conserve food energy. In a modern environment of plentiful food, widespread mechanization, and diminished activity, however, "thrifty genes" can lead to easy weight gain. This helps explain, for example, why today, 90 percent of Pima Indians are overweight and 75 percent are obese.

Women have a tendency to burn fewer calories than men due to their higher level of essential body fat and lower ratio of lean body mass to fat mass. Because muscle cells burn more energy, and because men usually have more muscle tissue than women, men burn 10 to 20 percent more calories than women do, even at rest. Monthly hormonal cycles and pregnancy also increase the likelihood of weight fluctuation and gain. Significantly, though, adult men are more likely to be overweight than adult women.

Source:
1. C. A. Schoenborn, P. F. Adams, and J. A. Peregoy, National Center for Health Statistics, "Health Behaviors of Adults: United States, 2008 -2010,"*Vital Health Statistics* 10, no. 257 (2013).

casestudy

MARIA

"I was never overweight as a kid, and I gained a normal amount of weight during my pregnancy, but now I'm considered overweight. My parents, grandparents, and two older sisters are all on the heavy side, so I wonder if my "heavy" genes just decided to kick in! While I was pregnant, I got used to eating more food than before, and after giving birth to Anna, I guess I just didn't cut back. I spend a lot of time running around after Anna, but otherwise, I drive everywhere and don't set aside special time to exercise. Anna is a picky eater right now—she'll only eat macaroni and cheese, chicken strips, and pizza—so we end up eating those most of the time. That makes it really hard to diet!"

THINK! Do you share any of Maria's eating and exercise habits? Is she like any of your friends?

ACT! Write down your current BMI. Does it represent underweight, healthy weight, overweight, or obesity? List aspects of your lifestyle that may have contributed to your current BMI.

HEAR IT! ONLINE

Additional lifestyle choices also influence body weight. Drinking alcohol is associated with weight gain over time, as is watching television, smoking and then quitting, and getting less than six hours of sleep per night or more than eight hours.[32]

How Does My Body Weight Affect My Wellness?

A leading nutritionist has written that body weight sits at the center of an intricate web of health and disease.[33] Indeed, research shows: You are more likely to remain healthy throughout life if (1) your BMI is between 21 and 23 if you are a woman and 22 and 24 if you are a man; (2) you maintain approximately the same BMI and the same waist size throughout your adult life; and (3) your body's fat deposits tend to occur around the hips and thighs rather than the abdomen. High BMIs and abdominal fat (indicated by a large waist size) are associated with higher risk for several chronic diseases.[34]

Being underweight is an important but far less common problem. Fewer than 5 percent of Americans have a BMI under 18.5.[35] Underweight carries its own significant health risks and can be the result of an unusually fast metabolism, excessive dieting, extreme levels of exercise, eating disorders, smoking, or illness.

Body Weight Can Promote or Diminish Your Fitness

A stable, healthy-range BMI goes hand in hand with regular exercise and physical activity. Maintaining weight and BMI within recommended ranges leads to increased energy and reduced likelihood of injury during fitness activities.

Overweight and underweight can contribute to poor fitness. Overweight can lead to a downward fitness spiral: An overaccumulation of body fat can strain bones, joints, and muscles and make exercising harder and injury more likely. Resulting stiffness and pain in the hands, feet, knees, and back, in turn, make exercising even more difficult. They also make work, employment, and activities of daily living—walking up stairs, carrying books or grocery bags, shoveling snow, getting in and out of automobiles, and so on—harder.

Underweight can lead to muscle wasting as the body breaks down muscle tissue for energy when fat stores are low. Muscle wasting, in turn, can lead to weakness and declining ability to exercise and accomplish daily tasks. These inevitably reduce both fitness and wellness.

Body Weight Can Have Social Consequences

Being overweight can subject a person to significant discrimination in education, employment, health care, and social interactions, starting in childhood.[36] "Weight stigma," or prejudice against overweight and obese people, is widespread in society and often starts with parents and teachers of overweight youngsters. Researchers have discovered, for example, that parents spend less money sending their overweight children to college than they do their thinner children, even when money isn't a limiting factor and the children have equivalent grades.[37] And adult attitudes rub off on children. Preschoolers are more likely to describe over-weight kids their own age as "mean, ugly, or stupid."[38]

Weight stigma is also quite common among employ-ers. Overweight job applicants suffer discrimination, get hired less often, and get fired more often than thinner individuals with similar qualifications.[39] In one study, job applicants standing near obese people were less likely to get hired, even if they were strangers![40] Weight stigma is even pronounced among health professionals, includ-ing specialists who treat the obese.[41]

Negative self-images and beliefs can lead to dis-couragement, shame, hopelessness, and in many, to eating "comfort foods" that temporarily boost mood but cause more weight gain.[42] Weight stigma scholars con-sider antifat bias to be a serious societal issue in need of more study and creative solutions. Awareness that weight management can boost energy, positive self-esteem, and physical wellness is a good starting place.

Body Weight Can Influence Your Risk for Chronic Disease

Researchers have confirmed that people with excess body fat have higher levels of several serious chronic diseases, including heart disease, stroke, type 2 diabetes, sleep apnea, arthritis, and cancer (**Figure 8.5**).[43] Specific cancers linked to high BMI include cancers of the pros-tate, colon, rectum, esophagus, pancreas, kidney, gall-bladder, ovary, cervix, liver, breast, uterus, and stomach.[44]

Accumulation of fat around the waist (a 40-inch waistline or higher for a man, or a 35-inch waistline or higher for a woman) increases the risk for developing metabolic syndrome. This serious medical condition is a combination of high blood cholesterol, high blood pressure, abdominal fat deposits, and insulin resistance or full-fledged type 2 diabetes.[45] A weight loss of just 10 pounds can bring measurable health benefits, even to an obese individual.[46]

Body Weight Can Affect Your Life Expectancy

You can expect to live longer if your body weight and BMI are within recommended ranges than you can if they fall under the categories for obesity or underweight. As **Figure 8.6** on page 293 shows, being fit significantly reduces mortality risk, especially when combined with healthy weight. Being obese (having a BMI of

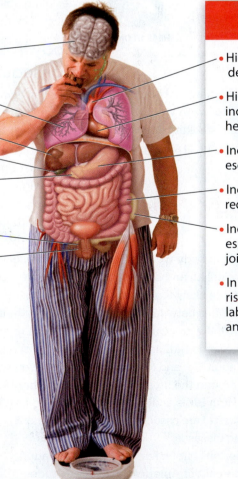

Negative health effects

- Increased risk of stroke
- Increased risk of sleep apnea and asthma
- Increased risk for kidney cancer
- Increased risks for gallbladder cancer and gallbladder disease
- Increased risks for type 2 diabetes and pancreatic cancer
- Higher rates of sexual dysfunction
- Increased risks for prostate, endometrial, ovarian, and cervical cancer
- Increased risk of breast cancer in women

Negative health effects

- Higher triglyceride levels and decreased HDL levels
- High blood pressure and increased risk for all forms of heart disease
- Increased risks for stomach and esophageal cancer
- Increased risks for colon and rectal cancer
- Increased risk of osteoarthritis, especially in weight-bearing joints, such as knees and hips
- In pregnant women, increased risks of fetal and maternal death, labor and delivery complications, and birth defects

FIGURE **8.5** Body weight can influence the risks for chronic disease.

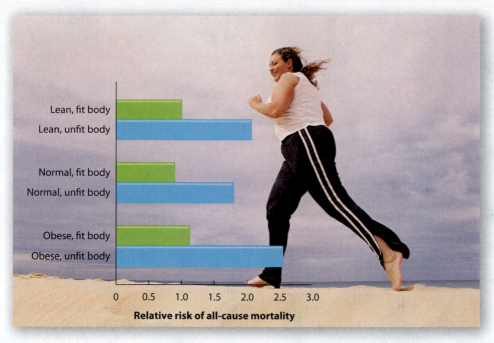

FIGURE **8.6** Being fit significantly reduces your mortality risk in any given year, regardless of your degree of body fat.

Source: Chong Do Lee et al., "Cardiorespiratory fitness, body composition and all-cause and cardiovascular disease mortality in men," *American Journal of Clinical Nutrition* 69, no. 3 (1999): 373–80. Used by permission of the American Society for Nutrition.

30 or above) cuts an average of six to seven years from the life of a nonsmoker and 13 to 14 years from a smoker.[47] Research indicates that Americans' average life expectancy may begin to decline because obesity is so prevalent and can shorten life so dramatically.[48]

Underweight people have a shorter life expectancy than normal-weight or overweight people.[49] In fact, some studies indicate that underweight people may have more than 18 times the risk of dying of cancer, and four times the risk of CVD death.[50] The statistics for early deaths among the underweight reflect the fact that a low BMI is characteristic of patients with illnesses such as cancer, uncontrolled diabetes, and disordered eating. Some researchers argue that people who are underweight but *not* ill and who are careful to get complete daily nutrition may actually realize greater longevity.[51] Underweight associated with poor nutrition, however, can lead to life-shortening conditions such as anemia, susceptibility to disease and infection, slower recovery from illness, muscle wasting and weakness, and osteoporosis and bone fractures.

Why Don't Most Diets Succeed?

Overweight or obese Americans face a discouraging cultural phenomenon. Most media images, such as television and magazines, show slim people or buffed-up athletes. This leads to high levels of body dissatisfaction and, in turn, fuels a $30 billion per year diet industry. Many people are

SEE IT! ONLINE
Best Diet Plan

convinced that they will successfully lose weight if they can simply find the right diet. They bounce from one highly publicized diet to another: low-fat, high carbohydrate; low carbohydrate, high protein; and so on. Experts tend to agree that any calorie-cutting diet can produce weight loss in the short term, often through water-weight loss. They also acknowledge that most diets are ineffective and that most people's attempts at weight loss will fail in the long run unless they change their eating habits permanently and make sustained exercise and activity part of their daily lives. Let's look more closely at dieting and why most diets fail.

Diets Often Lead to Weight Cycling

Do you know someone who is dieting? A recent survey by the American College Health Association indicated that almost 40 percent of college students dieted to lose weight over the past 30 days.[52] Dismayingly, three-quarters of dieters will regain their weight within two years (or sooner) after a major diet. Most will wind up in a process called **weight cycling**—a pattern of repeatedly losing and regaining weight.

Weight experts refer to this pattern as **yo-yo dieting** (**Figure 8.7**). Yo-yo dieting may have significant health

weight cycling The pattern of repeatedly losing and gaining weight, from illness or dieting

yo-yo dieting A series of diets followed by eventual weight gain

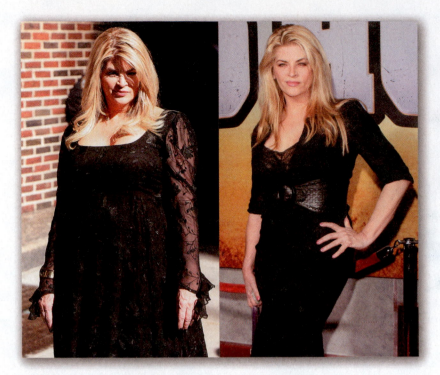

FIGURE **8.7** Actress Kirstie Alley, who was a contestant on *Dancing with the Stars*, has long struggled with "yo-yo dieting" or weight cycling.

consequences. Some studies show a link to high blood pressure and other chronic diseases, but experts are not sure whether weight cycling in itself leads to physical health problems.[53] It is a common misconception that yo-yo dieting slows down your metabolism and makes each new diet harder and less likely to succeed.[54] Studies of weight cycling do not generally reveal increases in fat tissue, decreases in muscle tissue, or decreased metabolic rate solely as a result of weight cycling. However, weight cycling can lead to feelings of depression or failure.

Marketers of diet plans and foods often promise quick weight loss with no hunger and very little effort. These diets usually backfire. One major reason they do is that they are rigid. **Rigid diets** specify rules like "eat only cabbage soup and grapefruit," or "never eat after 6:00 PM." Because rigid diets are unpleasant and restrictive, people seldom stick with them. People on rigid diets tend to have a higher percentage of body fat than people on more flexible plans.[55] The followers of rigid diets tend to exhibit more depression, anxiety, and binge eating as well.

rigid diets Weight-loss regimens that specify strict rules on calorie consumption, types of foods, and eating patterns

flexible diets Weight-loss regimens that focus on portion size and make allowances for variations in daily routine, appetite, and food availability

In contrast to rigid diets, **flexible diets** are based on energy balancing of calories eaten and burned. They focus on portion size and make allowances for variations in daily routine, appetite, and food availability. For example, if you go to a party and overeat, a flexible diet allows you to cut extra calories tomorrow and increase your exercise regimen to compensate. As a result, people tend to stay on flexible diets longer and, in the process, learn better long-term eating habits.

LIVE IT! ONLINE

Worksheet 21
All-or-Nothing
Thinking

Everyone who diets will experience some degree of lowered metabolism during a period of calorie restriction as the body "defends" its fat stores. That's why even in a sensible diet, weight loss tends to slow down after an initial quick drop and why the long-held rule that you must cut 3,500 calories to lose a pound of fat is not strictly correct.[56] It's also part of the reason successful weight maintenance requires permanent changes to your old eating habits.

Our Built-In Appetite Controls Make Diets Less Effective

Our bodies have a complicated set of internal chemical signals and control mechanisms that tell us when to eat, how much to eat, how much fat our bodies should store, and how we should respond when those fat stores start to shrink.[57] Researchers have learned, for example, that we produce powerful appetite stimulants such as leptin and ghrelin. Fat cells make the hormone leptin. The levels of this hormone fall when your body uses stored fat. This stimulates your appetite—and contributes to the difficulty of dieting. Before a meal, your stomach and small intestines make more of a hormone called ghrelin that stimulates food consumption. When leptin levels fall or ghrelin levels climb, your nervous system stimulates food seeking and eating behaviors. Ghrelin also explains the link between sleep and weight gain: Sleeping less than six hours per night can increase ghrelin levels, which increases appetite.[58]

Our bodies do make natural compounds that suppress appetite and signal a feeling of fullness. These compounds help diminish our appetites and get us to stop eating when full. They are less powerful than the factors that increase appetite, though, so they are much easier for most people to tolerate or ignore.[59] Thus, the biology of appetite control works against dieting.

Most Diet Products and Plans Are Ineffective

Most over-the-counter products—"fat burners," "starch blockers," muscle stimulators, diet plans, diet supplements, weight-loss program memberships, meal replacements, and other diet aids—are ineffective, and some are even dangerous. The prescription diet drugs available to date are only modestly effective and can have serious side effects.[60] The box Do Drastic Weight Loss Methods Work? explains more about prescription diet drugs and bariatric surgery, which are viable options for only a minority of overweight and obese people.

Q&A Do Drastic Weight Loss Methods Work?

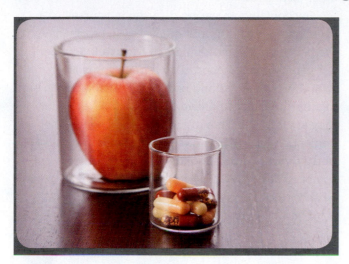

Millions of people think to themselves, "I hate diets and exercise, and they don't work for me, anyway. Why can't I just take drugs or have surgery to get thin?" The answers are complicated. Prescription diet drugs are expensive, have relatively small effectiveness, and cause numerous side effects. Over-the-counter diet drugs can be dangerous and are even less effective. And weight loss surgical procedures are expensive, carry significant risks, and are generally reserved for the severely obese or those with uncontrolled weight-related diseases like diabetes or high blood pressure.

The prescription drug Xenical (orlistat) partially blocks digestion of fats. Users lose an average of 13 pounds in a year (about 4 ounces per week), but side effects include oily stools and spotting, gas with fecal discharge, and urgent elimination. Phentride (phentermine) and Tenuate (diethylpropion) suppress appetite, but are addictive and prescribed only for short periods.[1] While prescription diet drugs can provide a small physical or psychological boost, people must still change their eating and exercise habits permanently for long-term success.[2]

Harmful side effects and health risks have led the FDA to ban many other drugs and supplements (e.g., drugs containing ephedra or phenylpropanolamine, also called *fen-phen*) and to issue safety alerts for others (such as Meridia) that led to their withdrawal from the market.[3] Over-the-counter diet remedies, including *Hoodia gordonii*, St. John's wort, herbal laxatives, bitter orange, ginseng and ginkgo, and green tea extracts, have not proven to be effective and can be harmful as well.

Surgery for weight loss (known as bariatric surgery) grew more than tenfold over the past 20 years, from about 16,000 procedures per year in the 1990s to an estimated 220,000 in 2008 and every year since.[4] During *gastric banding*, the surgeon partitions the stomach into two parts using an inflatable band that acts like a belt. The patient then eats far less before feeling full and stays full longer. This procedure is surgically reversible. In *gastric bypass*, the surgeon creates a permanent small stomach pouch that connects to the small intestine. This drastically reduces the amount a person can eat as well as the nutrients he or she can absorb—vitamins and minerals as well as calories. This irreversible surgery poses many medical risks but it has been shown to improve type 2 diabetes in obese patients and can lead to significant weight loss.[5] The high cost of bariatric surgery ($15,000 and up) and its ongoing medical risks restrict access for most people. About half of surgical patients regain most or all of their original weight within four years.[6] About half also experience medical complications or nutrient deficiencies.[7] The outlook for medical and surgical treatments could change with future research and development.

Questions to consider: Does the risk of using diet drugs and surgery outweigh the gains? If you answer yes, what are your reasons? If you answer no, why do you think this? What would you advise a loved one trying to decide how best to approach overweight or obesity?

Sources:
1. D. Rucker et al., "Long-Term Pharmacotherapy for Obesity and Overweight: Updated Meta-Analysis," *British Medical Journal* 335, no. 7631 (2007): 1194–99.
2. J. M. Nicklas et al., "Successful Weight Loss among Obese U.S. Adult," *American Journal of Preventive Medicine* 42, no. 5 (2012): 481–5.
3. U.S. Food and Drug Administration, "FDA Drug Safety Communication, FDA Recommends against the Continued Use of Meridia (sibutramine)," October 8, 2010, www.fda.gov
4. V. S. Elliott, "Bariatric Surgery Maintains, Doesn't Gain," *American Medical News*, April 23, 2012, www.amednews.com
5. F. Rubino et al., "Metabolic Surgery to Treat Type 2 Diabetes: Clinical Outcomes and Mechanisms of Action," *Annual Review of Medicine* 61 (2010): 393–411.
6. D. O. Magro et al., "Long-term Weight Regain after Gastric Bypass: A 5-Year Prospective Study," *Obesity Surgery* 6, no. 18 (2008): 648–51.
7. G. J. Service et al., "Hyperinsulinemia Hypoglycemia with Nesidioblastosis after Gastric-Bypass Surgery," *New England Journal of Medicine* 353, no. 3 (2005): 249–54.

What about commercial diet plans and programs? One comprehensive study revealed that none of the nationally known programs—Weight Watchers, Jenny Craig, Optifast, eDiets.com, and Overeaters Anonymous—deliver much weight loss.[61] Equally ineffective are commercial diets that promise easy, permanent weight loss; invoke spurious factors such as your blood type or food allergies; or prescribe extreme diets. For example, the Paleolithic diet concentrates on foods that hunter-gatherers ate such as fish, meat, fruits, vegetables, and nuts, and eliminates farmed foods such as legumes, dairy products, grains, and oils. Diets that cut out carbohydrates, dairy products, or other whole food groups may promote initial weight loss, but often result in nutrient deficiency, as well.[62]

What, then, should a would-be dieter do? If you are shopping for diet plans, look for one that advocates balanced nutrients and regular exercise. If you are joining a program, low-cost support groups are probably the best alternative for most people. They provide one important component: encouragement and support, either in person, online, or through weekly groups. Campus health centers can usually help students find group support for dieting. It's also important to enlist the personal encouragement of friends, roommates, and family members. If people undermine your diet efforts, tell them firmly that you need a different approach. We consider more tools for effective weight loss and management later in this chapter.

---

disordered eating Atypical, abnormal food consumption that diminishes wellness but is usually neither long-lived nor disruptive to everyday life

eating disorders Disturbed patterns of eating, dieting, and perceptions of body image that have psychological, environmental, and possibly genetic underpinnings and that lead to consequent medical issues

body dysmorphic disorder A psychological syndrome characterized by unrealistic and negative self-perception focusing on a perceived physical defect

anorexia nervosa A persistent, chronic eating disorder characterized by deliberate food restriction and severe, life-threatening weight loss

---

What Are Eating Disorders?

Skipping meals, going on diet after diet, and binging on junk food are all forms of disordered eating: atypical, abnormal food consumption that is common in the general public. **Disordered eating** diminishes your wellness but is usually neither long lived nor disruptive to everyday life. **Eating disorders** are long-lasting, disturbed patterns of eating, dieting, and perceptions of body image that have psychological, environmental, and possibly genetic underpinnings. Eating disorders can disrupt relationships, emotions, and concentration and can lead to physical injury, hospitalization, and even death. They require diagnosis and treatment from a psychiatrist or other physician.

SEE IT! ONLINE
EDNOS:
A Dangerous
Eating Disorder

Recognizing an eating disorder in yourself or a loved one can lead to treatment that improves or stops the behavior. The statements in **Figure 8.8** on page 297 can help you recognize abnormal or disordered thoughts about food and body image. People with eating disorders often believe they look fat even when they are rail thin. This unrealistic and negative self-perception can be part of a related syndrome called **body dysmorphic disorder** (BDD), in which a person becomes obsessed with a physical "defect" such as nose size or body shape.

The three most common types of eating disorders are anorexia nervosa, bulimia nervosa, and binge eating disorder. About 20 million American women and 10 million American men meet the criteria for one of these disorders during their lifetimes.[63]

LIVE IT! ONLINE
Worksheet 25
Out of Control or
Overcontrol?

Eating Disorders Have Distinctive Symptoms

Anorexia nervosa is a persistent, chronic eating disorder characterized by deliberate food restriction and severe, life-threatening weight loss (**Figure 8.9**, page 298). People with anorexia first restrict their intake of high-calorie foods, then of almost all foods, and then purge what they do eat through vomiting or using laxatives. They sometimes fast or exercise compulsively as well. The symptoms of anorexia include refusal to maintain a BMI of 18.5 or more; intense fear of gaining weight; disturbed body perception; and in teenage girls and women, amenorrhea (cessation of menstruation) for three months or more. Five to 20 percent of anorexics eventually die from medical conditions brought on by vitamin or mineral deficiencies or physiological results of starvation. This gives anorexia the highest death rate of any psychological illness.[64]

Eating disordered	Disruptive eating patterns	Food preoccupied/ obsessed	Concerned well	Food is not an issue
• I regularly stuff myself and then exercise, vomit, use diet pills or laxatives to get rid of the food or calories. • My friends/family tell me I am too thin. • I am terrified of eating fat. • When I let myself eat, I have a hard time controlling the amount of food I eat. • I am afraid to eat in front of others.	• I have tried diet pills, laxatives, vomiting, or extra time exercising in order to lose or maintain my weight. • I have fasted or avoided eating for long periods of time in order to lose or maintain my weight. • I feel strong when I can restrict how much I eat. • Eating more than I wanted to makes me feel out of control.	• I think about food a lot. • I feel I don't eat well most of the time. • It's hard for me to enjoy eating with others. • I feel ashamed when I eat more than others or more than what I feel I should be eating. • I am afraid of getting fat. • I wish I could change how much I want to eat and what I am hungry for.	• I pay attention to what I eat in order to maintain a healthy body. • I may weigh more than what I like, but I enjoy eating and balance my pleasure with eating with my concern for a healthy body. • I am moderate and flexible in goals for eating well. • I try to follow Dietary Guidelines for healthy eating.	• I am not concerned about what others think regarding what and how much I eat. • When I am upset or depressed I eat whatever I am hungry for without any guilt or shame. • Food is an important part of my life but only occupies a small part of my time.

Body hate/ dissociation	Distorted body image	Body preoccupied/ obsessed	Body acceptance	Body ownership
• I often feel separated and distant from my body—as if it belongs to someone else. • I don't see anything positive or even neutral about my body shape and size. • I don't believe others when they tell me I look OK. • I hate the way I look in the mirror and often isolate myself from others.	• I spend a significant amount of time exercising and dieting to change my body. • My body shape and size keeps me from dating or finding someone who will treat me the way I want to be treated. • I have considered changing or have changed my body shape and size through surgical means so I can accept myself.	• I spend a significant time viewing my body in the mirror. • I spend a significant time comparing my body to others. • I have days when I feel fat. • I am preoccupied with my body. • I accept society's ideal body shape and size as the best body shape and size.	• I base my body image equally on social norms and my own self-concept. • I pay attention to my body and my appearance because it is important to me, but it only occupies a small part of my day. • I nourish my body so it has the strength and energy to achieve my physical goals.	• My body is beautiful to me. • My feelings about my body are not influenced by society's concept of an ideal body shape. • I know that the significant others in my life will always find me attractive.

FIGURE **8.8** Thought patterns associated with healthy and disordered eating habits exist on a continuum, as do thought patterns associated with positive and negative body image.

Adapted from Smiley/King/Avery: Campus Health Service. Original continuum, C. Schislak: *Preventive Medicine and Public Health*. Copyright 1996 Arizona Board of Regents. Used with permission.

Bulimia nervosa is characterized by frequent bouts of binge eating followed by purging (self-induced vomiting), laxative abuse, or excessive exercise. Bulimics tend to consume much more food than most people would during a given time period and feel a loss of control over it. Binging and purging are often done secretly. A medical diagnosis includes binging and purging at least twice a week for three months. People with bulimia are also obsessed with their bodies, weight gain, and their appearance to others. Unlike those with anorexia, however, people with bulimia are often normal weight. Treatment appears to be more effective for bulimia than for anorexia.

Binge eating disorder (BED), a variation of bulimia, involves binge eating but usually no purging, laxatives, exercise, or fasting. Individuals with BED often wind up significantly overweight or obese but tend to binge much more often than does the typical obese person.

bulimia nervosa An eating disorder characterized by frequent bouts of binge eating followed by purging (self-induced vomiting), laxative abuse, or excessive exercise

binge eating disorder (BED) A variation of bulimia that involves binge eating but usually no purging, laxatives, exercise, or fasting

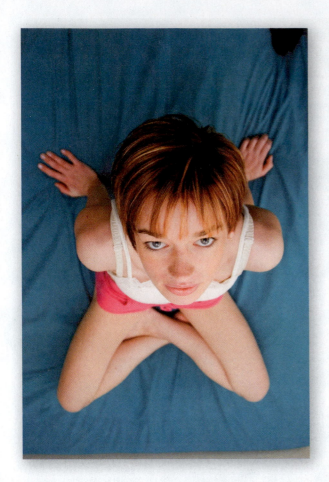

FIGURE **8.9** Anorexia nervosa is characterized by severe, life-threatening weight loss.

Eating Disorders Can Be Treated

Because eating disorders have complex physical, psychological, and social causes that unfold over many years, there are no quick or simple solutions for them. Still, eating disorders *are* treatable. The primary goal of treatment is usually to reduce the threat to the patient's life posed by his or her eating behaviors and the physical damage they can cause to the bones, teeth, throat, esophagus, stomach, intestines, heart, and other organs. Once the patient is stabilized medically, long-term therapy can begin. Often, the affected individual comes from a family that places undue emphasis on achievement, body weight, and appearance. Genetic susceptibility can also play a role.[65] Therapy focuses on the psychological, social, environmental, and physiological factors that have contributed. Therapy is aimed at helping the patient develop new eating behaviors, build self-confidence, deal with depression, and find constructive ways of dealing with life's problems. Eating disorder support groups can be pivotal as well.

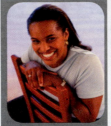
What Concepts Must I Understand to Achieve My Weight Goals?

Understanding the role of metabolic rates, recognizing your body's set point, and understanding the energy balance equation are all important weight management tools. Taking lessons from successful weight maintainers can help you set and achieve realistic weight goals. And balancing your energy equation by keeping track of your calorie intake and by adding or continuing a regular exercise program can help you maintain a healthy weight over time.

SEE IT! ONLINE
Keeping It Off

Recognize the Role of Your Metabolic Rate

As much as 60 to 70 percent of your daily calorie intake—typically between 900 and 1800 calories per day—is consumed as your body sustains functions such as heartbeat, breathing, and maintenance of body temperature.[66] The rate at which your body consumes food energy to sustain these basic functions is your **basal metabolic rate (BMR)**. Your **resting metabolic rate (RMR)** is slightly higher, because it includes the energy you expend to digest food. BMR can be influenced by your activity level and your body composition. The more lean tissue you have, the greater your BMR; the more fat tissue you have, the lower your BMR. The higher your fitness level, the greater your ratio of lean tissue to fat mass is likely to be, and the more energy you will burn while exercising and at rest. Cardiovascular and strength-building exercises contribute most directly to speeding up BMR.

basal metabolic rate (BMR) Your baseline rate of energy use, dictated by your body's collective metabolic activities

resting metabolic rate (RMR) Basal metabolic rate plus the energy expended in digesting food

set point A preprogrammed weight that your body returns to easily when you gain or lose a few pounds

negative caloric balance A state in which the amount of calories consumed in food falls short of the amount of calories expended through metabolism and physical activity

Recognize Your Body's Set Point

Perhaps you've noticed that your body is programmed around a certain weight or **set point** that it returns to fairly easily when you gain or lose a few pounds. Many dieters reach a plateau after a certain amount of weight loss and can't seem to trim off more pounds. This plateau is due, in part, to a downshifted metabolism balancing out lower calorie intake: The person's energy balance is now at a weight-maintenance, not a weight-loss, level. To "outsmart" and reset one's set point, a dieter must lose weight slowly and increase exercise.

Balance Your Energy Equation

Long-term weight management relies on balancing your energy equation—that is, reaching a balance where the calories you eat equal the calories you burn over time. To lose or gain weight, you must deliberately "unbalance" that equation for a while. If you expend more calories than you consume over time, you'll lose weight due to a **negative caloric balance** (**Figure 8.10**). Consume more calories than

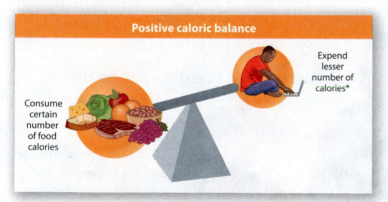

(a) Energy intake < Energy expenditure ⟶ Weight loss

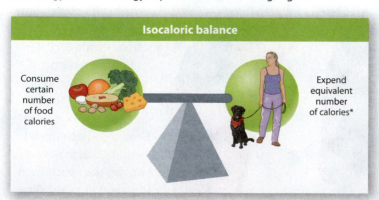

(b) Energy intake > Energy expenditure ⟶ Weight gain

(c) Energy intake = Energy expenditure ⟶ Weight maintenance

FIGURE **8.10** On any given day, each of us has a personal energy equation with either a negative caloric balance, a positive caloric balance, or an isocaloric balance. Over time, this equation helps determine our body weight.

*You expend calories through metabolism, activity, and exercise.

you expend and you'll gain weight due to a **positive caloric balance**. Consume and expend approximately the same number of calories over a period of time and you'll reach an **isocaloric balance**—and with it, be able to maintain your weight.

Learning to accurately approximate your daily calorie consumption and expenditure is important! Dieters often fail to lose weight because they underestimate how many calories they consume and overestimate how many they burn off with exercise.[67] **Lab 8.1** can help you calculate your current energy balance and set goals for a better balance. Alternatively, you can log on to www.ChooseMyPlate.gov to get a target number for calorie consumption based on your age, sex, and level of daily moderate or vigorous activity. The SuperTracker feature provides calorie counts for specific foods and portions so you can keep track of how many calories you consume each day. You can also get calorie-counting programs for smartphones, or find them online at websites such as www.caloriecontrol.org.

DO IT! ONLINE

How Can I Create a Behavior Change Plan for Weight Management?

Let's look at the steps you can take to manage your weight.

Assess Your Current Weight and Choose a Realistic Goal

Figure 8.11 shows healthy weight and BMI ranges based on height. If your body fat percentage is low and your muscle development is high, your healthy weight and your BMI will be on the higher end of the range. The same is also true if your frame size is large. If your body fat percentage is high and your muscle development is

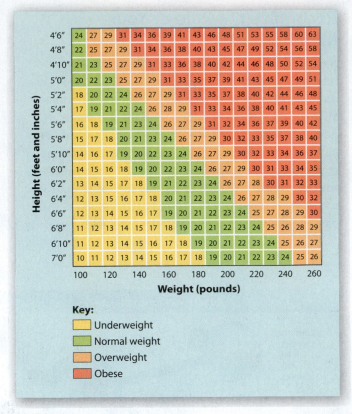

FIGURE **8.11** Locate your height, read across to find your weight, and then read up to determine your BMI. Note that BMI values have been rounded off to the nearest whole number.

low, your healthy weight will be in the middle-to-low end of the range. This is also true if your frame size is medium or small. Knowing these factors will help you calculate a realistic weight goal.

Contemplate Weight Management

If you are satisfied with your current weight, you can simply pursue and refine your application of good nutritional principles and regular exercise. If you are in the dissatisfied majority, use the assessment of your current weight and BMI from Figure 8.11 to choose a realistic weight goal based on no more than a 10 percent initial loss or gain. Even if you don't need weight change now, you can use the specifics in this section to stabilize your current weight and maintain it for the next few decades. Readiness requires motivation, commitment, goals, and a positive attitude. **Lab 8.2** helps you assess your readiness for weight change.

DO IT! ONLINE

Prepare for Better Weight Management

- *Think about your beliefs and attitudes.* Do you see yourself as a hopeless victim of "bad genes," overwork, or low budget? Think you are too young to worry about deliberate weight management? Believe that you *can* take effective control of your body composition and weight largely through eating intelligently, limiting your calorie intake, and establishing a program of regular exercise? Talk with others or write in your journal to clarify your attitudes in preparation for making an effective weight management plan.

- *Consider your goals.* Motivating goals are usually personal and extended, such as looking good, feeling fit and capable, and staying well over a period of years. Avoid one-shot goals that can lead to weight cycling. If your reason for losing weight is a specific upcoming event (e.g., looking good for a beach trip or a sports match), find additional long-term goals such as increasing self-esteem, relief from the stress of college life, and having more energy. You can write out your specific goals in **Lab 8.3**.

DO IT! ONLINE

- *Identify barriers to change.* What keeps you from changing or maintaining your weight? A lack of information about good weight management techniques? Poor nutrition and eating habits? Eating triggers that encourage overconsumption? Lack of social or emotional support? Lack of exercise? Identify your

---

TOOLS FOR CHANGE

Tips for Weight Management

Try these ideas for reframing weight loss in your mind, rather than jumping right in to a diet regimen unprepared:

LIVE IT! ONLINE
Worksheet 22
It Doesn't Last
If You Fast

- Think substitution. Instead of cookies or ice cream at snack time, substitute fresh fruit. Instead of chips or fries, substitute unbuttered popcorn, nuts, or vegetable sticks and low-fat dip.

- Consider yourself successful if you lose ½ to 1 pound per week. Faster weight loss stimulates too much hunger, slows down metabolism, and loses lean tissue.

- Avoid feeling famished by choosing high-volume, nutrient-dense foods. Items such as veggie-packed clear soups, salads with light dressing, whole grains, fruits, vegetables, and beans fill you more quickly and control hunger longer.

- Avoid rigid dieting. Strictly limiting calorie counts or forbidding yourself certain foods can trigger binging and weight gain, not loss. Flexible dieting works better and emphasizes portion control and lower-calorie, higher-volume foods.

- Don't drink "empty" calories. Drinks sweetened with sugar or corn syrup contribute disproportionately to weight gain. Alcoholic drinks pack a lot of calories and stimulate the appetite.

- Sleep well. Get seven to nine hours of sleep each night. Sleep deprivation triggers greater levels of hunger and eating.

- Increase the physical activity in your life. Take the stairs instead of the elevator. Walk the last mile to class instead of riding in a car or bus. Turn off the TV and go play Frisbee with a friend.

- Join a support group. Support groups help most people lose at least a small amount of weight and keep it off.

- Use an online or smartphone application to track calories, keep food diaries, calculate body fat and fat grams in foods, log in your weight to a social site, and so on. These high-tech tools can't substitute for your own motivation and adherence, but they can make tracking your information and getting support easier and more fun!

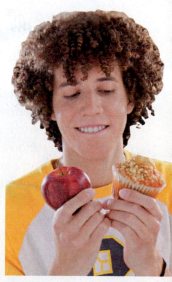

barriers and brainstorm solutions to them. **Lab 8.4** will help you get started by identifying and eliminating junk food from your diet.

DO IT! ONLINE

- *Visualize new behaviors.* What specific new behaviors will you adopt to improve your BMI and body composition? Here are some good choices: Choose only nutritious foods. Avoid junk food. Track the numbers of servings you eat from each food group. Plan for exercise most days of the week. Keep a log of your daily and weekly exercise. Ask friends to support you in planning new behaviors.

Take Action

- *Commit to your goals.* Behavior change requires commitment. Thinking and talking about your commitment with friends is helpful; so is writing it down and showing it to someone.

- *Set up support.* Solicit the help of people you can trust to support your efforts. Let's say it is 9:30 P.M., you've finished studying and you're hungry, but you've already eaten the 1800 calories on your day's food plan. A supportive friend might say, "Well, you can always eat some raw vegetables to fill up. You'll be glad you stuck with your program. Just think, once you've lost weight, you can add back some extra calories each day—and that won't be so long from now!"

- The GetFitGraphic Weight Loss Mythbusters on page 303 illustrates several specific ways to improve your action plan, based on common weight loss myths.

Establish a Regular Exercise Program

Along with monitored and controlled eating, physical activity is crucial both to weight change (loss or gain) and to weight maintenance. In addition to following a healthy diet, you may need to add at least half an hour or more per day of extra activity. The good news is that activity amounts are cumulative: Add seven minutes of stair-climbing here, plus eleven minutes of brisk walking across campus there, plus twenty minutes of stationary biking, and so on. Aerobic exercise is the best way to burn calories and lose fat and body weight.[68]

The greater the frequency, intensity, and time spent on an activity, the more energy you use and the more calories you burn. There are other considerations for choosing types of fitness exercise as well. The larger the muscle groups you use, the more you boost your metabolism and, in turn, your calorie expenditure. Kick boxing, for example, uses the thigh, calf, and gluteus muscles as well as those that move and support your torso. By contrast, lifting small hand weights works mainly the smaller muscles of the hand, wrist, and lower arms. **Table 8.1** lists the caloric expenditures for several

TABLE **8.1** Calories Burned through Activity			
Activity, Sport, or Exercise	Calories You Expend per Minute if You Weigh…		
	110 lb	150 lb	190 lb
Aerobics, 10" step	7.0	9.5	12.0
Basketball, pick-up	7.0	9.5	12.0
Biking, slow	5.3	7.1	9.0
Bowling	2.6	3.6	4.5
Dancing, moderate pace	4.2	5.7	9.0
Downhill skiing, moderate pace	5.5	7.5	9.5
Driving	1.8	2.4	3.0
Frisbee, casual	2.6	3.6	4.5
Golf, walking and pulling clubs	4.4	6.0	7.5
Grocery shopping	3.1	4.2	5.3
Hiking, hills	5.3	7.1	9.0
Jogging, moderate pace	5.3	7.1	9.0
Kickboxing	8.8	12.0	14.7
Office work	1.3	1.8	2.3
Ping-pong	3.5	4.8	6.0
Reading	0.9	1.2	1.5
Soccer, noncompetitive	6.1	8.3	10.5
Softball	4.4	6.0	7.5
Stair climbing, 40 stairs/minute	6.1	8.3	10.2
Stretching	3.5	4.8	5.8
Swimming	~8	~10	~13
Tennis, singles, recreational	7.0	9.5	12.0
Watching TV	1.0	1.4	1.8

Source: Adapted from F. I. Katch, V. L. Katch, and W. D. McArdle, *Calorie Expenditure Charts,* (Ann Arbor, MI: Fitness Technologies Press, 1996).

WEIGHT LOSS MYTHBUSTERS

FACT OR FICTION? Most freshman gain weight when they start college.

FACT

66% gained weight during their first year of school
average gain = 6 lbs

31% lost weight during their first year of school[1]
average loss = 4.4 lbs

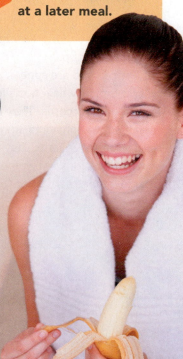

THE REASONS[2]

70% ate fewer than 5 servings of fruits and vegetables per day

50% ate fried foods 3 or more times per week

29% reported getting no exercise

YES OR NO: Smarter eating habits equal greater weight loss.

YES

IN ONE WEIGHT LOSS STUDY, THOSE WHO[3]

skipped meals and ate lunch out more than once a week

LOST LESS.

kept a daily food journal

LOST MORE.

FACT OR FICTION? Choosing popcorn over potato chips can help you eat less later.

FACT

SNACK ON THIS:
IN ONE STUDY[4]
STUDENTS WHO
SNACKED ON

6 CUPS OF AIR-POPPED POPCORN (100 calories) → **ate** **739 CALORIES** at a later meal.

1 CUP OF POTATO CHIPS (150 calories) → **ate** **803 CALORIES** at a later meal.

YES OR NO: A large piece of food will fill you up faster than several smaller ones.

NOT SO

AFTER BEING SERVED[5]

a single bagel weighing 82 grams, more students were still hungry and **ate more** at the next meal.

4 or 5 pieces of bagel weighing 82 grams total, fewer students were still hungry and on average they **ate less** at the next meal.

TRUE OR FALSE: Sleep doesn't affect appetite and eating.

FALSE

In a study where male students estimated their **ideal portion sizes of foods and snacks,**[6]

after sleeping **8 HOURS** and eating a full breakfast, they wanted **smaller** portions of additional food.

after sleeping **<6 HOURS** and eating a full breakfast, they wanted **larger** portions of additional food.

popular activities, sports, and exercises for adults of different weight levels.

Achieve Weight Maintenance

Weight maintenance is similar in principle to weight change. The tools are the same; but with weight maintenance, your daily calorie goal for weight management will be isocaloric. Tracking your calories is important, as is a weekly weigh-in. Many people plateau at a particular body weight and need to maintain that level for a few months before resuming more weight change. The skills you employ during an interim phase of weight maintenance will be excellent practice for the rest of your life! Once sustaining and tracking good nutrition and performing daily exercise and activity become your normal routine, it should become easier for you to change and maintain your body weight.

Take Lessons from Successful Weight Maintainers

Most people who sustain a normal, healthy weight over years or decades engage in a physically active lifestyle, averaging an hour per day of moderate to vigorous physical activity.[69] They don't skip meals; they eat breakfast every day. They eat a nutritious diet that is low in saturated fats and high in complex carbohydrates, has moderate levels of protein, and has a high volume but a low calorie density—even on weekends! They avoid sodas and juice drinks sweetened with sugar, corn syrup, or artificial sweeteners.

Successful weight maintainers stay conscious of situations that trigger overeating and they apply strategies to prevent overeating. They are motivated to stay at a healthy weight, and they respond quickly by cutting back calories and increasing activity when their weight starts to creep up.[70]

People who are successful at maintaining a healthy weight typically have tools for coping with problems and handling life stresses. They assume responsibility for their lifestyle behaviors, know where to seek help, and tend to be self-reliant. They have a good social support system, both for their weight maintenance and for their lives in general.[71]

casestudy

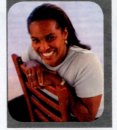

MARIA

"We moved to a new apartment recently, and after living there for a month, it's gotten easier to climb up and down the three flights of stairs. I guess I'm getting used to it! I know this isn't enough exercise to make me lose weight, but at least I'm a little more active. I can see that I need to change daily habits—eating and exercising—instead of just 'going on a diet.' Because I'll regain everything I lose as soon as I go off of it, right? So I need to figure out more ways to be active—ways that feel natural, like taking the stairs; not forced, like doing push ups!

"I weigh 155 right now. I need to lose 35 pounds to get back to my prepregnancy weight of 120. For now, I'm just going to try losing 10 pounds, at least to start off with. I've heard about weight-loss groups that help you plan meals, control how much you eat, and get regular exercise. I think a group might be a good approach for me."

THINK! You've just read about several tools for effective weight management. Which tools is Maria considering? Which tools do you already use? Which others could you use?

ACT! Write down some steps you can take to begin a regular exercise program, to improve the one you already have, or just to fit more physical activity into your day.

HEAR IT! ONLINE

Maintaining recommended weight and BMI confers so many benefits upon your appearance, energy level, and overall wellness that once you master the needed skill set, you'll rarely miss the junk food you used to eat, nor will you miss the few minutes it will take each day to track energy consumed and expended. The rewards in lifelong wellness are easily worth the trade-offs!

CHAPTER IN REVIEW

MasteringHealth™

Build your knowledge—and wellness!—in the Study Area of MasteringHealth with a variety of study tools.

SEE IT! ONLINE

videos

Best Diet Plan

EDNOS: A Dangerous Eating Disorder

Keeping It Off

HEAR IT! ONLINE

audio tools

Audio case study

MP3 chapter review

REVIEW IT! ONLINE

chapter review

Chapter reading quizzes

Glossary flashcards

LIVE IT! ONLINE

programs & behavior change

Customizable four-week exercise program for weight management

Take Charge of Your Health! Worksheets:

Worksheet 21 All-or-Nothing Thinking and "Safe Foods" versus "Forbidden Foods"

Worksheet 22 It Doesn't Last if You Fast

Worksheet 23 Why Do You Eat?

Worksheet 25 Out of Control or Overcontrol?

Behavior Change Log Book and Wellness Journal

DO IT! ONLINE

labs

Lab 8.1 Calculating Energy Balance and Setting Energy Balance Goals

Lab 8.2 Are You Ready to Jump-Start Your Weight Loss?

Lab 8.3 Your Weight Management Plan

Lab 8.4 Junk Food Detective

reviewquestions

1. The World Health Organization coined the term *globesity* to promote an understanding of
   a. global hunger.
   b. rising obesity rates in underdeveloped countries.
   c. rising obesity rates in developed countries.
   d. the epidemic of obesity in the global population.

2. Indicate the body system least likely to be affected negatively by excess body weight.
   a. Cardiovascular system (heart and lungs)
   b. Digestive system (gallbladder, kidneys, colon)
   c. Musculoskeletal system (bones and joints)
   d. Integumentary system (skin and hair)

3. At more than 20 percent above the recommended weight range, a person who is 5'8" tall is considered
   a. overweight.
   b. obese.
   c. at ideal weight.
   d. at his or her set point.

4. A BMI of 16 in a woman indicates
   a. overweight.
   b. underweight.
   c. normal weight.
   d. obesity.

5. Getting up, walking around, and jiggling your feet when seated are all examples of
   a. energy conservation.
   b. appetite control.
   c. non-exercise activity.
   d. depression.

6. To lose weight, you must establish a(n)
   a. negative caloric balance.
   b. isocaloric balance.
   c. positive caloric balance.
   d. set point.

7. Weight cycling is
   a. a pattern of repeatedly losing and regaining weight.
   b. characterized by rigid diets.
   c. characterized by flexible diets.
   d. uncommon.
8. Anorexia nervosa is characterized by
   a. frequent bouts of binge eating followed by self-induced vomiting.
   b. deliberate food restriction and severe, life-threatening weight loss.
   c. going on diet after diet.
   d. obesity.
9. The rate at which your body consumes food energy to sustain basic functions is your
   a. basal metabolic rate.
   b. resting metabolic rate.
   c. BMI.
   d. set point.
10. Successful weight maintainers are most likely to do which of the following?
    a. Indulge in junk food on weekends
    b. Skip meals
    c. Drink diet sodas
    d. Eat a diet that has a high volume and a low calorie density

critical thinkingquestions

1. How do height, physical build, and musculature affect recommended weight and BMI?
2. What do you see as the greatest contributor to "globesity"? Defend your answer.
3. List several effective tools for successful weight management. Is one more important than the others? If so, discuss.
4. Why do most diets fail?

references

1. First Lady Michelle Obama, Introduction of New Plan to Combat Overweight and Obesity, Press Conference, Alexandria, Virginia, January 28, 2010.
2. K. M. Flegal et al., "Prevalence of Obesity and Trends in the Distribution of Body Mass Index among U.S. Adults, 1999–2010," *Journal of the American Medical Association* 307, no. 5 (2012): 491–7.
3. Ibid.
4. C. L. Ogden et al., "Prevalence of Obesity in the United States, 2009–2010," NCHS Data Brief, No. 82 (Hyattsville, MD: National Center for Health Statistics. 2012).
5. C. D. Fryar and C. L. Ogden, "Prevalence of Underweight among Adults Aged 20 and Over: United States, 1960–1962 through 2007–2010." Health E-Stat, National Health and Nutrition Examination Survey, Updated September 2012, www.cdc.gov
6. M. Ogden and M. Carroll, "NCHS Health E-Stat: Prevalence of Obesity among Children and Adolescents: United States, Trends 1963–1965 through 2009–2010, Updated September 2012, www.cdc.gov
7. Ibid.
8. J. S. Morrell et al., "Metabolic Syndrome, Obesity, and Related Risk Factors among College Men and Women," *Journal of American College Health* 60, no. 1 (2012).
9. Ibid.
10. International Union of Nutritional Scientists, "The Global Challenge of Obesity and the International Obesity Task Force," IUNS 2012, www.iuns.org
11. World Health Organization, "Fact Sheet No. 311: Obesity and Overweight," Updated March 2013, www.who.int
12. World Health Organization, "Controlling the Global Obesity Epidemic," 2013, www.who.int
13. International Union of Nutritional Sciences, "The Global Challenge," IUNS 2012.
14. M. Ogden and M. Carroll, "NCHS Data Brief No. 82: Prevalence of Obesity in the United States, 2009–2010," National Center for Health Statistics, 2012.
15. U.S. Department of Agriculture Economic Research Service, "U.S. Food Consumption Up 16 Percent Since 1970," *Amber Waves*, November 2005, www.ers.usda.gov
16. D. Mozaffarian et al., "Changes in Diet and Lifestyle and Long Term Weight Gain in Women and Men," *New England Journal of Medicine* 364, (2011): 2392–404, doi: 10.1056/NEJMoa1014296, Available at www.nejm.org
17. B. Wamsink, J. E. Painter, and J. North, "Bottomless Bowls: Why Visual Cues of Portion Size May Influence Intake," *Obesity Research* 13, no. 1 (2005): 93–100.
18. J. C. Spence et al., "Relation between Local Food Environments and Obesity among Adults," *BMC PublicHealth* 9 (2009): 192; M. Wang et al., "Changes in Neighbourhood Food Store Environment, Food Behaviour, and Body Mass Index, 1981–1990,"*PublicHealth Nutrition* 11, no. 9 (2008): 963–70.
19. B. Wansink, "Environmental Factors That Increase the Food Intake and Consumption Volume of Unknowing Customers," *Annual Review of Nutrition* 24 (2004): 455–79.
20. C. D. Fryar and R. B. Ervin, "Caloric Intake from Fast Food among Adults: United States, 2007–2010." NCHS Data Brief No. 144, February 2013. National Center for Health Statistics, 2013.
21. G. Block et al., "Foods Contributing to Energy Intake in the U.S.: Data from NHANES III and NHANES 1999–2000," *Journal of Food Chemistry and Analysis* 17, no. 3–4 (2004): 439–47.
22. S. A. French, "Public Health Strategies for Dietary Change: Schools and Workplaces," *Journal of Nutrition* 135, no. 4 (2005): 91–2.
23. National Center for Health Statistics, "NCHS Health E-Stat: Prevalence of Sedentary Leisure-Time Behavior among Adults in the United States," Updated February 2010, www.cdc.gov
24. L. D. Frank et al., "Objective Assessment of Obesogenic Environments in Youth: Geographic Information System Methods and Spatial Findings from the Neighborhood Impact on Kids Study," *American Journal of Preventive Medicine* 42, no. 5 (2012): e47-55.
25. M. Papas et al., "The Built Environment and Obesity," *Epidemiological Reviews* 29, no. 1 (2007): 129–43; M. Rao et al., "The Built Environment and Health," *The Lancet* 370, no. 9593 (2007): 1111–13.
26. I. S. Farooqi and S. O'Rahilly, "Genetic Factors in Human Obesity," *Obesity Reviews* 8, Supp. 1 (2007): 37–40.
27. Centers for Disease Control and Prevention, "Obesity and Genetics," CDC Features, Updated January 2010, www.cdc.gov
28. J. A. Levine et al., "Interindividual Variation in Posture Allocation: Possible Role in Human Obesity," *Science* 307, no. 5709 (2005): 584–86.
29. Centers for Disease Control and Prevention, U.S. Physical Activity Statistics, "1988–2008 No Leisure-Time Physical Activity Trend Chart," Updated February 2010, www.cdc.gov
30. NCHC: Prevalence of Sedentary Leisure-time Behavior, Updated February 2010.
31. Ibid.
32. D. Mozaffarian, "Changes in Diet," 2011.

33. W. Willett, *Eat, Drink, and Be Healthy: The Harvard Medical School Guide to Healthy Eating* (New York: Free Press, 2003): 35.

34. D. Canoy et al., "Body Fat Distribution and Risk of Coronary Heart Disease in Men and Women in the European Prospective Investigation into Cancer and Nutrition in Norfolk Cohort: A Population-Based Prospective Study," *Circulation* 116, no. 25 (2007): 2933–43.

35. C. D. Fryar and C. L. Ogden, "Prevalence of Underweight among Adults Aged 20 Years and Over: United States, 1960–1962 through 2007–2010," 2012.

36. R. Puhl and K. D. Brownell, "Bias, Discrimination, and Obesity," *Obesity Research* 9, no. 12 (2001): 788–805.

37. D. R. Musher-Eizenman et al., "Body Size Stigmatization in Preschool Children: The Role of Control Attributions," *Journal of Pediatric Psychology* 29, no. 8 (2004): 613–20; S. H. Thompson and S. Digsby, "A Preliminary Survey of Dieting, Body Dissatisfaction, and Eating Problems among High School Cheerleaders," *Journal of School Health* 74, no. 3 (2004): 85–90.

38. D. R. Musher-Eizenman et al., "Body Size Stigmatization in Preschool Children," 2004.

39. R. Puhl and K. D. Brownell, "Bias, Discrimination, and Obesity," 2001; M. R. Hebl and L. M. Mannix, "The Weight of Obesity in Evaluating Others: A Mere Proximity Effect," *Perspectives in Social Psychology Bulletin* 29, no. 1 (2003): 28–38.

40. M. R. Hebl and L. M. Mannix, "The Weight of Obesity in Evaluating Others," 2003.

41. M. B. Schwartz et al., "Weight Bias among Health Professionals Specializing in Obesity," *Obesity Research* 11, no. 9 (2003): 1033–39.

42. S. S. Wang et al., "The Influence of the Stigma of Obesity on Overweight Individuals," *International Journal of Obesity* 28, no. 10 (2004): 1333–37.

43. Centers for Disease Control and Prevention, "Halting the Epidemic by Making Health Easier: At a Glance 2011," May 2011, www.cdc.gov

44. E. Calle et al., "Overweight, Obesity, and Mortality from Cancer in a Prospectively Studied Cohort of U.S. Adults," *New England Journal of Medicine* 348, no. 17 (2003): 1625–38.

45. N. Pandey and V. Gupta, "Trends in Diabetes," *Lancet* 369, no. 9569 (2007): 1256–57.

46. Mayo Clinic Staff, "Metabolic Syndrome," November 2009, www.mayoclinic.com

47. C. C. Mann, "Provocative Study Says Obesity May Reduce U.S. Life Expectancy," *Science* 307, no. 5716 (2005): 1716–17.

48. S. J. Olshansky et al., "A Potential Decline in Life Expectancy in the United States in the 21st Century," *New England Journal of Medicine* 352, no. 11 (2005): 1138–45.

49. K. Flegal et al., "Excess Deaths Associated with Underweight, Overweight, and Obesity," *Journal of the American Medical Association* 298, no. 17 (2007): 2028–37; K. M. Flegal and B. I. Graubard, "Estimates of Excess Deaths Associated with Body Mass Index and Other Anthropometric Variables," *American Journal of Clinical Nutrition* 89, no. 4 (2009): 1213–19.

50. Y. Takata et al., "Association between Body Mass Index and Mortality in an 80-Year-Old Population," *Journal of the American Geriatric Society* 55, no. 6 (2007): 913–17.

51. L. Fontana et al., "Long-Term Calorie Restriction Is Highly Effective in Reducing the Risk for Atherosclerosis in Humans," *Proceedings of the National Academy of Sciences* 101, no. 17 (2004): 6659–63.

52. American College Health Association, *American College Health Association-National College Health Assessment II: Reference Group Executive Summary Fall 2012*, 2013

53. U.S. Department of Health and Human Services, National Institute of Diabetes and Digestive and Kidney Diseases (NIDDK), "Weight Cycling," NIH Publication No. 01-3901, May 2008, www.win.niddk.nih.gov

54. NIDDK, "Weight Cycling," 2008.

55. C. F. Smith et al., "Flexible versus Rigid Dieting Strategies: Relationship with Adverse Behavioral Outcomes," *Appetite* 32, no. 3 (1999): 295–305.

56. K. D. Hall et al., "Quantification of the Effect of Energy Imbalance on Bodyweight," *The Lancet* 378, no. 9793 (2011): 826–37.

57. S. Stock et al., "Ghrelin, Peptide YY, Glucose-Dependent Insulinotropic Polypeptide, and Hunger Responses to a Mixed Meal in Anorexic, Obese, and Control Female Adolescents," *Journal of Clinical Endocrinology and Metabolism* 90, no. 4 (2005); E. T. Poehlman, "Reduced Metabolic Rate after Caloric Restriction," *Journal of Clinical Endocrinology and Metabolism* 88, no. 1 (2003): 14–15.

58. R. Leproult and E. Van Cauter, "Role of Sleep and Sleep Loss in Hormonal Release and Metabolism," *Endocrine Development* 17, (2010): 11–21.

59. D. Rucker et al., "Long-Term Pharmacotherapy for Obesity and Overweight: Updated Meta-Analysis," *British Medical Journal* 335, no. 7631 (2007): 1194–99; ConsumerSearch, "Diet Pills: Reviews," Updated August 2009, www.consumersearch.com

60. Ibid.

61. A. Tsai and T. Wadden, "Systematic Review: An Evaluation of Major Commercial Weight Loss Programs in the U.S.," *Annals of Internal Medicine* 142, no. 1 (J2005): 56–66.

62. J. B. Calton, "Prevalence of Nutrient Deficiency in Popular Diet Plans," *Journal of the International Society of Sports Nutrition* 7, no. 24 (2010); M. Metzgar et al., "The Feasibility of a Paleolithic Diet for Low-Income Consumers," *Nutrition Research* 31, no. 6 (2011): 444–51.

63. National Eating Disorder Association, "What Are Eating Disorders?" 2011, www.nationaleatingdisorders.org

64. K. Beals and A. Hill, "The Prevalence of Disordered Eating, Menstrual Dysfunction, and Low Bone Mineral Density among US Collegiate Athletes," *International Journal of Sport Nutrition and Exercise Metabolism* 16, no. 1 (2006): 1–23; American Psychiatric Association, "DSM-5 Development: Proposed Revision: 307.1 Anorexia Nervosa," Updated October 2010, www.dsm5.org

65. T. K. Clarke, et al., "The Genetics of Anorexia Nervosa," *Clinical Pharmacology and Therapeutics* 2, no. 91 (2012): 181–8; C. M. Bulik et al., "The Genetics of Anorexia Nervosa," *Annual Review of Nutrition* 27, (2007): 263–75.

66. Mayo Clinic Staff, "Metabolism and Weight Loss: How You Burn Calories," October 2011, www.mayoclinic.com

67. Loyola Medicine, "4 Top Reasons Why Dieters Do Not Lose Weight," January 2013, www.loyolamedicine.com; D. M. Thomas et al., "Why Do Individuals Not Lose More Weight from an Exercise Intervention at Defined Dose? An Energy Balance Analysis," *Obesity Research* 10, no. 13 (2012): 835–47.

68. L. H. Willis et al., "Effects of Aerobic and/or Resistance Training on Body Mass and Fat Mass in Overweight and Obese Adults," *Journal of Applied Physiology* 12, no. 113 (2012): 1831–7.

69. R. R. Wing and S. Phelan, "Long-Term Weight Loss Maintenance," *American Journal of Clinical Nutrition* 82, no. 1 (2005): 222S–25S.

70. K. Elfhag and S. Rossner, "Who Succeeds in Maintaining Weight Loss?" *Obesity Review* 6, no. 1 (2005): 67–85.

71. Ibid.

getfitgraphic references

1. S. S. Gropper et al., "The Freshman 15—A Closer Look," *Journal of American College Health* 58, no. 3 (2009): 223-31.

2. S. B. Racette et al., "Weight Changes, Exercise, and Dietary Patterns During Freshman and Sophomore Years of College," *Journal of American College Health* 53, no. 6 (2005): 245-51.

3. A. Kong et al., "Self-Monitoring and Eating-Related Behaviors Are Associated with 12-Month Weight Loss In Postmenopausal Overweight-to-Obese Women," *Journal of the Academy of Nutrition and Dietetics* 122, no. 9 (2012): 1428-35.

4. V. Nguyen et al., "Popcorn is More Satisfying Than Potato Chips in Normal-Weight Adults," *Nutrition Journal* 11, no. 1 (2012): 71-6.

5. D. Wadhera, Research presented at the Annual Meeting of the Society for the Study of Ingestive Behavior, July 2012, Reported by *Science Daily*, Available at www.sciencedaily.com

6. P. S. Hogenkamp et al., "Acute Sleep Deprivation Increases Portion Sizes and Affects Food Choice in Young Men," *Psychoneuroendocrinology*, (2013): S0306-4530, doi: 10.1016/j.psyneuen.2013.01.012. [Epub ahead of print]

Name: _____   **Date:** _____

Instructor: _____   **Section:** _____

Materials: Calculator, access to Internet (optional)

Purpose: To learn how to calculate energy balance and set realistic goals for calorie intake and energy expenditure.

Directions: Complete the following sections.

SECTION I: CALCULATING BMR AND ENERGY EXPENDITURE

Your basal metabolic rate (BMR) is the rate at which you burn calories to sustain life functions at rest at a normal room temperature. Your activities, fitness level, stress level, and many other things will affect your BMR.

1. **Calculate your BMR (the method shown here uses the Harris-Benedict formula):**

Men

1. BMR = 66 + (6.3 × weight in pounds) + (12.9 × height in inches) − (6.8 × age in years)

2. BMR = 66 + (   ) + (   ) − (   )

3. BMR = _____ calories

Women

1. BMR = 655 + (4.3 × weight in pounds) + (4.7 × height in inches) − (4.7 × age in years)

2. BMR = 655 + (   ) + (   ) − (   )

3. BMR = _____ calories

2. **Estimate your total energy expenditure (EE):**
Total energy expenditure takes into account your amount of activity within a 24-hour period. You can calculate your energy expenditure by keeping an activity log and adding up the calories expended during any nonsleep time. To do this, use the physical activity tracking tool on the ChooseMyPlate website (www.choosemyplate.gov). Another way to estimate total energy expenditure is to use the following calculations. Choose your level of activity on *average* and use that formula to calculate your energy expenditure (EE).

Multiply your BMR by the appropriate activity factor, completing ONE equation that follows:

- If you are **sedentary** (little or no exercise):

    EE = _____(BMR) × **1.2** = _____ calories

- If you are **lightly active** (light exercise/sports 1–3 days/week):

    EE = _____(BMR) × **1.375** = _____ calories

- If you are **moderately active** (moderate exercise/sports 3–5 days/week):

    EE = _____(BMR) × **1.55** = _____ calories

- If you are **very active** (hard exercise/sports 6–7 days/week):

    EE = _____(BMR) × **1.725** = _____ calories

- If you are **extra active** (very hard daily exercise/sports & physical job or 23-day training):

    EE = _____(BMR) × **1.9** = _____ calories

SECTION II: CALCULATING ENERGY BALANCE

1. Estimated **calorie INTAKE**

_____ calories

2. Estimated **calorie EXPENDITURE** (EE from Section I)

_____ calories

3. Subtract your EXPENDITURE (#2) from your INTAKE (#1) to get:

Out-of-balance calories = _____ calories

SECTION III: TOOLS FOR YOUR WEIGHT MANAGEMENT PLAN

1. What was your caloric intake from your dietary analysis? _____ What was your energy expenditure? _____ What was your overall energy balance? _____

- **Energy balance** (±200 calories): You are supplying your body with its energy needs and maintaining current weight.
- **Negative energy balance** (−201 calories): You are expending more energy than you are eating and should be losing weight.
- **Positive energy balance** (+201 calories): You are eating more energy than you are expending and should be gaining weight.

2. Do you want or need to lose body fat? **YES or NO**

3. What is your **goal** for your body fat percentage? _____

4. Complete the following calculations to figure out how many **pounds of fat** you need to lose in order to reach this goal:

- Find your **current fat weight:**

  _____ (current weight, lb) × _____ (current % body fat, expressed as a decimal) = _____ current fat weight (lb)

- Find your **lean body mass (LBM):**

  _____ (weight, lb) − _____ (fat weight, lb) = _____ LBM (lb)

- Find your **target body weight:**

  _____ (LBM) ÷ (1 − goal % body fat expressed as a decimal) = _____ target body weight (lb)

- Find the **lb of fat loss** needed to reach your body fat percentage goal:

  _____ (current weight, lb) − _____ (target weight, lb) = _____ fat loss needed (lb)

5. If you lose 1 pound of fat per week (500 calorie deficits per day), how many weeks will you take to lose your desired fat weight? _____

6. Brainstorm ways that you can get to a −500 calorie deficit per day through diet and exercise/activity changes.

DIET CHANGE (lower by 250 calories)

_____

_____

_____

_____

ACTIVITY CHANGE (increase by 250 calories)

_____

_____

_____

_____

Name: _____ Date: _____

Instructor: _____ Section: _____

Materials: None

Purpose: (1) To assess factors that that may predispose you to excess weight and make weight loss more challenging, and (2) to help you determine your readiness to begin losing weight right now.

Directions: If you are overweight or obese, complete each of the following questions by circling the response(s) that best represents your situation or attitudes, then total your points for each section.

SECTION I: FAMILY WEIGHT CHARACTERISTICS AND PERSONAL DIET HISTORY

1. How many people in your immediate family (parents or siblings) are overweight or obese?

a. No one is overweight or obese (0 points)

b. One person (1 point)

c. Two people (2 points)

d. Three or more people (3 points)

2. During which periods of your life were you overweight or obese? (circle all that apply)

a. Birth through age 5 (1 point)

b. Ages 6 to 11 (1 point)

c. Ages 12 to 13 (1 point)

d. Ages 14 to 18 (2 points)

e. Ages 19 to present (2 points)

3. To the best of your memory, how many times in the last year have you made a concerted effort to lose weight but have had little or no success?

a. None; I've never thought about it. (0 points)

b. I've thought about it, but I've never tried hard to lose weight. (1 point)

c. I have tried 2-3 times. (1 point)

d. I have tried at least once a month. (2 points)

e. I have tried so many times, I can't remember. (3 points)

Total points: _____

Scoring

If you scored higher than 3, you may have challenges ahead as you begin a weight-loss program. The higher your score, the greater the likelihood of challenges.

If your family includes overweight or obese members, your own weight problems may be related, at least in part, to the eating habits and preferences you learned at home. Ingrained habits tend to feel perfectly normal, so changing them may require a conscious effort. If your past weight-loss efforts ended in a return to your old behaviors, you may have to re-frame your thinking and approach.

SECTION II: READINESS TO CHANGE

1. Attitudes and Beliefs About Weight Loss

A. What is/are your main reason(s) for wanting to lose weight? (circle all that apply)

a. I want to please someone I know or attract a new person. (0 points)

b. I want to look great and/or fit into smaller size clothes for an upcoming event (wedding, vacation, date, etc.). (1 point)

    c. Someone I know has had major health problems because of being overweight/obese. (1 point)

    d. I want to improve my health and/or have more energy. (2 points)

    e. I was diagnosed with a health problem (pre-diabetes, diabetes, high blood pressure, etc.) because of being overweight/obese. (2 points)

B. What do you think about your weight and body shape? (circle all that apply)

    a. I'm fine with being overweight, and if others don't like it, tough! (0 points)

    b. My weight hurts my energy levels and my performance and holds me back. (1 point)

    c. I feel good about myself, but think I will be happier if I lose some of my weight. (1 point)

    d. I'm self-conscious about my weight and uncomfortable in my body. (1 point)

    e. I'm really worried that I will have a major health problem if I don't change my behaviors now. (2 points)

2. Daily Eating Patterns

A. Which of the following statements describes you? (circle all that apply)

    a. I think about food several times a day, even when I'm not hungry. (0 points)

    b. There are some foods or snacks that I can't stay away from, and I eat them even when I'm not hungry. (0 points)

    c. I tend to eat more meat and fatty foods and never get enough fruits and veggies. (0 points)

    d. I've thought about the weaknesses in my diet and have some ideas about what I need to do. (1 point)

    e. I haven't really tried to eat a "balanced" diet, but I know that I need to start now. (1 point)

B. When you eat or binge on things you know you shouldn't consume, what are you likely to do? (circle all that apply)

    a. Not care and go off of my diet. (0 points)

    b. Feel guilty for a while but then do it again the next time I am out. (0 points)

    c. Fast for the next day or two to help balance the high consumption day. (0 points)

    d. Plan ahead for next time and have options in mind so that I do not continue to overeat. (1 point)

    e. Acknowledge that I have made a slip and get back on my program the next day. (1 point)

C. On a typical day, what are your eating patterns? (circle all that apply)

    a. I skip breakfast and save my calories for lunch and dinner. (0 points)

    b. I never really sit down for a meal. I am a "grazer" and eat whatever I find that is readily available. (0 points)

    c. I try to eat at least 5 servings of fruits and veggies and restrict saturated fats in my diet. (1 point)

    d. I eat several small meals, trying to be balanced in my portions and getting foods from different food groups. (1 point)

3. Commitment to Weight Loss and Exercise

A. How would you describe your current support system for helping you lose weight? (circle all that apply)

    a. I believe I can do this best by doing it on my own. (0 points)

    b. I am not aware of any sources that can help me. (0 points)

    c. I have 2-3 friends or family members I can count on to help me. (1 point)

    d. There are counselors on campus with whom I can meet to plan a successful approach to weight loss. (1 point)

    e. I have the resources to join Weight Watchers or other community or online weight loss programs. (1 point)

B. How committed are you to exercising? (circle all that apply)

    a. Exercise is uncomfortable, embarrassing, and/or I don't enjoy it. (0 points)

    b. I don't have time to exercise. (0 points)

    c. I'd like to exercise, but I'm not sure how to get started. (1 point)

    d. I've visited my campus rec center or local gym to explore my options for exercise. (2 points)

    e. There are specific sports or physical activities I do already, and I can plan to do more of them. (2 points)

C. What statement best describes your motivation to start a weight loss/lifestyle change program?

    a. I don't want to start losing weight. (0 points)

    b. I am thinking about it sometime in the distant future. (0 points)

    c. I am considering starting within the next few weeks; I just need to make a plan. (1 point)

    d. I'd like to start in the next few weeks, and I'm working on a plan. (2 points)

    e. I already have a plan in place, and I'm ready to begin tomorrow. (3 points)

Total points: _____

Scoring

A score higher than 8 indicates that you are ready to change; the higher your score above 8, the more successful you may be. If you scored lower than 8, consider your stages of change (using the model discussed in Chapter 1).

SECTION III: REFLECTION

One of the first steps in making a plan to lose weight is recognizing your strengths and weaknesses and being ready to anticipate challenges.

1. Do your current thoughts and attitudes about weight and dieting reflect a good foundation for starting a successful weight-loss program, and if so, in what ways?

_____

_____

2. Which long-term motivations will you need to successfully lose weight?

_____

_____

3. Which benefits of losing weight motivate you most strongly?

_____

_____

4. Which behavioral changes are you ready to make to address your weight issues?

_____

To lose weight permanently, you will need to change your daily eating habits. Overeating (or eating poorly) may be a response to your food attitudes rather than to physical hunger. Poor eating may also reflect your emotional responses toward food, and/or unhealthy dietary choices.

5. To increase your commitment to weight loss and exercise, list friends or family who can support your efforts to stick to your plan.

_____

_____

6. Explore the wealth of available resources (web materials, support groups, counselors) both on and off campus where you can get assistance. Research and record one resource per day for the next five days. After you research, contact at least two sources, plan your program, and begin. Having a plan and sticking to it will be key as you begin your weight loss journey!

_____

_____

_____

_____

LAB 8.3

PLAN FOR CHANGE
YOUR WEIGHT MANAGEMENT PLAN

MasteringHealth™

Name: _____ Date: _____

Instructor: _____ Section: _____

Materials: None

Purpose: To create an appropriate weight management goal, you must apply behavior change tools and make a plan to implement your goals.

Directions: Complete the following sections.

SECTION I: SHORT- AND LONG-TERM GOALS

1. Short-Term Goals

- My three-month *or* six-month (circle one) % body fat goal is _____%.
- My three-month *or* six-month (circle one) weight goal is _____ lb.
- My three-month *or* six-month (circle one) BMI goal is _____ kg/m^2.

2. Long-Term Goals

a. Based on my current weight, BMI, % body fat, and the tools gained in Lab 8.2:

- My one-year % body fat goal is _____%.
- My one-year weight goal is _____ lb.
- My one-year BMI goal is _____ kg/m^2.

b. I plan to reach that goal by consuming about _____ calories per day and adding _____ activity calories per day.

SECTION II: DIET OBSTACLES AND STRATEGIES

1. Negative Food and Eating Triggers

Eating and food preferences can be triggered by emotions, social situations, and the sights and smells around you.

a. Fill out the following table exploring your negative food and eating triggers. For example, a situational trigger for you eating sugary foods may be "attending holiday parties."

Diet Behavior	Emotional Triggers	Social Triggers	Situational Triggers
Eating More Food			
Eating Late at Night			
Eating More Often			
Eating Sugary Foods			
Eating Fatty Foods			
Eating Fast Foods			
Eating Out			
Others:			

b. List three strategies to overcome or manage your food and eating triggers:

(1) _____

(2) _____

(3) _____

2. **Changing Food Patterns**

a. I will eat LESS of the following foods and beverages:

_____

_____

b. For good nutrition and weight management goals, I will replace the above foods and beverages with the following:

_____

_____

SECTION III: EXERCISE AND ACTIVITY OBSTACLES AND STRATEGIES

1. **Reducing Sedentary Behaviors**

a. Evaluate your sedentary activities in the space below. List your top three sedentary activities (not including time spent in class), the number of days per week you do them, and how many minutes per day.

	Sedentary Activity	Days/Wk	Min/Day
1			
2			
3			

b. Which sedentary activity could you replace with physical activity or even supplement with physical activity (such as exercising while you watch TV, or stretching while on your cell phone)? Write down three ideas for replacing sedentary activities with more active ones.

(1) _____

(2) _____

(3) _____

2. **Listing Activity Obstacles**

List a few of the obstacles to replacing sedentary activity with more energy-intensive physical activity, along with strategies for overcoming these obstacles.

Activity Obstacle	Strategy to Overcome
(1) _____	_____
(2) _____	_____
(3) _____	_____

SECTION IV: GETTING SUPPORT

1. I feel supported in my weight goals by these people:

_____

Here's what they do that assists me:

_____

2. I need additional support from these people:

_____

Here's what I need to ask for:

_____

3. **If I need group or medical support**, here are a few places to seek it: student health service, family physician, local hospital, local Weight Watchers chapter, online groups. If needed, I would be inclined to use _____ for support.

SECTION V: REWARDS

1. When I make the **short-term** behavior change described earlier, my reward will be:

_____

Target date _____

2. When I make the **long-term** behavior change described earlier, my reward will be:

_____

Target date _____

LAB
8.4

ASSESS YOURSELF
JUNK FOOD
DETECTIVE

MasteringHealth™

Name: _____   **Date:** _____

Instructor: _____   **Section:** _____

Materials: Paper, pen, access to Internet

Purpose: To investigate your typical snack and fast foods and find better substitutes.

Directions: Complete the following list of instructions.

SECTION I: FAVORITE SNACK AND FAST FOODS

1. Make a list of six snack or fast foods that you like to eat.

a. _____

b. _____

c. _____

d. _____

e. _____

f. _____

SECTION II: INVESTIGATE YOUR FAVORITES

1. Using nutrition labels or Internet information (e.g., nutritional sites on the websites of fast-food franchises), analyze *your typical serving* of each food and record in the blanks provided.

Note: On ingredient lists, added sugars may be called *sucrose, evaporated cane juice, concentrated grape juice, fructose, high fructose corn syrup, corn syrup, mannitol, sorbitol, xylitol, hydrogenated starch hydrosylates.*

Refined grains may be called *enriched wheat flour, white flour, bleached wheat flour, durum wheat semolina, de-germed cornmeal, enriched rice (white rice).* (If the label doesn't list 100% whole wheat, rice, oats, and so on, it's probably refined grain.)

Snack/ Fast Food	Total Calories	Saturated Fat (calories)	*Trans* Fat (grams)	Sodium (milligrams)	Cholesterol (grams)	Refined Grain Carbohydrates (grams)	Added Sugars (grams)

SECTION III: RATE YOUR JUNK FOOD

The USDA choosemyplate.gov website recommends these criteria for the nutrients you just analyzed:

Calories from saturated fat: Less than 10 percent of total calories (plug in your daily calorie allowance based on Lab 8.1)

***Trans* fat:** Avoid

Sodium: For certain adults (everyone over 51, African Americans, everyone with high blood pressure, diabetes, or kidney disease) less than 1,500 milligrams of sodium per day; for all other adults, less than 2,300 milligrams per day

Cholesterol: Less than 300 milligrams per day

Grains: Half of daily total should be whole grains, half or less refined grains

Added sugars: Minimize

1. Using these criteria, analyze your typical serving of your six favorite snacks or fast foods against these recommendations. Rate your list in order from 1 to 6, with 1 having the fewest negatives and the least impact on your daily quotients, 2 the next least, and so on, up to 6, the junk food with the most negatives and the highest impact on your nutritional quotients.

Snack/Junk Food	Rating (1–6)
a. _____	_____
b. _____	_____
c. _____	_____
d. _____	_____
e. _____	_____
f. _____	_____

SECTION IV: FIND NEW FAVORITES

1. Take the three foods on your list with the highest scores (4, 5, and 6), and for each, name a lower-calorie, more nutritious substitute.

Snack/Junk Food	Nutritious Substitute
a. _____ →	_____
b. _____ →	_____
c. _____ →	_____

Have fun trying these new foods! (If you are on a weight loss or maintenance diet, don't forget portion control.)

SECTION V: REFLECTION

1. Changes to your diet begin with motivation. Name three personal reasons why you would be better off by permanently reducing the amount of junk food in your diet.

a. _____

b. _____

c. _____

2. Rewards are another important part of behavior change. Name three noncaloric rewards you could give yourself for avoiding junk foods on three occasions.

a. _____

b. _____

c. _____

Activate, Motivate, & ADVANCE YOUR FITNESS

A WEIGHT MANAGEMENT EXERCISE PROGRAM

SCAN TO SEE IT
ONLINE!

ACTIVATE!

With weight management, progression is the key. Don't make the mistake of doing too much too soon. That is a leading cause of injury and will set you back even further from your goals. Start slowly and go at your own pace, building up stamina and strength; start where you are. Eventually, you will progress and increase the time or the intensity of your workouts (or both) as you become stronger and the sessions become easier. Follow these programs to gradually increase the number of minutes you train each week, the intensity of each session, and the calories you burn with each workout.

What Do I Need?

SHOES AND CLOTHING: The right shoes and clothes can go a long way toward keeping you comfortable and injury free as you begin a complete weight management program. Refer to the cardiorespiratory programs in this book (Chapter 3) for details and tips to consider when choosing shoes and exercise clothing that are right for you.

How Do I Start?

TECHNIQUE: Safe and effective training really depends on proper technique. This is true whether you are just starting to become active or whether you are incorporating more vigorous activities into your program. Be sure to read through each of the previous chapters for detailed exercise descriptions and to learn proper technique and form. If you are unable to maintain good form, simply decrease the weight, the speed of the movement, the number of repetitions, or the length of your workout session.

Where Do I Start?

AT HOME: Walking is the best place to start. Whether it is a walk inside your home or around the campus or neighborhood, walking is the easiest way to add more activity to your day. Start with flat and forgiving surfaces and as you progress, add inclines or increase your pace or your overall minutes each week.

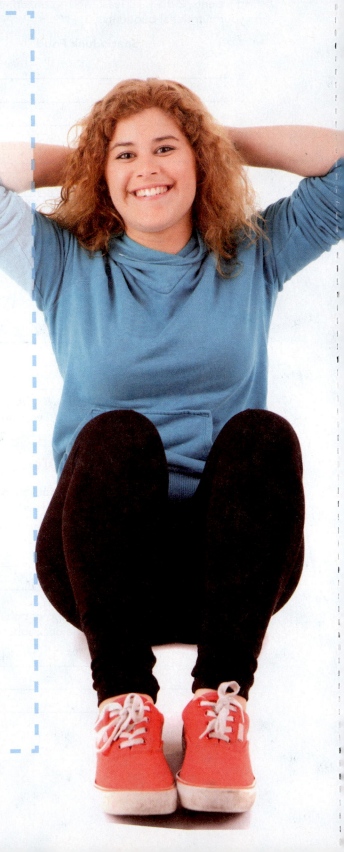

Although walking may be the best way to get started and increase your cardiorespiratory fitness, you will need to incorporate some resistance training to increase your muscular fitness, begin to change your body composition, and assist with increasing your overall weekly calorie expenditure. In the beginning weeks, you can complete your weight management resistance training program by using your own body weight against gravity to increase muscular endurance and strength. However, a few key items might help your motivation by keeping you comfortable and interested: a sturdy chair, a towel or a mat, and maybe a few household items (e.g., books in your backpack). As you progress, you can add pieces of equipment to provide more resistance and increase your intensity (bands or tubing, a good stability ball, and even medicine balls).

AT THE GYM: Here, too, walking is the best way to start a weight management program. The treadmill is a great option and offers less impact than cement and asphalt. An elliptical machine is another good option that reduces the stress placed on hips, knees, ankles, and feet. If your gym has a pool, make use of it. Water walking (shallow or deep) is a great way to move your body without placing stress on your joints. Water also adds resistance to your workout and, of course, the pool can help you stay cool!

For resistance training sessions, a gym provides access to the wide variety of equipment. You will be able to incorporate the use of barbells (long bars with weights attached or slots to add weight plates), dumbbells (smaller, handheld weights), benches (flat, incline, decline), plus cable stations and the latest the industry has to offer. All of these will help you progress, reducing your chances of boredom and increasing your likelihood of continued exercise.

Warm-Up and Cool-Down

A good warm-up and cool-down consists of simply doing your activity of choice at a slower pace and easing into and out of your training session. Break a light sweat as you slowly increase both your respiratory rate and your heart rate. Include a few dynamic range-of-motion exercises. After you finish your workout session, cool-down slowly, bringing your heart rate and respiratory rate back to your starting point. Once you have cooled down, include a few more dynamic moves or try a bit of foam rolling. Then begin to perform your static stretches for improved flexibility. (Be sure to review the programs in Chapter 5 for more ideas and descriptions of each of the stretches.)

Four-Week Weight Management Programs

If you are just beginning, if you have a BMI of 30 or greater, or if you have been sedentary for more than three months, start slowly and build gradually with the Beginner Program. Doing this will help you increase your overall calorie expenditure while helping to keep you injury free. Adjust intensity, volume, and training days to suit your personal fitness level and schedule.

BEGINNER

PROGRAM   **GOAL:** Increase cardiorespiratory exercise frequency to three days a week and time to 15 minutes continuously per session, 100+ minutes/week; also incorporate resistance training two days a week.

	Mon	Tue	Wed	Thurs	Fri	Sat	Sun
Week 1	Cardio, 10 min × 3	Resistance, 1 circuit	Cardio, 10 min × 3	Resistance, 1 circuit	Cardio, 10 min × 3		
	Cardio workout: Walk 10 minutes continuously 3× (morning, afternoon, evening) *Resistance circuit workout: Do each exercise for 60 seconds with 15-second rests between exercises.*						
Week 2	Cardio, 10 min × 3	Resistance, 2 circuits	Cardio, 10 min × 3	Resistance, 2 circuits	Cardio, 10 min × 3	Cardio, 10 min × 3	
	Cardio workout: Walk 10 minutes continuously, 3× (morning, afternoon, evening) *Resistance circuit workout: Do each exercise for 60 seconds with 15-second rests between exercises, 60-second rests between circuits.*						
Week 3	Cardio, 15 min × 3	Resistance, 2 circuits	Cardio, 15 min × 3	Resistance, 2 circuits	Cardio, 15 min × 3		
	Cardio workout: Walk 15 minutes continuously, 3× (morning, afternoon, evening) *Resistance circuit workout: Do each exercise for 60 seconds with no rest between exercises, 60-second rests between circuits.*						
Week 4	Cardio, 15 min × 3	Resistance, 3 circuits	Cardio, 15 min × 3	Resistance, 3 circuits	Cardio, 15 min × 3	Cardio, 15 min × 3	
	Cardio workout: Walk 15 minutes continuously, 3× (morning, afternoon, evening) *Resistance circuit workout: Do each exercise for 45 seconds with 10-second rests between exercises, 60-second rests between circuits.*						

Order of Resistance Circuit Exercises for Home Workout

Squat
Push-Up or Modified Push-Up
Lunge
Plank or Modified Plank
Row with Resistance Band or Dumbbell
Lat Pull-Down with Resistance Band
Side Bridge (each side)
Back Extension

Order of Resistance Circuit Exercises for Facility Workout

Chest Press
Squat or Leg Press Machine
Upright Row
Leg Extension
Rows
Overhead Press
Lat Pull-Down
Biceps Curl
Triceps Extension
Plank

MOTIVATE!

Create an exercise log to track your own weight management exercise program—make note of days, actual exercises, sets, reps, load amounts, rest intervals—or use the one on the mobile website. Here are a few tips to get you moving:

MOTIVATING MEASUREMENTS: Whether you use a scale, a tape measure, or simply your favorite jeans, be sure to check your progress each week. This can encourage and motivate you, and it will serve as a good catch to help you get back on track if you are not maintaining your nutrition and exercise program.

BAN THE NEGATIVE BODY-TALK: Stop your negative self-talk and start anew! Surround yourself with only positive comments, upbeat training partners, and true supporters of your new healthy behaviors and lifestyle. Stay focused. Remember your goals. Be patient with yourself and be sure to acknowledge how much you have already accomplished!

TAKE A LITTLE "YOU" TIME: Make fitness and nutrition a priority. Take time for you—schedule your favorite fitness activity (a stroll, your yoga DVD, pool time) and keep the appointment as you would for any other priority.

KEEP A DIGITAL PHOTO LOG: Take a "before" picture, and take a new picture each week. It may sound like the last thing you want to do at first. However, it can remind you of just how far you've come and keep you motivated to continue. This also works for your meals (especially when you eat out). Take pictures of your meals and gain a different perspective on what you are eating, how much, and when.

ADVANCE!

Now that you have established your exercise and weight management program, challenge yourself. Follow the Intermediate Program if you already exercise at least two days a week, if you have a BMI of 25 to 29, or if you simply want to take your weight management program to the next level.

INTERMEDIATE

PROGRAM **GOAL:** Increase cardiorespiratory exercise frequency to five days a week and time to 30 minutes continuously per session, 300+ minutes/week; also incorporate resistance training three days a week.

	Mon	Tue	Wed	Thurs	Fri	Sat	Sun
Week 1	Walk/jog 15 min continuously, × 3 (morning, afternoon, evening)	Resistance, 2 circuits	Walk/jog 15 min continuously, × 3 (morning, afternoon, evening)	Resistance, 2 circuits	Walk/jog 15 min continuously, × 3 (morning, afternoon, evening)	Walk/jog 20 min continuously, × 2 (morning, evening)	
	Resistance circuit workout: Do each exercise for 60 seconds with 10-second rests between exercises, 60-second rests between circuits.						

	Mon	Tue	Wed	Thurs	Fri	Sat	Sun
Week 2	Walk/jog 20 min continuously, × 3 (morning, afternoon, evening)	Walk/jog 15 min + Resistance, 2 circuits	Walk/jog 20 min continuously, × 3 (morning, afternoon, evening)	Walk/jog 15 min + Resistance, 2 circuits	Walk/jog 20 min continuously, × 3 (morning, afternoon, evening)	Walk/jog 25 min continuously, × 2 (morning, evening)	
	Resistance circuit workout: Do each exercise for 60 seconds with 10-second rests between exercises, 60-second rests between circuits.						
Week 3	Walk/jog 25 min continuously, × 3 (morning, afternoon, evening)	Walk/jog 15 min + Resistance, 3 circuits	Walk/jog 25 min continuously, × 3 (morning, afternoon, evening)	Walk/jog 15 min + Resistance, 3 circuits	Walk/jog 25 min continuously, × 3 (morning, afternoon, evening)	Walk/jog 30 min continuously, × 2 (morning, evening)	
	Resistance circuit workout: Do each exercise for 60 seconds with 10-second rests between exercises, 60-second rests between circuits.						
Week 4	Walk/jog 30 min continuously, × 3 (morning, afternoon, evening)	Walk/jog 15 min + Resistance, 3 circuits	Walk/jog 30 min continuously, × 3 (morning, afternoon, evening)	Walk/jog 15 min + Resistance, 3 circuits	Walk/jog 30 min continuously, × 3 (morning, afternoon, evening)	Walk/jog 15 min + Resistance, 3 circuits	
	Resistance circuit workout: Do each exercise for 60 seconds with 10-second rests between exercises, 60-second rests between circuits.						

Order of Resistance Circuit Exercises for Home Workout

Squat + Overhead Press with Resistance Band or Dumbbells
Push-Up or Modified Push-Up
Lunge + Biceps Curl with Resistance Band or Dumbbells
Row with Resistance Band or Dumbbells
Lat Pull-Down with Resistance Band
Triceps Extension with Resistance Band or Dumbbells
Oblique Curl
Plank or Modified Plank
Back Extension

Order of Resistance Circuit Exercises for Facility Workout

Squats or Leg Press Machine
Chest Press
Leg Extension
Overhead Press
Leg Curl
Upright Row
Lunge + Biceps Curl with Resistance Band or Dumbbells
Rows
Lat Pull-Down
Pullover
Plank
Abdominal Curl
Back Extension

9 Managing Stress

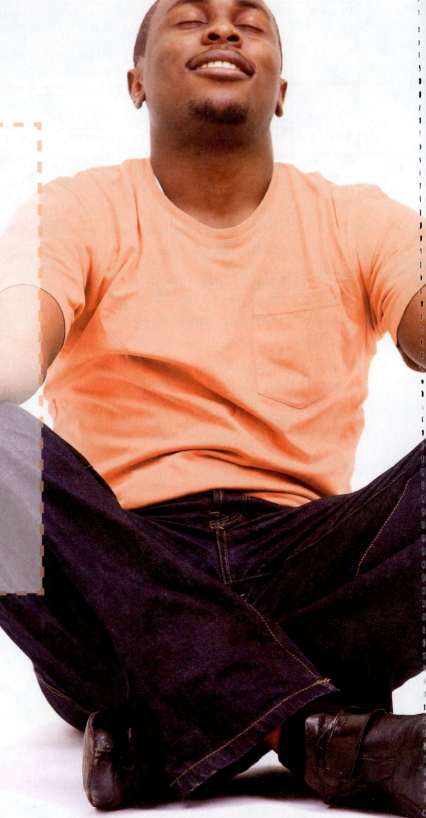

MasteringHealth™

Go online for chapter quizzes, interactive assessments, videos, and more!

casestudy

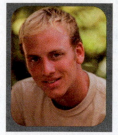

CORY

"Hi, I'm Cory. I'm a junior, majoring in biology. I'm from Denver, Colorado, and just transferred schools in August to be closer to my dad, who lives alone and has diabetes. I take five classes, I work part time as a lab assistant, and I'm up late every night studying so that I can keep up my grades for applying to medical school. I've always been able to work under pressure, but I have to admit, these past few months have been rough. I am constantly worn out, worried about my dad, and I can barely stay awake in class sometimes. I know that medical school will be even harder, so maybe I should just get used to living like this! But I am so tired of feeling dragged out."

HEAR IT! ONLINE

E veryone feels stress at least some of the time, be it from traffic, competition for the courses you need, job hunting, fast-changing technology, or a hectic pace that seems to accelerate yearly. Over time, stress can diminish not only our enjoyment of life, but it can also wreak havoc on our health and well-being, too.[1] Thus, learning effective stress-management techniques is an important part of any complete wellness program.

This chapter explains the stress response, details the ways accumulated stress can affect your health, and proposes several helpful strategies you can use to counteract stress. Using the stress-management tools in this chapter, you can better face the pressures of college life and beyond.

What Is Stress?

In a recent national survey, college students reported stress as the biggest impediment to their academic success, with a greater impact on achievement than colds, flu, sleep difficulty, relationship issues, and all other concerns.[2] But what, exactly, *is* stress?

The term **stress** is commonly used in many different ways. In this book, we'll define stress as a disturbance in an individual's physical and/or emotional state due to a real or perceived threat, aggravation, or excitement that disturbs the person's "normal" physiological state and to which the body must try to adapt. Any event that disrupts your body's "normal" state is a **stressor**. A stressor can be physical, such as an uncomfortably heavy backpack. It can also be emotional, like the anxiety you feel before you take a major exam. The term for the physical effect of a stressor is the **stress response**: the set of physiological changes initiated by your body's nervous and hormonal signals. The stress response prepares the brain, heart, muscles, and other organs to respond to a perceived threat or demand.

A more traditional view of stress includes the concepts of both positive stress and negative stress. Positive stress, or **eustress**, presents an opportunity for personal growth, satisfaction, and enhanced well-being. Eustress can invigorate us and motivate us to work harder and achieve more. Entering college, starting a job, and developing a new relationship are all challenges that can produce eustress. Negative stress, or **distress**, can result from negative stressors such as academic pressures, relationship discord, or money problems. It can even result from an overload of positive stressors such as graduating from college, getting married, moving to a new state, and starting a new job all in the same week. Distress can reduce wellness by promoting cardiovascular disease, impairing immunity, or causing mental and emotional dysfunction.

How Does My Body Respond to Stress?

As you sit down in the lecture hall to take your hardest midterm exam, you realize your heart is pounding, your breathing has quickened, your hands are sweating, you

> **stress** A disturbance in physical and/or emotional state due to a real or perceived threat, aggravation, or excitement that disturbs the body's "normal" physiological state and to which the body must try to adapt
>
> **stressor** A physical, social, or psychological event or circumstance to which the body tries to adapt; stressors are often threatening, unfamiliar, disturbing, or exciting
>
> **stress response** A set of physiological changes initiated by your body in response to a stressor
>
> **eustress** Stress based on positive circumstances or events; can present an opportunity for personal growth
>
> **distress** Stress based on negative circumstances or events, or those perceived as negative; can diminish wellness

have "butterflies" in your stomach, and you feel a sense of dread. You are experiencing a stress response: a reaction involving nervous and hormonal activities that prepare both body and mind to deal with the disturbance to your normal state.

The Stress Response

Here's what happens during the seconds that the body initiates a stress response and in the minutes and hours as the response continues (**Figure 9.1**):

1. Your senses perceive and your brain interprets something as a threat; in the preceding example, an exam that will determine half your grade.

2. The threat triggers a region of your brain called the *hypothalamus* to release a hormone that in turn triggers your pituitary gland to secrete **adrenocorticotropic hormone (ACTH)** into your blood.

3. ACTH travels through the bloodstream and reaches the outer zone of each adrenal gland (located on top of each kidney). ACTH causes the adrenal glands to secrete **cortisol**, your body's main stress hormone.

   At the same time, nerve signals from your brain and spinal cord reach and stimulate the central zone of each adrenal gland. Both adrenals

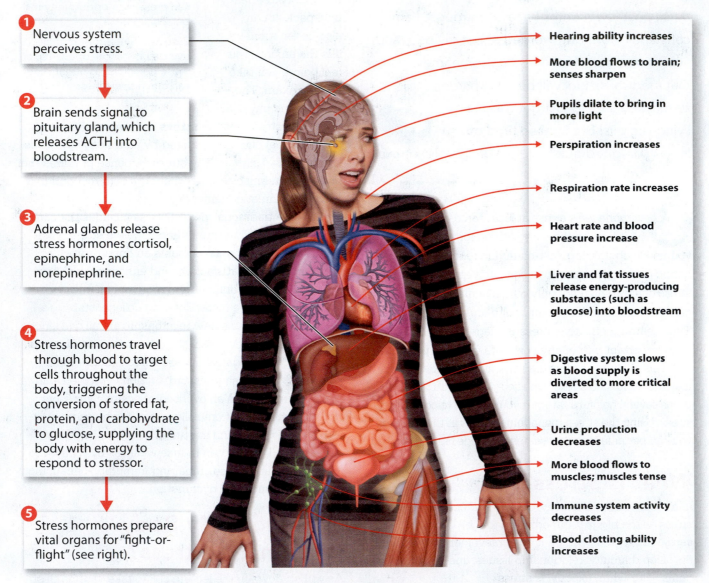

1 Nervous system perceives stress.

2 Brain sends signal to pituitary gland, which releases ACTH into bloodstream.

3 Adrenal glands release stress hormones cortisol, epinephrine, and norepinephrine.

4 Stress hormones travel through blood to target cells throughout the body, triggering the conversion of stored fat, protein, and carbohydrate to glucose, supplying the body with energy to respond to stressor.

5 Stress hormones prepare vital organs for "fight-or-flight" (see right).

Hearing ability increases

More blood flows to brain; senses sharpen

Pupils dilate to bring in more light

Perspiration increases

Respiration rate increases

Heart rate and blood pressure increase

Liver and fat tissues release energy-producing substances (such as glucose) into bloodstream

Digestive system slows as blood supply is diverted to more critical areas

Urine production decreases

More blood flows to muscles; muscles tense

Immune system activity decreases

Blood clotting ability increases

FIGURE **9.1** The stress response.

respond by releasing two additional stress hormones that ready the body for quick action: **epinephrine** (also called **adrenaline**) and **norepinephrine** (or **noradrenaline**).

4. Traveling inside the bloodstream, cortisol reaches specific *target cells* within the body fat and within several organs, including the liver and intestines. Cortisol quickly triggers target cells to convert stored fat, protein, and carbohydrate molecules into glucose. Soon, more glucose is circulating in the blood, supplying the whole body—especially the brain and skeletal muscles—with the extra energy needed to respond to the stressor.

5. The epinephrine and norepinephrine released into the blood rapidly reach target cells in the heart, lungs, stomach, intestines, sense organs, and muscles. Along with signals from sympathetic nerves, these additional stress hormones ready the vital organs in ways that promote survival: fleeing from or confronting the threat. This physiological reaction is called the **fight-or-flight response**.

If you have ever jammed on your car or bicycle brakes to avoid an accident, you have probably felt a jolt of epinephrine. As part of the fight-or-flight response, your pupils dilate, enabling you to see more clearly. The air passages in your lungs also dilate, allowing more oxygen to enter. Your heart beats faster and pumps more blood into your muscles and brain. Your sweat glands release more sweat, and blood is directed away from your hands and feet toward your large muscles and body core; this can make your hands feel cold and clammy. Your digestive action slows down or stops, and your bladder function slows down, since neither process is crucial to short-term survival. Primed in all these ways, your body is ready to handle the stressor, at least in the short term.

After a perceived stressor subsides, your nervous system returns the body to its "normal" state with slower heartbeats, normal breathing rate, normal digestion, and so on. The stress-reduction techniques you will learn later deliberately encourage the body's return to this more relaxed state.

Why Does Stress Cause Harm?

Why is chronic stress harmful? After all, if a truck is speeding toward you, your fight-or-flight response could save your life. However, if you are faced with financial hardship or excessive work pressures for years on end, your stress response can become chronic and start to harm your health. Two insightful models help explain how *sustained* stress can cause damage over time.

The General Adaptation Syndrome

LIVE IT! ONLINE
Worksheet 8
Stress Reaction

In the 1930s, biologist Hans Selye studied the response of laboratory rats to painful physical or emotional stressors. He discovered that a wide variety of stressors—such as extreme heat, extreme cold, forced exercise, or surgery—all seemed to provoke the same general set of changes in the rats' bodies. Selye proposed a model he called the **general adaptation syndrome (GAS)**, based on the reactions of the rats he observed (**Figure 9.2**, page 326).[3]

Central to Selye's GAS model is the idea that stress disrupts the body's stable internal environment, or *steady state*. Physiological mechanisms work to keep internal conditions (e.g., body temperature, blood-oxygen content, blood pH, and blood sugar levels) within certain "normal" ranges. Life scientists use the term **homeostasis** to describe the body's steady state. Selye's general adaptation syndrome characterizes the stages of the body's response to stress as follows:

1. In the *alarm stage*, a stressor disrupts the steady state and triggers a fight-or-flight response. The body starts adapting to the stressor, but the effort can lower one's resistance to injury or disease.

2. In the *resistance stage*, a person's physiology and behavior adjust, and resistance builds to the stressor. The body establishes a new level of homeostasis, despite the continued presence of the stressor.

epinephrine (adrenaline) One of two stress hormones released by adrenal glands that readies your body for quick action by stimulating sympathetic nerves

norepinephrine (noradrenaline) One of two stress hormones secreted by adrenal glands that readies your body for quick action by increasing arousal

fight-or-flight response A physiological reaction induced by nervous and hormonal signals that readies the heart, lungs, brain, muscles, and other vital organs and systems in ways that promote survival: fleeing from or confronting a threat

general adaptation syndrome (GAS) A historical model proposed by Hans Selye; it attempts to explain the body's stress response with three stages called alarm, resistance, and exhaustion

homeostasis A state of physiological equilibrium wherein various physiological mechanisms maintain internal conditions (e.g., pH, salt concentration, and temperature) within certain viable ranges

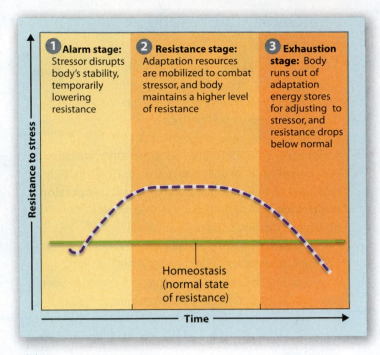

① **Alarm stage:** Stressor disrupts body's stability, temporarily lowering resistance

② **Resistance stage:** Adaptation resources are mobilized to combat stressor, and body maintains a higher level of resistance

③ **Exhaustion stage:** Body runs out of adaptation energy stores for adjusting to stressor, and resistance drops below normal

Resistance to stress

Homeostasis (normal state of resistance)

Time

FIGURE **9.2** Hans Seyle's general adaptation syndrome.

remain in the bloodstream. It can also develop when your body releases too *few* stress hormones and cannot mount an adequate stress response.[5] And it can build up if you experience a sustained string of stressful events over a long period of time. A classic example of a consequence of allostatic load is the development of stress-induced high blood pressure (hypertension.) As you will see shortly, chronically high blood pressure can damage arteries and increase one's risk of developing cardiovascular disease.[6]

A person's behavior and choices can also result in allostatic load. For example, some people respond to stress by exercising more, meditating, getting extra sleep, and avoiding drugs and alcohol—all behaviors that can help minimize allostatic load. Others respond by exercising less, staying up late, drinking more, or starting to smoke or take drugs. Such counterproductive measures can result in allostatic load and increase one's susceptibility to developing illness.

3. In the hypothetical *exhaustion stage,* the body runs out of resources to successfully adapt to the stressor, resulting in physiological harm in the form of reduced immunity and increased susceptibility to physical or mental illness.

The general adaptation syndrome recognized that sustained stress can take a toll on wellness. However, scientists have since modified Selye's concept of an "exhaustion stage" and the idea that illness results from running out of resources to adapt to a stressor. Rather, they now believe that over time, the stress response *itself* can damage the body and increase one's risk of developing illness, as we will see in the next section.

Allostatic Load

Today's stress researchers use the term **allostasis** to describe the many simultaneous changes that occur in the body to maintain homeostasis, and they use the term **allostatic load** to refer to the long-term wear and tear on the body caused by prolonged allostasis.[4]

Allostatic load can result if your body's ability to shut off the stress response (after a stressor has disappeared) is impaired, allowing high levels of stress hormones to

allostasis The many simultaneous changes that occur in the body to maintain homeostasis

allostatic load The long-term wear and tear on the body that is caused by prolonged allostasis

casestudy

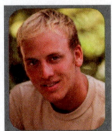

CORY

"I knew this year was going to be a challenge—transferring to a new school and taking upper-level classes. The first month actually went okay. I liked my classes, my dad seemed to be doing better, and I got used to getting by on five hours of sleep each night. Then sometime in September I caught a cold that didn't go away for four weeks! I was coughing all night, could barely pay attention in class, and did badly on one of my midterms. Now I have to work even harder to make up for the bad grade."

THINK! List Cory's main sources of stress. Which would you classify as *eustress* and which would you classify as *distress*? How might the allostatic load model explain what is happening with Cory?

ACT! Make a list of your own major sources of stress, organizing them into eustress and distress. How does stress affect your body and mind? What do you do when you feel stressed out? If you typically choose unhealthy responses to stress, list some alternative healthy responses you'd like to try.

HEAR IT! ONLINE

What Kinds of Harm Can Stress Cause?

Studies indicate that 40 percent of deaths and 70 percent of disease in the United States are related, in whole or in part, to stress.[7] The list of ailments related to chronic stress includes heart disease, diabetes, cancer, headaches, ulcers, low back pain, depression, and the common cold.

SEE IT! ONLINE

Stress Can Damage Women's Health

Stress and Cardiovascular Disease

Perhaps the most studied and documented health consequence of unresolved stress is cardiovascular disease (CVD). Research on this topic has demonstrated the impact of chronic stress on heart rate, blood pressure, heart attack, and stroke.[8] Historically, the increased risk of CVD from chronic stress has been linked to increased plaque buildup due to elevated cholesterol, hardening of the arteries, alterations in heart rhythm, and increased and fluctuating blood pressure. Recent research also points to metabolic abnormalities, insulin resistance, and inflammation in blood vessels as major contributors to heart disease.[9] In the past 15 to 20 years, researchers have identified direct links between the incidence and progression of CVD and stressors such as job strain, caregiving, bereavement, and natural disasters.[10] Whatever the mechanism, the evidence is clear that stress is a significant contributor to illness or death from CVD.

Stress and the Immune System

A growing area of scientific investigation known as **psychoneuroimmunology (PNI)** explores the intricate relationship between the mind's response to stress and the immune system's ability to function effectively. Research suggests that too much stress over a long period can negatively impact various aspects of the cellular immune response.[11] Whereas a short-term fight-or-flight response is usually protective, prolonged stress depresses the immune system. During prolonged stress, elevated levels of adrenal hormones (e.g., cortisol) destroy or reduce the ability of certain white blood cells, known as killer T cells, to aid the immune response.[12] When killer T cells don't work correctly, the body becomes more susceptible to illness.

Stress and Other Physical Effects

Prolonged periods of stress can have other physical effects, as well:

- *Weight gain* Evidence from animal and human studies shows that stress hormones can increase food consumption—particularly high-fat and high sugar foods—as well as the tendency to store belly fat.[13]

- *Hair and skin problems* Stress can worsen psoriasis and trigger hair loss, either temporarily or permanently.[14]

- *Diabetes* People under stress often eat poorly, drink alcohol to excess, take drugs, eat junk food, or get too little sleep. All of these can alter blood sugar levels and aggravate preexisting cases of type 2 diabetes or promote their development. Because the stress response itself increases the amount of glucose circulating in the blood, it also contributes directly to type 2 diabetes.[15]

- *Digestive problems* People under stress can experience nausea, vomiting, stomach pain, intestinal pain, or diarrhea. Stress hormones can cause existing digestive problems to flare. A classic example is irritable bowel syndrome.[16]

- *Loss of libido* Even in young people, stress can alter normal levels of sex hormones and this, in turn, can lead to erectile dysfunction, emotional swings, and loss of sex drive.[17]

If you experience any of these problems, a trip to the student health center may help you discover links to stress and solutions to the problems.

Stress and the Mind

Stress may be one of the single greatest contributors to mental impairment and disability and to emotional dysfunction in industrialized nations. One of the most common impairments is disrupted short-term memory, including memory functions during spatial tasks and a person's ability to remember words as quickly as he or she could before the period of stress.[18] Animal studies show that stress hormones can actually shrink the brain's memory center (the *hippocampus*) and negatively impact verbal and other memory functions.[19] Stress can lead to mental disorders, as well. Studies have shown that environmental stressors, including money and work pressures, family responsibilities, relationship conflict, and health issues, can aggravate or affect the onset of mental disorders, particularly depression and anxiety (see the box Can Stress Cause Depression? on page 328).[20]

In severe cases, an individual's response to stress may develop into **post-traumatic stress disorder (PTSD)**.

psychoneuroimmunology (PNI) Science of the interaction between the mind and the immune system

post-traumatic stress disorder (PTSD) An acute stress disorder caused by experiencing an extremely traumatic event

Q&A Can Stress Cause Depression?

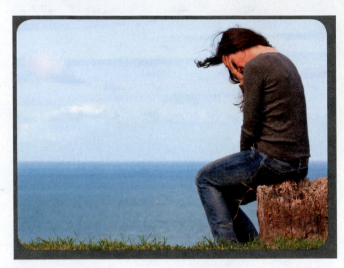

Stress and depression have complicated interconnections based on emotional, physiological, and biochemical processes. Prolonged stress can trigger depression in susceptible people, and prior periods of depression can leave individuals more susceptible to stress.[1]

The physical links between stress and depression are strong. During the stress response, the body is flooded with cortisol and with chemicals called *cytokines*. These factors promote inflammation as part of the body's immune response. Researchers think that exposure to both kinds of chemicals can damage or kill neurons in a part of the brain called the *hippocampus,* can alter nerve transmission within the brain, and can block connections (synapses) between neurons.[2] One result of hippocampal damage is impaired learning and memory.[3] Another is the onset of depression symptoms in genetically susceptible individuals.[4] Research confirms that loss of hippocampal neurons is present in many who suffer from depression.[5]

Realizing the important interconnections between stress and depression can help you take appropriate steps to handling one or both. Because stress and depression symptoms overlap, applying the stress-management techniques outlined in this chapter may help alleviate depression.

Physical activity is a particularly potent tool. A survey or more than 43,000 college students revealed that students who exercise or engage in physical activity each week have fewer feelings of depression, hopelessness, and suicidal behavior than do inactive students.[6]

If depression symptoms become severe enough to interfere with studying or other aspects of daily life, you should seek help. Potential sources for help are the student health service, the campus counseling center, a doctor or mental health professional in your community, and your local depression or suicide hotline.

Sources:
1. M. A. Ilgen and K. E. Hutchison, "A History of Major Depressive Disorder and the Response to Stress," *Journal of Affective Disorders* 86, no. 2 (2005): 143–50.
2. H. J. Kang et al., "Decreased Expression of Synapse-Related Genes and Loss of Synapses in Major Depressive Disorder," *Nature Medicine* 18, (2012): 1413–17, doi: 10.1038/nm.2886.
3. F. A. Scorza et al., "Neurogenesis and Depression: Etiology or New Illusion?" *Review of Brazilian Psychiatry* 27, no. 3 (2005): 249–53.
4. M. A. Ilgen and K. E. Hutchison, "A History of Major Depressive Disorder and the Response to Stress," 2005.
5. P. Price, "Stress and Depression," Updated June 2010, www.allaboutdepression.com
6. L. Taliaferro et al., "Associations between Physical Activity and Reduced Rates of Hopelessness, Depression, and Suicidal Behavior among College Students," *Journal of American College Health* 57, no. 4 (2009): 427–36.

Traumas that can trigger PTSD include wartime experiences, rape, near-death experiences in accidents, witnessing a murder or death, being caught in a natural disaster, or a terrorist attack.

What Are the Major Sources of Stress?

The American Psychological Association reports that young adults (ages 18 to 33) experience the highest stress levels of any adult group, and are most bothered by issues related to work, money, or job stability.[21] More than half of those surveyed report lying awake during the past month due to stress.[22]

Young adults in college can experience a flood of new stressors. Around 30 percent of freshmen report feeling frequently overwhelmed by all they have to do.[23] Female students also tend to report dieting and weight gain as stressful, while male students worry more about being underweight, relationship issues, and substance use (drugs, alcohol).[24] Nontraditional and foreign students may experience additional sources of stress, as described in the box International Student Stress on page 329.

Sources of Stress Can Be Internal or External

Interactions with others, expectations we and others have for ourselves, and the social and environmental conditions we live in force us to readjust constantly. Examining the causes of stress may help you identify

DiVeRSiTY
International Student Stress

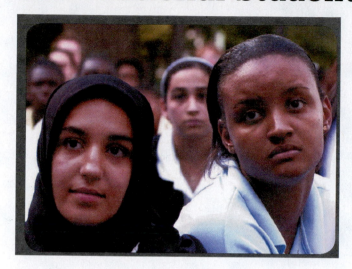

International students experience unique adjustment issues related to homesickness, language barriers, cultural barriers, and a lack of social support, among other challenges.[1] Academic stress may pose a particular problem for the more than 765,000 international students who left their native countries to study in the United States in 2011–2012. Accumulating evidence suggests that seeking emotional support from others can be one effective way to cope with stressful and upsetting situations. Yet, many international students refrain from doing so because of cultural norms, feelings of shame, and the belief that seeking support is a sign of weakness that calls inappropriate attention to both the individual and the respective ethnic group. This reluctance, coupled with the language barriers, cultural conflicts, and other stressors, can lead international students to suffer significantly more stress-related illnesses than their American counterparts. A recent study of Chinese international students at Yale, for example, revealed that 45 percent report symptoms of depression and 29 percent report symptoms of anxiety.[2] Even if we can't solve the many problems international students encounter, we can each share companionship and communication and lend a helping hand. To paraphrase a popular Hindu proverb: "Help thy neighbor's boat across and thine own boat will also reach the shore."

Sources:
1. C. A. Thurber and E. A. Walton, "Homesickness and Adjustment in University Students," *Journal of American College Health* 60, no. 5 (2012): 415–19, doi: 10.1080/07448481.2012.673520.
2. X. Han et al., "Report of a Mental Health Survey among Chinese International Students at Yale University," *Journal of American College Health* 61, no. 1 (2013): 1–8, doi: 10.1080/07448481.2012.738267.

your sources of stress and learn new ways to cope with them (**Figure 9.3**, page 330).

LIVE IT! ONLINE
Worksheet 9
Stress
Tolerance Test

Change Anytime change, whether good or bad, occurs in your normal routine, you experience stress—the more changes and adjustments you must make the more likely stress will impact your health. For example, leaving home to start college, adjusting to a new schedule, and learning to live with strangers in unfamiliar housing can all cause sleeplessness and anxiety and keep your body in a continual fight-or-flight mode.

Performance Demands We experience stress when we must meet higher standards or unfamiliar demands. In college, competition for grades, athletic positions, club memberships, internships, graduate school acceptance, and job interviews can exert considerable pressure. We can lessen the impact of such demands by setting priorities and realistic deadlines.

Inconsistent Goals and Behaviors The negative effects of stress can be magnified when we don't match our goals with our actions. For instance, you may want good grades. But if you party and procrastinate throughout the term, your goals and behaviors are inconsistent. Behaviors that are consistent with your goals—for example, studying harder and partying less to achieve good grades—can help alleviate stress.

Overload and Burnout Time pressure, responsibilities, course work, tuition, and high expectations for yourself and those around you—coupled with a lack of support—can lead to *overload:* a state of feeling overburdened, unable to keep up, and longing for escape. Overload pushes some students toward depression or substance abuse; others respond by using stress-management tools to alleviate tension before it piles up. Unrelieved overload can lead to *burnout,* a state of stress-induced physical and mental exhaustion. Teachers, nurses, and law enforcement officers, for example, experience high levels of burnout, and highly pressured professionals often use stress-management techniques to avoid reaching this point.

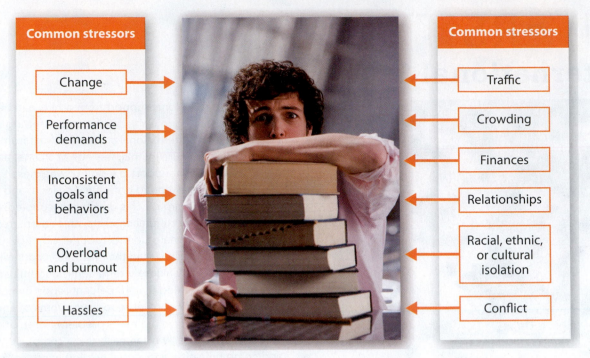

Common stressors		Common stressors
Change		Traffic
Performance demands		Crowding
Inconsistent goals and behaviors		Finances
Overload and burnout		Relationships
Hassles		Racial, ethnic, or cultural isolation
		Conflict

FIGURE **9.3** Which of these stressors impact you?

Hassles Petty annoyances and frustrations may seem unimportant if taken one by one: getting stuck in a long line at the bookstore, for example, or finding out that a school administrator has misplaced your paperwork. However, minor hassles can build to major stress if you perceive them negatively and let the feelings mount.[25] Regular release through stress management can counter this buildup.

Environmental Sources of Stress Environmental stress results from events occurring in the physical environment. People living in crowded urban environments, especially neighborhoods with lower socioeconomic status, tend to experience stress from things such as crime, traffic, housing density, and a high cost of living.[26] Meanwhile, people living in rural areas may experience different stresses such as limited employment opportunities and decreased services.

Relationships Relationships with friends, partners, family members, and co-workers can be important sources of strength and support, but they can also exert stress in our lives. These relationships can inspire and encourage us to achieve our highest goals and give us hope for the future. Staying connected can improve our mental, emotional, and physical health. Sometimes, though, relationships can diminish our self-esteem and leave us reeling from a destructive interaction. This kind of stress can diminish our wellness.

Racial, Ethnic, or Cultural Isolation Those who act, speak, or dress differently sometimes face additional pressures that do not affect more "typical" students. Students perceived as different—whether due to race,

ethnicity, religious affiliation, age, physical handicap, or sexual orientation—may become victims of subtle and not-so-subtle forms of bigotry, insensitivity, harassment, or hostility and this can increase the other forms of stress inherent in going to college.

Conflict Conflict occurs when we have to choose between competing motives, behaviors, or impulses, or when we must face incompatible demands, opportunities, needs, or goals. For example, what if your best friend wanted you to help her cheat on an exam, but you didn't feel right about it? College students often experience stress because their own developing set of beliefs conflicts with the values they learned from their parents.

What stresses do you face, and how are they affecting you? **Lab 9.1** charts many common sources of stress for college students and others. Completing this lab

DO IT! ONLINE

will help you measure your current stress level. Reading through the next section will then supply a series of helpful stress-reduction strategies and tools for using them.

What Effective Strategies Can I Use to Manage Stress?

Most young adults (62 percent) do try to reduce their stress levels, but studies show their techniques are often ineffective at alleviating stress and sometimes add to rather than help resolve their problems.[27] **Figure 9.4** on page 331 summarizes a low-key, multipronged approach to stress management, which can effectively help college students manage their stress.

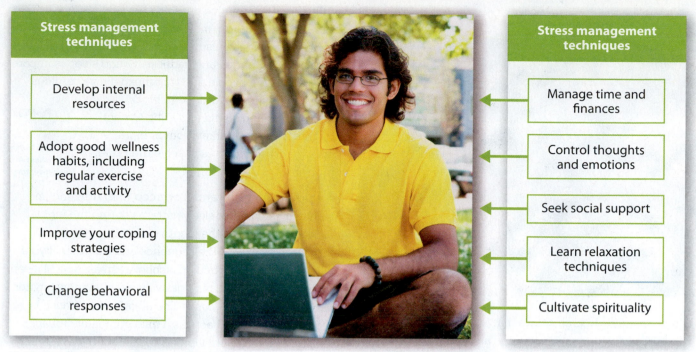

Stress management techniques

- Develop internal resources
- Adopt good wellness habits, including regular exercise and activity
- Improve your coping strategies
- Change behavioral responses

Stress management techniques

- Manage time and finances
- Control thoughts and emotions
- Seek social support
- Learn relaxation techniques
- Cultivate spirituality

FIGURE **9.4** There are many effective techniques for helping you manage stress.

Internal Resources for Coping with Stress

When you perceive that your personal resources are sufficient to meet life's demands, you experience little or no stress. By contrast, when you perceive that life's demands exceed your coping resources, you are likely to feel strain and distress.

Self-Esteem and Self-Efficacy Several coping resources influence your stress **appraisal**, how you appraise the stress in your life. Two of the most important are *self-esteem* and *self-efficacy*. Self-esteem is a sense of positive self-regard, or how you feel about yourself. Self-efficacy is a belief or confidence in personal skills and performance abilities. Researchers consider self-efficacy as one of the most important personality traits that influence psychological and physiological stress responses.[28] Low self-esteem or low self-efficacy can heighten your self-perception of stress, can increase your feelings of helplessness in coping with the stress in your life brought on by studying or work, and can contribute to depression.[29] Conversely, if you work to build your self-esteem and self-efficacy, you will add the benefit of less stress in your life!

Hardiness So-called Type A personalities are characterized as hard-driving, competitive, time-driven perfectionists. "Type B" personalities, in contrast, are more relaxed, noncompetitive, and more tolerant of others. Historically, researchers believed that people with Type A characteristics were more prone to heart attacks than their Type B counterparts.[30] Researchers today believe that personality types are more complex than previously thought—most people are not one personality type all the time, and other variables must be explored.

appraisal The interpretation and evaluation of information provided to the brain by the senses

psychological hardiness Personal characteristics of control, commitment, and an embrace of challenge that help individuals cope with stress

Psychological hardiness may negate self-imposed stress associated with Type A behavior. Psychologically hardy people are characterized by control, commitment, and a willingness to embrace challenge.[31] People with a sense of control are able to accept responsibility for their behaviors and change those that they discover to be debilitating. People with a sense of commitment have good self-esteem and understand their purpose in life. People who embrace challenge see change as an opportunity for personal growth. The concept of hardiness has been studied extensively, and many researchers believe it is the foundation of an individual's ability to cope with stress and remain healthy.[32]

Exercise, Fun, and Recreational Activity

Improving your overall level of fitness may be the most helpful thing you can do to combat stress. The GetFitGraphic Exercising to Improve Mental Health on page 333 illustrates some important connections.

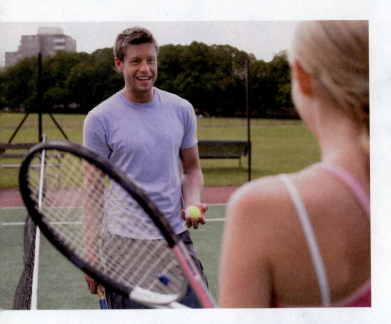

Interestingly, research shows that exercise actually stimulates the stress response, but that a well-exercised body adapts to the *eustress* of exercise, and as a result is able to tolerate greater levels of *distress* of all kinds.[33] Compared to an unfit person, a fit person develops a milder stress response to any given stressor.[34] Research also shows that exercise reduces both psychosocial stress and metabolic disturbances leading to belly fat, high blood pressure, high blood cholesterol, and vascular disease.[35]

Many physical activities relieve the feeling of stress and tension, while others—especially those that involve competition, high skill levels, or physical risk—may add to your stress load. Some activities are high in one value and low in the other, but many can build fitness and promote relaxation at the same time. The trick is to balance exercise, fun, and recreational activities in your free time so that you can stay fit and reduce chronic stress.

Basic Wellness Measures

Many of the habits you cultivate to improve your wellness can also fight the negative effects of stress.

Eating Well Eating nutrient-dense foods rather than fast foods and junk foods gives you more mental and physical energy, improves your immune responses, and helps you stay at a healthy weight. Undereating, overeating, or eating nutrient-poor foods can contribute to your stress levels and potential for depression. Many venders make claims about vitamins and supplements that reduce stress, but most of these are unsupported. Vitamin and mineral supplementation beyond your daily requirements may only add to your stress—financial stress, that is!

Getting Enough Sleep Sleep is a central wellness component. As explained in the box How Does Sleep Affect My Performance and Mood? on page 334, sleep loss hinders learning, memory, academic work, and body performance. It can also depress mood and prompt feelings of stress, anger, and sadness. *Sound* sleep is important, too. Some people find that inexpensive earplugs or eye masks from a drugstore block sleep-disturbing sound and light. Others require a quieter, darker room or more considerate roommates to solve their sleep problems.

LIVE IT! ONLINE
Worksheet 4
Sleep Inventory

Avoiding Alcohol and Tobacco Both drinking and smoking can disrupt sleep patterns during the night. Alcohol can disrupt the length of time it takes you to fall asleep as well as the sequence and duration of your sleep states.[36] In particular, alcohol decreases REM sleep and dreaming, and can negatively affect memory, motor skills, and concentration.[37] The nicotine in tobacco is highly addictive and acts as a mild stimulant. Tobacco use also impairs normal breathing and diminishes your ability to fight off colds and other infections.

Change Your Behavioral Responses

Realizing that stress is harming your fitness, wellness, relationships, or productivity is often the first step toward making positive changes. Start by assessing all aspects of a stressor, examining your typical response, determining ways to change it, and learning to cope. Often, you cannot change the stressors you face: the death of a loved one, the stringent requirements of your major, stacked-up course assignments, and so on. You can, however, change your reactions to them and better manage your stress.

Assess the Stressor List and evaluate the stressors in your life. Can you change the stressor itself? If not, you can still change your behavior and reactions to reduce the levels of stress you experience. For example, if you have a heavy academic workload, such as five term papers due for five different courses during the same quarter or semester, make a plan to start the papers early and space your work evenly so you can avoid panic over deadlines and all-night sessions to finish papers on time.

Change Your Response If something causes you distress—a habitually messy roommate, for example—you can (1) express your anger by yelling; (2) pick up the mess yourself but then leave a nasty note; (3) use humor to get your point across; or (4) initiate an even-tempered, matter-of-fact conversation about the problem. Before you respond, think through the most effective choice. Humor and laughter are surprisingly good ways to deescalate tense situations and to benefit your wellness generally. Laughter can boost your immune response, not to

EXERCISING TO IMPROVE MENTAL HEALTH

Can exercise help students stave off stress & beat the blues?

How does exercise help improve MENTAL HEALTH?

1. Increased stress ▶ Increased cortisol (linked to depression)

2. Increased exercise ▶ Increased serotonin, dopamine, and norepinephrine levels (associated with antidepressant effects) in stressed subjects with elevated cortisol levels [4]

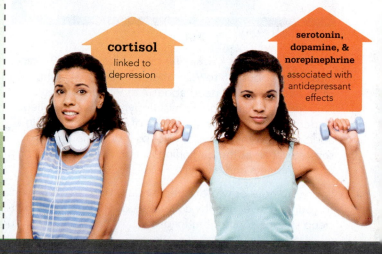

cortisol
linked to depression

serotonin, dopamine, & norepinephrine
associated with antidepressant effects

College students are STRESSED OUT.

Who feels **OVERWHELMED** by all they have to do?[1]

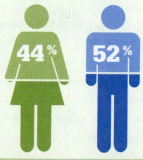

90% 74%

Who did the recommended amount of **EXERCISE** within the last week?*[2]

44% 52%

Exercise can help **REDUCE STRESS** and **DEPRESSION**, but within the last week an average of only 48% of students **EXERCISED MODERATELY** on 5+ days or **VIGOROUSLY** on 3+ days. [3]

*Recommended by the American College of Sports Medicine and the American Heart Association

FITTER IN 5!

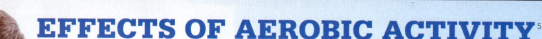

Exercising for as little as 5 minutes can improve mental health, and the more you exercise, the more positive the effects.

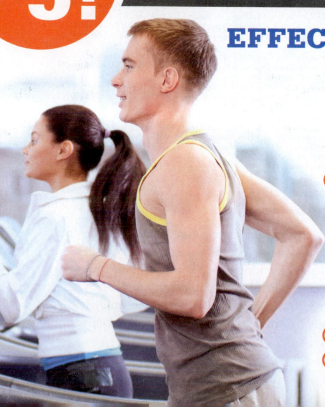

EFFECTS OF AEROBIC ACTIVITY [5]

5 MINS
- ⏱ Relieves anxiety

20 MINS
3x per week
- ⏱ Elevates mood
- ⏱ Improves your ability to deal with psychological stress

30 MINS
3x per week for 12+ weeks
- ⏱ Lessens symptoms of PMS (premenstrual syndrome)
- ⏱ Improves fitness
- ⏱ Increase your body's physiological response to stress
- ⏱ Improves your self-esteem, especially related to sports competence, fitness, strength, and appearance

Q&A How Does Sleep Affect My Performance and Mood?

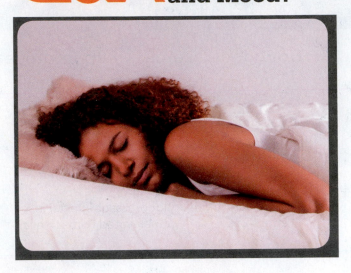

Sleep experts suggest that 18-to 20-year-olds need about 8.5 to 9.25 hours of sleep per night, while adults over 21 need about 7 to 9 hours of sleep (depending on individual physiology).[1] However, college students average 6 and 6.9 hours of sleep per night. In addition, the typical student sleeps less at the end of a semester than at the beginning due to the accumulation of assignments and exams.

Losing an hour or two of sleep actually does matter, even to young, active, healthy college students. Numerous sleep studies confirm the following:

- Sleep loss degrades learning and memory; students who stay up later at night and get less sleep tend to have lower grade point averages than earlier, longer sleepers.[2]

- Longer sleep benefits physical performance. A study of Stanford University men's basketball players showed that extending sleep by an hour or two for several weeks improved their shooting accuracy, reaction time, and sprinting speed.[3] Conversely, physical activity benefits sleep; those who exercised regularly got better sleep and felt less sleepy during the day.[4]

- Sleep loss degrades appearance. Sleeping less than 5.5 hours per night is linked to increased snacking, weight gain, and subjective judgments of a less healthy, less attractive, more tired appearance.[5]

- Sleep affects the immune system. In one study, healthy but sleep-deprived young men showed declining activity in the white blood cells needed to help fend off infections.[6]

- Sleep affects mood. Sleep deprivation can increase feelings of stress, anger, anxiety, and sadness.[7] These emotional states can, in turn, make sleeping even harder. Feeling extremely stressed out and having a negative emotional response to that stress is, in fact, the best predictor that a student will have sleep problems.[8]

Poor sleep is defined as getting fewer-than-recommended hours of sleep, having irregular bedtimes and rising times, and experiencing interrupted sleep. To improve your sleep and adopt better sleep habits:

- go to bed and wake up at as regular a time as possible;

- sleep in a room that is quiet, dark, cool (not cold), and ventilated (but not too drafty);

- get regular exercise, but not too close to bedtime;[9]

- avoid caffeine in the afternoon or evening;

- avoid excess alcohol.

Sources:
1. National Sleep Foundation, "How Much Sleep Do We Really Need?" (2011), www.sleepfoundation.org
2. J. Peszka, D. Mastin, and J. Harsh, "Sleep Hygiene, Chronotype, and Academic Performance during the Transition from High School through Four Years of College," Presented at the 2011 (25th Annual) meeting of the Associated Professional Sleep Societies (SLEEP) in Minneapolis, Minnesota.
3. C. D. Mah et al., "The Effects of Sleep Extension on the Athletic Performance of Collegiate Basketball Players," *Sleep* 34, no. 7 (2011): 943–50, doi: 10.5665/SLEEP.1132.
4. P. D. Loprini and B. J. Cardinal, "Association between Objectively Measured Physical Activity and Sleep, NHANES 2005–2006," *Mental Health and Physical Activity* 4, no. 2 (2011): 65–69, doi: 10.1016/j.mhpa.2011.08.001.
5. A. V. Nedeltcheva et al., "Sleep Curtailment Is Accompanied by Increased Intake of Calories from Snacks," *American Journal of Clinical Nutrition* 89, no. 1 (2009) 126–33, doi: 10.3945/ajcn.2008.26574; S. Patel et al., "Sleeping Less Linked to Weight Gain," *American Thoracic Society* (2006); J. Axelsson et al., "Beauty Sleep: Experimental Study on the Perceived Health and Attractiveness of Sleep Deprived People," *British Medical Journal* 341 (2010): c6614, doi: 10.1136/bmj.c6614.
6. K. Ackermann et al., "Diurnal Rhythms in Blood Cell Populations and the Effect of Acute Sleep Deprivation in Healthy Young Men," *Sleep* 36, no. 7 (2012): 933–40, doi: 10.5665/sleep.1954.
7. B. A. Marcks, "Co-Occurrence of Insomnia and Anxiety Disorder: A Review of the Literature," *American Journal of Lifestyle Medicine* 3, no. 4 (2009): 300–9, doi: 10.1177/1559827609334681.
8. L. A. Verlander, J. O. Benedict, and D. P. Hanson, "Stress and Sleep Patterns of College Students," *Perceptual Motor Skills* 88, no. 3 (1999): 893–8.
9. M. Burman and A. King, "Exercise as Treatment to Enhance Sleep," *American Journal of Lifestyle Medicine* 4, no. 6 (2010): 500–14, doi: 10.1177/1559827610375532.

mention lightening your mood and even bringing extra oxygen into your lungs![38] A calm, rational conversation can work well, too.

Improve Your Coping Strategies Good coping strategies can help relieve stress; poor ones can actually

contribute to stress and depression. In one study, coping strategies that helped college students under age 31 to better tolerate stress included deliberately relaxing; exercising in an extracurricular sport or activity; listening to music; and getting (or feeling) support from family, friends, or teachers.[39] Coping strategies which neither helped with stress nor contributed to it included taking a trip, reading a book, sitting quietly, surfing the Internet, writing in a journal, singing, or playing an instrument. Coping strategies that actually led to more stress included cleaning a room or apartment, calling a friend or Mom, spending time on an Internet social network, taking a study break, going shopping, eating, using drugs or alcohol, or watching a movie. A separate study showed that students who applied many different coping strategies were more likely to have positive outcomes when confronted with traumatic life events.[40]

Prepare Before Stressful Events Thinking things through before a potentially stressful event may help you avoid destructive or ineffective responses and tolerate increasingly higher stress levels. For example, practicing for a speaking event in front of friends may help you find and correct rough spots, and in turn, lower your levels of stress during the actual speech.

Downshift You may experience stress because you want to "have it all": a college diploma, a successful career, a family, a wide circle of friends, possessions, status in the community, and so on. But many people are **downshifting**: stepping back to a simpler life by, for example, moving from a large urban area to a smaller town, changing from a hectic high-pressure career to a low-key one, or scaling back to fewer, less-expensive possessions.

Consider some immediate and longer-term steps for simplifying your life:

- Avoid unnecessary spending.
- Choose a career that you enjoy for itself, not primarily for the salary it commands. Some lower-paying jobs are less stressful and allow for more free time for relaxation.
- Clear out clutter. Having fewer unnecessary, unused items means keeping track and taking care of that much less.

Managing Your Time and Finances

The world presents us with plenty of stressors. We create some of our own through ineffective time and finance management habits. Habits are learned behaviors, and you can *unlearn* bad habits or replace them with new habits that serve you better in managing stress. Here is what to aim for.

Manage Your Time Time—or our perceived lack of it—is one of our biggest stressors. If you learn to handle demands in a more streamlined, efficient way, you can

leave more time for other things, such as studying and having fun. To get a handle on time management, try working through **Lab 9.2**. The following tips can also help:

DO IT! ONLINE

- *Use a calendar.* A calendar can help you keep track of due dates, events, commitments, and the like. Pick out a calendar that fits your life. If you're constantly on the go, use an electronic calendar with built-in reminders rather than a desk calendar.

- *Multitask only when it's truly appropriate.* Save multitasking for things that take less concentration, such as doing the laundry and paying bills.

- *Break up big tasks.* Divide big tasks like finishing a term paper into smaller segments and then allocate a certain amount of time to each piece. If you find yourself floundering in a task, move on and come back to it when you are refreshed.

- *Clean your desk.* Periodically weed out unneeded papers and file the useful ones in separate folders. Promptly read, respond to, file, or toss mail into the recycle bin.

- *Accommodate your natural rhythms.* If you are a morning person, study and write papers in the morning, and take breaks when you start to slow down.

- *Avoid overcommitment.* Set your school and personal priorities and don't be afraid to say no to things you cannot or should not agree to do.

- *Avoid interruptions.* When you have a project that requires total concentration, schedule uninterrupted time. Go to a quiet room in the library or student union where no one will find you. Turn off your cell phone.

- *Remember that time is precious.* Many people learn to value their time only when they face a terminal illness. Try to value each day. Time spent not enjoying life is a tremendous waste!

Manage Your Finances Higher education can impose a huge financial burden on parents, students, and communities. In recent studies, nearly two-thirds of students indicated that they have "some" or "major" concerns regarding their ability to pay for their education.[41] The economic downturn of the past few years is pushing already financially stressed students and their families further toward the breaking

downshifting Forging new values that include stepping back to a simpler life

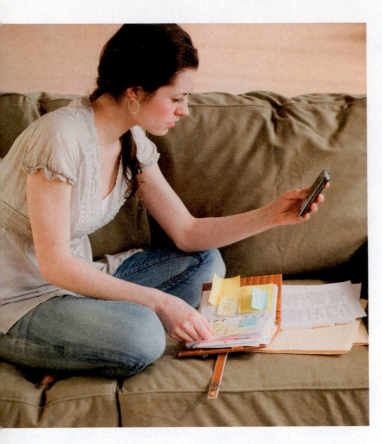

point. Many students must work part or full time in addition to carrying heavy class loads, and some have increasing levels of credit card debt.

Here are a few tips for easing your financial stress:

- Develop a realistic budget of monthly expenses and what you really need.
- Pay bills immediately and consider online banking to avoid late fees.
- Take money-management seminars and courses.
- Avoid unsolicited credit card offers.
- Take on as little new debt as possible.

Managing Your Thoughts and Emotions

Just as we can manage our time and finances, we can learn to manage how we think and react to events and to our emotions.

Manage Your Thinking Our "negative scripts" about ourselves contribute to our stress. When we see ourselves as unable to cope (i.e., when we have low self-efficacy), we tend to handle life's problems and stresses more poorly. You can change negative scripts to more positive ones, however, and in the process reduce your stress responses. Successful stress management involves developing and practicing self-esteem skills, such as applying positive thinking and examining self-talk to reduce negative and irrational responses. Focus on your current capabilities rather than on past problems.

Here are specific actions you can take to develop better mental skills for stress management:

- *Worry constructively.* Don't waste time and energy worrying about things you can't change or events that may never happen.

- *Perceive life as changeable.* If you accept that change is a natural part of living and growing, the jolt from changes will become less stressful.

- *Consider alternatives.* Remember, there is seldom only one appropriate action. Anticipating options will help you plan for change and adjust more rapidly.

- *Moderate your expectations.* Aim high but be realistic about your circumstances and motivation.

- *Don't rush into action.* Think before you act. Tolerate mistakes by yourself and others. Rather than getting angry and stressed by mishaps, evaluate what happened, learn from them, and plan to avoid future occurrences.

- *Take things less seriously.* Try to keep the real importance of things in perspective. Ask yourself: How much will this matter in two weeks? Six months?

Manage Negative Emotions and Anger Stress management involves learning to identify emotional reactions that are based on irrational beliefs and negative self-talk. Identifying those can allow you to deal with the belief or emotion in a healthy and appropriate way.

LIVE IT! ONLINE
Worksheet 11
Anger Log

Learning anger management is particularly important. Anger can be constructive if it mobilizes us to stand up for ourselves or to accomplish something others think we are incapable of. However, a habit of responding angrily when our wants or desires are thwarted can be destructive. The inverse is also true: A habit of boiling with anger inside but not showing it on the outside is linked with high levels of anxiety.[42]

Hotheaded, short-fused people are at risk for health problems. Numerous studies show that anger can significantly increase the risk of heart disease. Stress hormones released during anger may constrict blood vessels in the heart or actually promote clot formation, which can trigger a heart attack.[43] Strategies for controlling and redirecting anger include practicing problem-solving techniques in place of complaining, seeking objective opinions and constructive advice from friends, anticipating situations that trigger your anger and brainstorming solutions in advance, learning to express your feelings constructively, learning to de-escalate from anger by taking deep breaths or counting to 10, and keeping a journal to observe your own reactions and progress in controlling anger.

Seeking Social Support

Making, keeping, and spending time with supportive friends is a central stress-management tool that helps protect you against harmful stressors.[44] Social interactions are important buffers against the effects of stress: A person who is well integrated socially is only half as likely to die from any cause at any age than is a person with few or no sources of social support.[45] Social networking—through Facebook and Twitter, for example—has been an enormously popular way to stay connected. When used obsessively, however, social networking can become its own source of stress.[46] In fact, the larger the network, the greater the incidence of stress-induced colds (upper respiratory infections)![47] In addition, some research suggests that smoking, obesity, and other behaviors may tend to spread through networks of friends.[48] Clearly, social connectedness—pursued thoughtfully and with intelligent choices made toward eating, smoking, and other socially influenced behaviors—is important to wellness. And supportiveness is key; reaching out to friends or relatives who knock you down emotionally becomes a stressor in itself.

The flip side of social connectedness is social isolation, and it, too, has important health implications. Compared to students with a network of friends, isolated students experience more stress, poorer moods, and lower quality sleep.[49] Studies have found deleterious changes to the cardiovascular, immune, and nervous systems in chronically lonely people and these changes may help explain the increased risks for heart disease, infection, and depression in isolated individuals.[50] This research also suggests that a person's actual number of social contacts is less important to wellness than the subjective experience of being unpopular or lonely.[51]

While friends can be important stress reducers, people sometimes need the help of a counselor or support group. Most colleges and universities offer counseling services at no cost for short-term crises. Clergy, instructors, and dorm supervisors also may be helpful resources. If university services are unavailable or if you are concerned about confidentiality, most communities offer low-cost counseling through mental health clinics. You may be able to find and join a stress-reduction program or stress support group through one of these professional resources. Many individual counselors and classes teach stress-reduction techniques to help you manage your stress.

Relaxation Techniques

Deliberate relaxation techniques can be beneficial tools for coping with stress. These techniques tend to focus the mind and breathing. Here are some of the most popular examples.

Relaxation Breathing When we're tense, we often breathe shallowly in the upper chest or even hold our breath, but this kind of breathing can increase anxiety.[52] **Relaxation breathing**—inhaling deeply and rhythmically and involving the abdominal muscles—can help relieve tension and increase oxygen levels in

> **relaxation breathing** Inhaling deeply and rhythmically, expanding and then relaxing the abdomen; this breathing technique can help relieve tension and increase oxygen intake

Progressive Muscle Relaxation

Progressive muscle relaxation involves systematically contracting and relaxing different muscle groups in your body. The standard pattern is to begin with the feet and work your way up your body, contracting and releasing as you go. With practice, you can quickly identify tension in your body when you are facing stressful situations and consciously release that tension to calm yourself.

Sit or lie down in a comfortable position and follow the steps below: Start with one foot. Inhale to the count of five, contracting the muscle of your foot. Hold for three seconds and notice the feeling of tension. Exhale to the count of eight, slowly releasing the muscles. Notice the feeling of tension flowing away. Repeat the same steps contracting and releasing your foot and lower leg, then your entire leg.

Follow the same sequence with your other foot and leg. Starting with one hand, follow the same sequence for both arms. Continue these isolations as you progress up your body, contracting and then relaxing your abdomen, then chest, followed by neck and shoulders, and ending with your face.

Hint: When you isolate and tense a muscle group, be sure not to contract too tightly. This can cause cramping, especially in your toes, feet, calves, and neck. You may want to record the steps of PMR beforehand. Some prefer to memorize the sequence of muscle groups and repeat the instructions mentally. Alternatively, ask another person to read the instructions out loud.

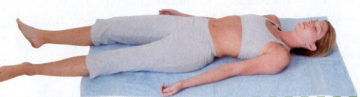

the blood. This, in turn, can boost energy and sharpen thinking. Relaxation breathing, also called *diaphragmatic breathing,* is easy and can be done sitting in a chair or lying down, alone or in a small group, and for a few minutes or longer. The object is to expand the lungs fully by drawing downward with the diaphragm and outward with the abdomen, then releasing fully.

Progressive Muscle Relaxation **Progressive muscle relaxation (PMR)** releases tension in the muscles, muscle group by muscle group. To do PMR, lie down in a quiet, comfortable place and devote 10 or 20 minutes to gradually letting go of accumulated stiffness and tension in the affected muscles. The box Progressive Muscle Relaxation shows you how. You can do this alone or in a group as a way to relax and refresh yourself fully. Some people also use it as a means of falling asleep.

Meditation There are dozens of forms of meditation. Most involve sitting quietly for 15 to 30 minutes and focusing on breathing, body sensations, and detaching from stray thoughts and worries. Researchers have confirmed that meditation reduces the stress response, cuts symptoms of inflammation, boosts the immune response, and improves mental functioning.[53] Meditation also shifts brain activity from the right prefrontal lobe, associated with unhappiness, anger, and distress, and toward the left prefrontal lobe, associated with happiness and enthusiasm. See Activate, Motivate, and Advance: A Meditation Program at the end of this chapter for guidance on beginning a meditation practice.

SEE IT! ONLINE
Meditating to Happiness

Yoga Yoga, a set of stretching, relaxation, and breathing movements based on ancient Indian practices, has both physiological and psychological effects. Researchers have documented physical benefits to flexibility and muscular strength as well reductions in stress, anxiety, and chronic pain, and even increased adherence to other kinds of physical exercise programs.[54] The Activate, Motivate, and Advance: Yoga Program at the end of this chapter will guide you through some yoga routines.

SEE IT! ONLINE
Beginner's Guide to Yoga

Biofeedback **Biofeedback** involves monitoring physical stress responses such as brain activity, blood

progressive muscle relaxation (PMR) A stress-management technique that identifies tension stored in the muscles and releases it, one muscle group at a time

biofeedback A stress-management technique that teaches you to alter automatic physiological responses such as body temperature, heart rate, or sweating

pressure, muscle tension, and heart rate with a special machine and then learning to consciously alter these responses. Biofeedback is effective for several stress-related conditions, including high blood pressure, headaches, irritable bowel syndrome, and asthma.[55]

Hypnosis **Hypnosis** trains people to focus on one thought, object, or voice and to become unusually responsive to suggestion. A qualified hypnotherapist can implant a suggestion that directs a patient to resist habits such as smoking or overeating or to lessen phobias such as fear of snakes or air travel. The patient then learns to induce a state of self-hypnosis as a way to relax deeply and reinforce the behavioral changes.

casestudy

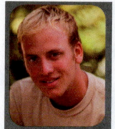

CORY

"This semester was getting out of control. I was exhausted but would have trouble falling asleep, so that was a vicious cycle. I stopped working out—which I used to do twice a week but just didn't have the time for anymore. And I caught another cold at the end of October. My dad started joking that he was healthier than I was! I had to cut out something so I dropped my only elective, Spanish, even though I liked it. I used the extra time to start going back to the gym, and that actually seemed to give me back some energy. I honestly think just those two things alone helped me to get through the rest of the semester. Now, I just need to ace my MCATs …"

THINK! What kinds of stress-related problems was Cory exhibiting? Review the section on stress-management tools. Which strategies did Cory employ?

ACT NOW! Today, make a list of the stress-management strategies you use. Using that same list, put a check by the techniques that seem to be the most effective for you. This week, start observing your periods of stress and ways of coping more carefully. Keep a simple diary of when you feel more stressed and what to do when this happens. Do you see patterns in the timing of your stress periods and how you respond? In two weeks, take one pattern—let's say a recurrent stress associated with commuting to campus—and note three ways you could improve this pattern and your response to it. Over the next few days, try each of your ways for coping with the stressor.

HEAR IT! ONLINE

People who exercise regularly and practice one or more of these relaxation methods—relaxation breathing, progressive muscle relaxation, meditation, yoga, biofeedback, and hypnosis—can achieve effective relief from stress symptoms. Many will also see improvement in medical conditions that are worsened by stress.

hypnosis A medical and psychiatric tool that trains people to focus on one thought, object, or voice and to become unusually responsive to suggestion

Spiritual Practice

Several medical studies have discovered correlations between spirituality and wellness. Prayer, for example, elicits the same relaxation response attained through other stress-management techniques: lowered blood pressure, heart rate, breathing and metabolism, and a more vigorous immune response.[56] Spirituality is also correlated with a reduced *perception* of stress in one's life.

Developing one's spirituality can be more than just an internal process. It can also be a social process that enhances your relationships with others. The abilities to give and take, speak and listen, and forgive and move on are integral to any process of spiritual development.

LIVE IT! ONLINE
Worksheet 7
Developing Your
Spirituality

How Can I Create My Own Stress Management Plan?

Tools such as self-assessment, drawing up a behavior change contract, and journaling can help you reduce your stress levels. Lab 9.1 helps you assess situations that may leave you susceptible to chronic stress. Using this information, target for change one or more behaviors that contribute to your increased stress.

Then, evaluate the behavior(s) you have chosen. Identify your stress-producing behavior patterns. What can you change now? What can you change in the near future? Select one stress-producing behavior pattern that you want to change. Devise an action plan and create a behavior change contract using **Lab 9.3**. As you learned earlier, your behavior change contract should include your long-term goals for change, your short-term goals, the rewards you

DO IT! ONLINE

will give yourself for reaching these goals, potential obstacles along the way, and strategies for overcoming these obstacles.

Chart your progress in your journal. At the end of a week, evaluate how successful you were in following your plan. What helped you to be successful? What obstacles to change did you encounter? What will you do differently next week? After you assess yourself, make a plan and revise it as needed. Are your short-term goals attainable? Are the rewards satisfying? Do you need to go beyond your own self-efforts and enlist the help of your peers or professionals? If you think you need professional support, start by consulting the student health service for advice and direction on finding suitable counselors, therapists, or stress-management support groups.

CHAPTER IN REVIEW

MasteringHealth™

Build your knowledge—and wellness!—in the Study Area of MasteringHealth with a variety of study tools.

SEE IT! ONLINE

videos

Stress Can Damage Women's Health

Meditating to Happiness

Beginner's Guide to Yoga

HEAR IT! ONLINE

audio tools

Audio case study

MP3 chapter review

REVIEW IT! ONLINE

chapter review

Chapter reading quizzes

Glossary flashcards

LIVE IT! ONLINE

programs & behavior change

Customizable four-week starter and intermediate meditation programs

Customizable four-week starter and intermediate yoga programs

Take Charge of Your Health! Worksheets:

Worksheet 4 Sleep Inventory

Worksheet 7 Developing Your Spirituality

Worksheet 8 Stress Reaction

Worksheet 9 Stress Tolerance Test

Worksheet 11 Anger Log

Behavior Change Log Book and Wellness Journal

labs

Lab 9.1 How Stressed Are You?

Lab 9.2 Managing Your Time

Lab 9.3 Your Personal Stress Management Plan

DO IT! ONLINE

reviewquestions

1. Graduating from college and moving to a new city can create stress as well as provide an opportunity for growth. This type of stress is called
   a. strain.
   b. distress.
   c. eustress.
   d. adaptive response.

2. The physiological instinct to flee from or confront a threat is called
   a. homeostasis.
   b. the fight-or-flight response.
   c. allostasis.
   d. allostatic load.

3. *Homeostasis* describes
   a. the body's "normal" or "steady state."
   b. long-term wear-and-tear on the body.
   c. sustained stress.
   d. the exhaustion stage of the general adaptation syndrome.

4. Contemporary researchers have modified one stage of Hans Selye's general adaptation syndrome. Which one is it?
   a. The alarm stage
   b. The resistance stage
   c. The allostasis stage
   d. The exhaustion stage

5. Which of the following statements is true?
   a. Stress reduces the risk of cardiovascular disease.
   b. Stress improves immune system function.
   c. Stress alleviates depression and anxiety.
   d. Stress reduces overall health and wellness.

6. Change, hassles, performance demands, and burnout are all examples of
   a. psychosocial sources of stress.
   b. environmental sources of stress.
   c. internal sources of stress.
   d. homeostasis.

7. *Allostatic load* refers to
   a. changes that occur in the body to maintain homeostasis.
   b. long-term wear-and-tear on the body caused by stress.
   c. the first stage of the general adaptation syndrome.
   d. eustress.

8. Effective stress management includes
   a. getting by on little sleep.
   b. reducing exercise and physical activity to allow more time for studying.
   c. eating fast food and junk food to save money and provide comfort.
   d. avoiding alcohol and tobacco.

9. *Relaxation breathing* refers to
   a. inhaling deeply and rhythmically to relieve tension and increase oxygen levels in the blood.
   b. progressive muscle relaxation.
   c. monitoring physical stress responses and then consciously working to alter those responses.
   d. biofeedback.

10. What stress-fighting technique allows people to become unusually responsive to suggestion?
    a. Meditation
    b. Massage
    c. Biofeedback
    d. Hypnosis

critical thinkingquestions

1. Compare and contrast distress and eustress. In what ways are both types of stress potentially harmful?
2. Describe the body's physiological response to stress.
3. What are some of the health risks that result from chronic stress? Summarize the main points of the general adaptation syndrome and the allostatic load model.
4. What major factors seem to influence the nature and extent of a person's susceptibility to stress? Explain how social support, self-esteem, personality, and coping strategies may make a person more or less susceptible.

references

1. American Psychological Association, "Stress in America: Our Health at Risk," *Monitor on Psychology* 43, no. 3 (2012): 18, www.apa.org.
2. American College Health Association, *American College Health Association–National College Health Assessment II (ACHA-NCHA II) Reference Group Executive Summary Fall 2012* (Hanover, MD: American College Health Association, 2013).
3. H. Selye, "The General-Adaptation-Syndrome," *Annual Review of Medicine* 2 (1951): 327–42.
4. B. McEwen and T. Seeman, "Allostatic Load and Allostasis," John D. and Catherine T. MacArthur Research Network on Socioeconomic Status and Health, University of California at San Francisco (revised 2009).
5. Ibid.
6. A. Steptoe and M. Kivimaki, "Stress and Cardiovascular Disease," *Nature Reviews Cardiology* 9, no. 6 (2012): 360–70, doi: 10.1038/nrcardio.2012.45.
7. A. Mokdal et al., "Actual Causes of Death in the United States 2000," *Journal of the American Medical Association* 291, no. 10 (2004): 1238–45.
8. E. Backe et al., "The Role of Psychosocial Stress at Work for the Development of Cardiovascular Disease: A Systematic Review," *International Archives of Occupational and Environmental Health* 85, no. 1 (2011): 67–79, doi: 10.1007/s00420-011-0643-6; A. Steptoe, A. Rosengren, and P. Hjemdahl, "Introduction to Cardiovascular Disease, Stress, and Adaptation," in *Stress and Cardiovascular Disease*, eds. A. Steptoe, A. Rosengren, and P. Hjemdahl (New York: Springer, 2012), 1–14.
9. S. Cohen et al., "Chronic Stress, Glucocorticoid Receptor Resistance, Inflammation, and Disease Risk," *Proceedings of the National Academy of Sciences for the United States of America* (2012), doi: 10.1073/pnas.1118355109.
10. M. Kivimaki et al., "Job Strain as a Risk Factor for Coronary Heart Disease: A Collaborative Meta-Analysis of Individual Participants," *The Lancet* 380, no. 9852 (2012): 1491–97, doi: 10.1016/S0140-6736(12)60994-5; E. Mostofsky et al., "Risk of Acute Myocardial Infarction after the Death of a Significant Person on One's Life. The Determinants of Myocardial Infarction Onset Study," *Circulation* 125, no. 3 (2012): 491–96, doi: 10.1161/CIRCULATIONAHA.111.061770.
11. J. Campisi et al., "Acute Psychosocial Stress Differentially Influences Salivary Endocrine and Immune Measures in Undergraduate Students," *Physiology and Behavior* 107, no. 3 (2012): 317–21, doi: 10.1016/j.physbeh.2012.09.003; G. Marshall, ed., "Stress and Immune-Based Diseases," *Immunology and Allergy Clinics*

of North America 31, no. 1 (2011): 317–21; M. L. Hanke et al., "Beta Adrenergic Blockade Decreases the Immunomodulatory Effects of Social Disruption Stress," *Brain, Behavior & Immunity* 26, no. 7 (2012): 1150–59, doi: 10.1016/j.bbi.2012.07.011.

12. S. C. Segerstrom and G. E. Miller, "Psychological Stress and the Human Immune System," *Psychological Bulletin* 130, no. 4 (2004): 601–30, doi: 10.1037/0033-2909.130.4.601.

13. B. C. Finger et al., "High-Fat diet Selectively Protects against the Effects of Chronic Social Stress in the Mouse," *Neuroscience* 192 (2011): 351–60, doi: 10.1016/j.neuroscience.2011.06.072; V. Michopoulos, "Social Stress Interacts with Diet History to Promote Emotional Feeding in Females," *Psychoneuroendocrinology* 37, no. 9 (2012): 1479–90, doi: 10.1016/j.psyneuen.2012.02.002; V. Vicennati et al., "Cortisol, Energy Intake, and Food Frequency in Overweight/Obese Women," *Nutrition* 27, no. 6 (2011): 677–80, doi: 10.1016/j.nut.2010.07.016; K. Scott, S. Melhorn, and R. Sakai, "Effects of Chronic Social Stress on Obesity," *Current Obesity Reports Online First* 1, no. 1 (2012): 16–25, doi: 10.1007/s13679-011-0006-3.

14. K. Thorslund et al., "The Expression of Serotonin Transporter Protein Correlates with the Severity of Psoriasis and Chronic Stress," *Archives of Dermatological Research* 305, no. 2 (2013): 99–104, doi: 10.1007/s00403-012-1303-8; D. K. Hall-Flavin, "Stress and Hair Loss: Are They Related?" MayoClinic.com, 2012, www.mayoclinic.com

15. T. Morris et al., "Stress and Chronic Illness: The Case of Diabetes," *Journal of Adult Development* 18, no. 2 (2011): 70–80, doi: 10.1007/s10804-010-9118-3.

16. National Digestive Diseases Information Clearinghouse (NDDIC), "What I Need to Know about Irritable Bowel Syndrome," NIH Publication No. 12–4686, Last updated August 2012, www.digestive.niddk.nih.gov

17. V. Bitsika, C. Sharpley, and R. Bell, "The Contribution of Anxiety and Depression to Fatigue among a Sample of Australian University Students: Suggestions for University Counselors," *Counseling Psychology Quarterly* 22, no. 2 (2009): 243–53.

18. M. Agnieszka et al., "Chronic Stress Impairs Prefrontal Cortex-Dependent Response Inhibition and Spatial Working Memory," *Behavioral Neuroscience* 126, no. 5 (2012): 605–19, doi: 10.1037/a0029642; L. Schwabe, T. Wolf, and M. Oitzl, "Memory Formation under Stress: Quantity and Quality," *Neuroscience and Biobehavioral Reviews* 34, no. 4 (2009): 584–91, doi: 10.1016/j.neubiorev.2009.11.015.

19. M. Marin et al., "Chronic Stress, Cognitive Functioning and Mental Health," *Neurobiology of Learning and Memory* 96, no. 4 (2011): 583–95, doi: 10.1016/j.nlm.2011.02.016; E. Dias-Ferreira et al., "Chronic Stress Causes Frontostriatal Reorganization and Affects Decision-Making," *Science* 325, no. 5940 (2009): 621–5, doi: 10.1126/science.1171203.

20. American Psychological Association, "Missing the Mark on Stress Management," in *The Impact of Stress*, 2012, www.apa.org

21. American Psychological Association, "Stress at Any Age Is Still Stress." *Stress by Generation: 2012*, www.apa.org

22. Ibid.

23. J. H. Pryor et al., *The American Freshman: National Norms Fall 2012* (Los Angeles: Higher Education Research Institute, 2012), Available at http://heri.ucla.edu

24. D. Pedersen, "Stress Carry-Over and College Student Health Outcomes," *College Student Journal* 46, no. 3 (2012): 620–27.

25. D. J. Maybery and D. Graham, "Hassles and Uplifts: Including Interpersonal Events," *Stress and Health* 17, no 2 (2001): 91–104, doi: 10.1002/smi.891; R. Blonna, *Coping with Stress in a Changing World*, 4th ed. (New York: McGraw-Hill, 2006).

26. C. E. Chloe et al., "Neighbourhood Socioeconomic Status and Biological 'Wear and Tear' in a Nationally Representative Sample of US Adults," *Journal of Epidemiology and Community Health* 64, no. 10 (2010): 860–65, doi:10.1136/jech.2008.084814.

27. APA, Stress by Generation, 2012; H. W. Bland et al., "Stress Tolerance: New Challenges for Millennial College Students," *College Student Journal* 46, no. 2 (2012): 362–75.

28. S. Abraham, "Relationship between Stress and Perceived Self-Efficacy among Nurses in India," International Conference on Technology and Business Management, 2012, www.ictbm.org; Seaward, *Managing Stress*, 2012.

29. J. S. Lee et al., "Perceived Stress and Self-Esteem Mediate the Effects of Work-Related Stress on Depression," *Stress & Health: Journal of the International Society for the Investigation of Stress* 29, no. 1 (2013): 75–81, doi: 10.1002/smi.2428; C. Eisenbarth, "Does Self-Esteem Moderate the Relations among Perceived Stress, Coping, and Depression?" *College Student Journal* 46, no. 1 (2012): 149–57.

30. M. Friedman and R. H. Rosenman, *Type A Behavior and Your Heart* (New York: Knopf, 1974).

31. S. Kobasa, "Stressful Life Events, Personality, and Health: An Inquiry into Hardiness," *Journal of Personality and Social Psychology* 37 (1979): 1–11.

32. B. J. Crowley et al., "Psychological Hardiness and Adjustment to Life Events in Adulthood," *Journal of Adult Development* 10 (2003): 237–48.

33. L. Poole et al., "Associations of Objectively Measured Physical Activity with Daily Mood Ratings and Psychophysiological Stress Responses in Women," *Psychophysiology* 48, no. 8 (2011): 1165–72, doi: 10.1111/j.1469-8986.2011.01184.x; A. Leal-Cerro et al., "Mechanisms Underlying the Neuroendocrine Response to Physical Exercise," *Journal of Endocrinological Investigation* 26, no. 9 (2003): 879–85.

34. U. Rimmele et al., "Trained Men Show Lower Cortisol, Heart Rate, and Psychological Responses to Psychosocial Stress Compared with Untrained Men," *Psychoneuroendocrinology* 32, no. 6 (2007): 627–35.

35. A. Tsatsoulis and S. Fountoulakis, "The Protective Role of Exercise on Stress System Dysregulation and Comorbidities," *Annals of the New York Academy of Sciences* 1083 (2006): 196–213.

36. National Institute of Alcohol Abuse and Alcoholism, "Alcohol and Sleep," *Alcohol Alert* 41, http://pubs.niaaa.nih.gov (1998).

37. I. Ebrahim et al., "Alcohol and Sleep I: Effects on Normal Sleep," *Alcoholism: Clinical and Experimental Research* 37, no. 4 (2013): 539–49, doi: 10.1111/acer.12006.

38. G. Colom et al., "Study of the Effect of Positive Humour as a Variable That Reduces Stress. Relationship of Humour with Personality and Performance Variables," *Psychology in Spain* 15, no. 1 (2011): 9–21.

39. H. W. Bland et al., "Stress Tolerance: New Challenges for Millennial College Students," 2012.

40. I. R. Galatzer-Levy et al., "Coping Flexibility, Potentially Traumatic Life Events, and Resilience: A Prospective Study of College Student Adjustment," *Journal of Social and Clinical Psychology* 31, no. 6 (2012): 542–67.

41. J. H. Pryor et al., *The American Freshman: National Norms Fall 2012*, 2012.

42. S. S. Deschenes et al., "The Role of Anger in Generalized Anxiety Disorder," *Cognitive Behaviour Therapy* 41, no. 3 (2012): 261–71, doi: 10.1080/16506073.2012.666564.

43. L. D. Kubzansky et al., "Shared and Unique Contributions of Anger, Anxiety, and Depression to Coronary Heart Disease: A Prospective Study in the Normative Aging Study," *Annals of Behavioral Medicine* 31, no. 1 (2006): 21–9.

44. P. A. Bovier, E. Chamot, and T. V. Perneger, "Perceived Stress, Internal Resources, and Social Support as Determinants of Mental Health among Young Adults," *Quality of Life Research* 13, no. 1 (2004): 161–70; A. M. McLaughlin et al., *Determinants of Minority Mental Health and Wellness* (New York: Springer, 2009); L. Crockett et al., "Acculturative Stress, Social Support and Coping: Relations to Psychological Adjustment among Mexican American College Students," *Cultural Diversity and Ethnic Minority Psychology* 13, no. 4 (2007): 347–55; J. Ruthig et al., "Perceived Academic Control: Mediating the Effects of Optimism and Social Support on College Students' Psychological Health," *Social Psychology of Education* 12, no. 7 (2009): 233–49, doi: 10.1007/s11218-008-9079-6.

45. S. Levine, D. M. Lyons, and A. F. Schatzberg, "Psychobiological Consequences of Social Relationships," *Annals of the New York Academy of Sciences* 89, no. 7 (1999): 210–8.

46. A. Lenhart et al., "Social Media and Young Adults," Pew Internet and American Life Project, 2010, www.pewinternet.org

47. J. Campisi et al., "Facebook Stress, and Incidence of Upper Respiratory Infection in Undergraduate College Students," *CyberPsychology, Behavior, and Social Networking* 15, no. 12 (2012): 675–81, doi: 10.1089/cyber.2012.0156.

48. J. Couzin, "Friendship as a Health Factor," *Science* 323, no. 5913 (2009): 454–7, doi: 10.1126/science.323.5913.454.

49. J. T. Cacioppo and L. C. Hawkley, "Social Isolation and Health, with an Emphasis on Underlying Mechanisms," *Perspectives in Biology and Medicine* 46, no. 3 Suppl (2003): S39–52.

50. G. Miller, "Why Loneliness Is Hazardous to Your Health," *Science* 331, no. 6014 (2011): 138–40, doi: 10.1126/science.331.6014.138.

51. Ibid.

52. A. Conrad et al., "Psychophysiological Effects of Breathing Instructions for Stress Management," *Applied Psychophysiology and Biofeedback* 32, no. 2 (2007): 89–98.

53. M. A. Rosenkranz et al., "A Comparison of Mindfulness-Based Stress Reduction and an Active Control in Modulation of Neurogenic Inflammation," *Brain, Behavior, and Immunity* 27, no. 1 (2013): 174–84, doi: 10.1016/j.bbi.2012.10.013; Y. Singh, R. Sharma, and A. Talwar, "Immediate and Long-Term Effects of Meditation on Acute Stress Reactivity, Cognitive Functions, and Intelligence," *Alternative Therapies in Health & Medicine* 18, no. 6 (2012): 46–53; S. Jain et al., "A Randomized Controlled Trial of Mindfulness Meditation versus Relaxation Training: Effects on Distress, Positive States of Mind, Rumination, and Distraction," *Annals of Behavioral Medicine* 33, no. 1 (2007): 11–21; R. J. Davidson et al., "Alterations in Brain and Immune Function Produced by Mindfulness Meditation," *Psychosomatic Medicine* 65, no. 4 (2003): 564–70.

54. A. W. Li and C. A. Goldsmith, "The Effects of Yoga on Anxiety and Stress," *Alternative Medicine Review* 17, no. 1 (2012): 21–35; A. Bussing et al., "Effects of Yoga Interventions on Pain and Pain-Associated Disability: A Meta-Analysis," *Journal of Pain* 13, no. 1 (2012): 1–9, doi: 10.1016/j.jpain.2011.10.001; S. Bryan, G. Pinto Zipp, and R. Parasher, "The Effects of Yoga on Psychosocial Variables and Exercise Adherence: A Randomized, Controlled Pilot Study," *Alternative Therapies in Health and Medicine* 18, no. 5 (2012): 50–9.

55. Mayo Clinic Staff, "Biofeedback: Using Your Mind to Improve Your Health," January 2013, www.mayoclinic.com

56. D. K. Reibel et al., "Mindfulness-Based Stress Reduction and Health-Related Quality of Life in a Heterogeneous Patient Population," *General Hospital Psychiatry* 23, no. 4 (2001): 183–92; R. Sethness et al., "Cardiac Health: Relationships among Hostility, Spirituality, and Health Risk," *Journal of Nursing Care Quality* 20, no. 1 (2005): 81–9; L. E. Carlson et al., "Mindfulness-Based Stress Reduction in Relation to Quality of Life, Mood, Symptoms of Stress and Levels of Cortisol, Dehydroepiandrosterone Sulfate (DHEAS) and Melatonin in Breast and Prostate Cancer Outpatient," *Psychoneuroendocrinology* 29, no. 4 (2004): 448–74.

getfitgraphic references

1. American College Health Association, *American College Health Association–National College Health Assessment II (ACHA-NCHA II) Reference Group Executive Summary Fall 2012*, 2013.

2. Ibid.

3. Ibid.

4. S. B. He et al., "Exercise Intervention May Prevent Depression," *International Journal of Sports Medicine* 33, no. 7 (2012): 525-30, doi: 10.1055/s-0032-1306325.

5. D. Scully et al., "Physical Exercise and Psychological Well Being: A Critical Review," *British Journal of Sports Medicine* 32, no. 2 (1998): 111–20.

Name: _____   Date: _____

Instructor: _____   Section: _____

Purpose: To uncover your major stressors and your stress levels during the past year.

Directions: Learning to "de-stress" starts with an honest examination of your life experiences and your reactions to stressful situations. Respond to each section, assigning points as directed. Total the points from each section, then under scoring, add them and compare to the life-stressor scale.

SECTION I: RECENT HISTORY

In the last year, how many of the following major life events have you experienced? (Give yourself **five points** for each event you experienced; if you experienced an event more than once, give yourself **ten points**, etc.)

1. Death of a close family member of friend	_____
2. Ending a relationship (whether by your own choice or not)	_____
3. Major financial issue(s) jeopardizing your ability to stay in college	_____
4. Major move, leaving friends, family, and past activities behind	_____
5. Serious illness (your own)	_____
6. Serious illness (of someone close to you)	_____
7. Marriage or entering a serious relationship	_____
8. Loss of a beloved pet	_____
9. Involvement in a legal dispute or issue	_____
10. Involvement in a hostile, violent, or threatening relationship	_____
Total Points	_____

SECTION II: SELF-REFLECTION

For each of the following, indicate where you are on the scale of 0 to 5 then add up the points.

	Strongly Disagree					Strongly Agree
1. I have a lot of worries at home and at school.	0	1	2	3	4	5
2. My friends or family members put too much pressure on me.	0	1	2	3	4	5
3. I am often distracted and have trouble focusing on schoolwork.	0	1	2	3	4	5
4. I am highly disorganized and do assignments at the last minute.	0	1	2	3	4	5
5. My life seems to have far too many crisis situations.	0	1	2	3	4	5
6. I spend a lot of time sitting; I don't have time to exercise.	0	1	2	3	4	5
7. I don't have enough control in decisions that affect my life.	0	1	2	3	4	5
8. I wake up most days feeling tired/like I need a lot more sleep.	0	1	2	3	4	5
9. I often feel that I am alone and don't fit in very well.	0	1	2	3	4	5
10. I have few friends or people with whom to share thought/feelings.	0	1	2	3	4	5

(Continued)

	Strongly Disagree					Strongly Agree
11. I am uncomfortable in my body and wish I could change my looks.	0	1	2	3	4	5
12. I'm unsure of whether my major will lead to a job after graduation.	0	1	2	3	4	5
13. If I have to wait, I quickly become irritated and upset.	0	1	2	3	4	5
14. I get upset with myself unless I'm the best in activities and classes.	0	1	2	3	4	5
15. World events upset me and I'm angry about people's behavior.	0	1	2	3	4	5
16. I'm overloaded and there are never enough hours in the day.	0	1	2	3	4	5
17. I feel uneasy when I'm caught up, relaxing, or doing nothing.	0	1	2	3	4	5
18. I often check emails/tweets/text messages during the night.	0	1	2	3	4	5
19. I seldom get enough alone time each day.	0	1	2	3	4	5
20. I worry about whether or not others like me.	0	1	2	3	4	5
21. I am struggling in my classes and worry about failing.	0	1	2	3	4	5
22. My relationship with my family is distant and unsupportive.	0	1	2	3	4	5
23. I tend to be critical and think negatively about the people I observe.	0	1	2	3	4	5
24. Most people are selfish and distrustful and I'm careful around them.	0	1	2	3	4	5
25. Life is basically unfair and most of the time, I can't change things.	0	1	2	3	4	5
26. I give more than I get in relationships with people.	0	1	2	3	4	5
27. What I do is often not good enough and I should do better.	0	1	2	3	4	5
28. My friends would describe me as highly stressed and quick to react to people and events with anger and/or frustration.	0	1	2	3	4	5
29. My friends are always telling me I "need a vacation to relax."	0	1	2	3	4	5
30. Overall, the quality of my life right now isn't all that great.	0	1	2	3	4	5
Total Points	0	1	2	3	4	5

SECTION III: SCORING

Total your points from Sections I and II: _____

The following scores are not meant to be diagnostic, but they do serve as an indicator of potential problem areas. If your scores are:

0-50, your stress levels are low. It is still worth examining areas where you did score points and taking action to reduce your stress levels further.

51-100, your stress levels are moderate, and you may need to reduce certain stresses in your life. Long-term stress and pressure can be counterproductive. Consider what you can do to change your perceptions, your behaviors, or your environment.

100-150, your stress levels are high, and you are probably quite stressed. Examine your major stressors and begin making a plan right now to reduce your stress levels. Delaying this action could lead to significant stress-related problems that affect your wellness, your grades, your social life, and your future!

151-200, you are carrying very high stress and without some significant changes, you could be heading for some serious difficulties. Locate a campus counselor with whom you can share the major issues you just identified as causing stress. Aim to get more sleep and exercise and find time to relax. Surround yourself with people who are supportive and make you feel safe and competent.

SECTION IV: REFLECTION

Were you surprised by your total stress score? Go back over the list of stressors and find two that you could eliminate with simple actions. Jot them here along with the action for each.

Stressor _____ Action _____

Stressor _____ Action _____

Name: _____ Date: _____

Instructor: _____ Section: _____

Purpose: Learn a concrete way to manage your time so you can accomplish the things you want to.

SECTION I: ANALYZING YOUR TIME

Every evening for a week fill out the following table, listing how much time you spent doing each activity that day.

Activity	Monday	Tuesday	Wednesday	Thursday	Friday	Saturday	Sunday	Total Hours
Getting ready								
On the road								
In class								
Working for pay								
Exercising								
Eating								
Studying								
Watching TV or movies								
Using computer (school)								
Using computer (recreational)								
Spending time with friends								
Leisure activities								
Sleeping								
Other (specify)								

At the end of the week, total the hours for each activity. Are there any activities that you would like to do more or less frequently? You can use the rest of this lab to clarify your goals and set up your calendar so that you accomplish the things that you want to accomplish.

SECTION II: CLARIFY YOUR GOALS AND CREATE YOUR TASK LIST

1. On a piece of paper or in a journal, list your goals down the left side. Goals can be anything from "go to nursing school" to "learn to play racquetball." Make the goals specific. Instead of "be more musical," come up with a concrete goal such as "learn to play guitar."

2. On the right side of the paper, break each of your goals down into specific tasks. For example, as part of the nursing school goal, you might add "make a list of possible schools" to the task list.

3. Next, prioritize the tasks by numbering them in order of importance.

SECTION III: ENTER YOUR TASKS ONTO YOUR CALENDAR

In your calendar, write the commitments you already have—classes, job, exercise, rehearsals, and so on. Be sure to look at the schedule you filled out in Section I. Now is your chance to think about what activities you want to continue and which you would like to curb.

When you have all of your commitments written in, you'll be able to see windows of free time in your schedule. Now review your task list from Section II and choose the most important tasks to put in your free time. Make sure these tasks are things that are really important to you to accomplish.

SECTION IV: MAKE IT HAPPEN

Go over your schedule at the start of each day. This gives you a chance to prepare for the day and remember things that you need to take with you. At the end of the day, cross off tasks you were able to accomplish and rearrange (or delete) tasks that you didn't do.

SECTION V: REFLECTION AND EVALUATION

1. Describe any times you found yourself procrastinating. What do you think caused that? Were you bored? Were you overwhelmed? What specific thing could you do next time to get back on track quicker? For example, if you were overwhelmed, is there an advisor you could talk to who could help you prioritize?

_____

_____

_____

2. Did you check your schedule each morning, write in tasks, check them off, and do weekly planning? If not, what got in the way? What could you do differently next time?

_____

_____

_____

3. Did you find other people encroaching on your time? What happened? How could you handle that differently next time?

_____

_____

_____

4. Review your goals and tasks for the next week, adjust the list to reflect tasks you've accomplished or any other changes, and then block off time on your calendar for the most important items. Remember that time management is an ongoing exercise. Spend at least 20 minutes at the start of your week planning for the upcoming week, then stay focused on the goals you want to accomplish!

Name: _____   Date: _____

Instructor: _____   Section: _____

Purpose: To develop a stress-management plan that targets the key sources of stress in your life.

SECTION I: EXAMINE YOUR BEHAVIOR AND ATTITUDES

1. Enter your results from the Scoring section of Lab 9.1 here:

Score: _____   Stress level: _____

Suggested actions: _____

2. Do you feel that stress is a problem in your life right now?   ☐ Yes   ☐ No

If your score indicated high levels of stress in Lab 9.1, and yet you don't see stress as an issue to address, consider your readiness for change.

SECTION II: IDENTIFY MAJOR SOURCES OF STRESS

After reviewing your entries in the stress survey in Lab 9.1, describe your main sources of stress, grouping them into the following categories:

College

_____

_____

Family

_____

_____

Fitness/Wellness Issues

_____

_____

Social Issues

_____

_____

Money Matters

_____

_____

Time-Management Issues

_____

_____

SECTION III: SET REALISTIC GOALS

Use this chart to rank your top five stressors from Section II, in order of urgency. Note ways to modify or eliminate each stressor. Note stress-reduction techniques that you can apply when the stressor arises.

	Stressors	Can I Modify or Eliminate the Stressor? Y/N	Can I Reduce Stress Symptoms? Y/N
Most urgent	1.		
⇓	2.		
⇓	3.		
⇓	4.		
Least urgent	5.		

SECTION IV: DEVISE A STRATEGY AND AN ACTION PLAN

Use this section to target the most urgent source of stress in your life first, and then address additional stressors as you feel ready to work on them.

1. Stressor:_____

2. Is it possible that I will need help from others?   ☐ Y   ☐ N

If yes, ask yourself the following:

What professional resources are available where I live, work, or go to school? _____

_____

_____

How can I get my friends or family involved? _____

_____

3. List general strategies for modifying or eliminating environmental stressors that apply to more than one of your most urgent examples: _____

_____

4. What stress-management techniques can I use to relieve my own ongoing or recurrent symptoms of stress? (Consider relaxation breathing, progressive muscle relaxation, visual imagery, meditation, yoga, improved fitness, improved diet, better time-management skills, and enhanced spiritual connectedness.)

_____

_____

5. How can I plan ahead to avoid this stressor in the future?

_____

_____

6. How will I reward myself for sticking to my plan? _____

_____

SECTION V: CREATE A BEHAVIOR CHANGE CONTRACT

Use the information from Section IV to develop a behavior change contract that targets the stressor(s) you selected. A basic behavior change contract is included at the front of this book.

SECTION VI: REFLECTION

How will you be better off by reducing the top stressors in your life?

_____

_____

Activate, Motivate,
& ADVANCE YOUR WELL-BEING

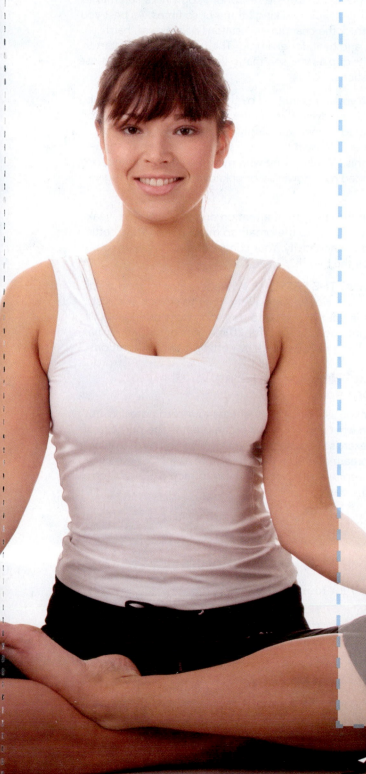

A MEDITATION PROGRAM

SCAN TO SEE IT
ONLINE!

ACTIVATE!

Meditation is a popular relaxation and centering activity. We all experience tension from worrying about or anticipating our problems. Meditation can help us relax and compose ourselves. It instills a sense of well-being that improves many aspects of life. People who meditate regularly often enjoy a realistic sense of optimism, enhanced intimacy, more satisfying social relations, and a stronger ability to pay attention. In short, meditation brings physical, emotional, and intellectual enhancement.

What Do I Need?

LOCATION: You may meditate in your own living space, but be on the lookout for quiet places to meditate on campus, indoors or out. If you meditate at home, be sure to put your living space in order before you start. A clean, tidy place in which to meditate invites the mind to settle down.

TIME: If you live with others, plan to sit at a quiet time of the day, perhaps before your roommates get up or after they leave for the morning. Turn off your cell phone. For the period of time that you meditate you are not available. Place a silent timer, such as a watch or digital alarm clock, in your meditation area so that you can set it and not have to be concerned with keeping track of time while you meditate.

POSTURE: Sitting on the floor with crossed legs is by far the best posture for meditation. Place your hands in your lap or on your thighs, whichever is comfortable for you. Sit on a firm cushion that supports your spine and lifts your buttocks higher than your knees. The height of the cushion is a very individual matter based on comfort.

The first advantage of this posture is its stability. The broad base supports you, inviting relaxation at the physical and mental level. Second, the spine is self-supporting, not resting against anything. This discourages sleepiness and promotes balanced energy. Meditation is very much a physical activity.

If sitting on the floor is too uncomfortable, use a kneeling bench or sit on a firm chair such as a folding chair or a dining room chair. Sit toward the forward edge of the chair—don't lean against the backrest.

CLOTHING: Loose-fitting pants allow the abdomen to relax and allow room for the thighs to rotate outward. Bare feet are most comfortable for sitting cross-legged. It's a good idea to wear a long-sleeved shirt for warmth.

How Do I Start?

BEGIN BY FOCUSING YOUR ATTENTION ON YOUR BREATH: Close your eyes and draw your attention to the area of your abdomen where you find the sensations of breathing most obvious; follow the sequence of sensations occurring as you inhale and exhale. As you mindfully observe the rising and falling of the abdomen, make soft mental notes, "rising" and "falling." Noticing the breath is the primary activity of meditation, and it helps to sharpen and strengthen your attention.

Don't exaggerate the breath, let it be natural. Don't use your imagination to create an image of the breath, just attend to the sensations that are actually occurring.

You may find that your mind wanders off. Gently reapply your attention to your breath. Your mind may wander, and you cannot control it with your will power. Relax! Make a mental note, "wandering, wandering," and aim your focus on the breath again. Already you are learning about stress and how to let go. Try to notice every breath. Watch each breath from the beginning, through the middle, to the end. As a beginner you won't be able to be present with every breath, but you must try. To be patient about this wandering, appreciate how passive your attention is generally. Your attention is drawn to stimulating things and is held there by the excitement. Think about the opening moments of a movie. Does it excite your interest? Must you make a special effort to stay with it, or are you swept along?

By contrast, in meditation you focus inward, on your breath. To avoid boredom, sleepiness, and wandering thoughts you attend to your breath. Through noticing the breath and the sensations of the rising and falling of the abdomen—stretching, tightness, swelling; then softness, cascading, and deflation—you will feel stress leave you.

As you become more skilled, your attention will become sustained and steadier for longer periods of time. Gradually your mind will settle down and your body will relax.

This composure of mind and body is energizing, bright, and pleasant.

FOCUSING ATTENTION ON THE FELT SENSE OF DISCOMFORT: Physical pain or mental pain can be difficult for the body and mind. In trying to push them away, you may experience tension and stress. Try to turn toward what you have been avoiding. The rewards will be immediate.

When physical pain or mental displeasure arises for you, track and scrutinize the sensation, applying a soft mental label "pain" or "disliking" three or so times. As best you can, track the changing sensations of pressure, hardness, and heat, for example. The fear of pain will start to lose its grip as you see that pain is a collection of intense sensations.

When you are disturbed by thinking about someone you dislike, try saying this mantra: "If I have hurt, harmed, or offended anyone knowingly or unknowingly, may I be forgiven." Repeat that several times and then continue with this: "And anyone who may have hurt, harmed, or offended me knowingly or unknowingly, I freely forgive them."

When the strength of attention on the discomfort weakens, turn back to the breath to make a fresh start, setting aside the negativity. Your composure will grow as you focus on the breath.

ENDING THE SESSION: When it is time to stop meditating, move slowly. Take a little time to stretch and rest, write in your journal, and transition from quiet and stillness into activity. Wait for 20 minutes or so before making phone calls, texting, or getting into conversations.

Four-Week Beginning Meditation Program

After you sit, take a few minutes to record notes. Write down what you observed of the breath. The purpose of this exercise is to enhance your ability to pay attention to the breath as it is, in the same spirit as if you were an artist who kept a sketchbook in which to record things seen during the day.

BEGINNER

PROGRAM **GOAL:** Sit for 15 minutes every other day for four weeks.

	Mon	Tue	Wed	Thurs	Fri	Sat	Sun
Week 1	15 min		15 min		15 min		15 min
Week 2		15 min		15 min		15 min	
Week 3	15 min		15 min		15 min		15 min
Week 4		15 min		15 min		15 min	

MOTIVATE!

Create a journal—or use the log on the mobile website—to keep track of your meditation sessions and become aware of the changing quality of your meditation experiences. Here are some other things to bear in mind and potential motivators to consider as you progress in your meditation practice:

ACCEPT THE CHALLENGE: Meditation can bring the benefits of centeredness, relaxation, and brightness of mind. Learning to meditate is a lifelong endeavor. To sit still, watch the breath, focus attention, and calm down sound simple, but they are a challenge! To do them, one must meet and overcome doubt, boredom, desire, irritability, and restlessness in turn.

FACE DISTRACTIONS: When you find yourself stopped by doubt, remember that being able to meet life's challenges with a calm mind is a valuable thing—worth working for. If you keep wanting to get up and eat something or check for text messages, then observe each mental interruption, acknowledge it, and let it go.

ENJOY THE FREEDOM: It is usually a great relief to detach from discomfort and from taking things personally. It is uplifting to be able to relax in the face of annoyances that previously would have provoked resistance and retaliation. When you truly attend to displeasure, annoyances don't dominate or push you

around as they used to. Introspection gives rise to insight and inner freedom.

JOIN A GROUP: Beginners can find it motivating to join a meditation class with a teacher. You may be able to find such a meditation class through a yoga center, through your fitness instructor, or in a local alternative newspaper. If you sit with a group you will enjoy the inspiration and support of the group energy and can begin to feel confident about the benefits of daily practice. If you can't find an established group, you may form your own group of people with similar goals. In a quiet setting, you may want to read a book together, selecting an interesting passage to precede the sitting, or listen to a recorded talk from the Internet before you sit.

ATTEND A RETREAT: In addition to a weekly sitting group, you may want to deepen your learning by going on a silent retreat. Retreats may be for a weekend or for as long as three months! Some retreats are specifically for young people.

ADVANCE!

Meditation is a lifelong affair. When you learn how to meditate, you learn how to be attentive and reflective all the time. You will want to mediate every day. People often find that 45 minutes to an hour daily is enough to see real effects in personality, friendships, and ability to concentrate on work.

INTERMEDIATE

PROGRAM

GOAL: Sit for 20 minutes five days a week, working up to sitting daily for a minimum of 20 minutes.

	Mon	Tue	Wed	Thurs	Fri	Sat	Sun
Week 1	20 min	20 min	20 min	20 min	20 min		
Week 2	20 min	20 min	20 min	20 min	20 min		
Week 3	20 min	20 min	20 min	20 min	20 min	20 min	
Week 4	20 min	20 min	20 min	20 min	20 min	20 min	20 min

Activate, Motivate, & ADVANCE YOUR WELL-BEING

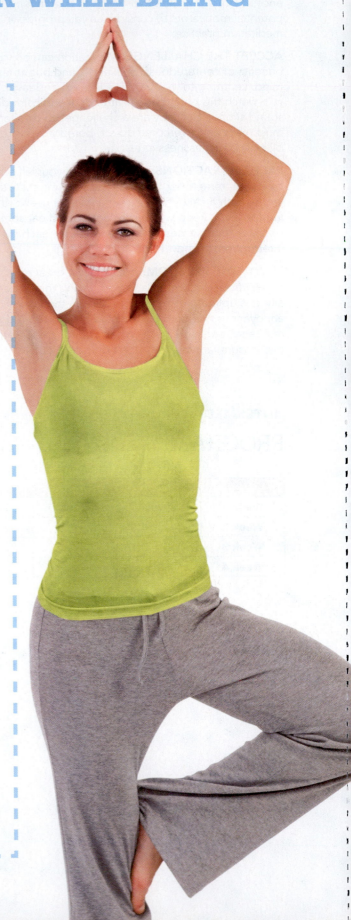

A YOGA PROGRAM

SCAN TO SEE IT
ONLINE!

A C T I V A T E !

Yoga is a fun physical and psychological practice that incorporates stretching, relaxation, and breathing movements to bring greater balance to our body and mind. Yoga's benefits range from enhancing flexibility and muscular strength to reducing tension and stress. The postures can renew, invigorate, and heal the body through stretching and strengthening. Breathing techniques can release tension and stress and bring an overall calmness of mind and spirit. These programs will help you learn how to get started with basic yoga.

What Do I Need?

MATERIALS: Choose a mat at least 1/8 of an inch thick—the thicker the mat the more cushion it will provide for your body. You may also want to use blocks and straps. They aid in supporting the body for postures that might be challenging, especially in the beginning.

LOCATION: You can practice yoga anywhere big enough to lay down a mat. Choose a space that is calm, quiet, and comfortable in light and temperature.

CLOTHING: Wear comfortable clothing that allows you to freely move your body.

How Do I Start?

BREATH: Your breath (referred to as *pranayama* in yoga exercises) is the most important part of yoga. Aim for deep breaths, inhaling and exhaling from the belly. Never force or strain your breathing.

The most common breath used during yoga is called *ujjayi* (pronounced *ooo-ja-i-aa*). Practice this breath while in a seated position. Once you can sustain your ability to breathe in this manner, begin using it during yoga practice.

To perform ujjayi breathing, inhale and exhale slowly and deeply through the nose. You will begin to slightly constrict the passage of air. Your breathing will sound like Darth Vader or like you are fogging up a pair of glasses.

During your yoga practice, every time you lift your chest, inhale, and when you drop your chest, exhale. If you are holding a pose, breathe deeply and slowly so you can hear yourself breathe.

TECHNIQUES: Yoga postures focus on aligning the body. Follow these techniques as you're practicing the different poses:

Maintain an active back extension using core strength, with a neutral spine and pelvis.

During forward bending, hinge from the hips, engaging the abdominal muscles, and keep your knees soft to maintain length and strength in the spine. Avoid bending from the lumbar spine. When returning to a neutral spine from a forward bend, soften your knees and use the muscles in your legs to push you back to a neutral position.

Keep your shoulders relaxed down away from your ears to avoid tension in your neck and shoulders. In most poses, it is safest for your neck to keep your head in line with the spine. You can look up, center, or down, as long as your head remains a natural extension of the spine.

To avoid unnecessary stress to the low back when coming into and out of forward bending in standing poses, sweep your arms out to the sides instead of bringing your arms out in front of you.

To prevent joint injuries and muscular imbalances, distribute your weight evenly into your hands and/or feet when setting the foundation of a pose. Always keep your knees in line with your toes.

Four-Week Beginning Yoga Program

If you're new to yoga or if you've practiced yoga in the past but have taken a break, start with the beginning program. Examples of the poses you'll perform are on pages 357–358. Start each session with corpse pose for 1 minute, which means you will simply lie down, close your eyes, and scan your body for any tension. Breathe with slow, deep inhales and exhales; if you notice any tension in some area of your body, release it as you exhale. For greater relaxation and meditation, end each session with the corpse pose for 5–10 minutes. Hold each pose for 1 count of breath as you inhale and 1 count of breath as you exhale.

BEGINNER

PROGRAM **GOAL:** Practice a basic yoga sequence two to four times a week, building to a total of 120 minutes by week four.

	Mon	Tue	Wed	Thurs	Fri	Sat	Sun
	T	T	T	T	T	T	T
Week 1	20			20			
Week 2	25		25		25		
Week 3	30		30		30		
Week 4	30		30		30		30

T = Total time of session in minutes.

Order of Poses

Corpse Pose
Cat/Cow
Spinal Balance
Downward Facing Dog
Warrior 1 (left foot forward, right foot back, and anchored to the floor)
Triangle
Warrior 2
Extended Angle

Downward Facing Dog
Warrior 1 (right foot forward, left foot back, and anchored to the floor)
Triangle
Warrior 2
Extended Angle
Downward Facing Dog
Cat/Cow
Corpse Pose

MOTIVATE!

The entire yoga practice is about relaxing and listening inwardly to reduce tightness, anxiety, and mind chatter. Keeping a yoga journal of how you feel when doing each pose can help you become aware of your own practice. Here are some other motivators to keep you going when your mind and body want to quit:

NO TIME? NEVERMIND! If you are having difficulty committing to longer practices, start with some deep breathing, neck circles, and then reach your arms up and stretch long. You're already on your way to feeling the benefits of stretching and breathing!

FIND A FRIEND: Find a friend who will encourage you to stick with your yoga program or even join with you. Use the power and motivation of holding each other accountable and committed to the practice.

TRY A NEW STYLE: There are many different styles of yoga. Seek out classes at your school, gym, or local yoga studio that specialize in yoga types that sound fun to you. *Bikram* yoga is done in a very hot room, *Iyengar* emphasizes alignment and perfecting poses, and *vinyasa* is a flowing series that warms and energizes the body in an aerobic practice.

ADVANCE!

Now that you've laid the foundation for beginning yoga, become even more present with your breath and dedicate yourself to building a healthier body and a calmer mind. As in the Beginner program, you will end each session by sustaining corpse pose for pose for 5–10 minutes. (If you want to start with corpse pose at the beginning of your practice, just add on an extra minute.)

ADVANCED

PROGRAM **GOAL:** Practice a basic yoga sequence three to five times a week, building to 250 minutes of yoga per week and 6 counts of breath per pose by week four.

	Mon		Tue		Wed		Thurs		Fri		Sat		Sun	
	T	B	T	B	T	B	T	B	T	B	T	B	T	B
Week 1	40	1I 1E			40	1I 1E			40	1I 1E				
Week 2	40	1I 1H 2E			40	1I 1H 2E			40	1I 1H 2E			40	1I 1H 2E
Week 3	40	2I 1H 2E			40	2I 1H 2E	40	2I 1H 2E	40	2I 1H 2E			40	2I 1H 2E
Week 4	50	2I 2H 2E			50	2I 2H 2E	50	2I 2H 2E	50	2I 2H 2E			30	2I 2H 2E

T = Total time of session in minutes.
B = Counts per breath (or for holding the breath) for each pose. For example,
1I = inhale for 1 count; 1H = hold the breath for 1 count; 1E = exhale for 1 count.

Order of Poses

Repeat this sequence the more your body adjusts to the added time.

Cat/Cow
Spinal Balance
Downward Facing Dog
Warrior 1 (left foot forward, right foot back and anchored to the floor)
Warrior 2
Triangle
Extended Angle
Triangle
Warrior 2
Warrior 1
Extended Angle
Downward Facing Dog
Cat/Cow

Downward Facing Dog
Warrior 1 (right foot forward, left foot back and anchored to the floor)
Warrior 2
Triangle
Extended Angle
Triangle
Warrior 2
Warrior 1
Extended Angle
Downward Facing Dog
Cat/Cow
Corpse Pose

POSES BREAKDOWN

Cat/Cow

Strengthens: Core stabilizers, neck, and shoulders

Stretches: Core stabilizers

Getting into the pose: From all fours, with your wrists on the floor directly under your shoulders and your knees directly un-

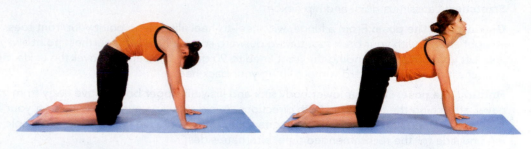

der your hips, exhale and round your back up toward the sky into Cat pose. As you inhale, arch your back so your tailbone, chest, and chin are turning upwards into Cow pose.

Holding the pose: Move with the breath, alternating Cat pose (rounding) and Cow pose (lengthening).

Spinal Balance

Strengthens: Back of body and core stabilizers

Getting into the pose: From all fours, with your wrists on the floor directly under your shoulders and your knees directly under your hips, extend one arm forward and lift the opposite leg backward, so your arm, torso and leg form one straight line.

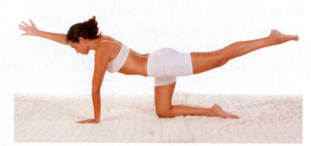

Holding the pose: Keep your core stabilizer muscles active to support your midsection. Look toward the ground and focus on lengthening, instead of lifting higher. Avoid collapsing into the supporting shoulder. After holding one side for the recommended time, alternate sides.

Downward Facing Dog

Strengthens: Upper body

Stretches: Shoulders, hamstrings, calves, and lats

Getting into the pose: Start in Child's pose on the floor, face down, with your legs tucked under you (so you are sitting on your heels) and your arms extended outwards. From Child's pose, with your palms flat on the floor, shoulder width apart, come up onto all fours, tucking your toes under and pressing your hips high and back away from your hands. Straighten your legs (if appropriate), and lift your knee caps upward while pressing your heels down.

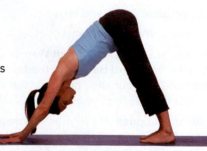

Holding the pose: Lift your tailbone while pushing your palms forward and your heels back and down. Let your chest, shoulders, head, and neck sink toward the floor, and breathe into your back. Make sure your weight is equally distributed across your hands and into your thumbs and fingers.

Warrior 1

Strengthens: Quads and gluts

Stretches: Latissimus dorsi and hip flexors

Getting into the pose: From a lunge, with heel-to-heel alignment, point your front toes straight ahead, with your back foot turned outward so your heel is the furthest point away from you. Lift your arms up, bending the front knee to 90 degrees, keeping it over the ankle. Bring your chest and naval forward without lifting your back heel.

Holding the pose: Let your lower body sink and lift your upper body. Move away from your navel, stretching the mat out in both directions. Avoid moving your front knee past your front ankle. Bring your arms behind your ears and draw your chin back gently. After holding one side for the recommended time, alternate sides.

Warrior 2

Strengthens: Quads and gluts

Stretches: Chest and adductors

Getting into the pose: From a wide stance, float your arms out at shoulder height. Point your front toes straight ahead, keeping your back heels flat and pushed out so they are the furthest point away from you. Bend your front knee to 90 degrees and keep it over your front ankle. Keep your hips level and point your navel toward the side.

Holding the pose: The focal point is your front fingertips. Continue stretching away from the center of your body so your lower body drops and your upper body lifts. Maintain your front knee to ankle alignment. Relax your shoulders and collarbones down. After holding one side for the recommended time, alternate sides.

Triangle

Strengthens: Torso and legs

Stretches: Waist and hamstrings

Getting into the pose: From Warrior 2, straighten your forward leg, reaching forward with your hand and back with the hips. Hinging over towards your front leg, rest your front hand on your shin, ankle, or the floor. Revolve your chest toward the sky, imagining your body is flat between two panes of glass and in line with the heels.

Holding the pose: Press your feet away from one another, and expand away from the center. Roll your lower hip under and avoid letting your torso, neck, and head fall out of alignment with your heels. After holding one side for the recommended time, alternate sides.

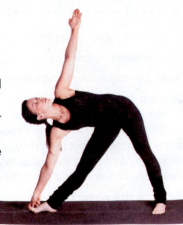

Extended Angle

Strengthens: Quads and gluts

Stretches: Groin, adductors, waist

Getting into the pose: From a wide stance (such as a lunge), turn your front toes straight ahead with your back toes turned in slightly. Bend your front knee, and bring down your front arm until your hand is inside the front foot, lining your arm up with your lower leg. Extend your top arm to the sky, and if comfortable, look up.

Holding the pose: Your chest revolves upwards as your shoulder presses into your knee. Drop your hips down and press them forward, keeping them in alignment with your heels. There should be a straight line from your back heel to your fingertips. After holding one side for the recommended time, alternate sides.

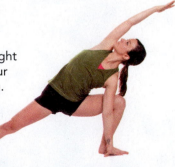

10 Reducing Your Risk of Cardiovascular Disease

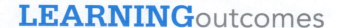

LEARNINGoutcomes

1 Define cardiovascular disease (CVD), explain why a college student should be concerned about CVD, and list the human and economic impacts of CVD.

2 Explain how CVD affects the heart and blood vessels and the symptoms it produces. Describe various forms of CVD, including hypertension, atherosclerosis, stroke, heart disease, and others.

3 Outline the main risk factors for CVD, including those you can and cannot control.

4 Create a plan and apply behavior-change skills to lower your own risk of CVD.

MasteringHealth™

Go online for chapter quizzes, interactive assessments, videos, and more!

casestudy

DARYL

"Hi, I'm Daryl. I'm a junior, majoring in education. I'm also a jazz pianist and I play at clubs around town about three times a week. I love jazz, and the gigs help me pay my college tuition.

"I think I'm pretty healthy—I've never been hospitalized for anything in my life—but I do have a family history of heart disease. Both of my grand-fathers died from heart attacks when they were in their 40s. My dad died of a stroke when I was 10, and my mom is currently taking pills for high blood pressure and high cholesterol. I know I'm still young, but given the family history, I'm worried. Are there things I can be doing to protect myself? And how can I help my mom?"

HEAR IT! ONLINE

Cardiovascular disease (CVD) is the term commonly used to describe diseases of the heart and the blood vessels brought on by a buildup of fatty, waxy accumulations that restrict or block blood flow. CVD can induce potentially devastat-ing consequences such as a heart attack and stroke, which are the number one and number four lead-ing causes of death in America (cancer and lung diseases being number two and three, respectively).[1] You may think that cardiovascular problems strike only older people but in fact, 9 to 15 percent of women and men under age 40 have some form of CVD.[2] The prevalence rises to about 40 percent in middle-aged adults of both sexes and then climbs sharply after age 60, involving about three-quarters or more of older Americans.[3] Among Americans of all age groups, approximately one out of every three has some form of cardiovascular disease.[4]

cardiovascular disease (CVD)
A disease of the heart and/or blood vessels

Why Should I Worry about Cardiovascular Disease?

As a college student, your most pressing concerns are probably things like getting good grades, paying tuition, and landing a job. Cardiovascular disease could be the furthest thing from your mind. However, it is not too early to start learning about CVD. For many people, the earliest manifestations of heart and blood vessel diseases take root during childhood and early adulthood, especially if they are overweight or obese.[5] While genetic predisposition plays an important role, lifestyle choices that you make now—such as whether to smoke, how often to exercise, your stress level, and what you eat—can also greatly influence your risk for developing cardiovascular disease later.

LIVE IT! ONLINE
Worksheet 39 Healthy Heart I.Q.

Cardiovascular Disease Is America's Biggest Killer

Cardiovascular disease and stroke account for about 29 percent of all deaths in the United States each year—more than any other single cause of death in America.[6] In fact, cardiovascular disease has been the leading cause of death in the United States every year since 1900, except in 1918, when a worldwide flu killed more Americans. If we completely eliminated CVD in the United States, experts estimate our average life expec-tancy would rise by almost seven years.[7] Together, heart disease and strokes kill more Americans each year—both men *and* women and people of various races—than cancer or any other cause (**Table 10.1**; also, see the box Men, Women, and Cardiovascular Disease on page 362).

TABLE 10.1 Five Leading Causes of Death in the United States

Cause	Number of deaths
Heart disease and stroke	787,931
Cancer	567,628
Chronic lower respiratory diseases	137,353
Accidents (unintentional injuries)	118,021
Alzheimer's disease	79,003

Data from A. S. Go et al., "Heart Disease and Stroke Statistics 2013 Update: A Report from the American Heart Association," *Circulation* 127 (2013): e6–245, doi: 10.1161/ CIR.0b013e31828124ad

The GetFitGraphic on page 363 illustrates the impact of CVD on society. It shows the prevalence of CVD throughout the United States and around the world, where it is the number one cause of death in most countries. The GetFitGraphic also pictures CVD's costs in direct care and lost productivity—both in today's economy and by 2030, when the impact on American consumers could reach $818 billion per year.[8]

Cardiovascular Disease Can Greatly Decrease Your Quality of Life

The potential of cardiovascular disease to cause death is obviously its most serious consequence, but even when it is not fatal, it can seriously impact daily life. Heart attack and stroke survivors may lose their ability to walk, talk, read, exercise, or carry out other daily activities normally. Cardiovascular disease can cause chest pain, shortness of breath, and damage to internal organs. It can also require expensive drugs, which have their own negative side effects.

Cardiovascular Disease Can Begin Early in Life

Childhood and early adolescence are often the time when people first start experiencing the risk factors for cardiovascular disease—poor diet, lack of exercise, BMI above 25, and smoking.[9] These, in turn, can trigger physical processes that initiate the start of cardiovascular disease itself surprisingly early in life. A recent study by Dutch public health researchers found that in a group of obese children under age 13, nearly two-thirds already had one or more physiological markers for CVD, including type 2 diabetes, high blood pressure, high LDL ("bad") cholesterol levels, and high blood sugar levels.[10]

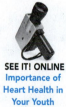

SEE IT! ONLINE
Importance of Heart Health in Your Youth

A now-classic study of blood vessel tissue from 3,000 young people between the ages of 15 and 34 who had died of accidents, homicides, or suicides discovered glistening streaks of fat and fatty, waxy buildup in some of the vessel specimens—deposits that marked the unmistakable beginnings of cardiovascular disease. The researchers found early signs of CVD in 2 percent of males aged 15 to 19. They also observed advanced markers of CVD in 20 percent of 30- to 34-year-old males, and 8 percent of females in the same age group. In examining the individual health records of those young people with blood vessel deposits, the researchers found a higher incidence of poor

diet, lack of exercise, high BMI, and smoking than in healthier young people lacking those deposits.[11] These same habits continue to contribute to cardiovascular disease in middle-aged and older adults. More recent studies reflect the result of those early risk factors and blood vessel deposits: A 2011 CDC study revealed that stroke-related hospitalizations rose dramatically in 15- to 44-year-olds between the years 1994 and 2007.[12] Among 15- to 34-year-old men, they found a 51 percent jump in stroke hospitalizations, and among boys and girls aged 5 to 14, a 30 percent rise. The actual numbers of young people who suffer strokes are small but the trend is clear; CVD prevention must begin in childhood.

SEE IT! ONLINE
Stroke In Young Adults

How Does Cardiovascular Disease Affect the Body?

Learning about how cardiovascular disease affects your body is useful for understanding why it causes the symptoms it does and what you can do to keep your cardiovascular system healthy.

Cardiovascular Disease Affects the Heart and Blood Vessels

Your body contains trillions of living cells, all needing a continuous supply of oxygen and energy compounds. The cardiovascular system—the heart and blood vessels—does the critical work of delivering that oxygen and energy *to* your cells. It also removes carbon dioxide and other wastes *from* your cells. (To review the anatomy of the cardiovascular, or circulatory, system, see Chapter 3.)

In a healthy 10-year-old, the heart is almost adult size. The blood vessel walls are smooth inside and out. The walls of the arteries are strong and elastic, while the walls of the veins are thinner and more fixed in diameter. Blood can flow freely down the long narrow opening in the middle of each vessel. The ventricles fill smoothly and forcibly push blood out. Tight-closing valves help prevent blood from flowing backward. The circulating blood reaches all the distant capillary beds in the brain, limbs, kidneys, skin, and other organs. It then returns quickly through the venous system.

Atherosclerosis Starting at age 10 or even earlier, abnormal accumulations inside the blood vessels can begin to restrict blood flow. The process of accumulation and restriction in blood vessels is known as

DIVeRSiTY

Men, Women, and Cardiovascular Disease

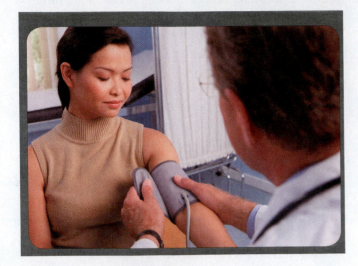

Many people are aware that cardiovascular disease is the leading cause of death in men in the United States. Few realize, however, that cardiovascular disease is the leading cause of death in American women as well—and in fact kills more women than men each year; in 2009, heart disease claimed 292,188 female victims and stroke added 76,769 more. Adding deaths from all forms of CVD, over 400,000 women died of CVD in 2009, compared to about 385,000 men.[1] The figure for women is higher than the number of female lives lost in 2009 due to cancer, Alzheimer's, diabetes, and accidents *combined*.

Even physicians can harbor misconceptions about women and cardiovascular disease. In one study, fewer than one doctor in five knew that CVD kills more women than men annually.[2] Another study has shown that doctors are more likely to screen male patients for heart disease and make recommendations for intervention than they are to screen or treat female patients for the same.[3]

Researchers have also found significant differences in the ways men and women tend to express patterns and symptoms of cardiovascular disease. For example:

- Men tend to develop heart disease 10 to 15 years earlier than women. Women rarely have heart attacks before menopause (early 50s); they show rates of CVD two or three times higher after menopause than before.

- While having a heart attack, men tend to experience the classic "squeezing" sensation in the chest, pain in the chest or arm, and/or shortness of breath. Women, however, are less likely to feel these symptoms. Instead, they are more likely to experience shortness of breath, weakness or fatigue, a cold sweat, or dizziness. If they feel any localized pressure, it tends to be between the shoulder blades rather than in the chest or arm. Women are also more likely than men to have early warning symptoms up to one month before, including unusual fatigue, sleep disturbances, shortness of breath, indigestion, and anxiety.[4] However, because they don't recognize these symptoms as a heart attack, they are more likely than men to delay treatment and die from the initial attack.

- Looking at cardiovascular disease as a whole, men are more likely to have heart attacks, while women with CVD are more likely to have strokes. This is perhaps based on the smaller size of blood vessels throughout the body, including the brain.[5]

- Doctors have long prescribed daily aspirin to both sexes as a way to prevent heart attacks. Some studies, however, have shown that aspirin seems to prevent some heart attack deaths in men and some stroke deaths in women but does not seem to prevent stroke deaths in men or heart attack deaths in women.[6]

Sources:
1. Statistical Fact Sheet, 2013 Update, "Women & Cardiovascular Diseases," American Heart Association, 2013, www.heart.org
2. L. Mosca et al., "National Study of Physician Awareness and Adherence to Cardiovascular Disease Prevention Guidelines," *Circulation* 111, no. 4 (2005): 499–510.
3. J. H. Mieres, "Review of the American Heart Association's Guidelines for Cardiovascular Disease Prevention in Women," *Heart* 92, Supp. 3 (2006): iii10–3.
4. J. Canto, W. Rogers, and R. Goldberg et. al., "Association of Age and Sex With Myocardial Infarction Symptom Presentation and in Hospital Mortality," *Journal of the American Medical Association* 307, no. 8 (2012): 813-22, doi: 10.1001/jama.2012.199.
5. T. Kurth et al., "Healthy Lifestyle and the Risk of Stroke in Women," *Archives of Internal Medicine* 166, no. 13 (2006): 1403–9.
6. J. S. Berger et al., "Aspirin for the Primary Prevention of Cardiovascular Events in Women and Men: A Sex-Specific Meta-Analysis of Randomized Controlled Trials," *Journal of the American Medical Association* 295, no. 3 (2006): 306–13.

atherosclerosis Hardening or stiffening of the arteries as plaque accumulates, often at injury sites, in the inner linings of arteries

atherosclerosis (from the Greek words *athero*, meaning "gruel," and *sclerosis*, meaning "hardness").

Atherosclerosis is a major factor in many forms of cardiovascular disease. Both lifestyle and genetic factors can cause deposits of fatty, waxy, yellowish, sludgelike debris called *atheromas* to accumulate inside arteries and smaller arterioles. Other substances such as calcium salts, cholesterol, cellular waste, blood clotting

WHAT IS THE IMPACT OF CARDIOVASCULAR DISEASE ON SOCIETY?

CVD takes a huge toll on the U.S. and globally: it affects over 80% of Americans over the age of 80 and costs billions of dollars in annual medical expenses. Here are a few figures and facts about the impact of CVD on society.

HOW COMMON IS CVD IN THE U.S.?

The prevalence of CVD increases with age, affecting 4 out of 5 Americans by the age of 80.[1]

	Male	Female
20-39 years old	12.8%	10.1%
40-59 years old	40.0%	34.4%
60-79 years old	70.2%	70.9%
80 years & older	83.0%	87.1%

What are the annual MEDICAL COSTS of CVD in the U.S.?

Coronary heart disease	$108.9
Hypertension	$93.5
Stroke	$53.9
Heart failure	$34.4
TOTAL	**$290.7**

Estimated costs in billions, 2010 [2]

How will the MEDICAL COSTS of CVD in the U.S. INCREASE IN THE FUTURE?

Estimated annual costs in billions [3]

- 2015 $358
- 2020 $470.3
- 2025 $621.6
- 2030 $818.1

What is the global burden of annual CVD DEATHS?

Estimates rounded to the nearest thousand [4]

- Europe **4,584,000**
- Western Pacific **4,735,000**
- South East Asia **3,616,000**
- The Americas **1,944,000**
- Africa **1,254,000**
- Eastern Mediterranean **1,195,000**
- World (total) **17,327,000**

WHAT CAN I DO TO PREVENT CVD?

Although there are some risk factors that you cannot control (such as heredity, age, gender, and race), taking these steps may lessen your CVD risk:

- ☑ **Don't smoke**
- ☑ **Eat a nutritious diet**
- ☑ **Exercise regularly**
- ☑ **Maintain a healthy weight**
- ☑ **Reduce stress**
- ☑ **Control diabetes**
- ☑ **Avoid abusing drugs & alcohol**

plaques A pinpoint area of fatty, waxy debris that accumulates at a site along the inner wall of an artery or arteriole

arterial stenosis A narrowing of the inner channel of arteries and smaller arterioles due to the buildup of a sludge-like layer of fatty, waxy debris

proteins, and white blood cells can accumulate around the atheromas, enlarging and solidifying the yellowish deposits into hardened blockages called **plaques**. These plaques, in turn, tend to bulge inward and cause a narrowing of the vessels' inner channels. This narrowing is called **arterial stenosis**. Plaques can eventually grow large enough to block blood passage through the vessel (see **Figure 10.1**) or even cause the vessel to rupture. The buildup process can take decades, but atherosclerosis can start in childhood, especially in the overweight and obese.[13]

Arteries with plaques that cause a narrowed channel or inward-bulging side walls transport less blood and are stiffer and less flexible. Just as the pressure builds up in a hose if you prevent normal water flow with your thumb, channel narrowing and plaque buildup can increase pressure within the blood vessels. Unhealthy lifestyle characteristics, including smoking, chronic stress, inactivity, high alcohol consumption, high blood sugar, high blood pressure, obesity, and unfavorable levels of certain fats and cholesterol in the blood can all increase the speed and severity of atherosclerosis and, in turn, contribute to CVD.[14] Atherosclerotic cardiovascular disease is America's leading cause of death and disability.[15]

In recent years, medical researchers have studied the role of *inflammation* in atherosclerosis.

Inflammation is an immune response that causes redness and swelling in response to injury. Researchers think that low-grade inflammation inside a blood vessel can contribute to plaque buildup. Eventually, inflammation can cause a rupture in a bulging plaque deposit that leads to a blood clot, which, in turn, can cause a heart attack or stroke.[16]

Several factors can injure the inner walls of blood vessels and promote inflammation at the injury site.[17] These include high blood levels of LDL (low-density lipoprotein) cholesterol, smoking, hypertension, diabetes mellitus, poor diet, alcohol consumption, and disease-causing bacteria and viruses. The latter include *Chlamydia pneumoniae* (a common cause of respiratory infections), *Helicobacter pylori* (which causes ulcers), herpes simplex virus (which the majority of Americans are exposed to by the age of 5), and cytomegalovirus (another herpes virus transmitted through body fluids and infecting most Americans before the age of 40).

Several natural substances within the body serve as links between unhealthy lifestyle habits, inflammation in blood vessel walls, and cardiovascular disease. Stored fat and associated immune cells in a person's adipose tissue spew out proteins called *C-reactive proteins* (CRPs), as well others—the more stored fat, the more CRPs. Alcohol consumption and diets low in whole grain, fruits, and green leafy vegetables can lead to higher levels of an amino acid called *homocysteine*.[18] Both CRPs and homocysteine appear to promote inflammation and plaque formation. Doctors are now using high blood levels of these substances as markers in the prediction and diagnosis of atherosclerosis.[19] Lifestyle changes such as regular exercise, weight management,

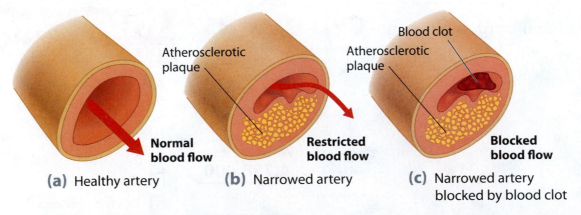

Blood clot

Atherosclerotic plaque

Atherosclerotic plaque

Normal blood flow

Restricted blood flow

Blocked blood flow

(a) Healthy artery

(b) Narrowed artery

(c) Narrowed artery blocked by blood clot

FIGURE **10.1** (a) Cross-section of a healthy artery, allowing normal blood flow. (b) Cross-section of an artery with plaque buildup narrowing the channel and restricting blood flow. (c) Cross-section of a blood clot that blocks the flow of blood.

Figures (a) and (b) from J. S. Blake, *Nutrition and You*, 1st Edition, © 2008. Reprinted and electronically reproduced by permission of Pearson Education, Inc., Upper Saddle River, New Jersey.

smoking cessation, moderation of alcohol intake, eating less saturated fat and cholesterol, and consuming more whole grains and fruits and vegetables appear to reduce inflammation and its markers in the blood.

Cardiovascular Disease Takes Many Forms

Table 10.2 identifies the most common forms of cardiovascular disease and their prevalence in American adults. Let's look at each of these forms of CVD in more detail.

Hypertension **Hypertension**, or sustained high blood pressure, is the most common form of cardiovascular disease. It is also considered a risk factor for other forms of CVD. About 30 percent of all Americans have hypertension.[20] Because it has no initial symptoms, many are unaware they have the condition.[21] In fact, some experts refer to hypertension as a "silent killer."[22] Hypertension causes blood vessel damage and promotes plaque development.[23] As mentioned earlier, plaque deposits and vessel-channel narrowing can in turn increase resistance to blood flow throughout the circulatory system and can cause blood pressure to rise further, creating a damaging vicious cycle. In addition to leading to other forms of CVD, hypertension can cause your thinking to slow down or make you more susceptible to dementia later in life.[24]

You may think of high blood pressure as an older person's disease. Among all American adults aged

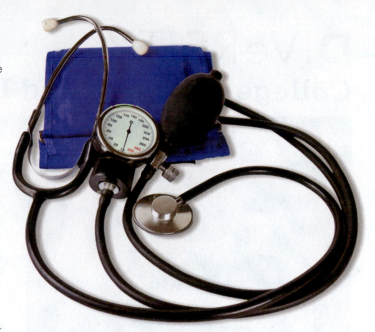

18 to 44, however, 10.5 percent have diagnosed hypertension and in some groups, the percentages are much higher.[25] Hypertension can result from consuming too much sodium in the diet, leading to water retention and increased blood volume. Other causes of hypertension include kidney or heart abnormalities, aging, inherited tendencies, obesity, sleep apnea, stress, or certain kinds of tumors. Could hypertension be impacting you? See the box College Students and Hypertension on page 366 to find out more.

A blood pressure device can help diagnose hypertension. Such devices measure your blood pressure in two parts, expressed as a fraction—for example, 120/80. Both values are measured in millimeters of mercury (mm Hg). The first number refers to **systolic pressure**, or the pressure being applied to the walls of the arteries when the heart contracts, pumping blood to the rest of the body. The second value is **diastolic pressure**, or the pressure applied to the walls of the arteries during the heart's relaxation phase. During this phase, blood is reentering the heart's chambers, preparing for the next heartbeat.

Normal blood pressure varies, depending on an individual's weight, age, physical condition, gender, and ethnic background. Systolic blood pressure tends to increase with age, while diastolic blood pressure tends to increase until age

TABLE **10.2** Major Types of Cardiovascular Disease and Prevalence of Each	
Type of Cardiovascular Disease	Prevalence in the United States
Hypertension	77.9 million
Coronary heart disease (including heart attack)	15.4 million
Angina pectoris	7.8 million
Arrhythmia	2.2 million
Congestive heart failure	5.1 million
Congenital cardiovascular defects	Eight defects per 1,000 live births
Stroke	6.8 million; 795,000 new or recurrent cases of stroke each year

Data from A. S. Go et al., "Heart Disease and Stroke Statistics 2013 Update: A Report from the American Heart Association," *Circulation* 127 (2013): e6–245, doi: 10.1161/ CIR.0b013e31828124ad

hypertension Sustained blood pressure over 130/85 mm Hg

systolic pressure The pressure applied to the walls of the arteries when the heart contracts

diastolic pressure The pressure applied to the walls of the arteries during the heart's relaxation phase

DIVeRSiTY
College Students and Hypertension

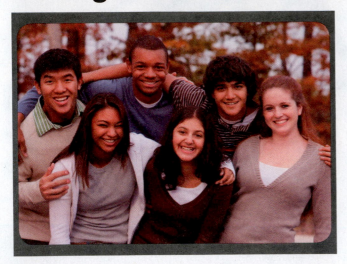

Our discussion of increased hospitalizations for stroke among young people is part of a bigger trend: increased hypertension in people from 20 to 44. A revealing study of 800 students at the University of New Hampshire, for example, showed that one-third were overweight or obese and that fully 60 percent of male students had high blood pressure.[1] Other reports have shown that more than 4 million young adults (about 4 percent) are now taking anti-cholesterol medications, while 8.5 million (8 percent) are now taking medications to combat high blood pressure (hypertension).[2]

As with the general U.S. adult population, college students of both sexes are at risk of hypertension based on the prevalence of obesity, poor diet, and sedentary lifestyles in our culture. But young men, particularly young African American men, seem to be at highest risk (we'll explore this further in the chapter).[3] In general, men under age 35 are more likely to ignore early symptoms and delay return visits to doctors after a preliminary discussion about their high blood pressure. Depression and high alcohol consumption can also increase the risk for hypertension, and both are common among college students of both sexes.[4]

Hypertension can have devastating long-term effects on nearly every organ of the body. Among the many health problems that they may encounter, men with prehypertension and hypertension are nearly three times as likely to experience erectile dysfunction as men without these cardiac problems. Reducing sodium consumption, losing weight, and exercising, among other measures, can make a huge difference in risk reduction and help you avoid the need for medical intervention.

Sources:
1. University of New Hampshire, "New Nutritional Research Indicates College Students Face Obesity, High Blood Pressure, Metabolic Syndrome," June 14, 2007, www.unh.edu
2. J. T. Flynn, "Pediatric Hypertension Update," *Current Opinion in Nephrology and Hypertension* 19, no. 3 (2010): 292–7.
3. B. Rosner, "Blood Pressure Differences by Ethnic Group among United States Children and Adolescents," *Hypertension* 54, no. 3 (2009): 502–8; D. T. Lackland, "High Blood Pressure: A Lifetime Issue," *Hypertension* 54, no. 3 (2009): 457–8.
4. S. B. Patten et al., "Major Depression as a Risk Factor for High Blood Pressure: Epidemiologic Evidence from a National Longitudinal Study," *Psychosomatic Medicine* 71, no. 3 (2009): 273–9.

55, and then decline. Generally, men have a greater risk for high blood pressure than women until age 55; at that point, the risks become about equal. After age 75, women are more likely to have high blood pressure than men.[26]

For a healthy adult, normal systolic blood pressure is less than 120 mm Hg, and normal diastolic blood pressure is less than 80 mm Hg.[27] A physician may diagnose *prehypertension* or the potential beginnings of hypertension when blood pressure is above normal, but not yet in the hypertensive range (see **Table 10.3** on page 367). *High blood pressure* (HBP) is usually diagnosed when systolic pressure is 140 or above. When only systolic

coronary artery disease (CAD) or **coronary heart disease (CHD)** Atherosclerosis (the buildup of plaque deposits) in the main arteries that supply oxygen and other materials to the heart muscle

pressure is high, the condition is known as *isolated systolic hypertension* (ISH), the most common form of high blood pressure in older Americans.

If you are diagnosed with high blood pressure in college, you can do something about it. Lifestyle modifications are helpful in reducing or preventing hypertension in early adulthood. These include losing weight, exercising, reducing stress, and reducing dietary salt and sugar (see the box Do Salt and Sugar Increase My Risk of Cardiovascular Disease? on page 366).[28] You may also need to work with your physician to lower your blood pressure through prescription drugs.

Coronary Heart Disease When atherosclerosis occurs in the heart's main blood vessels, it is called **coronary artery disease (CAD)** or **coronary heart disease (CHD)**. When it occurs in the feet, ankles, calves, hands, or forearms, it is called *peripheral artery disease*. Of all the

TABLE 10.3 Blood Pressure Readings

Classification	Systolic Reading (mm Hg)	Diastolic Reading (mm Hg)
Normal	Less than 120	Less than 80
Prehypertension	120–139	80–89
Hypertension		
Stage 1	140–159	90–99
Stage 2	160 or higher	100 or higher

Note: If systolic and diastolic readings fall into different categories, treatment is determined by the highest category. Readings are based on the average of two or more properly measured, seated readings on each of two or more health care provider visits.

Source: National Heart, Lung, and Blood Institute, *Seventh Report of the Joint National Committee on Prevention, Detection, Evaluation, and Treatment of High Blood Pressure* (NIH Publication No. 03-5233) (Bethesda, MD: National Institutes of Health, May 2003).

types of cardiovascular disease, CHD is the greatest killer. Each year, an estimated 1.25 million Americans suffer a new or recurrent heart attack.[29] The American Heart Association calculates that approximately every *minute*, somewhere in the United States, someone dies of a first or subsequent heart.

A heart attack, also called a **myocardial infarction (MI)**, occurs when an area of the heart suffers permanent damage after its normal blood supply has been blocked. The blockage can be caused by a blood clot in a coronary artery or by atherosclerotic narrowing. When blood flow slows down dramatically or stops, the surrounding tissue is deprived of oxygen. If the blockage is extremely minor, an otherwise healthy heart will adapt over time as small blood vessels reroute needed blood through other areas.

When heart blockage is more severe, a person can experience the symptoms of a heart attack and will require life-saving support. The box In the Event of a Heart Attack, Stroke, or Cardiac Arrest (on page 369) describes how you should respond if you recognize such symptoms in someone else or yourself.

Angina Pectoris Atherosclerosis and other circulatory impairments may reduce the heart's blood and oxygen supply and cause a condition called **ischemia**. People with ischemia often suffer from varying degrees of chest pain, also called **angina pectoris**. The American Heart Association estimates that more than 9 million Americans suffer from angina.[30] Many people experience short episodes of angina whenever they exert themselves physically. Symptoms may range from slight indigestion to a feeling that the heart is being crushed. Generally, the more serious the oxygen deprivation, the more severe the pain.

Doctors currently use several methods of treating angina. In mild cases, they prescribe rest. To treat more serious chest pain, they may recommend nitroglycerin tablets to relax veins and lessen the heart's workload. Calcium channel blockers can also relieve angina caused by spasms of the coronary arteries. Drugs called *beta-blockers* can control potential overactivity of the heart muscle.

Arrhythmias An **arrhythmia**, or irregular heartbeat, is relatively common: More than 2.2 million Americans experience it each year.[31] The disturbance of heartbeat rhythm can take several forms: a racing heart in the absence of exercise or anxiety (called *tachycardia*); an abnormally slow heartbeat (called *bradycardia*); or a sporadic, quivering pattern called *fibrillation*. **Fibrillation** renders the heart extremely inefficient at pumping blood through the vessels. If a fibrillation incident or series of incidents go untreated, the condition may be fatal. Even without cardiovascular disease, you may feel heart arrhythmias from drinking too much caffeine or from the nicotine in tobacco. Mild cases like this are seldom life-threatening. If you develop a severe case due to disease, you may require drug therapy or a pacemaker.

myocardial infarction (MI) Medical term for a heart attack; involves permanent damage to an area of the heart muscle brought on by a cessation of normal blood supply

ischemia A damaging reduction in the blood (and therefore the oxygen supply) to a region of the heart, brain, or other organ

angina pectoris Chest pain due to ischemia, or reduction in blood flow to the heart muscle and surrounding tissues

arrhythmia Irregular heartbeat; can involve abnormally fast or slow heartbeat or the disorganized, sporadic beat of fibrillation

fibrillation A sporadic, quivering heartbeat pattern that results in inefficient pumping of blood

Q&A Do Salt and Sugar Increase My Risk of Cardiovascular Disease?

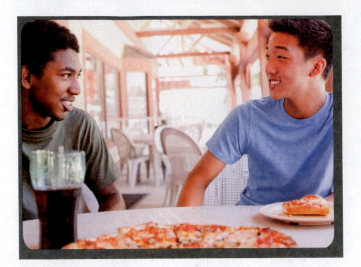

The average American adult consumes 3,466 mg of sodium per day in salt (NaCl)—more than twice the USDA-recommended level of 1,500 mg for those over 50, African Americans, and those who have high blood pressure.[1] The 2010 Federal Dietary Guidelines recommend that all other adults consume below 2,300 mg per day (the American Heart Association recommends a more conservative limit of 1,500 mg per day for adults and children of all ages). These health organizations advocate limiting salt because excess sodium induces fluid retention. This, in turn, elevates blood pressure and contributes to hypertension and CVD. To get below 2,300 mg, most adults would have to cut overall salt consumption by about half a teaspoon.

Most of the salt in our national diet comes from foods high in processed grains (for example, pizza and cookies) and from meats, poultry, and lunch meats.[2] Researchers estimate that a population-wide average drop in dietary salt by 1,200 mg/day would annually cut new cases of cardiovascular disease by 60,000 to 120,000 and prevent 32,000 to 66,000 new strokes, 54,000 to 99,000 new heart attacks, and 44,000 to 92,000 deaths. They have also projected that this trend would save $10 to $24 billion in annual health care costs.[3] A recent Harvard study projects that in 2010, 15 percent of the world's 2.3 million cardiovascular deaths (or 345,000 of them) can be attributed to eating too much salt. By extension, this many people could be saved each year by eating less salt.[4]

What about sugar? The average American consumes more than 150 pounds of caloric sweeteners (sugar, corn syrup, brown sugar, honey, agave syrup, concentrated fruit juice, and so on) each year. That's almost three pounds per week![5] Most of this extra sugar comes from sweetened sodas, sports drinks, energy drinks, coffee drinks, and tea drinks. Like salt, sugar takes a toll on our cardiovascular health by increasing weight gain and by raising both glucose and triglyceride levels in the blood. Consuming an extra 2.6 ounces per day of corn syrup (the amount in two or three sweetened drinks) doubles a person's risk for high systolic blood pressure.[6] In one large study, women who consumed two sweetened drinks per day had a 20 percent greater risk of heart disease over those who drank sugary drinks only about once per month.[7] In another, men who drank one 12-ounce sugary drink per day increased their heart disease risk by 20 percent over men who never choose those beverages.[8] Dietary sugar, in other words, increases the risks of CVD, just as salt does.

Sources:
1. Centers for Disease Control and Prevention, "CDC Survey Find Nine in Ten U.S. Adults Consume Too Much Sodium," Press Release June 24, 2010, www.cdc.gov.
2. Ibid.
3. K. Bibbins-Domingo et al., "Projected Effect of Dietary Salt Reductions on Future Cardiovascular Disease," *The New England Journal of Medicine* 362, no. 7 (2010): 590–9.
4. American Heart Association Meeting Report, "Eating too much salt led to nearly 2.3 million heart-related deaths worldwide in 2010," American Heart Association, March 21, 2013, http://newsroom.heart.org
5. USDA, "Chapter 2: Profiling Food Consumption in America," *Agricultural Fact Book 2001–2002*, (2002) www.usda.gov.
6. D. I. Jalal et al., "Increased Fructose Associates with Elevated Blood Pressure," *Journal of the American Society of Nephrology* 21, no. 9 (2010): 1543–9.
7. T. T. Fung et al., "Sweetened Beverage Consumption and Risk of Coronary Heart Disease in Women," *American Journal of Clinical Nutrition* 89, no. 4 (2009): 1037–42.
8. Lawrence de Koning et al., "Sweetened Beverage Consumption, Incident Coronary Heart Disease, and Biomarkers of Risk in Men," *Circulation* 125, no. 14 (2012): 1735–41, doi: 10.1161/CIRCULATIONAHA.111.067017

Congestive Heart Failure More than 5 million Americans suffer from **congestive heart failure (CHF)** each year.[32] In CHF, the heart muscle is damaged or overworked, the pumping chambers are often taxed to the limit, and the heart lacks the strength to keep blood circulating normally through the body. The weakened heart pumps less blood out through the arteries. As a result, the "return" blood can't flow back through the veins to the heart in normal amounts. As the blood begins to back up, it causes congestion in body tissues. Blood pooling enlarges the heart, making it even less efficient, and fluid accumulates in the legs, ankles, or lungs, where it can cause swelling or difficulty in breathing. Causes for CHF include defects, infection, heart attack,

congestive heart failure (CHF) A cardiovascular disease in which the heart muscle is damaged or overworked, and the heart lacks the strength to keep blood circulating normally through the body

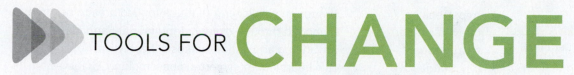
In the Event of a Heart Attack, Stroke, or Cardiac Arrest

Knowing what to do in a cardiovascular emergency could save a friend's life—or your own.

Warning Signs of a Heart Attack

- Uncomfortable pressure, fullness, squeezing, or pain in the center of the chest (more likely in men) or between the shoulder blades (more likely in women), lasting two minutes or longer

- Jaw pain and/or shortness of breath

- Pain spreading to the shoulders, neck, or arms

- Dizziness, fatigue, fainting, sweating, and/or nausea

Not all of these warning signs occur in every heart attack. For instance, a woman's heart attack may show up as shortness of breath, fatigue, and jaw or shoulder blade pain or pressure, stretched out over hours rather than minutes. If any of these symptoms appear, don't wait. Get help immediately!

Warning Signs of a Stroke

- Sudden numbness or weakness, especially on one side of the body, affecting face, arm, and/or leg

- Sudden mental confusion, especially trouble speaking or understanding words

- Sudden vision problems in one or both eyes

- Sudden dizziness, loss of balance, lack of coordination, or trouble walking

- Sudden severe headache without apparent cause

Warning Signs of a Cardiac Arrest

- Sudden loss of responsiveness (won't respond if tapped on either shoulder)

- Cessation of normal breathing (tilt head up; check for breathing for 5 seconds)

Know What to Do before an Emergency Strikes

- Find out which hospitals in your area have 24-hour emergency cardiac care.

- Determine (in advance) the hospital or medical facility that is nearest your home, school, and office and tell your family and friends to call this facility in an emergency.

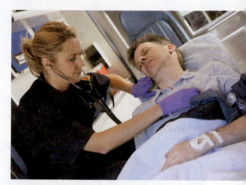

- Keep a list of emergency rescue service numbers next to your telephone and in your pocket, wallet, or purse. Remember 911 if you don't have time to call emergency rescue numbers.

- If you have chest or jaw discomfort that lasts more than two minutes, call the emergency rescue service or 911. Do not drive yourself to the hospital unless there is no other alternative.

Be a Lifesaver during a Crisis

- If you are with someone who is showing signs of a heart attack or stroke and the warning signs last for two minutes or longer, act immediately.

- Expect a denial. It is normal for a person with chest discomfort to deny the possibility of anything as serious as a heart attack. Don't take no for an answer. Insist on taking prompt action.

- Call 911 or an emergency rescue service, or get to the nearest hospital emergency room that offers 24-hour emergency cardiac care.

- If you are with someone in cardiac arrest and if you are properly trained, give chest compressions and mouth-to-mouth breathing. Continual chest compressions appear to be more important for adult heart attack victims; combined compressions and breathing (CPR or cardiopulmonary resuscitation) seem to be more important for children having a heart, stroke, or breathing-related emergency. Get instructions on which to use from a 911 operator, emergency medical technician, or other rescue personnel if possible.

- An automated external defibrillator (AED) may save a person during cardiac arrest. These devices are increasingly common in public places—workplaces, restaurants, health clubs, sports stadiums, schools, shopping centers, airports, hotels, and so on. Try to cultivate the habit of noticing their location in case of emergency.

Source: Adapted from American Heart Association, "Heart Attack, Stroke, and Cardiac Arrest Warning Signs," Accessed March 18, 2011, www.americanheart.org.

hypertension, or even cancer treatments.

Congestive heart failure can be fatal if undiagnosed and untreated, but most cases respond well to drug treatment. Diuretics (water pills) increase urination and reduce fluid accumulation, drugs such as digitalis increase the heart's pumping action, and vasodilators expand blood vessels so blood can flow through more easily and reduce the heart's workload.

Congenital Heart Disease

Congenital heart disease, meaning heart disease present at birth, affects 9 out of every 1,000 live births.[33] A baby may be born with a slight *heart murmur,* an audible sound based on an irregular heart valve that allows turbulent blood flow through the heart. Some children outgrow such heart murmurs and have no further problems. Others, however, can have more serious congenital irregularities with heart anatomy or function that require surgical repair. Causes may include hereditary factors, a mother's case of rubella or certain other infections during pregnancy, or the mother's use of alcohol or drugs during fetal development. Advances in treatment continually improve the prospects for children with congenital heart defects.

Stroke

The American Heart Association's most recent statistics show that approximately 7 million Americans alive today have suffered a stroke at some point in their lives. Each year more than 795,000 people experience a new or recurrent stroke, and 129,000 of them die, making stroke the third leading cause of death after heart disease and cancer.[34] In recent years, the incidence of stroke has been rising in adults aged 15 to 44.[35]

We saw that a heart attack can occur when a blocked vessel prevents a region of the heart from getting enough oxygenated blood. In a similar way, a **stroke** is a sudden loss of function in a region of the brain caused by blockage in or rupture of a blood vessel, leading to oxygen deprivation and cell damage or death. *Ischemic* strokes are the result of a plaque-blocked vessel or a floating blood clot that lodges in a vessel and cuts off blood supply to a brain region. *Hemorrhagic* strokes occur when a blood vessel bursts, spilling oxygenated blood rather than transporting it to a distal brain region, allowing that unsupplied area to become damaged through oxygen deprivation. Family history, advancing age, atherosclerosis, heart disease, congestive heart failure, hypertension, smoking, diabetes, inactivity, overweight, heavy drinking, stimulant drug use, and other factors can all contribute to triggering strokes.[36]

Some strokes are mild and cause only temporary dizziness or slight weakness or numbness. If an affected area is large or in a crucial part of the brain, stroke may cause speech impairments, memory problems, loss of motor control, or death. About 1 in 10 major strokes is preceded days, weeks, or months earlier by *transient ischemic attacks (TIAs),* brief interruptions of the blood supply to the brain that cause only temporary dizziness, weakness, paralysis, numbness, or other symptoms.[37] Deaths due to strokes have decreased in recent years thanks to better diagnosis, better surgical options, new clot-busting drugs that can be injected immediately after a stroke has occurred, better aftercare for stroke patients, and campaigns to teach awareness and avoidance of risk factors.

What Are the Main Risk Factors for Cardiovascular Disease?

The prevalence of cardiovascular disease is an unfortunate reality. However, we can modify many of our individual risk factors. By identifying your risks and understanding which are controllable (see **Lab 10.1**), you can learn to modify risk-promoting behaviors and lower your chances of developing CVD.

DO IT! ONLINE

Risks You Can Control

Experts have identified at least 10 significant risk factors for CVD: tobacco use, hypertension, high blood fats, obesity/overweight, physical inactivity, type 2 diabetes, metabolic syndrome, heavy alcohol consumption, poor diet, and uncontrolled stress. Since lifestyle choices underlie many of these risk factors, changes to daily habits can often reduce the chances of developing cardiovascular disease. Many people have multiple risk factors for CVD; the more risk factors they have, the greater their chances of experiencing a heart attack, stroke, angina, atherosclerosis, and other specific forms of CVD.[38] Let's look at each of these risk factors more closely.

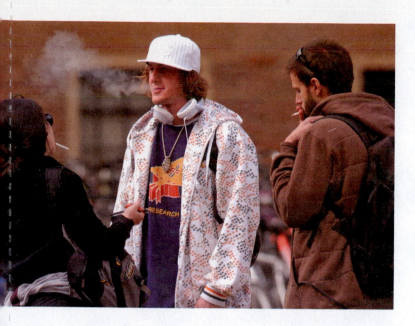

Tobacco Use In 1964, the Surgeon General of the United States asserted that smoking was the greatest risk factor for heart disease. Today, more than 46,000 annual deaths from CVD are directly related to smoking.[39] Cigarette smokers are two to four times more likely to develop CHD than nonsmokers.[40] Evidence also indicates that an estimated 46,000 *non*smokers die from cardiovascular disease each year as a result of chronic exposure to environmental tobacco smoke.[41]

How does tobacco use damage the heart? There are two plausible explanations. One is that nicotine increases heart beat rate, heart output, blood pressure, and oxygen use by heart muscles. The heart is forced to work harder to obtain sufficient oxygen. The other explanation is that chemicals in smoke damage and inflame the lining of the coronary arteries, allowing cholesterol and plaque to accumulate more easily, increasing blood pressure, and forcing the heart to work harder. In addition, chemicals in smoke increase blood clotting and the chance of heart attack.

Hypertension We have seen that hypertension can damage artery walls and lead to atherosclerosis. It can also weaken artery walls and lead to an *aneurysm,* an abnormal, blood-filled bulge in a blood vessel that has the potential to rupture. Hypertension can damage coronary arteries, enlarge the heart, or weaken the heart muscle. By affecting blood vessels in the brain, hypertension can cause strokes and TIAs, promote dementia, and impair cognitive functioning. By damaging delicate blood vessels in the kidneys and eyes, hypertension can lead to kidney damage or failure and to impaired vision or vision loss. In addition, hypertension can reduce

sexual function, disrupt sleep, and magnify the bone loss of osteoporosis.[42] Reducing dietary sodium and blood fats can help lower blood pressure, as can managing stress and taking certain prescription drugs. Maintaining a healthy weight is especially important: One recent study found that 25 percent of college students who gained 5 percent of their body weight (for example, 7.5 pounds in a 150-pound student) over one year saw increases in their blood pressure. For some female students, a gain of just 1.5 pounds raised blood pressure by three to five points. Luckily, weight *loss* can *lower* blood pressure.[43]

High Levels of Fats in Your Blood *Hyperlipidemia*— or high levels of cholesterol, triglycerides, and other fats in the blood—is correlated with increased risk of several cardiovascular diseases. According to one report, more than 50 percent of American men aged 65 and older and 40 percent of American women aged 65 or older are on some type of anti-hyperlipidemia prescription drug, including such medications as the "statins" (Lipitor, Crestor, Zocor) and other drugs designed to reduce blood fats.[44] Unfortunately, many of these medications carry significant risks of their own. Additionally, many people use these medications as "crutches" and continue to eat high-fat foods, assuming that the medications will keep any risks from CVD at bay.

Diets high in saturated fats and/or *trans* fats can raise blood cholesterol levels and contribute to atherosclerosis. They can also switch on the body's blood-clotting system, making the blood thicker and stickier. All of these blood changes increase the risk of heart attack or stroke. **Table 10.4** on page 372 shows recommended levels for blood cholesterol. People with several risk factors for CVD should follow the most stringent range of the guidelines for blood cholesterol.

Total cholesterol levels are just one measure of cardiovascular disease risks. Another is the ratio of "bad" to "good" cholesterol. Low-density lipoprotein (LDL), often referred to as "bad" cholesterol, contributes to plaque buildup on artery walls. High-density lipoprotein (HDL), or "good" cholesterol, removes plaque from artery walls, thus serving as a protector. In theory, if LDL levels get too high relative to HDL levels, plaque will tend to accumulate inside arteries and lead to cardiovascular problems. The LDL/HDL ratio can increase because of too much saturated fat in the diet, lack of exercise, high stress levels, or genetic predisposition.

A second type of blood fat, the *triglycerides,* also promote atherosclerosis. As people get older, heavier, or both, their triglyceride and cholesterol levels tend to

TABLE 10.4 LDL, Total, and HDL Cholesterol and Triglycerides (mg/dL) Levels for Adults

LDL Cholesterol	
Less than 100	Optimal
100–129	Near optimal/above optimal
130–159	Borderline high
160–189	High
190 or higher	Very high
Total Cholesterol	
Less than 200	Desirable
200–239	Borderline high
240 or higher	High
HDL Cholesterol	
Less than 40	Low
60 or higher	Desirable
Triglycerides	
Less than 150	Normal
150–199	Borderline high
200–499	High
500 or higher	Very high

Source: National Heart, Lung, and Blood Institute, "Detection, Evaluation, and Treatment of High Blood Cholesterol in Adults" (NIH Publication No. 02-5215), 2002, www.nhlbi.nih.gov

rise. No one has yet proved that high triglyceride levels cause atherosclerosis and thus underlie CVD. However, these blood fats may contribute to faster plaque development.

It can be useful to obtain an accurate assessment of your LDL, HDL, and total cholesterol levels as well as your triglyceride levels. This analysis requires a fasting blood test (no eating or drinking for 12 hours before the test) administered by a reputable health provider. You can compare your numbers to Table 10.4 and discuss their significance with your physician.

Overweight and Obesity Being overweight or obese can strain the heart, forcing it to push blood through "extra" miles of capillaries that supply each pound of fat. A heart that must continuously move blood through an overabundance of vessels has to work harder and

may become weakened or damaged. The same high-fat, high-sugar, and high-calorie diets that lead to overweight and obesity can also contribute to plaque formation.

Overweight people are more likely to develop heart disease and stroke even if they have no other CVD risk factors.[45] This is especially true for people who tend to store fat around the upper body and waist (an "apple" shape) as opposed to those who tend to store fat around the hips and thighs (a "pear" shape). Further, losing as little as 5 to 10 percent of your body weight can significantly lower blood cholesterol.[46]

SEE IT! ONLINE

Mediterranean Diet Could Help Reduce Heart Disease

Physical Inactivity A sedentary lifestyle is one of the most significant risk factors for CVD. Elevating the heart rate and blood flow through moderate to vigorous activity benefits the heart muscle and helps prevent plaque deposits on artery walls. Conversely, inactivity decreases the efficiency of the heart muscle and allows plaque buildup to occur more easily. Even modest levels of low-intensity physical activity—walking, gardening, housework, dancing—are beneficial if done regularly and over the long term. Despite the clear benefits of regular exercise, only 34.4 percent of Americans over age 18 engage in any regular physical activity.[47]

Diabetes Mellitus Chronic diseases are interrelated: People who have one tend to have others. This connection is especially clear when it comes to diabetes and CVD. Having diabetes significantly increases one's risk for CVD even if blood sugar levels are well controlled. When they're uncontrolled, the risks are even higher. People with diabetes have death rates from CVD that are two to four times higher than those of people without diabetes.[48] Some experts estimate that as many as 50 percent of people with diabetes eventually die of CVD.[49] In fact, the risk is so great, many physicians consider someone with pre-diabetes or with the early stages of diabetes to have the same risks as someone who has already had his or her first heart attack. Diabetics also tend to have elevated blood fat levels, increased atherosclerosis, and a tendency toward deterioration of small blood vessels, particularly in the eyes and extremities.

Metabolic Syndrome **Metabolic syndrome** refers to a cluster of obesity-related risk factors associated with CVD and type 2 diabetes.[50] People with metabolic

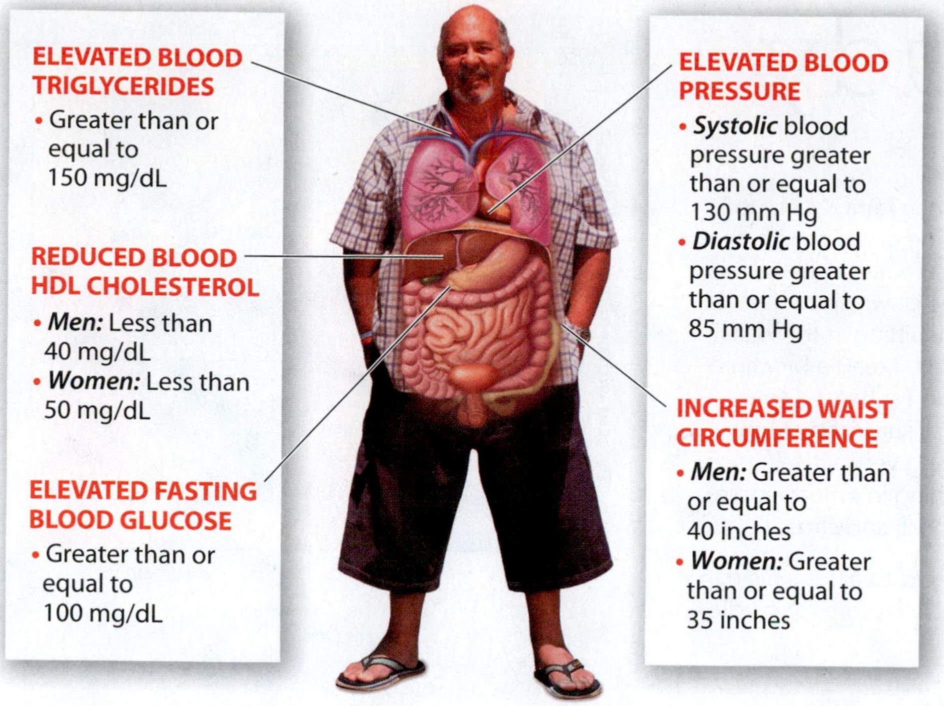

ELEVATED BLOOD TRIGLYCERIDES
- Greater than or equal to 150 mg/dL

REDUCED BLOOD HDL CHOLESTEROL
- *Men:* Less than 40 mg/dL
- *Women:* Less than 50 mg/dL

ELEVATED FASTING BLOOD GLUCOSE
- Greater than or equal to 100 mg/dL

ELEVATED BLOOD PRESSURE
- *Systolic* blood pressure greater than or equal to 130 mm Hg
- *Diastolic* blood pressure greater than or equal to 85 mm Hg

INCREASED WAIST CIRCUMFERENCE
- *Men:* Greater than or equal to 40 inches
- *Women:* Greater than or equal to 35 inches

FIGURE **10.2** Risk factors associated with metabolic syndrome.

syndrome have several characteristics in common (see **Figure 10.2**):

- Abdominal obesity, meaning a large waistline (more than 40 inches in men or 35 inches in women)
- Elevated levels of triglycerides in the blood (more than 150 mg/dL)
- Low levels of "good cholesterol" (HDLs below 40 mg/dL in men or 50 mg/dL in women)
- High blood pressure (greater than 130/85 mm Hg)
- High levels of the sugar glucose in the blood (more than 100 mg/dL after fasting)
- High levels of C-reactive protein (more than 10 mg/L), indicating inflammation

The National Heart, Lung, and Blood Institute estimates that 47 million American adults—fully one-quarter of our adult population—have metabolic syndrome.[51] By definition, they have multiple risk factors for CVD, and thus their overall risk of developing cardiovascular illness is high.

The prevalence of metabolic syndrome in adolescents and young adults is causing concern among many health professionals. Over 20 percent of people aged 20–39 meet the criteria for metabolic syndrome.[52] According to another study, 43 percent of college students had at least one of the indicators.[53] Poor nutrition (specifically low intake of fruits and vegetables and

high intake of sweetened beverages), poor fitness levels, and being overweight are all associated with higher risk for metabolic syndrome.[54] The message here is clear: Being young does not make you immune to metabolic syndrome and its multiple risk factors for cardiovascular disease.

Other Controllable Factors Stress can act as a risk factor for CVD. Your body's stress response can cause blood pressure to rise and can trigger blood-clotting and heart rhythm abnormalities.[55] Stress can also foster habits that promote CVD, such as overeating, smoking, or poor sleep. Disrupted sleep, insomnia, sleep apnea, and snoring have all been linked to higher CVD risk.[56]

Poor nutrition also increases CVD risk. Too much saturated fat, salt, and refined carbohydrates and too little fiber and too few fruits and vegetables all heighten risk, while improved nutrition lowers risk.

Although some studies have suggested that *moderate* amounts of alcohol may help lower the risk of cardiovascular disease, excessive alcohol consumption can raise blood triglycerides, trigger arrhythmias, raise blood pressure, promote obesity, and contribute to heart failure and strokes. Stimulant drugs, such as amphetamines or cocaine, can also trigger strokes—even in young people.[57]

Risks You Cannot Control

Unfortunately, there are risk factors for cardiovascular disease that you cannot control, but knowing about them can help you plan for the right kinds of action. The list includes:

Heredity A family history of cardiovascular disease—that is, CVD in several generations of an extended family—appears to increase risk

metabolic syndrome A group of metabolic conditions occurring together that increase a person's risk of heart disease, stroke, and diabetes

casestudy

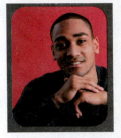

DARYL

"I took my mom in for a check-up the other day. The good news is that her blood pressure and cholesterol have both come down since her last visit. While I was sitting in the waiting room, though, I read a brochure about risk factors for heart disease. I knew genetics was a factor, but I was surprised at how many other risk factors I had: not being very active (unless you count playing the piano!), breathing in other people's smoke at jazz clubs, too much fast food, and stress."

THINK! What else could Daryl do to assess his risk for cardiovascular disease? What risk factors for cardiovascular disease do you have?

ACT NOW! Today, sort your risk factors by "controllable" and "non-controllable" and place them in order of greatest risk. This week, list ways you could change your lifestyle to reduce your vulnerability for the top three controllable risk factors. In two weeks, list ways to work on each listed item. These will overlap, so boil your lifestyle ideas down to one set and begin!

HEAR IT! ONLINE

FIGURE **10.3** Cardiovascular disease affects a disproportionate percentage of African Americans.

Data from American Heart Association, "Heart Disease and Stroke Statistics—2013 Update," *Circulation* 127 (2013): e6-e245. Comparable data on Hispanic American and Asian American populations were not available in this report.

---

significantly. Even subtle inherited traits like blood type can increase risk. In a recent study, people with type A blood had a risk of CVD 5 percent higher than those with type O. People with type B had an 11 percent higher risk, and those with type AB had a 23 percent risk![58] The increased risk may be due both to genetics, to your home environment and learned patterns of diet, exercise, and stress, and to the way these factors interact.

Age Seventy-five percent of all heart attacks occur in people over age 65. The risk for CVD increases with age for both sexes.[59] As we've seen, though, blood vessel plaques can begin in kids and teens.

Gender Men are at greater risk for CVD until about age 60, when risk equalizes between the sexes.[60] A man's risk, carried at least in part by the Y chromosome, is magnified in males with ancestors from Northern Europe.[61] In women, the age when menstruation starts and stops is correlated with greater risk for CVD: an earlier start (menarche) comes with higher risk, as does an earlier stop (menopause).[62] Regardless of menstrual

timetable, women under age 35 have a fairly low risk of CVD unless they have high blood pressure, kidney problems, or diabetes. The risks rise in all women over 35, especially those who smoke and also take oral contraceptives. In all women after menopause or after estrogen levels decline due to hysterectomy or ovary disease, LDL levels tend to rise and with them the risk for developing cardiovascular disease.[63]

Race Members of certain racial/ethnic groups may face increased cardiovascular disease risk (see **Figure 10.3**).[64] African Americans have the highest rates of cardiovascular disease, followed by Caucasian Americans and Mexican Americans. Rates for Asian Americans are below 25 percent.[65] A recent study revealed that black males have higher levels of aldosterone, a hormone produced by the adrenal glands on the kidneys and involved in the body's water and salt retention and excretion. Naturally higher levels of aldosterone cause increased sodium and water retention, higher blood pressure, and changes to the heart, even in black males aged 15 to 19.[66]

How Can I Avoid Cardiovascular Disease?

People often wait until they get a scary medical diagnosis before changing their habits. If you have risk factors for cardiovascular disease, the earlier you identify and confront them, the better your chances of avoiding CVD later.

LIVE IT! ONLINE

Worksheet 38 Cardiovascular Risk Assessment

Lower Your Controllable Risks

Here are specific behavioral tips for avoiding cardiovascular disease by reducing the risk factors you can control.

Don't Use Tobacco According to the American Heart Association, smoking is the greatest preventable cause of disease and death. Even light smoking—just two cigarettes per day—increases your CVD risk. When people stop smoking, regardless of how long or how much they have smoked, their risk of heart disease declines rapidly. Three years after quitting, the risk of death from heart disease and stroke for people who smoked a pack a day or less is almost the same as for people who never smoked. Women appear to recover lung function more fully than men.[67] Since secondhand smoke is a potent risk factor, avoid smoky places when possible. Avoid all forms of tobacco, since nicotine increases blood pressure, heart rate, blood clotting, and plaque buildup.

Eat Well There are numerous ways you can promote cardiovascular health through better nutrition. The American Heart Association recommends the following:[68]

- Aim to use up at least as many calories as you consume.

- Eat a wide variety of foods from all the basic food groups.

- Aim to have a diet that consists of mainly nutrient-rich foods such as vegetables, fruits, and whole-grain products. Fruits and vegetables are high in vitamins, minerals, and fiber and are low in calories. Individual studies on apples, raisins, citrus fruit, hot peppers, blueberries, and strawberries have each identified specific compounds that cut LDL levels, lower blood pressure, open blood vessels, or lower cardiovascular risks in other ways.[69] Meanwhile, the fiber in unrefined whole-grain foods can help lower cholesterol and help you feel full (which can help with weight management).

- Consume healthy oils. The omega-3 fatty acids in fish such as salmon and trout may help lower the risk of death from coronary artery disease. Nuts and vegetable oils also contain omega-3 and omega-6 fatty acids. Vegetable oils high in monounsaturated fats, such as canola oil, can actually help reduce belly fat.[70]

- Consume lean meats without skin, and cook them without added saturated and *trans* fat. Or substitute beans and legumes as a protein source instead of meats. Eating red meat is linked to higher risks of CVD and cancer.[71] Low-carbohydrate, high-protein diets that concentrate on animal proteins can significantly increase CVD risk.[72]

- Avoid high-fat dairy products, and instead consume fat-free, 1 percent fat, or low-fat dairy products.

- Reduce your consumption of foods containing partially hydrogenated vegetable oils to lower the amount of *trans* fat in your diet.

- Cut back on foods high in dietary cholesterol. Aim to eat less than 300 milligrams of cholesterol each day. Eating three or more egg yolks per week can accelerate plaque formation in blood vessels.[73]

- Cut back on beverages and foods with added sugars.

- Reduce your intake of sodium to 1,500 milligrams or less per day.

- Drink alcohol in moderation.

- Be aware of portion sizes, especially while dining out.

If you have (or are at risk of developing) hypertension, your physician may suggest that you adopt the DASH (Dietary Approaches to Stop Hypertension) diet. Following this diet can help lessen your risk of hypertension and other forms of cardiovascular disease. The box on the DASH Diet on the following page discusses the diet's specific recommendations.

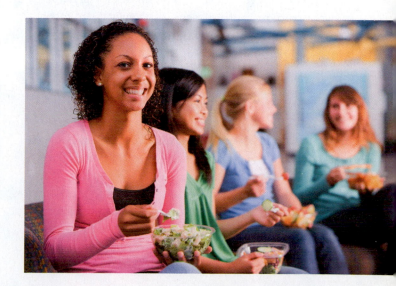

TOOLS FOR CHANGE

The DASH Diet

The DASH (Dietary Approaches to Stop Hypertension) diet is a set of nutritional guidelines designed to reduce blood pressure. Recommended by the National Heart, Lung, and Blood Institute and the American Heart Association, it is characterized by the following:

- Reduced consumption of saturated fat, total fat, red meats, sodium, sweets, added sugars, and sugar-containing beverages

- Increased consumption of fruits, vegetables, fat-free or low-fat dairy products, whole-grain foods, fish, poultry, and nuts

- Special care to consume recommended levels of potassium, magnesium, calcium, protein, and fiber

You can find the entire DASH eating plan—including nutrient goals and serving recommendations at different calorie levels for various food groups—online at www.nhlbi.nih.gov/health/public/heart/hbp/dash /new_dash.pdf.

In addition to these guidelines, the DASH diet provides tips for reducing sodium—often hidden in processed foods—that can benefit virtually everyone:

- Buy the low- or reduced-sodium versions of soups, condiments, crackers, and other packaged foods. Read labels carefully and watch for sodium in such items as breakfast cereals and salad dressings.

- Choose fresh or frozen vegetables. If buying canned foods, look for no-sodium or low-sodium versions.

- Watch out for canned, smoked, cured, or processed meats and brined foods such as pickles and olives, which are usually very high in sodium. Rinse when practical to wash away some of the salt.

- Some processed foods have so much sodium you may simply have to avoid them; examples include packaged cake and sauce mixes, pizzas, and frozen dinners.

Source: U.S. Department of Health and Human Services, National Institutes of Health, National Heart, Lung, and Blood Institute, *What Is the DASH Eating Plan?* Accessed July 02, 2012, www.nhlbi.nih.gov

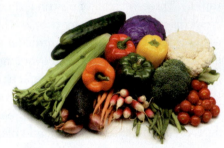

Exercise Regularly Regular cardiovascular exercise strengthens the heart muscles and helps keep the blood vessels resilient. Performing 30 to 60 minutes or more of moderate activity most days of the week will help prevent cardiovascular disease, especially if you reach your target heart rate. Strength training and flexibility are also important components of your exercise plan for cardiovascular wellness, helping you to maintain muscle mass, speed metabolism, control weight, and prevent injury.

Manage Your Stress The physiological stress response raises blood pressure, speeds the heart rate, and floods the bloodstream with glucose. All of these, in turn, can promote cardiovascular disease by damaging the blood vessels and directly contributing to atherosclerosis, and by weakening the heart through electrical and hormonal overstimulation. Learning specific techniques for stress reduction, relaxation, and anger management can give you important tools for lowering your risk of cardiovascular disease.

Control Diabetes Because elevated sugar levels in the blood greatly increase the risk for heart disease, stroke, and artery disease, people with diabetes are at tremendous risk. The very factors that contribute to the development of diabetes (obesity, hypertension, elevated blood cholesterol and triglycerides, inactivity) are additional risks for CVD. Careful diet, increased exercise, and medication help most diabetics control their condition and lower their CVD risk.

Avoid Alcohol and Drug Abuse If you drink, keep your consumption below one drink per day if you are a woman and two per day if you are a man. Greater consumption raises blood sugar and triglyceride levels. Avoid recreational drugs, especially stimulants.

CHAPTER IN REVIEW

MasteringHealth™

Build your knowledge—and wellness!—in the Study Area of MasteringHealth with a variety of study tools.

SEE IT! ONLINE

videos
Importance of Heart Health in Your Youth

Stroke in Young Adults

Mediterranean Diet Could Help Reduce Heart Disease

LIVE IT! ONLINE

programs & behavior change
Take Charge of Your Health! Worksheets:

Worksheet 38 Cardiovascular Risk Assessment

Worksheet 39 Healthy Heart I.Q.

Behavior Change Log Book and Wellness Journal

HEAR IT! ONLINE

audio tools
Audio case study

MP3 chapter review

DO IT! ONLINE

labs
Lab 10.1 Understand Your CVD Risk

REVIEW IT! ONLINE

chapter review
Chapter reading quizzes

Glossary flashcards

---

review questions

1. Cardiovascular disease and stroke are responsible for about _____ of deaths in the United States each year.
   a. one-half
   b. one-tenth
   c. one-sixth
   d. one-third

2. In annual medical care costs and lost productivity, CVD could cost Americans about _____ in 2030.
   a. $818,000
   b. $81.8 million.
   c. $818 million.
   d. $818 billion.

3. Which of the following is an example of cardiovascular disease (CVD)?
   a. Diabetes
   b. Low blood pressure
   c. Coronary heart disease
   d. Systolic pressure

4. Which of the following accurately describes *hypertension*?
   a. Sustained high blood pressure
   b. A thickening or hardening of the arteries
   c. Heart blockage
   d. Irregular heartbeat

5. Which of the following is characteristic of cardiovascular disease?
   a. Joint pain
   b. Feeling energized
   c. Having no symptoms at all
   d. Dry skin

6. When atherosclerosis occurs in the heart's main blood vessels, it is called
   a. peripheral artery disease.
   b. coronary artery disease.
   c. inflammation.
   d. homocysteine.

7. Which of the following is a significant risk factor for CVD?
   a. Regular exercise
   b. Managed stress
   c. Underweight
   d. Tobacco use

8. A person with metabolic syndrome is likely to have which one of the following?
   a. Abdominal obesity or a large waistline
   b. Depressed levels of triglycerides in the blood
   c. High levels of "good" cholesterol (HDLs)
   d. Hypoglycemia or low blood sugar

9. Which of the following statements is true?
   a. The earliest manifestations of cardiovascular disease often take root during childhood.
   b. Only seniors need to worry about cardiovascular disease.
   c. Heavy alcohol consumption is unrelated to your risks for developing cardiovascular disease.
   d. People who are skinny are protected against cardiovascular disease.

10. Low-density lipoprotein (LDL) is often referred to as
   a. "good" cholesterol.
   b. "bad" cholesterol.
   c. diabetes mellitus.
   d. metabolic syndrome.

critical thinkingquestions

1. List six different forms of CVD. Compare and contrast their risk factors, symptoms, and prevention.
2. Describe the atherosclerosis process and explain the medical term *atherosclerotic cardiovascular disease*.
3. Discuss the evidence that people in your age group are at risk for developing CVD.
4. Discuss specific ways that exercise and dietary changes can help prevent CVD.

references

1. National Center for Health Statistics (NCHS), "FastStats: Leading Causes of Death," Updated January 2013, www.cdc.gov
2. A. S. Go et al., "Heart Disease and Stroke Statistics 2013 Update: A Report from the American Heart Association," *Circulation* 127 (2013): e6–245, doi: 10.1161/ CIR.0b013e31828124ad
3. Ibid.
4. Ibid.
5. C. Friedemann et al., "Cardiovascular Disease Risk in Healthy Children and Its Association with Body Mass Index: Systematic Review and Meta-Analysis," *British Medical Journal* 2012; 345: e4759, doi: 10.1136bmj/e4759; A. S. Go et al., "Heart Disease and Stroke Statistics, 2013," 2013.
6. S. L. Murphy et al., "Deaths: Preliminary Data for 2010," *National Vital Statistics Reports* 60, no. 4 (Hyattsville, MD: National Center for Health Statistics, 2012).
7. American Heart Association, "American Heart Association Scientific Statement: Combined Behavioral Interventions Best Way to Reduce Heart Disease Risk," July 12, 2010, http://newsroom.heart.org.
8. A. S. Go et al., "Heart Disease and Stroke Statistics 2013," 2013.
9. H. C. McGill et al., "Origin of Atherosclerosis in Childhood and Adolescence," *American Journal of Clinical Nutrition* 72, no. 5 (2000): 1307S–15S.
10. N. M. van Emmerick et al., "High Cardiovascular Risk in Severely Obese Young Children and Adolescents," *Archives of Diseases in Children* 97, no. 9 (2012): 818–21, doi: 10.1136/archdischild-2012-301877
11. H. C. McGill et al., "Association of Coronary Heart Disease Risk Factors with Microscopic Qualities of Coronary Atherosclerosis in Youth," *Circulation* 102, no. 4 (2000): 374–9.
12. M. G. George et al., "Trends in Stroke Hospitalizations and Associated Risk Factors among Children and Young Adults, 1995–2008," *Annals of Neurology* 70, no. 5 (2011): 713–21.
13. Friedemann, 2012; P. Franks et al., "Childhood Obesity, Other Cardiovascular Risks, and Premature Death," *New England Journal of Medicine* 362, no. 6 (2010): 485–93; Y. M. Hong, "Atherosclerotic Cardiovascular Disease Beginning in Childhood," *Korean Circulation Journal* 40, no. 1 (2010): 1–9; R. E. Kavey et al., "American Heart Association Guidelines for Primary Prevention of Atherosclerotic Cardiovascular Disease Beginning in Childhood," *Circulation* 107, no. 11 (2003): 1562–6.
14. A. G. Mainous III et al., "Life Stress and Atherosclerosis: A Pathway through Unhealthy Lifestyle," *International Journal of Psychiatry in Medicine* 40, no. 2 (2010): 147–61; Mayo Clinic Staff, "Arteriosclerosis/Atherosclerosis: Causes," June 2012, www.mayoclinic.com.
15. Centers for Disease Control and Prevention, "Heart Disease: Frequently Asked Questions (FAQs)," Updated March 19, 2013, www.cdc.gov
16. B. Liebman, "Fighting Inflammation: It's Not as Simple as Some Claim," *Nutrition Action Healthletter*, November 2011, 9–11.
17. American Heart Association, "Inflammation and Heart Disease," Updated November 2012, www.heart.org
18. American Heart Association, "Homocysteine, Folic Acid, and Cardiovascular Disease," Updated January 2012, www.heart.org
19. Emerging Risk Factors Collaboration, "C-Reactive Protein, Fibrinogen, and Cardiovascular Disease Prediction," *New England Journal of Medicine* 367, no. 14 (2012): 1310–20, doi: 10. 1056/ NEJMoa1107477.
20. B. M. Egan, Y. Zhao, and R. N. Axon, "US Trends in Prevalence, Awareness, Treatment, and Control of Hypertension, 1988–2008," *Journal of the American Medical Association* 303, no. 20 (2010): 2043–50.
21. Mayo Clinic Staff, "High Blood Pressure (Hypertension)," August 2012, www .mayoclinic.com
22. "Why Blood Pressure Matters," American Heart Association, Updated August 2012, www.heart.org
23. Ibid.
24. S. I. Sharp et al., "Hypertension Is a Potential Risk Factor for Vascular Dementia: Systematic Review," *International Journal of Geriatric Psychiatry* 26, no. 7 (2011): 661–9; F. D. Testai and P. B. Gorelick, "Vascular Cognitive Impairment and Alzheimer's Disease: Are These Disorders Linked to Hypertension and Other Cardiovascular Risk Factors?" in V. Aiyagari and P. B. Gorelick (eds.) *Hypertension and Stroke: Pathophysiology and Management* (New York: Humana Press, 2011): 195–210.
25. N. L. Keenan and K. A. Rosendorf, "Prevalence of Hypertension and Controlled Hypertension—United States, 2005–2008," Centers for Disease Control and Prevention, *Morbidity and Mortality Weekly Report, Supplements* 60, no. 1 (2011): 94–97.
26. American Heart Association, "About High Blood Pressure," Updated January 2013, www.heart.org
27. Ibid.

28. J. Flynn, "Hypertension in the Young: Epidemiology, Sequelae, and Therapy," *Nephrology, Dialysis, Transplantation* 24, no. 2 (2009): 370–75.

29. A. S. Go et al., "Heart Disease and Stroke Statistics 2013," 2013.

30. Ibid.

31. American Heart Association, "About Arrhythmia," Updated May 2012, www.heart.org

32. American Heart Association, "About Heart Failure," Updated August 2012, www.heart.org

33. American Heart Association, "About Congenital Heart Defects," Updated January 2011, www.heart.org

34. A. S. Go et al., "Heart Disease and Stroke Statistics 2013," 2013.

35. Mary G. George et al., "Trends in Stroke Hospitalizations and Risk Factors in Children and Young Adults: 1995–2008," *Annals of Neurology* 70, no 5 (2011): 713–21, doi: 10.1002/ana.22539

36. Mayo Clinic Staff, "Stroke: Risk Factors," July 2012, www.mayoclinic.com.

37. Mayo Clinic Staff, "Transient Ischemic Attack (TIA)," March 2011, www.mayoclinic.com

38. National Heart, Lung, and Blood Institute, "What Are Coronary Heart Disease Risk Factors?" February 2011, www.nhlbi.nih.gov

39. Centers for Disease Control, Chronic Disease Prevention and Health Promotion, "Tobacco Use," Updated November 2012, www.cdc.gov

40. American Heart Association, "Heart Disease and Stroke Statistics," 2013; R. S. Shah and J. W. Cole, "Smoking and Stroke: The More You Smoke the More You Stroke," *Expert Review of Cardiovascular Therapy* 8, (2010): 917–32, doi: 10.1586/erc.10.56.

41. American Cancer Society, "Secondhand Smoke," Revised October 2012, www.cancer.org

42. Mayo Clinic Staff, "High Blood Pressure Dangers: Hypertension's Effects on Your Body," January 2011, www.mayoclinic.com

43. F. C. D. Andrade et al., "One-Year Follow-Up Changes in Weight Are Associated with Changes in Blood Pressure in Young Mexican Adults," *Public Health* 126, no. 6 (2012): 535, doi: 10.1016.j.puhe.2012.02.005

44. National Center for Health Statistics, *Health, United States, 2010: With Special Feature on Death and Dying* (Hyattsville, MD: U.S. Department of Health and Human Services, 2011) Table 95.

45. A. S. Go et al., "Heart Disease and Stroke Statistics 2013," 2013.

46. Mayo Clinic Staff, "Top 5 Lifestyle Changes to Reduce Cholesterol," September 2012, www.mayoclinic.com

47. National Center for Health Statistics, "National Health Interview Survey, 1997–2010, Leisure-Time Physical Activity," June 2011, www.cdc.gov

48. American Diabetes Association, "Diabetes Statistics: 2011 National Diabetes Fact Sheet," January 2011, www.diabetes.org

49. World Heart Federation, "Diabetes and Cardiovascular Disease," January 2011, www.world-heart-federation.org

50. A. S. Go et al., "Heart Disease and Stroke Statistics 2013," 2013.

51. National Heart, Lung, and Blood Institute, "What Is Metabolic Syndrome?" April 2011, www.nhlbi.nih.gov

52. A. S. Go et al., "Heart Disease and Stroke Statistics 2013," 2013.

53. T. L. Keown, C. B. Smith, and M. S. Harris, "Metabolic Syndrome among College Students," *The Journal for Nurse Practitioners* 5, no. 10 (2009): 754–9.

54. J. Schilter and L. Dalleck, "Fitness and Fatness: Indicators of Metabolic Syndrome and Cardiovascular Disease Risk Factors in College Students?" *Journal of Exercise Physiology* 13, no. 4 (2010): 29–39.

55. M. Esler et al., "Chronic Mental Stress Is a Cause of Essential Hypertension: Presence of Biological Markers of Stress," *Clinical and Experimental Pharmacology and Physiology* 35, no. 4 (2008): 498–502; A. Flaa et al., "Sympathoadrenal Stress Reactivity Is a Predictor of Future Blood Pressure: An 18-Year Follow-Up Study," *Hypertension* 52, no. 2 (2008): 336–41; T. Chandola et al., "Work Stress and Coronary Heart Disease: What Are the Mechanisms?" *European Heart Journal* 29, no. 5 (2008): 640–8.

56. Wageningen University, "Short and Bad Sleepers Have Increased Risk of Cardiovascular Disease," February 28, 2013, www.wageningenur.nl; European Society of Cardiology, "Treat Snoring to Avoid Deadly Heart Failure," Dec. 5, 2012, www.escardio.org

57. A. N. Westover, S. McBride, and R. W. Haley, "Stroke in Young Adults Who Abuse Amphetamines or Cocaine," *Archives of General Psychiatry* 64 (2007): 495–502.

58. M. He et al., "ABO Blood Group and Risk of Coronary Heart Disease in Two Prospective Cohort Studies," *Arteriosclerosis, Thrombosis and Vascular Biology* 32, no. 9 (2012): 2314–320, doi: 10.1161/%u200BATVBAHA.112.248757

59. A. S. Go et al., "Heart Disease and Stroke Statistics 2013," 2013.

60. Ibid.

61. F. J. Charchar et al., "Inheritance of Coronary Artery Disease in Men: An Analysis of the Role of the Y Chromosome," *The Lancet* 379, no. 9819 (2012): 915–22, doi: 10.1016/S0140-6736(11)61453-0.

62. S. Trikudanathan et al., "Association of Female Reproductive Factors with Body Composition: The Framingham Heart Study," *Journal of Clinical Endocrinology and Metabolism* 98, no. 1 (2012): 236–44, doi: 10.1210/jc.2012-1785; M. Wellons et al., "Early Menopause Predicts Future Coronary Heart Disease and Stroke: The Multi-Ethnic Study of Atherosclerosis," *Menopause* 19, no. 10 (2012): 1081–7, doi: 10.1097/gme.0b013e3182517bd0

63. National Heart, Lung, and Blood Institute, National Cholesterol Education Program, "High Blood Cholesterol: What You Need to Know," NIH Publication No. 05-3290, Revised June 2005, www.nhlbi.nih.gov

64. American Heart Association, "Heart Disease and Stroke Statistics 2013 Update," 2013.

65. Ibid.

66. D. G. Murro et al., "Aldosterone Contributes to Elevated Left Ventricular Mass in Black Boys," *Pediatric Nephrology* 28, no. 4 (2013): 2–12, doi: 10.1007/s00467-012-2367-6.

67. Centers for Disease Control and Prevention, "Tobacco Use: Targeting the Nation's Leading Killer—At A Glance 2011," Updated February 2011, www.cdc.gov

68. American Heart Association, "American Heart Association Supports New USDA/HHS Dietary Guidelines and Encourages Adherence: AHA Also Expresses Disappointment That Sodium, Saturated Fat Guidance Is Weak." Press Release January 2011, http://newsroom.heart.org

69. S. Zhao et al., "Intakes of Apples or Apple Polyphenols Decrease Plasma Values for Oxidized Low-Density Lipoprotein/beta2-glycoprotein I," *Journal of Functional Foods* 5, no. 1 (2013): 493–97, doi: 10.1016/j.jff.2012.08.010; Cardio Source, "Snacking on Raisins May Offer a Heart-Healthy Way to Lower Blood Pressure," American College of Cardiology, March 25, 2012, www.cardiosource.org; A. Cassidy et al., "Dietary Flavonoids and Risk of Stroke in Women," *Stroke*, (2012), doi: 10.1161/STROKEAHA.111.637835; American Chemical Society, "Hot Pepper Compound Could Help Hearts," March 27, 2012, http://portal.acs.org; A. Cassidy et al., "High Anthocyanin Intake Is Associated with a Reduced Risk of Myocardial Infarction in Young and Middle Aged Women," *Circulation* 127, no. 2 (2013): 188–96, doi: 10.1161/CIRCULATIONAHA.112.122408.

70. Pennsylvania State University, "Monounsaturated Fats Reduce Metabolic Syndrome Risk," March 29, 2013, http://news.psu.edu

71. An Pan et al., "Red Meat Consumption and Mortality," *Archives of Internal Medicine* 172, no. 7 (2012): 555–63, doi: 10.1001/archinternmed.2011.2287.

72. P. Lagiou et al., "Low Carbohydrate-High Protein Diet and Incidence of Cardiovascular Diseases in Swedish Women: Prospective Cohort Study," *British Medical Journal*, 2012; 344: e4026, doi: 10.1136/bmj.e4026; I. Johansson et al., "Associations among 25-Year Trends in Diet, Cholesterol and BMI from 140,000 Observations in Men and Women in Northern Sweden," *Nutrition Journal* 11, no. 40 (2012), doi: 10.1186/1475-2891-11-40, www.nutritionj.com

73. J. D. Spence et al., "Egg Yolk Consumption and Carotid Plaque," *Atherosclerosis* 224, no. 2 (2012): 469–73, doi: 10.1016/j.atherosclerosis.2012.07.032.

getfitgraphic references

1. A. S. Go et al., "Heart Disease and Stroke Statistics—2013 Update: A Report from the American Heart Association," *Circulation* 127 (2013): e6-e245.

2. Centers for Disease Control and Prevention, "Heart Disease and Stroke Prevention— Addressing the Nation's Leading Killers: At A Glance 2011," Updated July 2010, www.cdc.gov

3. A. S. Go et al., "Heart Disease and Stroke Statistics—2013 Update: A Report from the American Heart Association," 2013.

4. World Health Organization, "Causes of Death 2008 Summary Tables," May 2011, www.who.int

LAB 10.1

UNDERSTAND YOUR CVD RISK

MasteringHealth™

Name: _____ Date: _____

Instructor: _____ Section: _____

Purpose: To engage students in critical thinking about their own risk factors for CVD.

Directions: Complete each of the following questions about CVD risk and total your points in each section—the higher the score, the greater your risk. If you answered "don't know" for any question, talk to your parents or other family members as soon as possible to find out whether you have any unknown risks.

SECTION I: ASSESS YOUR FAMILY RISK FOR CVD

	Yes	No	Don't Know
1. Do any of your primary relatives (mother, father, grandparents, siblings) have a history of heart disease or stroke?	1	0	
2. Do any of your primary relatives (mother, father, grandparents, siblings) have diabetes?	1	0	
3. Do any of your primary relatives (mother, father, grandparents, siblings) have high blood pressure?	1	0	
4. Do any of your primary relatives (mother, father, grandparents, siblings) have a history of high cholesterol?	1	0	
5. During the time you lived at home, did your family consume red meat and high-fat dairy products several times per week?	1	0	
Total for Section I = _____			

SECTION II: ASSESS YOUR LIFESTYLE RISK FOR CVD

	Yes	No	Don't Know
1. Do you have high blood pressure?	1	0	
2. Is your total cholesterol level higher than recommended? (See Table 10.4)	1	0	
3. Have you been diagnosed as pre-diabetic or diabetic?	1	0	
4. Do you smoke three or more cigarettes per day?	1	0	
5. Would you describe your life as being highly stressful?	1	0	
Total for Section II = _____			

SECTION III: ASSESS YOUR ADDITIONAL RISKS FOR CVD

1. How would you best describe your current BMI?	
<8.5 (1 point)	25–29.9 (1 point)
18.5–24.9 (0 point)	≥30 (2 points)

2. How would you describe your level of exercise?	
Moderate activity for 30 to 60 minutes on fewer than three days per week, plus fewer than three cardio workouts per week and fewer than two strength-training workouts per week	1 point
Moderate activity for 30 to 60 minutes most days of the week, plus three cardio workouts and two strength-training workouts per week	0 points
Moderate activity for 60 minutes or more most days of the week, plus more than three cardio workouts and two strength-training workouts per week	0 points

3. How would you describe your dietary behaviors?	
I eat more than the recommended number of calories each day.	1 point
I eat about the recommended number of calories/day for my age, BMI, and activity level.	0 points
I eat fewer than the recommended number of calories each day.	0 points

4. Which of the following best describes your typical dietary behavior?	
I eat several servings of red meat per week and consume saturated fat from other meats and high-fat dairy products most days.	1 point
I eat from the major food groups, trying hard to get the recommended fruits and vegetables.	0 points
Whenever possible, I try to substitute olive oil or canola oil for other forms of dietary fat.	0 points

Total for Section III = _____

Scoring: Look at each section. If your total score for that section is 0, your CVD risk is minimal. Keep up the good work! If your score is between 1 and 3, your risk is moderate and you should initiate some change to lower it. If you score a 4 or 5, you should make substantial changes in those factors that you can control. Your behavior change plan for the chapter will help, and you can get additional advice from your instructor.

SECTION IV: REFLECTION

1. What are your risk factors for CVD? Identify any behaviors that put you at risk for CVD. What can you change right now? What can you change in the future to reduce your risk?

_____

_____

_____

_____

2. Which risk factors for CVD are outside your control? What can you do to reduce your risk of CVD, even though you have some uncontrollable risk factors?

_____

_____

_____

_____

11 Reducing Your Risk of Diabetes and Other Chronic Diseases

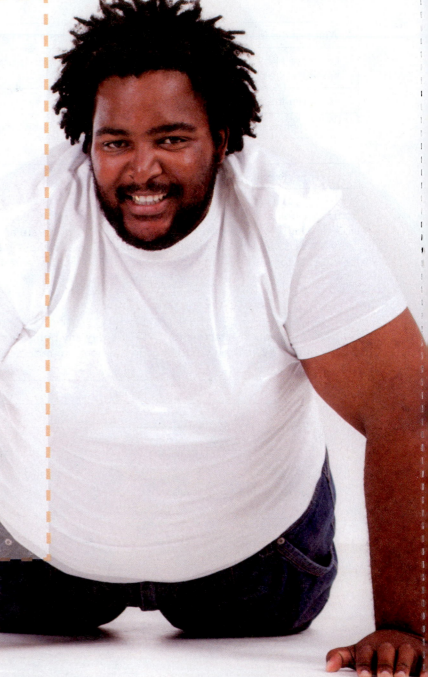

LEARNINGoutcomes

1 Define *chronic disease*, and explain why Americans should be concerned about chronic disease now and in the future.

2 Describe *type 2 diabetes* and list reasons why it is America's fastest-growing chronic disease.

3 Define *chronic lung disease* and explain why it is so common.

4 Define *osteoporosis* and explain how it heightens the risk for brittle and broken bones.

5 Provide details on *arthritis* and how it limits daily activity for millions of Americans.

6 For each major chronic disease, identify the common and specific risk factors. List several ways to lower your own risk of developing a chronic disease through exercise and other lifestyle factors.

MasteringHealth™

Go online for chapter quizzes, interactive assessments, videos, and more!

casestudy

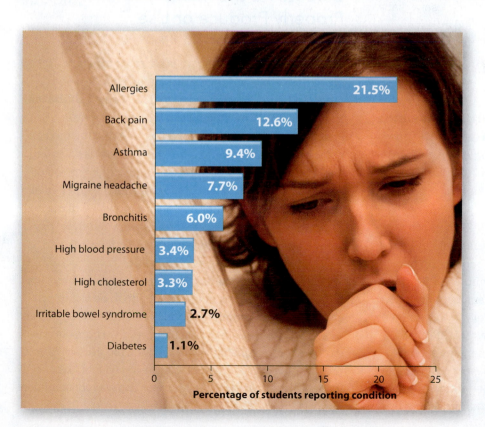

GRACE

"I'm Grace. I'm a nursing student and just found out that my blood sugar level is high enough to put me in the category for pre-diabetes. In class, I learned about patients with diabetes and other common diseases like emphysema, osteoporosis, and arthritis. Now it looks like I'm going to be a patient myself. Are some people more likely to develop diabetes than others? What can I do to keep my condition from getting any worse?"

HEAR IT! ONLINE

Y ou probably have a friend or family member with a **chronic disease**: a disease that tends to develop gradually and persist for months or years, often causing pain and disability. Generally, vaccines do not prevent chronic diseases and treatments do not provide a cure. However, lifestyle changes can often delay the onset of symptoms, and medications and treatments can relieve them. Common chronic diseases include cardiovascular disease (Chapter 10), cancer (Chapter 12), and the main topics of this chapter: diabetes, chronic lung diseases, osteoporosis, and arthritis. Chronic *conditions* are usually less severe medical issues and include allergies, back pain, migraine headaches, and irritable bowel syndrome.

Your chance of developing chronic diseases and conditions increases as you get older. College students are not immune, however, as **Figure 11.1** shows. The roots of many long-term diseases lie in poor health behaviors developed during childhood and in early adulthood. The U.S. Centers for Disease Control and Prevention (CDC) blames four behaviors—smoking, eating poorly, not exercising, and drinking too much alcohol— as causes for much of the illness and early death related to chronic diseases.[1] The CDC also warns that almost half of all American adults have at least one chronic disease and 7 out of 10 will die from one.[2] Learning about chronic disease now can inspire you to establish lifelong exercise, nutrition, and health care habits that may help you prevent or delay illness later in life.

Having one chronic disease can increase your susceptibility to developing other chronic diseases.[3] For example, having arthritis or osteoporosis makes exercise more difficult, which in turn may result in weight gain and exacerbate cardiovascular disease. And in people with diabetes, uncontrolled high levels of blood glucose can increase the risk of CVD and kidney disease, among others. By making plans for behavior change discussed in the earlier chapters of this textbook, you have already built a good foundation for lowering your risks of developing chronic

> **chronic disease** A medical condition that persists for a long period of time

FIGURE **11.1** Proportion of college students diagnosed with or treated for chronic conditions in the past 12 months.

Data are from American College Health Association, *American College Health Association—National College Health Assessment II (ACHA-NCHA II): Reference Group Data Report Fall 2012* (Hanover, MD: American College Health Association, 2013), www.acha-ncha.org

Percentage of students reporting condition

Condition	Percentage
Allergies	21.5%
Back pain	12.6%
Asthma	9.4%
Migraine headache	7.7%
Bronchitis	6.0%
High blood pressure	3.4%
High cholesterol	3.3%
Irritable bowel syndrome	2.7%
Diabetes	1.1%

TOOLS FOR CHANGE

Tips to Reduce Your Risk of Chronic Disease

The major risk factors for diabetes, chronic lung diseases, osteoporosis, and arthritis include obesity, inactivity, poor diet, and smoking. Fortunately, the same behavioral choices that increase overall wellness can also help you avoid chronic disease.

- Exercise daily
- Eat more fruits, vegetables, beans, nuts, whole grains, and heart-healthy fats
- Limit salt and sugar in your diet
- Maintain your recommended BMI
- Manage stress
- Avoid tobacco as well as drug and alcohol abuse
- Get enough sleep

Sleep aids in immune function and increased ability to ward off infection. Sleep deprivation can increase risks for diabetes, hypertension, obesity, depression, stress-related muscle aches and pains, and a host of other problems.[1]

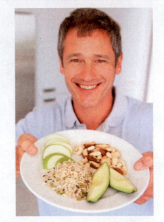

Sources:
1. Centers for Disease Control and Prevention, "Sleep and Sleep Disorders: Sleep and Chronic Disease," May 2012, www.cdc.gov; L. Rafalson et al., "Short Sleep Duration Is Associated with the Development of Impaired Fasting Glucose: The Western New York Health Study," *Annals of Epidemiology* 20, no. 12 (2010): 883–9, doi: 10.1016/j.annepidem.2010.05.002.

---

disease. Take a look at the box Tips to Reduce Your Risk of Chronic Disease for suggestions of other behaviors you might need to change to avoid chronic disease. The GetFitGraphic on page 387 illustrates how lifestyle choices can promote chronic disease. In the next sections, we examine four common chronic diseases more closely: diabetes, chronic lung disease, osteoporosis, and arthritis.

diabetes mellitus A disorder characterized by inadequate secretion or utilization of insulin, excessive urine production, excessive amounts of sugar in the blood and urine, and thirst, hunger, and weight loss

type 1 diabetes An autoimmune disease that destroys the insulin-producing cells of the pancreas, compromising the body's ability to make insulin and to properly regulate blood sugar

autoimmune disease A disorder in which the body's immune system creates antibodies that attack the person's own living cells

pre-diabetes A condition marked by blood glucose levels that are higher than normal but not yet diabetic

What Is Diabetes?

Diabetes mellitus is the fastest-growing chronic disease in America.[4] Today, diabetes affects 25.8 million Americans. By 2050, those numbers could more than double, with one-third of all Americans born after 2000 developing diabetes in their lifetimes.[5] Diabetes seems to be increasing more dramatically among younger adults than

among older Americans. One study by the CDC showed a rise in cases of almost 70 percent among people in their thirties.[6]

SEE IT! ONLINE

Young Adults and Diabetes

Diabetes Is the Inability to Properly Produce or Use Insulin

In healthy people, the pancreas secretes *insulin,* a hormone that is needed to convert sugar, starches, and other food into energy needed for life. **Type 1 diabetes** is an **autoimmune disease** in which the body's immune system creates antibodies that destroy the pancreas's ability to make insulin. The disease has a strong genetic basis and usually develops during childhood or adolescence. Type 1 diabetes represents 5 percent of all cases of diabetes mellitus.[7] People with type 1 diabetes depend on insulin injections or infusions and must pay careful attention to diet, exercise, and stress levels to control their blood glucose.

In people with **pre-diabetes**, blood glucose levels are higher than normal but not high enough to be classified as diabetes.[8] An estimated 57 million Americans age 20 or older have pre-diabetes.[9] If you're like Grace from our case study, you can probably halt or slow the progression of your pre-diabetes or type 2 diabetes by losing weight, exercising more, controlling stress, and avoiding overconsumption of alcohol.[10]

In **type 2 diabetes**, the pancreas may produce too little insulin, or it may secrete sufficient insulin but the body's cells are unable to use the hormone properly to convert glucose into cellular energy (**Figure 11.2**). This results in elevated glucose levels in the blood and urine, a condition known as *hyperglycemia*. Over time, high blood glucose levels can result in blindness, nerve damage, and significant circulatory system damage. In adults, type 2 diabetes represents 90 to 95 percent of all cases of diabetes mellitus.[11] It is most common in older Americans; one in four adults over age 65 has the disease.[12] Physicians used to refer to type 2 diabetes as *adult-onset diabetes*; now, however, they are diagnosing it in younger adults and even in teens and children. In the United States prior to the year 2000, only 1 to 2 percent of patients below age 18 diagnosed with diabetes had type 2. But recent reports indicate that as many as 33 percent of Americans born after the year 2000 could one day develop type 2 diabetes.[13] The disease has a weak genetic basis and is linked to obesity and inactivity, so people are often able to control their diabetes through weight loss, increased activity, improved diet, and sometimes medications.

type 2 diabetes A disease linked to obesity and inactivity in which the body loses its ability to respond to insulin and cannot properly regulate blood sugar

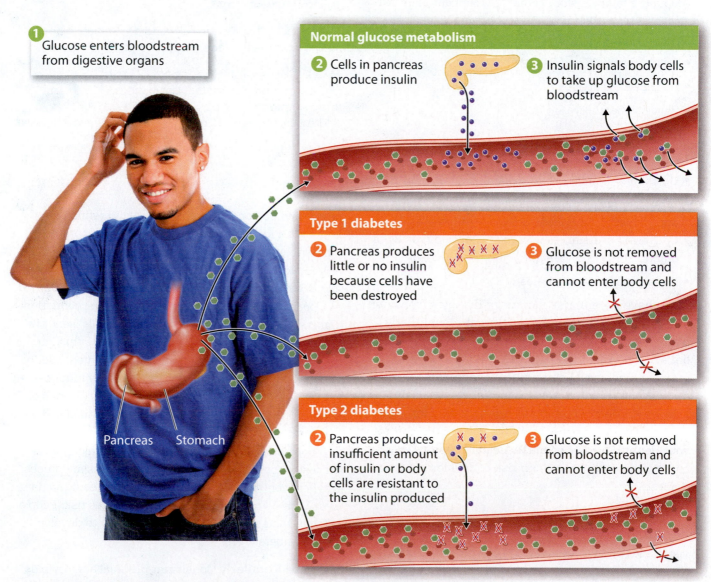

① Glucose enters bloodstream from digestive organs

Pancreas   Stomach

Normal glucose metabolism

② Cells in pancreas produce insulin

③ Insulin signals body cells to take up glucose from bloodstream

Type 1 diabetes

② Pancreas produces little or no insulin because cells have been destroyed

③ Glucose is not removed from bloodstream and cannot enter body cells

Type 2 diabetes

② Pancreas produces insufficient amount of insulin or body cells are resistant to the insulin produced

③ Glucose is not removed from bloodstream and cannot enter body cells

FIGURE **11.2** In type 1 diabetes, the pancreas produces too little insulin. In type 2 diabetes, either the pancreas doesn't produce enough insulin or the body cells have developed resistance to insulin so they cannot properly respond to it. Both diseases result in body cells lacking energy because they cannot take up glucose from the bloodstream. Glucose accumulates in the blood causing high blood sugar levels that can lead to damage of nerves, kidneys, eyes, and blood vessels.

A third form of diabetes, *gestational diabetes,* can develop in women during pregnancy. The condition usually disappears after childbirth but can leave the woman at greater risk of developing type 2 diabetes.[14] Gaining weight between pregnancies also increases the risk of type 2 diabetes.

Common symptoms of diabetes include excessive thirst and frequent urination. Physicians confirm a diagnosis of diabetes by measuring the levels of glucose in blood or urine.

You Can Lower Your Risk of Developing Diabetes

You may have an elevated risk for type 1 diabetes if you have a family history of diabetes or of autoimmune diseases.[15] Your risks for developing type 2 diabetes increase with the following factors:

- Age between 35 and 64
- High BMI (30 or above)
- Physical inactivity
- Poor diet
- A family history of type 2 diabetes
- Gestational diabetes during pregnancy
- Ethnic status (Native Americans, African Americans, and Hispanic Americans are twice as likely as Caucasian or Asian Americans to develop type 2 diabetes)
- A diagnosis of pre-diabetes

If you have several risk factors for diabetes, consult a physician and get your blood sugar tested. Early diagnosis of pre-diabetes or diabetes can allow earlier and better control of blood sugar and can help reduce blood vessel and nerve damage. If you are diagnosed with diabetes or pre-diabetes, closely follow your doctor's recommendations for diet, exercise, and drug treatments. While you cannot control your genetics, you can make lifestyle choices that can significantly lower your risk of developing type 2 diabetes.[16]

Eat a Healthy Diet You can lower your risk of type 2 diabetes by eating five to nine servings of fruits and vegetables and several servings of whole-grain foods each day.[17] One recent study showed that the beta carotene in yellow and orange fruits and vegetables is particularly protective for people with genetic risk of type 2 diabetes.[18] Choose proteins and dairy products low in saturated fat and consume heart-healthy

case study

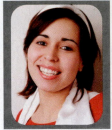

GRACE

"The doctor told me that several things put me at high risk of becoming diabetic: lack of exercise, a high BMI, being Hispanic, and my family medical history—my aunt has diabetes. He also said that pre-diabetes is pretty common and that to keep it from getting worse, I should lose weight and start exercising. I'll admit it—I hate to sweat, and I know I don't always eat the healthiest foods! But if that is what it takes to keep from getting diabetes, I'm willing to give it a try."

THINK! What are the risk factors for type 2 diabetes? Do any of these risk factors apply to you?

ACT! Make a list of your personal risk factors for type 2 diabetes. List two to three simple things you could do to start addressing the easiest one.

HEAR IT! ONLINE

mono- and polyunsaturated oils.[19] Avoid refined carbohydrates and sugars: white bread, white potatoes, white rice, sweets (candy, cookies, desserts, and so on), sodas, and sweetened juices.[20] Sugar has a twofold effect on the body with regards to diabetes. Surges in blood sugar followed by spikes in insulin production can stimulate appetite and reduce your cells' sensitivity to insulin. Recent research also suggests that sugars themselves—and not just the concentrated calories they provide or the blood sugar surges they induce—increase diabetes risk. Consuming just 150 calories of sugar per day (the amount in a 12-ounce can of soda) is enough to measurably increase the diabetes rate in a population.[21] Eating protein and fiber along with modest amounts of sugars (such as in fruits and juices) can help control blood sugar levels throughout the day. Even your eating speed can affect diabetes risk: People who eat their food quickly are more likely to develop type 2 diabetes.[22]

Exercise Regularly Consistent physical activity plus a healthy diet can cut your risk of developing type 2 diabetes by nearly 60 percent.[23] Exercise builds muscle tissue, which is more sensitive to insulin and uses it more efficiently than other tissue. Thus exercise

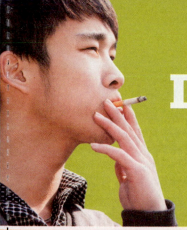

LIFESTYLE CHOICES
AND YOUR RISK OF CHRONIC DISEASE

The lifestyle choices you make now have a long-lasting impact on your future—including increasing or reducing your risks for chronic diseases.

HOW MUCH DO SMOKING, AN UNHEALTHY DIET, AND PHYSICAL INACTIVITY CONTRIBUTE TO CHRONIC DISEASES?

SMOKING

UNHEALTHY DIET

PHYSICAL INACTIVITY

Stomp out the cigarettes!

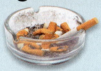

Each year smoking is a contributing factor in U.S. deaths from the following chronic diseases:[1]

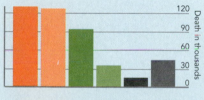

Death in thousands — 120, 90, 60, 30, 0

Lung cancer
128,900 deaths

Heart disease
126,000 deaths

COPD
92,900 deaths

Other cancers
35,300 deaths

Stroke
15,900 deaths

Other diagnoses
44,000 deaths

Forgo the fat!

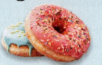

Adults who are at high risk for developing chronic diseases tend to exhibit poor eating habits:[2]

30% **eat fast food**
more than 3 times/week

29% **drink sugary drinks**
more than 3 times/week

22% **eat high-fat snacks**
more than 3 times/week

36% **eat desserts**
more than 3 times/week

11% **eat butter/meat fat**
every day

62% **eat fruits and veggies**
less than 2 times/day

Turn off the tube!

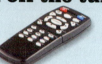

An average **lifetime of TV viewing reduces** the typical lifespan by **4.8 years**.

After age 25, every **1 hour of TV viewing** = a life expectancy shortened by **21.8 minutes**.[3]

CAN MINDFULNESS MEDITATION REDUCE THE RISKS FOR CHRONIC DISEASES?

Research shows that mindfulness meditation can **reduce symptoms** of rheumatoid arthritis, inflammatory bowel disease, and asthma, among other chronic conditions.[4]

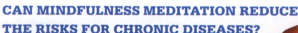
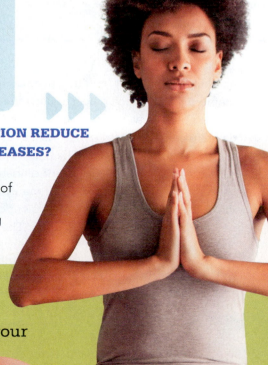

THE BOTTOM LINE?

Get regular physical activity, eat a healthy diet, don't smoke, and try meditation to sweep away some of your risk of chronic disease!

Q&A Does Exercise Reduce the Risk for Chronic Diseases?

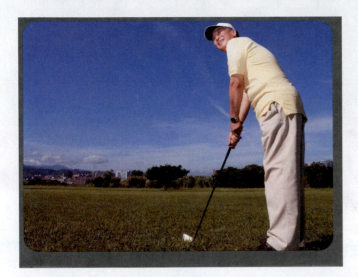

Compared to our predecessors in the first half of the twentieth century and before, we live longer lives and are safer, more amply fed, better housed, and better rested. But the news isn't all good: Researchers have documented a downhill trend from activity to inactivity, and the price we are now paying for this unprecedented leisure and sedentary lifestyle is a dramatic rise in chronic illness.[1] We can change this trend, though, and a growing body of research indicates that even small changes in daily activity can reap big rewards.

In one large national study, people at high risk for type 2 diabetes were able to lower their risk by 58 percent through a combination of losing weight and increasing both aerobic exercise and resistance training over a three-year period.[2]

For people with chronic lung disease, regular physical activity (particularly aerobic exercise) can improve circulation and oxygen use by tissues, strengthen the heart, and build lung capacity.[3] The best prevention remains avoiding smoking.

To prevent osteoporosis, the National Osteoporosis Foundation recommends getting enough calcium and vitamin D as well as performing regular weight-bearing and strengthening exercise such as running, field or court sports, and resistance training.[4] Studies show that bone responds to resistance training with slowed loss of mass and often increased mineral density.[5]

Finally, arthritis, too, responds to increased physical activity. The Centers for Disease Control and Prevention (CDC) reports that among adults with arthritis, 44 percent had no leisure-time activity, while among adults without arthritis, 36 percent had no exercise.[6] The CDC also reports that people with arthritic knees can reduce their disability by 47 percent by engaging in physical activity (experts often recommend swimming or riding a stationary bicycle submerged in a swimming pool) at least three times per week.[7]

Clearly, increased exercise is a good way to prevent chronic disease and to help alleviate it!

Sources:
1. G. Heath, "Physical Activity Transitions and Chronic Disease," *American Journal of Lifestyle Medicine* 3, no. 1 (2009): 27S–31S.
2. National Diabetes Information Clearinghouse, National Institute of Diabetes and Digestive and Kidney Diseases (NIDDK), "What Do I Need to Know About Physical Activity and Diabetes?" November 2012, http://diabetes.niddk.nih.gov
3. Cleveland Clinic, "COPD Exercise and Activity Guidelines."
4. National Osteoporosis Foundation, "Exercise for Strong Bones," www.nof.org
5. S. Going and M. Laudermilk, "Osteoporosis and Strength Training," *American Journal of Lifestyle Medicine* 3, no. 4 (2009): 310–9.
6. Centers for Disease Control and Prevention, "Arthritis-Related Statistics," Updated October 2010, www.cdc.gov
7. Ibid.

---

can help you prevent impaired glucose tolerance and maintain better blood glucose. Conversely, sitting for long periods at a stretch and for many hours in a day or week can increase your risks of both diabetes and heart disease.[24] Researchers have estimated that 43 percent of new cases of type 2 diabetes could be prevented if adults viewed fewer than 10 hours of television per week and did the equivalent of 30 minutes or more of brisk walking each day.[25] The box Does Exercise Reduce the Risk for Chronic Diseases? covers the role of exercise in preventing all forms of chronic disease.

asthma A condition in which air passages to and within the lungs "overreact" to smoke, allergens, or other triggers

What Is Lung Disease?

Lung disease is the third leading cause of death in the United States, after heart disease and cancer. In 2009, lung disease was responsible for one death in six, or more than 400,000 people. Today, tens of millions of Americans are living with chronic lung diseases such as asthma, emphysema, and bronchitis.[26]

Asthma Has a Wide Range of Triggers

Asthma is a chronic disease in which the lungs' airways swell, restricting airflow. Increased mucous makes breathing more difficult and tiny airways often

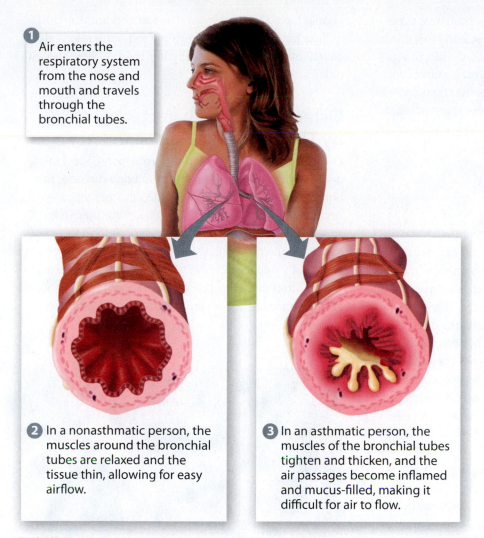

1 Air enters the respiratory system from the nose and mouth and travels through the bronchial tubes.

2 In a nonasthmatic person, the muscles around the bronchial tubes are relaxed and the tissue thin, allowing for easy airflow.

3 In an asthmatic person, the muscles of the bronchial tubes tighten and thicken, and the air passages become inflamed and mucus-filled, making it difficult for air to flow.

FIGURE **11.3** Asthma is an inflammation of the airways within the lungs.

react with spasms that lead to wheezing, coughing bouts, and shortness of breath (**Figure 11.3**). Air restriction can be so severe that an individual loses consciousness and can even die during a prolonged asthma attack. Controlling asthma requires medical care as well as avoiding or responding to triggers, such as cigarette smoke, wood smoke, dust mites, industrial pollution, vehicle exhaust, cockroaches, pets, mold, flu, strenuous exercise, and in some cases, stress and strong emotional responses. Researchers have even discovered that geophysical factors such as increased UV light near the equator and the hot, humid air in many regions can trigger more asthma, as can eating fast food three times or more per week in children.[27] If you have asthma, learn to anticipate and avoid its triggers. Carry asthma inhalers and other medications

LIVE IT! ONLINE
Worksheet 43
Check Your
Asthma I.Q.

and use them as prescribed by your physician to prevent serious asthma-related problems.

COPD

Chronic obstructive pulmonary disease (COPD) affects more than 12 million Americans—25 times more people than those affected with lung cancer.[28] COPD is the third leading cause of death in America.[29] COPD refers to two lung diseases that disrupt airflow and cause breathing problems: **emphysema** and **chronic bronchitis**.

Emphysema Emphysema begins when toxic substances such as those in tobacco smoke damage the millions of tiny air sacs (called *alveoli*) in the lungs. As alveoli are destroyed, emphysema patients find it more and more difficult to exhale. Their chest cavities can gradually begin to expand, producing a characteristic "barrel-shaped" chest. They may become winded by limited exertion and feel as though they are suffocating. Over time, the condition taxes the heart and can lead to hospitalization or death.

Chronic Bronchitis In **chronic bronchitis**, cigarette smoke, air pollution, mold, infectious agents, or other irritants cause the bronchial tubes to become inflamed. Symptoms of chronic bronchitis include chronic cough, increased mucus, frequent clearing of the throat, and shortness of breath that tend to persist and reoccur. Continued exposure to the irritants can cause scarring in

chronic obstructive pulmonary disease (COPD) Progressive lung disease that causes breathing difficulties; includes emphysema and chronic bronchitis

emphysema A type of COPD involving damage to the air sacs (alveoli) in the lungs

chronic bronchitis A type of COPD characterized by inflammation of the main air passages (bronchi) in the lungs

the bronchial tubes that leads to a chronically thicker mucus layer. A person with chronic bronchitis is more susceptible to pneumonia, cardiovascular diseases, and other medical conditions.[30]

You Can Reduce Your Risk of Developing COPD

In 85 to 90 percent of emphysema and chronic bronchitis cases, smoking is the primary risk factor.[31] So, don't smoke or spend time in smoky areas! Some chronic bronchitis and emphysema cases, however, can be attributed to poor urban air quality or to home and workplace air pollution, including frequent fireplace use or industrial exposures. Changing your habits or your home/work environments may be necessary to reduce your risks. This may include changing eating habits, as well; an Australian study shows that, for unknown reasons, people who drink more than half a liter of soft drinks per day have higher levels of both asthma and COPD.[32]

Respiratory infections can trigger some COPD cases and make existing cases worse. People with COPD or COPD risk factors should try to avoid colds and flu by getting flu shots, by observing general wellness behaviors, by washing hands regularly—particularly after being around crowds in confined spaces—and by keeping hands away from the mouth, nose, and eyes. People who are short of breath and feel as though they are suffocating are often reluctant to exert themselves by exercising. This reluctance, however, can lead to progressive physical deterioration and even disability.[33] Started slowly and built up gradually under medical supervision, exercise programs can give COPD patients more physical capacity and less fatigue and breathlessness. For people with risk factors for COPD but no current breathing problems, exercise is essential for maintaining lung function.[34]

What Is Osteoporosis?

Do you have a grandmother who looks a bit stooped forward or hunched around the shoulders, or perhaps has broken a bone during a fall? These symptoms describe a common condition of older Americans: **osteoporosis**. Fifty-five percent of all Americans over 50 have osteoporosis or early signs of it: 10 million people have the full-blown disease and another 30 million have *osteopenia* (diminished bone mass; also called low bone density), putting them at heightened risk for the disease.[35]

Osteoporosis Is Characterized by Thinning, Brittle Bones

Osteoporosis literally means "porous bone," and indeed, in this chronic degenerative bone disease, the bones become full of holes, brittle, and susceptible to breaking (see **Figure 11.4**). The thinning can be so extreme that a simple cough, sneeze, or bend can cause a bone to break. Osteoporosis develops over a period of years, beginning with diminished bone mass that is often rooted in the eating, smoking, drinking, and exercise habits of youth. Race, age, frame size,

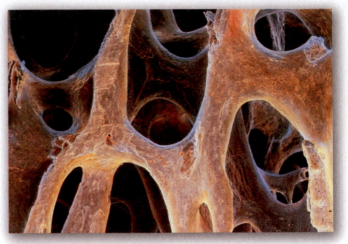

(a) Normal bone

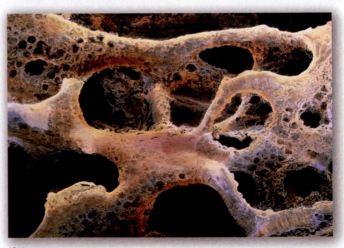

(b) Osteoporotic bone

FIGURE **11.4** Osteoporosis causes bones to become more porous.

family history, and other factors can increase your risk. In general, women are more susceptible than men but the incidence of osteoporosis is rising in males. Because most of your bone mass accumulates before adulthood, building strong bones during childhood and adolescence can help prevent osteoporosis later in life.[36]

Your body builds bone tissue in response to the physical demands you place on it. Weight-bearing exercise (during which you bear your body weight on your legs) and resistance exercise (e.g., weight lifting) are both conducive to building bone tissue. The body also stores excess calcium and phosphates in bone tissue and draws upon them when these minerals are needed elsewhere. Physical inactivity signals a diminished need for fortified bones, leading the body to release more minerals and resulting in decreased reserves.[37] In postmenopausal women, declining levels of certain hormones also cause the body to retain fewer minerals in bone tissue, making bones more vulnerable to osteoporosis.

A simple, noninvasive procedure called a *bone mineral density test* can evaluate your bone mass. Bone-density testing is important for people in high-risk groups for osteoporosis, because the disease is essentially symptom free.

You Can Reduce Your Risk for Developing Osteoporosis

You are at greater risk of osteoporosis if you are female, if you are thin or have a small frame, if you are over age 50 (**Figure 11.5**), if you are over age 50 and have broken a bone, or if you have a low bone mass reading. Beyond these factors, there are four groups of risk factors for osteoporosis: genetic, hormonal, nutritional, and lifestyle choices. Your wellness choices can lessen many of the individual risk factors within each group.

- *Genetic factors.* Having a close relative who has been diagnosed with osteoporosis or has suffered a fracture after age 50 increases your risk. You can't change these factors, but they can alert you to osteoporosis risk and inspire greater effort toward prevention.

- *Hormonal factors.* Diminishing estrogen levels in women—and to a lesser extent, testosterone in men—can lead to bone "dismantling," calcium release, osteopenia, or full-fledged osteoporosis. Women are particularly at risk after menopause, but women whose menstrual periods stop prematurely due to heavy exercise, extreme dieting, or illness are also at risk.[38]

- *Nutritional factors.* What you eat now can continue to support your bone health throughout life. We all need calcium in our daily diet to build strong bones. We also need vitamin D so that the body can transport calcium out of the digestive tract and deliver it to bone-building cells. Getting enough calcium (1,300 mg/day during adolescence; 1,000 mg/day from ages 19 to 50; and 1,200 mg/day after age 50) and enough vitamin D (400 to 800 IU/day) is important to stave off osteoporosis.[39] One recent study revealed that milk and yogurt are better sources of calcium for bone-building than are cream and cheese; another reported that the vitamin K in leafy green vegetables is crucial to bone repair.[40]

- *Lifestyle choices.* Your daily habits can increase or decrease osteoporosis risk. Try to get enough calcium and vitamin D each day. Avoid caffeine,

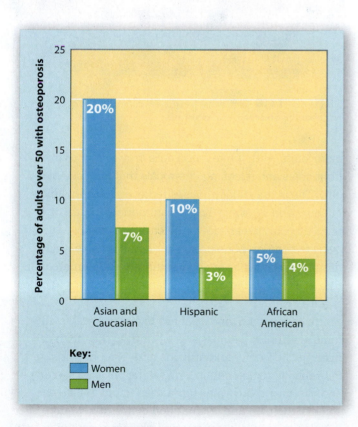

FIGURE **11.5** Osteoporosis is most prevalent among Asian and Caucasian females over age 50.

Data from National Osteoporosis Foundation, "Fast Facts on Osteoporosis," July 2005, www.nof.org

carbonated sodas, and too much salt. Make regular weight-bearing exercise and resistance exercise part of your fitness routine. Avoid smoking and drinking—both can reduce your body's ability to retain calcium. If you have risk factors for osteoporosis, get a bone-density test.

What Is Arthritis?

Arthritis is acute or chronic inflammation of a joint that can cause stiffness, aching, swelling, or permanent deformation and dysfunction. About one in five American adults or 50 million people have some form of the one hundred diseases and conditions that fall under the category of arthritis.[41] Arthritis limits daily activity such as walking, dressing, and bathing for millions of Americans, making it the leading cause of disability in the United States.[42]

The most common types of arthritis are *osteoarthritis,* caused by long-term wear and tear of cartilage, and *rheumatoid arthritis,* caused by autoimmune activity.[43]

Osteoarthritis

In a joint, two bones are attached by tendons and ligaments, allowing one or both bones to move relative to the other. A layer of *cartilage* (connective tissue) separates the bones, allowing smooth movement. **Osteoarthritis** is a slow, progressive joint disease that involves a breakdown of cartilage due to injury, too much or too little use, joint deformity, the physical strain of obesity, muscle weakness, and other causes. After years of wear and tear, bone can start grinding against bone, causing pain and sometimes creating detached bone, cartilage fragments, or little projections called *bone spurs.* Extra joint fluid builds up, acting like a buffer but also enlarging the joint in a way that restricts movement. Osteoarthritis usually affects the hips, knees, toes, fingers, or joints in the spine (**Figure 11.6**).

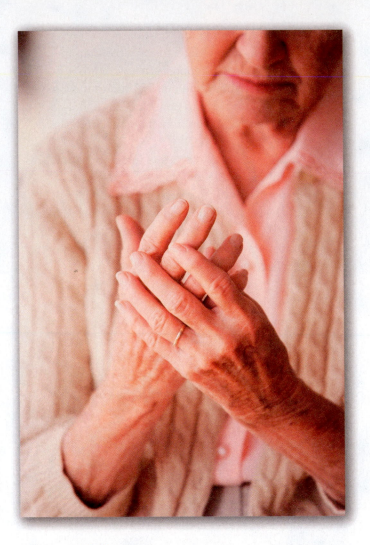

FIGURE **11.6** Stiff, aching joints are characteristic of both osteoarthritis and rheumatoid arthritis.

arthritis Inflammation of joints, typically accompanied by pain, swelling, and stiffness

osteoarthritis A type of arthritis characterized by stiffness, aching, swelling, or permanent deformation and dysfunction of a joint, caused primarily by wear and tear

rheumatoid arthritis A type of arthritis characterized by chronic inflammation, swelling, and pain in a joint brought about by an autoimmune attack

Rheumatoid Arthritis

Rheumatoid arthritis is a chronic inflammation of the joints that tends to appear between ages 25 and 40 and affects about 1.5 million Americans.[44] The body's immune system triggers an attack on one or more joints, with white blood cells crowding into the tight areas and releasing chemicals that increase blood flow. The influx usually causes redness, warmth, fluid buildup, and swelling. This inflammation, in turn, irritates the joint, wears down the cartilage, and eventually leads to bone-on-bone grinding. Hands with painfully misshapen knuckles are characteristic of rheumatoid arthritis, although the condition can affect knees and other joints as well.

Swelling, pain, and stiffness in a joint are all symptoms of arthritis; redness and warmth to the touch can distinguish rheumatoid arthritis from osteoarthritis. Pain-relieving medications, massage, physical therapy, and alternative therapies have been found to help ease some of the pain and dysfunction of arthritis. Many people use supplements such as glucosamine and chondroitin, but when tested in large, carefully designed scientific trials, these appear to be no more effective than placebos.[45]

You Can Reduce Your Risks of Developing Arthritis

Your likelihood of developing rheumatoid arthritis is only one-tenth as great as your chances of developing osteoarthritis, and the risk factors are quite different for the two conditions. Because rheumatoid arthritis is a genetically determined autoimmune disease, your risk for it rises if you or a close relative has had asthma, lupus, or type 1 diabetes. Your risk is higher if you are female because several of the susceptibility genes lie on the X chromosome and women have two Xs.[46] Your most controllable risk factor is body weight; overweight and obesity are both linked to increased likelihood of developing rheumatoid arthritis, possibly due to higher body levels of inflammation.[47]

There are more risk factors for osteoarthritis, some of which you can change:

- Advanced age (two-thirds of arthritis cases are in 40 to 65 year olds; by age 85, half of all adults have arthritic knees)[48]
- Genetics
- Race, ethnicity, and sex (African American women have the highest risk of knee osteoarthritis, men of all races the lowest)[49]
- Injuries (a single accident, or repeated stress)
- Obesity (extra weight adds pressure on weight-bearing joints and may cause premature wear and tear)
- Physical weakness (weak muscles, inactivity, or certain diseases can atrophy the muscles that surround and normally protect joints)
- Hormone deficiency (especially in women after menopause)
- Vitamin deficiency (vitamin D promotes healthy cartilage)

A good strategy is to avoid hard-hitting activities such as football and running long distances on hard pavement, or to at least alternate such activities with less percussive sports like swimming—especially if joint problems start to appear. The kinds of repetitive motions

that go into practicing and excelling at nearly any sport will eventually cause joint wear and tear. High-level and competitive sports performance is a choice people make for many reasons—including benefit to fitness and wellness—despite the inevitable costs. Good athletes, trainers, and coaches keep athletes' future joint problems in mind, including switching to milder forms of activity when the prospect of joint damage and future disability starts to emerge.

Finally, to avoid deficiencies, be sure to get the proper amount of vitamin D and to consult a doctor about potential hormonal deficiencies.

casestudy

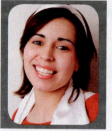

GRACE

"I have a cousin, Bart, who plays college football. He's been playing since junior high school, and his apartment is full of trophies. But his neck, back, and knees are already starting to bother him. In fact, he has to use ice and aspirin to get the swelling down in his joints after most of the practices and games. He's heard that college and professional athletes can wind up with arthritis later on, and he wants to keep that from happening. But football is Bart's life and if he could get into the pros he'd be ecstatic."

THINK! What steps could an athlete like Bart take to prevent arthritis? What steps could you take to reduce your risk?

ACT NOW! Today, make a list of your risk factors for arthritis. This week, make a list of 2–3 simple things you could do to start addressing the easiest of your risk factors, and get started on one of those solutions. In two weeks, start tackling other risk factors on your list with other solutions, and keep making changes until you have addressed all your risk factors. Which ones can you incorporate permanently?

HEAR IT! ONLINE

CHAPTER IN REVIEW

MasteringHealth™

Build your knowledge—and wellness!—in the Study Area of MasteringHealth with a variety of study tools.

SEE IT! ONLINE

videos
Young Adults and Diabetes

LIVE IT! ONLINE

programs & behavior change
Take Charge of Your Health! Worksheets:
Worksheet 43 Check Your Asthma I.Q.
Behavior Change Log Book and Wellness Journal

HEAR IT! ONLINE

audio tools
Audio case study
MP3 chapter review

DO IT! ONLINE

labs
Lab 11.1 Are You at Risk for Diabetes?

REVIEW IT! ONLINE

chapter review
Chapter reading quizzes
Glossary flashcards

---

reviewquestions

1. Which one of the following is true about chronic diseases?
   a. In the United States, chronic diseases cause 7 percent of deaths and kill 170,000 Americans per year.
   b. Chronic diseases are mainly a problem in the developing world.
   c. Getting one chronic disease usually gives you immunity from other chronic diseases.
   d. Smoking, poor diet, and physical inactivity are the underlying causes of more than 30 percent of chronic disease deaths in the United States.

2. Which one of these statements is true about chronic diseases?
   a. They tend to come on suddenly.
   b. They usually last for short periods and often resolve without treatment.
   c. Pharmaceutical companies have developed many effective vaccines for preventing chronic diseases.
   d. They have multiple causes.

3. Which one of the following can help you reduce your risk of type 2 diabetes and cardiovascular disease?
   a. Eating one serving of fruits and vegetables per day
   b. Eating more foods that contain saturated fat
   c. Maintaining a BMI above 25
   d. Avoiding drug and alcohol abuse

4. Which one of the following statements is true about type 2 diabetes?
   a. It is the fastest-growing chronic disease in America.
   b. It has a strong genetic basis and usually develops during childhood.
   c. Body cells can still use insulin properly, but the pancreas usually stops making insulin.
   d. Exercise is unimportant in its prevention and management.

5. The biggest risk factor for chronic obstructive pulmonary disease is
   a. allergies.
   b. genetics.
   c. smoking.
   d. physical inactivity.

6. Which one of the following statements about COPD is correct?
   a. A smoker's chances are far higher of developing lung cancer than COPD.
   b. A smoker's chances are far higher of dying from lung cancer than COPD.
   c. You can develop emphysema or chronic bronchitis but avoid COPD.
   d. Emphysema destroys alveoli and lung capacity.

7. Which of the following is a risk factor for developing osteoporosis?
   a. Regular weight-bearing exercise
   b. Being thin or having a small frame
   c. Getting excess calcium in the diet
   d. Having high levels of estrogen hormones

8. Diminished bone mass usually has its roots in behaviors established during
   a. childhood or young adulthood.
   b. menopause.
   c. middle age.
   d. old age.

9. Which of the following statements is true about osteoporosis?
   a. Women have to worry about it, but men don't.
   b. Getting enough protein in the diet can help prevent osteoporosis.
   c. Females needn't worry about osteoporosis until after menopause.
   d. More than half of all Americans over 50 have osteoporosis or osteopenia.

10. Which one of these will increase your risk of osteoarthritis?
    a. Maintaining a healthy BMI
    b. Regular weight-bearing exercise
    c. Regular resistance exercise
    d. Playing competitive football

critical thinking questions

1. Give an example of two interrelated chronic diseases. Explain how they are interrelated.

2. Identify five behaviors that can help you avoid chronic diseases, and explain why these behaviors can lower your risks.

references

1. Centers for Disease Control and Prevention, "Chronic Diseases and Health Promotion," Updated August 2012, www.cdc.gov
2. Ibid.
3. R. M. Merrill, *Introduction to Epidemiology* 6e (Sudbury, MA: Jones and Bartlett, 2012): 270.
4. Centers for Disease Control and Prevention, "Diabetes Successes and Opportunities for Population-Based Prevention and Control: At A Glance 2011," Updated August 2011, www.cdc.gov
5. "Call to Congress: A Volunteer's Story," American Diabetes Association, March 2011, www.diabetes.org
6. Centers for Disease Control and Prevention, "Diabetes Data & Trends," 2013, www.cdc.gov
7. Centers for Disease Control and Prevention, "Diabetes Successes and Opportunities for Population-Based Prevention and Control," 2011, www.cdc.gov
8. American Diabetes Association, "Diabetes Basics: Pre-Diabetes FAQs," www.diabetes.org
9. American Diabetes Association, "Living with Diabetes: Stress," June 2013, www.diabetes.org; C. Lindtner et al., "Binge

Drinking Induces Whole-Body Insulin Resistance by Impairing Hypothalamic Insulin Action," *Science Translational Medicine* 5, no. 170 (2013): 170ra14, doi: 10.1126/scitranslmed.3005123; National Diabetes Information Clearinghouse, National Institute of Diabetes and Digestive and Kidney Diseases (NIDDK), *National Diabetes Statistics*, 2011 (Bethesda, MD: National Institutes of Health, 2011) NIH Publication no. 11–3892.
10. Ibid.
11. Centers for Disease Control and Prevention, "Diabetes Successes and Opportunities for Population-Based Prevention and Control," 2011.
12. Ibid.
13. H. Rodbard, "Diabetes Screening, Diagnosis, and Therapy in Pediatric Patients with Type 2 Diabetes," *Medscape Journal of Medicine* 10, no. 8 (2008): 184.
14. Centers for Disease Control and Prevention, "Diabetes Successes and Opportunities for Population-Based Prevention and Control," 2011.
15. Ibid.
16. National Diabetes Education Program, *Small Steps. Big Rewards. Your GAME

PLAN to Prevent Type 2 Diabetes: Information for Patients* (Bethesda, MD: National Institutes of Health, 2006) NIH Publication no. 06-5334.
17. J. de Munter et al., "Whole Grain, Bran, and Germ Intake and Risk of Type 2 Diabetes: A Prospective Cohort Study and Systematic Review," *PLoS Medicine* 4, no. 8 (2007): e261; Robert E. Post et al., "Dietary Fiber for the Treatment of Type 2 Diabetes Mellitus: A Meta-Analysis," *Journal of the American Board of Family Medicine* 25, no. 1 (2012): 16–23, doi: 10.3122/jabfm.2012.01.110148.
18. C. J. Patel et al., "Systematic Identification of Interaction Effects Between Genome- and Environment Wide Associations in Type 2 Diabetes Mellitus," *Human Genetics* 132, no. 5 (2013): 495–508, doi: 10.1007/s00439-012-1258-z.
19. A. Wallin et al., "Fish Consumption, Dietary Long-Chain N-3 Fatty Acids, and the Risk of Type 2 Diabetes: Systematic Review and Meta Analysis of Prospective Studies," *Diabetes Care* 35, no. 4 (2012): 918–29, doi: 10.2337/dc11-1631; L. Djousse et al., "Dietary Omega-3 Fatty Acids and Fish Consumption and Risk of Type 2 Diabetes,"

American Journal of Clinical Nutrition 93, no. 1 (2011): 113–50, doi: 10.3945/ajcn 110.005603.

20. Linus Pauling Institute, "Glycemic Index and Glycemic Load," Updated April 2010, http://lpi.oregonstate.edu

21. Centers for Disease Control and Prevention, "Diabetes Successes and Opportunities for Population-Based Prevention and Control," 2011; S. Basu et al., "The Relationship of Sugar to Population-Level Diabetes Prevalence: An Econometric Analysis of Repeated Cross-Sectional Data," *PLoS ONE* 8, no. 2 (2013): e57873, doi: 10/10/1371/journal. pone.0057873.

22. L. Radzevičienė and R. Ostrauskas, "Fast Eating and the Risk of Type 2 Diabetes Mellitus: A Case-Control Study," *Clinical Nutrition* 32, no. 2 (2012): 232–5, doi: 10.1016/j.clnu.2012.06.013.

23. National Diabetes Education Program, 2006.

24. T. Yates et al., "Self Reported Sitting Time and Markers of Inflammation, Insulin Resistance, and Adiposity," *American Journal of Preventive Medicine* 42, no. 1 (2012): 1–7, doi: 10.1016/j. amepre.2011.09.022; E.G. Wilmot et al., "Sedentary Time in Adults and the Association with Diabetes, Cardiovascular Disease and Death: Systematic Review and Meta-Analysis," *Diabetologia* 55, no. 11 (2012): 2895–905, doi: 10.1007/ s00125-012-2677-z.

25. F. B. Hu et al., "Television Watching and Other Sedentary Behaviors in Relation to Risk of Obesity and Type-2 Diabetes Mellitus in Women," *Journal of the American Medical Association* 289, no. 14 (2003): 1785–91.

26. American Lung Association, "Lung Disease," www.lungusa.org

27. Vicka Oktaria et al., "Association between Latitude and Allergic Diseases: A Longitudinal Study from Childhood to Middle-Age," *Annals of Allergy Asthma & Immunology* 110, no. 2 (2013): 80–5, doi: 10.1016/j.anai.2012.11.005; D. Hayes et al., "Bronchoconstriction Triggered by Breathing Hot Humid Air in Patients with Asthma: Role of Cholinergic Reflex," *American Journal of Respiratory and Critical Care Medicine* 185, no. 11 (2012): 1190–6, doi: 10.1164/rccm.201201-0088OC; P. Ellwood et al., "Do Fast Foods Cause Asthma, Rhinoconjunctivitis and Eczema? Global Findings from the International Study of Asthma and Allergies in Childhood (ISAAC) Phase Three," *Thorax*, (2013), doi: 10.1136/ thoraxjnl-2012-202285.

28. National Heart, Lung, and Blood Institute, Diseases and Conditions Index, "What Is COPD?" June 2012, www.nhlbi.nih.gov

29. Ibid.

30. American Lung Association, "Chronic Obstructive Pulmonary Disease (COPD) Fact Sheet," February 2011, www.lungusa.org

31. Ibid.

32. Z. Shi et al., "Association Between Soft Drink Consumption and Asthma and Chronic Obstructive Pulmonary Disease Among Adults in Australia," *Respirology* 17, no. 2 (2012): 363–9, doi: 10.1111/j.1440-1843.2011.02115.x.

33. R. H. Dressendorfer et al., American College of Sports Medicine, "ACSM Current Comment: Exercise for Persons with COPD," www.acsm.org

34. Ibid.

35. National Osteoporosis Foundation, "Fast Facts," 2011, www.nof.org; NIH Osteoporosis and Related Bone Diseases National Resource Center, "What Is Osteoporosis: Fast Facts," January 2011, www.niams.nih.gov

36. L. Gracia-Marco et al., "Sedentary Behaviour and Its Association with Bone Mass in Adolescents: The HELENA Cross-Sectional Study," *BMC Public Health* 12, no. 1 (2012): 971, doi: 10.1186/14712458 -12-971; Centers for Disease Control and Prevention, "Calcium and Bone Health," 2011, www.cdc.gov; National Osteoporosis Foundation, "Fast Facts," 2011.

37. J. Postlethwait and J. L. Hopson, *Explore Life* (Pacific Grove, CA: Brooks/Cole Publishing Company, 2003): 516–7.

38. Cleveland Clinic, "Menopause and Osteoporosis."

39. Office of Dietary Supplements, National Institutes of Health, "Dietary Supplement Fact Sheet: Calcium," Reviewed August 2011, http://ods.od.nih.gov

40. S. Sahni et al., "Milk and Yogurt Consumption Are Linked with Higher Bone Mineral Density but Not with Hip Fracture: the Framington Offspring Study," *Archives of Osteoporosis* 8, (2013): 119, doi: 10.1007 /s11657-013-0119-2; A. A Poundarik et al., "Dilatational Band Formation in Bone." *Proceedings of the National Academy of Sciences* 109, no. 47 (2012): 19178, doi: 10.1073/pnas.1201513109.

41. Arthritis Foundation, "Understanding Arthritis: Get the Facts," 2013, www.arthritis .org/facts.php.

42. Centers for Disease Control and Prevention, "Arthritis: Meeting the Challenge of Living Well, At A Glance 2012" April 2012, www.cdc.gov

43. Arthritis Foundation, Disease Center, "Osteoarthritis," 2013, www.arthritis .org; Arthritis Foundation, Disease Center,

"Rheumatoid Arthritis", 2013, www .arthritis.org

44. CDC, "Rheumatoid Arthritis," Updated November 2012, www.cdc.gov

45. NIH National Center for Complementary and Alternative Medicine, "Questions and Answers: NIH Glucosamine/Chondroitin Arthritis Intervention Trial Primary Study," February 2012, http://nccam.nih.gov; A. D. Sawitzke, "Clinical Efficacy and Safety of Glucosamine, Chondroitin Sulphate, Their Combination, Celecoxib or Placebo Taken to Treat Osteoarthritis of the Knee: 2-Year Results from GAIT," *Annals of the Rheumatic Diseases* 69, no. 8 (2010): 1459–64.

46. Steve Eyre et al., "High-Density Genetic Mapping Identifies New Susceptibility Loci for Rheumatoid Arthritis," *Nature Genetics* 44, no. 12 (2012): 1336–40, doi: 10.1038/ng.2462.

47. Cynthia S. Crowson et al., "Contribution of Obesity to the Rise in Incidence of Rheumatoid Arthritis," *Arthritis Care & Research* 65, no. 1 (2013): 71–7, doi: 10.1002/acr.21660; Healthfinder.gov, "Extra Pounds Linked to Rheumatoid Arthritis Risk in Women," U.S. Department of Health and Human Services, Healthday, 2013.

48. Arthritis Foundation, "The Heavy Burden of Arthritis in the U.S.," 2011, www .arthritis.org; L. Murphy et al., "Lifetime Risk of Symptomatic Knee Osteoarthritis," *Arthritis and Rheumatism* 59, no. 9 (2008): 1207–13, doi: 10.1002/art.24021.

49. Arthritis Foundation, "Female Minorities Are at Most Risk of Knee Osteoarthritis," November 2012, www.arthritistoday.org

getfitgraphic references

1. Centers for Disease Control and Prevention, Morbidity and Mortality Weekly Report 57, no. 45 (2008): 1226-8.

2. N. D. Gaskins, et al., "Poor Nutritional Habits: A Modifiable Predecessor of Chronic Illness? A North Carolina Family Medicine Research Network (NC-FM-RN) Study," *Journal of the American Board of Family Medicine* 20, no. 2 (2007): 124-34.

3. J. L. Veerman et al., "Television Viewing Time and Reduced Life Expectancy: A Life Table Analysis," *British Journal of Sports Medicine* 46, no. 13 (2012): 927-30, doi:10.1136/bjsm.2011.085662.

4. M. A. Rosenkranz et al., "A Comparison of Mindfulness-Based Stress Reduction and an Active Control in Modulation of Neurogenic Inflammation," *Brain, Behavior, and Immunity* 27, no. 1 (2013): 174-84, doi: 10.1016/j.bbi.2012.10.013.

LAB 11.1

ARE YOU AT RISK FOR DIABETES?

MasteringHealth™

Name: _____ Date: _____

Instructor: _____ Section: _____

Purpose: To assess your personal risk factors for developing diabetes.

Directions: Answer the questions below.

1. Do you have a history of diabetes in your family?	☐ Yes	☐ No
2. Do any of your primary relatives (mother, father, sister, brother, or grandparents) have diabetes?	☐ Yes	☐ No
3. Are you overweight (BMI above 25) or obese (BMI above 30)?	☐ Yes	☐ No
4. Are you typically sedentary (seldom, if ever, engage in vigorous aerobic exercise)?	☐ Yes	☐ No
5. Have you noticed an increase in your craving for water or other beverages (not related to physical activity or summer heat)?	☐ Yes	☐ No
6. Have you noticed that you have to urinate more frequently than you used to during a typical day?	☐ Yes	☐ No
7. Have you noticed any tingling or numbness in your hands and feet, which might indicate circulatory problems?	☐ Yes	☐ No
8. Do you often feel a gnawing hunger during the day, even though you usually eat regular meals?	☐ Yes	☐ No
9. Have you noticed that you are losing weight without conscious dieting and/or increase in exercise?	☐ Yes	☐ No
10. Are you often so tired that you find it difficult to stay awake to study, watch television, or engage in other activities?	☐ Yes	☐ No
11. Have you noticed that you have skin irritations more frequently and that minor infections don't heal as quickly as they used to?	☐ Yes	☐ No
12. Have you noticed any unusual changes in your vision (blurring, difficulty in focusing, etc.)?	☐ Yes	☐ No
13. Have you noticed unusual pain or swelling in your joints?	☐ Yes	☐ No
14. Do you often feel weak or nauseated if you wait too long to eat a meal?	☐ Yes	☐ No
15. If you are a woman, have you had several vaginal (yeast) infections during the past year?	☐ Yes	☐ No

If you answer yes to three of more of these questions, consider seeking medical advice. Talk to health professionals at your student health center or make an appointment with your family physician.

REFLECTION

Based on what you read in the chapter and your answers to the questions above, what changes can you make right now to decrease your risk for developing diabetes? What changes can you make over the long term?

_____

_____

12 Reducing Your Risk of Cancer

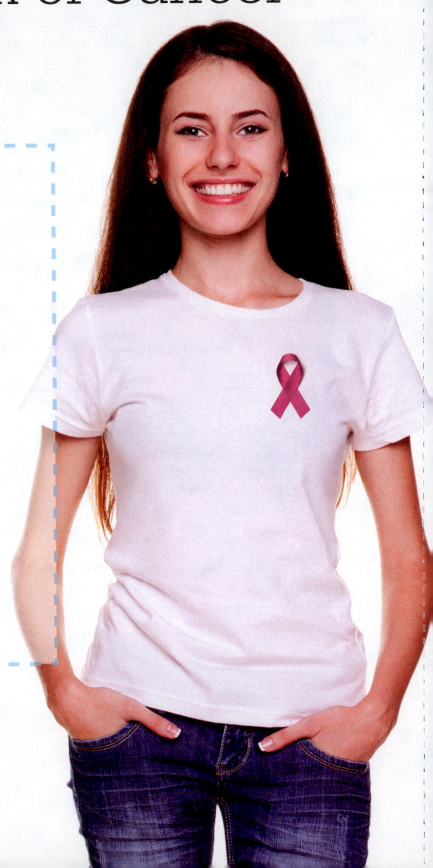

LEARNINGoutcomes

1 Define cancer and explain how it develops and spreads.

2 Discuss the causes of cancer.

3 List seven major types of cancer and the risk factors for each.

4 Describe the factors that affect an individual's risk of developing cancer, including lifestyle choices, biological factors, and environmental exposures.

5 Identify your own risk factors and make choices to reduce those risks.

6 Discuss approaches to cancer treatment and recovery.

MasteringHealth™

Go online for chapter quizzes, interactive assessments, videos, and more!

casestudy

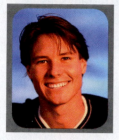

TIM

"I'm Tim. I'm in my second year of community college in Arizona and I work part time in the pro shop at the local golf course. I'm a recreation major; between my classes, labs, and job, I spend half of my time outside. I really like being outdoors, and I like having a tan. I know that I should use sunscreen, but I just get lazy about it. Anyway, skin cancer is mainly a problem for very light-skinned people, right?"

HEAR IT! ONLINE

Cancer is second only to cardiovascular disease as a cause of death in the United States; in 2013, cancer killed over an estimated 580,000 Americans.[1] Nearly half of all American males and one-third of all American females will develop cancer at some point during their lives.[2] Lifestyle choices have a dramatic impact on cancer risk: Scientific evidence suggests that tobacco use causes one-third of all cancer deaths, while another 20 percent of the deaths are related to overweight or obesity, and perhaps 10 percent more are due to physical inactivity and poor nutrition.[3] Overexposure to the sun's harmful rays and exposure to certain viruses and other infectious agents can also contribute to skin cancer and cancers at various other sites.[4] Advanced techniques for diagnosis and treatment are helping to reduce the death rate from cancer, but prevention remains the best strategy.[5] Understanding the relationships between cancer and lifestyle choices can help you identify unhealthy behaviors to avoid in order to reduce your risk of developing these potentially deadly diseases.

What Is Cancer?

Cancer is the name given to a large group of diseases characterized by the uncontrolled growth and spread of abnormal cells.

Cancer Is the Unchecked Growth of Abnormal Cells

Living cells contain biochemical instructions called DNA that control the cell's growth, division, and daily functions. Sometimes a segment of a DNA molecule inside a cell becomes damaged. This may cause a *mutation* or a change in the genetic instructions that can override the cell's normal cycle of growing and dividing. The offspring of that mutated cell can form a **tumor**—a mass of cells that serves no physiological function and that may grow and spread into other areas.

Most tumors are **benign** (noncancerous)—they are generally harmless unless their growth obstructs or crowds out normal tissue. A benign tumor is usually enclosed in a capsule of collagen that prevents it from spreading to other areas of the body (**Figure 12.1**).

Cancerous tumors may stay localized; these are called *in situ* carcinomas. Lacking a capsule, *in situ* carcinomas can grow in place and disrupt neighboring tissues. Or they can further mutate into malignant tumors. **Malignant** tumors invade surrounding tissue. *Metastases*, or clusters of malignant cells, can break off them and migrate to other parts of the body through the bloodstream in the process of **metastasis**

cancer The name given to a large group of diseases characterized by the uncontrolled growth and spread of abnormal cells

tumor A clumping of cells that grows more rapidly than surrounding tissue

benign Refers to a slow-growing, noninvasive, noncancerous tumor

malignant Very dangerous or harmful; refers to a cancerous tumor

metastasis Process by which cancer spreads from one area to different areas of the body

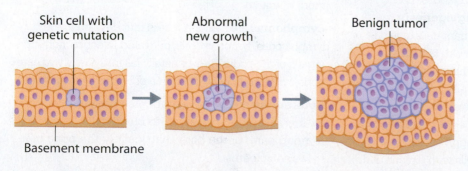

Skin cell with genetic mutation

Abnormal new growth

Benign tumor

Basement membrane

FIGURE **12.1** A mutation in the genetic material of a skin cell triggers abnormal cell division, resulting in a benign tumor. A capsule of normal cells keeps the tumor localized.

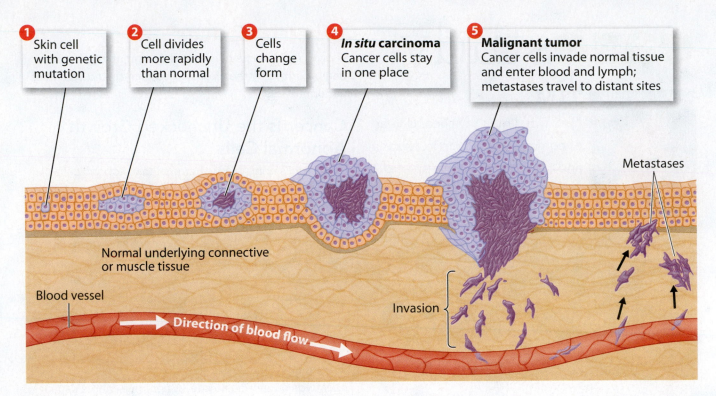

1 Skin cell with genetic mutation

2 Cell divides more rapidly than normal

3 Cells change form

4 *In situ* carcinoma Cancer cells stay in one place

5 **Malignant tumor** Cancer cells invade normal tissue and enter blood and lymph; metastases travel to distant sites

Metastases

Normal underlying connective or muscle tissue

Blood vessel

Direction of blood flow

Invasion

FIGURE **12.2** A mutation in the DNA of a skin cell triggers abnormal cell division and changes cell formation, resulting in a cancerous tumor. *In situ* cancer remains localized; malignant cancer spreads to neighboring tissues and can metastasize to other parts of the body.

(**Figure 12.2**). Once lodged in new places, metastases can disrupt normal cell functioning and lead to more mutations. As the invaded, now mutated cells divide and metastasize further, the cancer spreads. A **biopsy** (a surgical retrieval of cells, followed by microscopic or biochemical examination of their characteristics) can usually determine whether a given tumor is benign or malignant.

To grow much beyond the size of the tip of a ballpoint pen, a tumor must have its own blood supply.[6] In a process called **angiogenesis**, malignant cells give off growth factors that induce new blood capillaries to grow toward the tumor. The new capillaries supply the tumor cells with oxygen and nutrients and carry off wastes, allowing the tumor to grow much faster and larger. Some cancer treatments called angiogenesis inhibitors prevent the growth of new blood vessels and thus the growth of certain tumors as well.[7]

Cancers Are Assigned Classes and Stages

There are four different classes of cancerous tumors:

- **Carcinomas** are solid tumors that occur in epithelial tissue (the tissues covering body surfaces and lining most body cavities). Carcinomas are the most common class of tumors and include those of the breast, lung, intestines, skin, and mouth.

- **Sarcomas** are solid tumors that occur in middle layers of tissue—for example, in bones, muscles, and other connective tissue. Less common than carcinomas, sarcomas generally grow faster and become dangerous more quickly.

- **Lymphomas** are malignant cells that develop in the lymph nodes, lymph vessels, or related infection-fighting organs of the body. They generally fall into one of two categories: *non-Hodgkin's* lymphoma or *Hodgkin's* lymphoma.

- **Leukemias** are nonsolid cancers characterized by an increased number of white blood cells in blood-forming parts of the body, particularly the bone marrow and spleen.

biopsy Surgical retrieval of cells and microscopic examination of tissue to determine if a tumor is benign or malignant

angiogenesis Process in which malignant cells induce new blood capillaries to grow toward the tumor

carcinomas Solid tumors that occur in epithelial tissues (the tissues covering body surfaces and lining most body cavities)

sarcomas Solid tumors that occur in middle layers of tissue (e.g., in bones, muscles, and connective tissue)

lymphomas Tumors that develop in lymph nodes, lymph vessels, or related infection-fighting regions of the body

leukemias Nonsolid cancers characterized by an increase in the number of white blood cells, particularly in the bone marrow and spleen

A doctor who specializes in cancer treatment (called an **oncologist**) determines the class of a patient's tumor and rates its seriousness, assigning a stage number from 1 to 4 based on the size of the tumor(s), the number of lymph nodes involved, and the degree of spread (or metastasis). Stage 1 tumors are localized and often curable. Stage 2 to 4 cancers have spread farther and are less likely to be cured. **Table 12.1** shows the most common cancer sites and the number of annual deaths from each type.

What Causes Cancer?

Most research supports the idea that cancer is caused by both *external* factors, such as chemicals, radiation, viruses, and lifestyle, and *internal* factors, such as hormones, immune conditions, and inherited mutations.[8] These factors may act separately, together, or in sequence

oncologist A doctor who specializes in detection and treatment of cancer

TABLE **12.1** Leading Sites of New Cancer Cases and Deaths, 2013 Estimates

Estimated New Cases of Cancer		Estimated Deaths from Cancer	
Site	**Incidence (% of all cases)**	**Site**	**Mortality (% of all deaths)**
Male			
Prostate	238,590 (28%)	Lung and bronchus	87,260 (28%)
Lung and bronchus	118,080 (14%)	Prostate	29,720 (10%)
Colon and rectum	73,680 (9%)	Colon and rectum	26,300 (9%)
Urinary bladder	54,610 (6%)	Pancreas	19,480 (6%)
Melanoma of the skin	45,060 (5%)	Liver and intrahepatic bile duct	14,890 (5%)
Kidney and renal pelvis	40,430 (5%)	Leukemia	13,660 (4%)
Non-Hodgkin lymphoma	37,600 (4%)	Esophagus	12,220 (4%)
Oral cavity and pharynx	29,620 (3%)	Urinary bladder	10,820 (4%)
Leukemia	27,880 (3%)	Non-Hodgkin lymphoma	10,590 (3%)
Pancreas	22,740 (3%)	Kidney and renal pelvis	8,780 (3%)
All Sites	854,790 (100%)	All Sites	306,920 (100%)
Female			
Breast	232,340 (29%)	Lung and bronchus	72,220 (26%)
Lung and bronchus	110,110 (14%)	Breast	39,620 (14%)
Colon and rectum	69,140 (9%)	Colon and rectum	24,530 (9%)
Uterine corpus	49,560 (6%)	Pancreas	18,980 (7%)
Thyroid	45,310 (6%)	Ovary	14,030 (5%)
Non-Hodgkin lymphoma	32,140 (4%)	Leukemia	10,060 (4%)
Melanoma of the skin	31,630 (4%)	Non-Hodgkin lymphoma	8,430 (3%)
Kidney and renal pelvis	24,720 (3%)	Uterine corpus	8,190 (3%)
Pancreas	22,480 (3%)	Liver and intrahepatic bile duct	6,780 (2%)
Ovary	22,240 (3%)	Brain and other nervous system	6,150 (2%)
All Sites	805,500 (100%)	All Sites	273,430 (100%)

Data from: The American Cancer Society, *Cancer Facts and Figures* 2013 (Atlanta: American Cancer Society, 2013).

casestudy

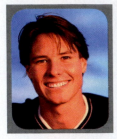

TIM

"One of my good friends, Kevin, was recently diagnosed with skin cancer. He's a surfer and a lifeguard, and I've never seen him without a tan. Fortunately, they caught it early and he's going to be OK. Ever since his diagnosis, he's been lecturing me about wearing sunscreen and about how I should learn from his mistakes. The other day, I counted up the number of hours I spend in the sun—it's at least ten hours each week."

THINK! How much time do you spend in the sun? Do you wear protective clothing and sunscreen with a SPF of at least 15?

ACT NOW! Today, count the number of hours per week you spend in the sun. This week, write down two things you could do differently to protect your skin and begin with one. In two weeks, make sure you are doing both protective measures. Remember to reapply sunscreen regularly while out-of-doors.

HEAR IT! ONLINE

---

to promote cancer development. Some mutations arise spontaneously during cell division. Other mutations are caused by **carcinogens** that damage a normal cell's DNA and reprogram the genetic information. Common carcinogens in the environment include the ultraviolet radiation in sunlight and the tar in cigarette smoke.[9] Cancer may also be caused by **oncogenes**—genes that researchers suspect play a role in uncontrolled cell growth. Oncogenes may initially be dormant but become activated by age, stress, viral infection, radiation, or exposure to other carcinogens, transforming healthy cells into cancerous ones. Women, for example, who inherit a mutation of oncogenes are significantly more likely to develop breast cancer.[10]

Most experts agree that many cancers are preventable through modifying environmental factors and avoiding risk-related behaviors. For example, at least 30 percent of all cancer deaths and 87 percent of lung cancer deaths are attributable to smoking.[11]

carcinogens Cancer-causing agents

oncogenes Suspected cancer-causing genes

malignant melanoma An invasive cancer of the pigment-producing cells of the skin

---

What Are the Most Common Types of Cancers?

There are many different types of cancers. This section surveys the most common types.

Skin Cancer Is the Most Common

More than 3.5 million cases of skin cancer are diagnosed in the United States each year.[12] Most skin cancer cases are *basal cell carcinoma* or *squamous cell carcinoma* and are highly curable. **Malignant melanoma** accounts for only about 5 percent of skin cancer cases, but causes most of the deaths from skin cancer each year. Once melanoma has spread, it is extremely difficult to treat. Malignant melanoma has been increasing at 4 percent per year since 1981 (faster than any other cancer) and occurs more frequently in young adults aged 15–29 than do other types of skin cancers (see the GetFitGraphic on page 405). Among Caucasian women aged 30–34, melanoma is second only to breast cancer.[13]

The risk of skin cancer is greatest for people with light skin; with blond, red, or light brown hair; and with blue, green, or gray eyes. A Caucasian's lifetime risk of melanoma is 23 times higher than an African American's risk.[14] You are also at risk if you burn easily, peel readily, and spend lots of time outdoors. High-altitude exposure, having a relative who has been treated for skin cancer, and inadequate use of sunscreen (e.g., using an SPF below 15 or failing to reapply every two hours) can further increase your risk.

Many people do not know what to look for when examining themselves for skin cancer. Basal and squamous cell carcinomas show up most commonly on the face, ears, neck, arms, hands, and legs as warty bumps, colored spots, or scaly patches (see **Figure 12.3a, b** on the following page). Many skin cancers begin in less obvious places, such as between the toes, near the genitals or anus, or on the scalp. Surgery may be necessary to remove the growths, but they are seldom life-threatening. By contrast, melanoma starts as a normal-looking mole but quickly develops abnormal characteristics (**Figure 12.3c**). Remember the simple "ABCD" guidelines to help you detect the warning signs of melanoma:

- **A**symmetry: One half of the mole does not match the other half.
- **B**order irregularity: The edges of the mole are uneven, notched, or scalloped.
- **C**olor: Pigmentation is not uniform. Melanoma may vary in color from tan to deeper brown, reddish black, black, or deep bluish black.

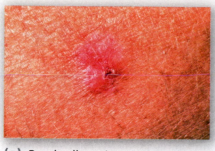
(a) Basal cell carcinoma

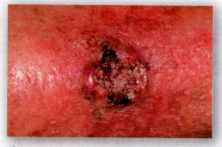
(b) Squamous cell carcinoma

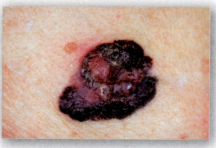
(c) Malignant melanoma

FIGURE 12.3 The three main types of skin cancers: (a) Basal cell carcinoma starts as a small bump, then develops a central crater that crusts and bleeds. (b) Squamous cell carcinoma is often a small nodule surrounded by inflamed tissue. (c) Malignant melanoma is usually irregular in shape, non-uniformly (and often darkly) pigmented, and larger than pea size.

- *Diameter:* The diameter of the mole is greater than 6 millimeters (about the size of a pea).

If you notice any of these symptoms, or if there is a rapid change in the size or color of a mole, skin tag, or area of the skin, consult a physician promptly.

Lung Cancer Is the Leading Killer

Lung cancer kills more men and women than any other cancer and accounts for 27 percent of all cancer deaths.[15] Although more women develop breast cancer each year, more die from lung cancer, and women now have the same rates of lung cancer from smoking as men.[16] The good news is that fewer Americans smoke today than in the past three decades, and lung cancer rates have declined in men and leveled off in women (**Figure 12.4**).[17] Most lung cancer patients are smokers or former smokers, but people who have only experienced secondhand smoke or no exposure to smoking may also develop the disease.[18]

Warning signs of lung cancer include pain, shortness of breath, persistent wheezing or hoarseness, repeated bouts of pneumonia or bronchitis, a cough that won't go away (or gets worse), weight loss, loss of appetite, coughing up blood, or fever. Treatments for lung cancer include surgery, radiation, or chemotherapy. Despite medical advances, only 16 percent of all lung cancer patients survive for five or more years after diagnosis.[19]

Breast Cancer Strikes Mainly Women

Breast cancer is the second leading cause of cancer death in American women, but it can also occur in men. Earlier diagnosis and better treatments help cut the death rate, especially in women under 50. Risk factors associated with breast cancer include a prior history of breast cancer, a primary relative with breast cancer, unusual cell growths in the breast confirmed by biopsy, obesity after menopause, never having children or having a first child after age 30, consuming two or more drinks of alcohol per day, higher education and socioeconomic status, and hormone replacement therapy after menopause. The box Do Birth Control Pills Increase Cancer Risk?

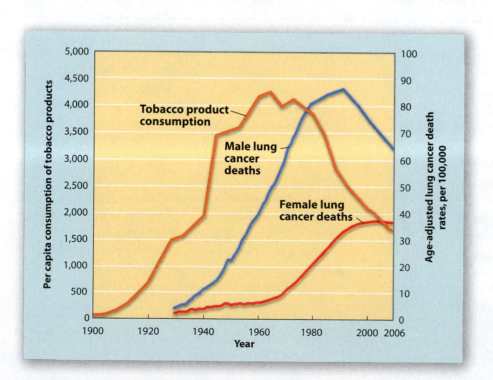

FIGURE 12.4 For decades, lung cancer was by far the biggest cancer killer of American men, but incidence has fallen along with smoking rates. Lung cancer deaths have also risen for women but have begun to plateau.

Data from: Death Rates: U.S. Mortality Files, National Center for Health Statistics, Centers for Disease Control and Prevention, 2010; Cigarette Consumption: U.S. Department of Agriculture, 1900–2006.

Q&A Do Birth Control Pills Increase Cancer Risk?

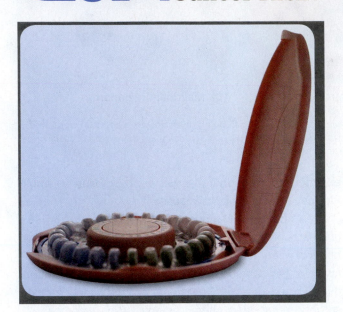

For decades, medical researchers
have tried to resolve the important question of whether using oral contraceptives increases the risk of cancer in women. In 1996, a large, widely publicized study concluded that women who took birth control pills had a slightly increased risk of developing breast cancer both while they were taking the pills and for 10 years after stopping use.[1] Many women in such long-term studies were taking traditional contraceptive formulations with higher doses of estrogen. So what about women taking newer low-dosage pills? A recent study of 116,000 nurses aged 24–43 found a small increased

risk of breast cancer in those who took oral contraceptives, but significantly, it was mainly in women who took "triphasic" birth control pills—a type with changing hormone levels during three phases of the menstrual cycle.[2] Some studies, however, have shown no increased risk of breast cancer. And to complicate matters further, several studies, including a major study published in 2008, concluded that oral contraceptives lower a woman's risk for ovarian cancer.[3] On their informational websites, both the American Cancer Society and the National Cancer Institute advise women that birth control pills appear to carry a small risk of breast cancer that diminishes 5 to 10 years after stopping. Medical researchers are continuing to probe other questions about oral hormones, including whether they increase the risk of strokes or other cardiovascular diseases, especially when used after menopause. Young women should consider such studies and the resulting advice given by ACS and NCI. After consulting with their doctors, they must weigh the very small but finite risks involved in taking birth control pills.

Sources:
1. Collaborative Group on Hormonal Factors in Breast Cancer, "Breast Cancer and Hormonal Contraceptives: Collaborative Reanalysis of Individual Data on 53,297 Women with Breast Cancer and 100,239 Women Without Breast Cancer from 54 Epidemiological Studies," *Lancet* 347, no. 9017 (1996): 1713–27.
2. D. J. Hunter et al., "Oral Contraceptive Use and Breast Cancer: A Prospective Study of Young Women," *Cancer Epidemiology Biomarkers and Prevention* 19, no. 10 (2010): 2496–502.
3. Collaborative Group on Epidemiological Studies of Ovarian Cancer, "Ovarian Cancer and Oral Contraceptives: Collaborative Reanalysis of Data from 45 Epidemiological Studies Including 23,257 Women with Ovarian Cancer and 87,303 Controls," *Lancet* 371, no. 9609 (2008): 303–14.

---

above presents the conflicting research studies on oral contraceptives and cancer risk. Other possible risk factors for breast cancer include a high-fat diet, genetic predisposition due to oncogenes such as *BRCA1* and *BRCA2*, exposure to pesticides and other chemicals, weight gain, and physical inactivity. Researchers recently discovered a protein (CtBP) that can increase the risk of breast cancer; significantly, metabolic imbalances such as obesity and diabetes cause the body to generate more of the protein. This protein provides one of the first direct links between diet, exercise, and breast cancer, as well as a possible target for new cancer drugs.[20]

SEE IT! ONLINE
Breast Cancer Patients Getting Younger

Regular breast self-examinations and medical check-ups (including *mammography*—breast X-rays) can detect cancer early, at its most treatable stage. The box Breast Awareness and Self-Exam on page 406 walks

you through performing breast self-exams. The American Cancer Society (ACS) recommends that women begin monthly breast self-examinations at age 20 with a clinical breast exam at least every three years. Beginning at age 40, women should have yearly clinical breast exams and mammograms.[21] The U.S. Preventive Services Task Force recommends mammograms every two years for women over 50 to minimize radiation exposure.[22] Keep in mind that most breast lumps are harmless cysts or fibrous tissue. A physician may investigate a lump with a biopsy, an ultrasound, or a noninvasive technique that measures the elasticity of a mass with pressure waves. If invasive cancer is discovered, treatments include surgery, radiation, and chemotherapy.

Female Reproductive Tract Cancers

Cancers of the female reproductive tract include ovarian, uterine, and cervical cancer.

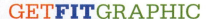

SHINING MORE LIGHT ON TO SKIN CANCER

Malignant melanoma is the most common form of cancer in young adults.[1] It also causes **75% of all skin cancer deaths**,[2] so it's crucial that you protect your skin from cancer.

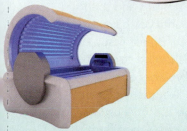

Using a tanning bed before age 35 increases your risk of:[3]

Melanoma by **75%**
Squamous cell carcinoma by **67%**
Basal cell carcinoma by **29%**

Of melanoma survivors,[4]

25% say they never use sunscreen
2% still use tanning beds

BLOCKING THE SUN FROM YOUR SKIN

The SPF of sunscreen stands for sun protection factor. The SPF rating shows what percentage of burning rays (*ultraviolet B* or *UVB*) the sunscreen can block out.[5]

% UVB BLOCKED

50%	93%	97%	98%	99%

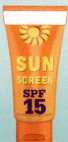 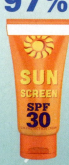 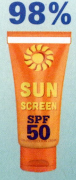 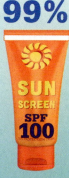

SUN SCREEN SPF 4 — SUN SCREEN SPF 15 — SUN SCREEN SPF 30 — SUN SCREEN SPF 50 — SUN SCREEN SPF 100

A "base" suntan won't protect you from the sun's burning rays: A deep tan offers no more protection than sunscreen with an **SPF 4**.

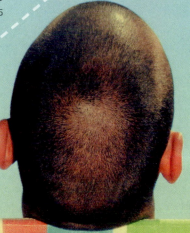

Experts recommend that you choose sunscreen with an **SPF 30 or higher**, apply it liberally, then reapply **every 2 hours** or more often if sweating. Waterproof sunscreens last about 90 minutes and then must be reapplied.

TIPS TO KEEP YOUR SKIN SAFE

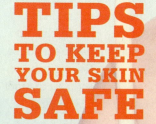

☀ Use sunscreen (SPF 30 or higher)
☀ Avoid tanning beds
☀ Wear long sleeves, hats, and sunglasses
☀ Limit UVB exposure, especially between 10 AM and 4 PM

Breast Awareness and Self-Exam

Women should know how their breasts normally look and feel and report any new breast changes to a health professional as soon as these changes are noted. It is best for a woman to examine her breasts when they are not tender or swollen.

To do a breast self-exam, inspect the breasts in a mirror, looking for their usual symmetry (**Figure a**). Some breasts are normally asymmetrical, and if this is not a change, it is okay. Raise and lower both arms while checking that the breasts move evenly and freely. Next, inspect the skin, looking for areas of redness, thickening, or dimpling, which might have the appearance of an orange peel. Look for any scaling on the nipple.

To feel for lumps, raise one arm above your head while either standing or lying. Using the index, middle, and fourth fingers of your opposite hand, gently push down on the breast tissue and move the fingers in small circular motions, varying pressure from lighter to firmer. Start at one edge of the breast and move upward and then downward, working your way across until you have covered all of the breast tissue (**Figure b**). Breast tissue often feels dense and irregular, and this can be completely normal. Regular self-exams can help you become familiar with what your breast tissue feels like; then you can notice more easily if there is a change. Cancers usually feel like a dense or firm little rock and are very different from the normal breast tissue.

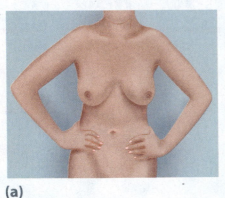

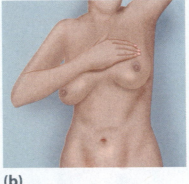

(a)   **(b)**

Next, lower the arm and reach into the top of the underarm and move fingers downward with gentle pressure, feeling for any enlarged lymph nodes. To complete the exam, squeeze the tissue around the nipple. If you notice discharge from the nipple and you have not recently been breastfeeding, consult your doctor. Likewise, if you notice any asymmetry, skin changes, scaling on the nipple, or new lumps in the breast, you should see your doctor for evaluation.

Ovarian Cancer Among reproductive tract cancers in women, ovarian cancer is the deadliest. It is also the fifth leading cause of cancer death among American women.[23] Because ovarian cancer has few overt signs (symptoms include feeling bloated, a constant feeling of fullness, changes in bowel or bladder activity, and pain in the pelvis, abdomen, or back), it often progresses to an advanced stage before it is discovered.[24]

A woman's risk of ovarian cancer increases if she has a prior history of (or has a close relative with) breast, colon, or ovarian cancer. The risk also increases if a woman is over 50 and has had few or no children. Other suspected risk factors are the use of fertility drugs before menopause and the use of hormone replacement drugs after menopause. Factors that appear to *lower* risk include eating a low-fat diet, consuming plenty of fruits and vegetables, effectively managing weight and stress levels, exercising regularly,

having full-term pregnancies, breastfeeding, using oral contraceptives, and having annual medical check-ups.[25]

Uterine and Cervical Cancer Most uterine cancers develop in the body of the uterus, usually in the endometrium (lining). The rest develop in the cervix, at the base of the uterus.

Risk factors for uterine (endometrial) cancer include increasing age, race (Caucasian women are at higher risk), endometrial tissue buildup due to hormone imbalances, estrogen replacement therapy, overweight or obesity, diabetes and high blood pressure, a history of other cancers, having few or no children, and menopause late in life.[26] Early symptoms of uterine cancer may include bleeding outside the normal menstrual period or after menopause, or persistent unusual vaginal discharge. Recent genetic studies of endometrial cancer have revealed four distinct genetic types, and this new classification is helping

Testicular Self-Exam

Most testicular cancers can be found at an early stage. The American Cancer Society (ACS) advises men to be aware of testicular cancer and to see a doctor right away if they find a lump in a testicle.

The testicular self-exam is best done after a hot shower, which relaxes the scrotum. Inspect for any changes in color or in the size of each testicle. It is common for one testicle to be larger than the other, and if this is not a change, it is okay.

Hold a testicle using the three middle fingers of one hand. Using small circular motions and light pressure, move the index and middle fingers of the second hand over the testicle until the whole surface has been covered. Feel for changes in texture or small nodules that may feel like a pea or a grain of rice.

Note if there are any painful areas. Along the back of each testicle is the epididymis, which contains the spermatic cord and the blood vessels serving the testicle. Feel this area with the index finger and the thumb, again looking for painful areas, changes in texture, or small lumps. Repeat the process for the second testicle. Consult your doctor for further evaluation if you find something of concern.

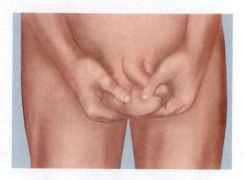

---

doctors treat uterine tumors more specifically and successfully than older methods.[27]

The main cause of cervical cancer is infection by the human papillomavirus (HPV).[28] Activities that increase the risk of acquiring HPV infection, such as early age at first intercourse and multiple sex partners, also increase the risk of cervical cancer, as do smoking and infection by the herpes virus.[29] The **Pap smear** is very effective for detecting early stage cervical cancer and has helped reduce the incidence of dangerous later-stage cancers. There are also new vaccines for females aged 9–26 that protect against HPV, which can in turn decrease the risk of developing cervical cancer.[30]

Screening for cervical cancer should begin at age 21 and continue with a Pap smear once every three years until age 65. Women aged 30–65 should have an additional test for the HPV once every five years. For endometrial cancer, women at menopause and of average risk should report unexpected bleeding to their physician.

SEE IT! ONLINE
Preventing Cervical Cancer

Male Reproductive Tract Cancers

Male reproductive tract cancers include those of the prostate and testicles.

Prostate Cancer Prostate cancer is the most common cancer in men and the second-most frequent cause of male cancer deaths. Symptoms may include weak or interrupted urine flow; difficulty starting or stopping urination; feeling the urge to urinate frequently; pain upon urination; blood in the urine; or pain in the low back, pelvis, or thighs. Prostate cancer can be slow-growing and symptom-free in the early stages, making testing and early diagnosis important.

Prostate cancer risk increases with age; 60 percent of cases occur in men over the age of 65; 97 percent in men over 50.[31] Race is also a significant factor: African American men and Jamaican men of African descent have the highest rates of prostate cancer in the world. Other risk factors include family history of prostate cancer, high BMI, and a diet high in processed meat and dairy products and low in fiber, fruits, and vegetables.[32] The ACS recommends that starting at age 50, men at average risk consult with their doctor to determine whether to have a *prostate-specific antigen test* with or without a digital rectal exam.

Testicular Cancer Unlike prostate cancer, testicular cancer tends to be diagnosed in younger men, mostly between the ages of 20 and 34.[33] It is also much less common than prostate cancer. Genetic predisposition may increase the risk of testicular cancer, as does having undescended testicles. The box Testicular Self-Exam explains how to perform a testicular self-examination to check for early symptoms.

> **Pap smear** A procedure in which cells taken from the cervical region are examined for abnormal cellular activity

Colon and Rectal Cancers

Cancers of the colon and rectum are the third most common cancer in both men and women.[34] In the early stages, colorectal cancer has no symptoms. Bleeding from the rectum, blood in the stool, and changes in bowel habits can signal later-stage colorectal cancer. Risk factors include being over age 50, race (African Americans appear to have the highest risk of colorectal cancer), obesity (with the highest risk in African American and Hispanic males), a personal or family history of polyps (benign growths) in the colon or rectum, or bowel problems such as colitis.[35] The risk due to family history extends from immediate family members to second- and third-degree relatives such as grandparents, cousins, and great-grandparents.[36] Women under age 50 who have had endometrial cancer also have a much higher risk of colon cancer.[37] Research suggests that the risk of developing colorectal cancer can be lowered significantly by eating less red meat and more high-fiber foods, including fruits and vegetables; exercising regularly; and getting regular colorectal screening—a simple blood test (*fecal occult blood test*) and *colonoscopy* after age 50. Polyp removal during these procedures can prevent a growth from progressing to cancer later. Treatment of a colorectal cancer often requires radiation or surgery. Medical researchers are currently developing a simple urine test for colon cancer that could one day replace the more invasive tests.[38]

Pancreatic Cancer and Leukemia

Two additional cancers are among the most-often diagnosed: pancreatic cancer and leukemia. Risk factors for pancreatic cancer include being male, being over age 45, smoking, eating a high-fat diet, having diabetes, and having a family history of cancer.[39]

Leukemia is a cancer of the blood-forming tissues, particularly the soft, spongy marrow of the bones. There are several types of leukemia; these can be acute or chronic and can strike both sexes and all age groups. Although it is the most common childhood cancer, over 90 percent of all leukemia cases occur in adults aged 20 and over.[40] Symptoms may include frequent infections, flu-like symptoms, headaches, vomiting, anemia, and pain or swelling in the joints.

How Can I Reduce My Risk of Cancer?

Lab 12.1 will help you assess yourself for risk factors associated with many common cancers, and the box Reduce Your Cancer Risk summarizes wellness behaviors that can lower your cancer risk. Completing **Lab 12.2** can help you plan for cancer prevention.

LIVE IT! ONLINE
**Worksheet 40
Cancer Risk
Assessment**

TOOLS FOR CHANGE

Reduce Your Cancer Risk

Here is a checklist of wellness behaviors that can lower your risk of developing cancer:

☐ Don't smoke or use tobacco.

☐ Limit alcohol consumption to one drink per day or less if you are a woman, and two drinks a day or less if a man.

☐ Limit consumption of grilled meats, blackened meats, processed meats, and fried foods.

☐ Limit intake of saturated and *trans* fats.

☐ Eat at least five servings per day or more of fruits and vegetables.

☐ Eat several servings per day of whole-grain foods.

☐ Engage in regular physical activity and exercise.

☐ Maintain your BMI within recommended levels (18.5 to 24.9).

☐ Practice stress management techniques.

☐ Limit environmental exposures to carcinogens, including infectious agents, radiation, and chemicals.

☐ Limit sun exposure by using sunscreen (SPF 15 or higher) and protective clothing and by staying out of the sun during the brightest midday hours.

☐ Learn to do regular self-exams for breast cancer, skin cancer, and testicular cancer.

☐ Get regular medical check-ups and the professional screenings recommended for your sex and age group.

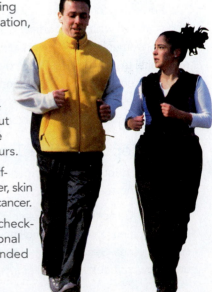

In addition to assessing and reducing your risks, being "in touch" with your body, and seeking medical attention when suspicious changes occur, can be critical to increasing the chances of successful intervention and treatment. There are seven general early warning signs of cancer, summarized by the acronym CAUTION:

*C*hange in bowel or bladder habits

A sore that does not heal

*U*nusual bleeding or discharge

*T*hickening or lump in breast or elsewhere

*I*ndigestion or difficulty in swallowing

*O*bvious change in a wart or mole

*N*agging cough or hoarseness

If you have what may be a warning sign of cancer, make an appointment with your doctor. If it is an indicator of cancer, your chances of full recovery are higher the earlier you detect it. If it isn't cancer, you can rest easier that much sooner.

Lifestyle Choices Can Reduce Your Cancer Risk

Your lifestyle choices can substantially affect your risk of developing cancer (**Figure 12.5**). **Lifetime risk** refers to the probability that you will develop cancer at some point during your life. **Relative risk** is a measure of how likely you are to develop cancer while engaging in a known risk behavior, compared to people who abstain from that behavior.

Quit Smoking, Drink Less, Avoid Drugs
Smoking, excessive alcohol use, or illegal drug use can increase cancer risk. If you are a smoker, your relative risk of developing lung cancer is about 18 to 23 times higher than that of a nonsmoker.[41] Drinking alcohol,

Being overweight or obese

Increases susceptibility to

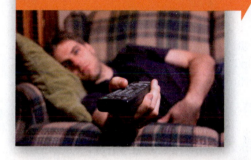

Breast, colon, thyroid, ovarian, cervical, prostate, endometrial, pancreatic, gallbladder, and kidney cancers; multiple myeloma; Hodgkin's disease; adenocarcinomas of the esophagus

Sedentary lifestyle

Increases susceptibility to

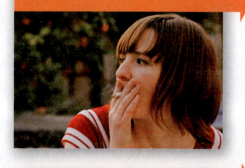

Colon cancer, breast cancer

Smoking, tobacco use

Increases susceptibility to

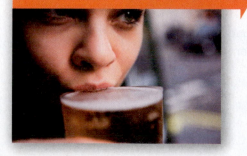

Lung, esophageal, pancreatic, uterine, cervical, kidney, bladder, stomach, and nasopharyngeal cancers; cancers of the nasal cavity, lip, and oral cavity

Alcohol

Increases susceptibility to

Liver, esophageal, and breast cancers; cancers of the mouth, pharynx, and larynx

lifetime risk The probability that a person will develop cancer at some point during his or her lifetime

relative risk A measure of how likely a person is to develop cancer while engaging in known risk behaviors compared to people who abstain from these behaviors

FIGURE **12.5** Lifestyle factors such as smoking, drinking alcohol, overeating, and too little physical activity can increase the risk of cancer.

especially in combination with smoking, increases the risk of oral and pancreatic cancers. Drinking more than one glass of alcohol daily is also associated with an increased risk of breast cancer among women.[42] Hepatitis, which can be contracted from contaminated needles, increases the risk of liver cancer, as does the use of anabolic steroids.[43]

Watch Your Weight, Move More, and Eat Right

Scientific evidence suggests that 30 to 40 percent of cancer deaths are related to overweight or obesity, poor nutritional habits, and lack of exercise.[44] This means that people could prevent a significant number of cancer deaths through their own weight control, healthier eating, and increased physical activity.

Several studies have shown reductions in cancer risk through physical exercise: The most physically active women had a 20 to 30 percent lower risk of breast cancer.[45] In other studies, leisure-time physical activity appeared to reduce the risk of colon cancer by more than 20 percent in men and women.[46] Physical activity also seems to lower a man's risk for the more aggressive forms of prostate cancer and his survival once prostate cancer is diagnosed.[47]

Certain food additives are suspected of causing cancer, particularly *sodium nitrate,* a chemical used to preserve and give color to red meat. High doses of beta-carotene, selenium, and folic acid taken as supplements increase cancer risk, as do high levels of dietary cadmium.[48] There is also evidence that consumption of grilled meats, deep fried foods, and processed lunch meats can increase the risk of some types of cancer.[49] High levels of blood sugar from eating excess sugar or from having diabetes or being

obese can also predispose a person to cancer.[50] At the same time, more than 40 plant-based compounds in fruits, grains, and vegetables including vitamins, flavonoids, and antioxidants can turn on genes that slow down cancer growth and spread.[51]

Manage Stress Stress has been implicated in increased susceptibility to several types of cancers.[52] People who are under chronic, severe stress or who suffer from depression or other persistent psychological disorders show higher rates of cancer than their healthy counterparts. Sleep disturbances, diet, or a combination of factors may weaken the body's immune system, increasing susceptibility to cancer.

Biological Factors Play a Role in Cancer Risk

Our genes, our internal hormonal environments, and our exposures to biological agents such as viruses can increase our risk of cancer.

Genetics Cancers of the breast, stomach, colon, prostate, uterus, ovaries, and lungs appear to run in families.[53] For example, a woman runs a much higher risk of breast cancer if her mother or sisters have had the disease. Hodgkin lymphoma and certain leukemias also seem to be hereditary.

Reproductive Hormones The effect estrogen has on breast cancer risk is well documented. A woman's risk of breast cancer increases a small but statistically significant amount if she begins menstruation early (before age 12), has no children or has her first child after age 30, uses birth control pills (within the past 10 years), or takes hormone replacement therapy after menopause—all of which increase the amount of estrogen a woman is exposed to over a lifetime. Conversely, the risk of breast cancer decreases slightly in women who experience late menstruation (after age 14), have their first child at a young age, have many children, breast feed, or experience early menopause (before age 45), all circumstances that reduce the amount of estrogen a woman is exposed to in her lifetime.[54]

Infectious Agents According to recent estimates, microbes and their by-products cause some 20 percent of new cancers worldwide.[55] Hepatitis B virus (HBV) and hepatitis C virus (HCV), for example, can damage DNA that leads to liver cancer. Meanwhile, virtually all women with cervical cancer have evidence of infection from certain strains of HPV, which also causes genital warts.[56]

Environmental Factors Can Increase Cancer Risk

Exposure to radiation, chemicals, and other carcinogens in the environment can increase your cancer risk. Limiting your exposure to such environmental factors can decrease the risk.

Radiation *Ionizing radiation (IR)*—such as radiation from X-rays, radioactive material, radon gas, cosmic rays, and ultraviolet radiation (UV) from sunlight—can cause cancer. IR can promote cancer in virtually any part of the body, but bone marrow and the thyroid gland are particularly susceptible. Routine diagnostic medical and dental X-rays are usually set at the lowest possible levels of radiation in order to minimize such risk. Radon, both in industrial settings and in homes, is the leading cause of lung cancer in nonsmokers and the second leading cause of lung cancer overall.[57] Exposure to ultraviolet radiation through sun-tanning and the use of tanning booths is a well-known risk for skin cancers (see the GetFitGraphic on page 405).

SEE IT! ONLINE
Extreme Tanning

Occupational Exposures Certain occupations expose workers to known carcinogens at a much higher level than the average person would ever encounter. For example, uranium miners, sewage workers, and petroleum refinery workers tend to encounter high levels of radon gas and have higher-than-average rates of lung cancer.[58]

What If I or Someone I Know Is Facing Cancer?

The emotional distress of facing cancer can cloud a person's critical health care decision making. Find a close friend or family member who will support you. After any cancer diagnosis, find out the type and stage of the cancer and the prognosis for recovery. Ask about the benefits, risks, and possible side effects of each treatment option. Seek out well-established hospitals and treatment centers that specialize in treating cancer of your kind and interview cancer specialists, surgeons, and chemo and radiation therapists. Surgical removal of tumors, radiation, chemotherapy, immunotherapies, and gene therapies are all possible treatment avenues.

Radiation and Chemotherapy **Radiation**, targeted beams of ionizing energy, works by destroying malignant cells or stopping cell growth. It is most effective in treating localized cancers. Unfortunately, radiation also destroys some healthy cells and increases the risk of other

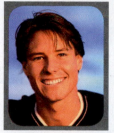
types of cancers. Nonetheless, radiation continues to be one of the most common and effective forms of treatment.

During **chemotherapy**, the patient receives intravenous doses of drugs capable of targeting and killing fast-growing cells throughout the body, including metastasized cancer cells. Because chemotherapy also kills the fast-dividing cells in normal hair follicles, it tends to cause hair loss. Damage to rapidly dividing digestive-tract cells explains the nausea and nutritional deficiencies so common to patients undergoing chemotherapy.

Radiation and chemotherapy can cause long-term damage to the heart, brain, and other organs, so the decision to undergo either treatment is a serious one. However, millions of people have gone on to live productive lives for years or decades after radiation or chemotherapy treatment.

New Approaches to Treatment Today, researchers are exploring treatments that target cancer as a genetic disease that is brought on by a mutation, either inherited or acquired. Potential treatments include *immunotherapies*, such as those

> **radiation** Powerful, targeted beams of ionizing energy that can kill cancerous cells
>
> **chemotherapy** The use of drugs to kill cancerous cells

that enhance the body's immune system to help control cancer, and *gene therapies,* such as those that manipulate genes to increase the patient's immune response to a cancerous tumor or that allow the patients' bone marrow to withstand stronger doses of chemotherapeutic drugs. Stem-cell research, though controversial, may also yield promising new cancer treatments.

CHAPTER IN REVIEW

MasteringHealth™

Build your knowledge—and wellness!—in the Study Area of MasteringHealth with a variety of study tools.

SEE IT! ONLINE

videos

Breast Cancer Patients Getting Younger
Preventing Cervical Cancer
Extreme Tanning

HEAR IT! ONLINE

audio tools

Audio case study
MP3 chapter review

REVIEW IT! ONLINE

chapter review

Chapter reading quizzes
Glossary flashcards

LIVE IT! ONLINE

programs & behavior change

Take Charge of Your Health! Worksheets:
Worksheet 40 Cancer Risk Assessment
Behavior Change Log Book and Wellness Journal

DO IT! ONLINE

labs

Lab 12.1 Assess Your Personal Risk of Cancer
Lab 12.2 Plan for Cancer Prevention

reviewquestions

1. Which of the following can help you decrease your risk of developing cancer?
   a. Smoking only a few cigarettes per day
   b. Drinking one to two drinks per day
   c. Maintaining a BMI over 25
   d. Getting 30 to 60 minutes of exercise five days a week

2. The difference between a benign tumor and a malignant tumor is that
   a. a benign tumor is cancerous; a malignant tumor is noncancerous.
   b. a benign tumor is inherited; a malignant tumor is caused by lifestyle factors.
   c. a benign tumor is noncancerous; a malignant tumor is cancerous.
   d. a benign tumor is caused by lifestyle factors; a malignant tumor is inherited.

3. Suspected cancer-causing genes are called
   a. carcinogens.
   b. oncogenes.
   c. phytochemicals.
   d. metastases.

4. A physician who specializes in cancer is an
   a. internist.
   b. oncologist.
   c. endocrinologist.
   d. epidemiologist.

5. Cancers characterized by an increased number of white blood cells are classified as
   a. leukemias.
   b. lymphomas.
   c. sarcomas.
   d. carcinomas.

6. You can lower your risk of lung cancer by reducing your exposure to
   a. UV radiation from sunlight.
   b. red meat.
   c. cigarette smoke.
   d. oncogenes.

7. In the "ABCD" warning signs of melanoma, the "A" stands for
   a. asymmetry.   c. angiogenesis.
   b. asbestos.   d. alcohol use.

8. Angiogenesis is
   a. a method of treating cancer.
   b. the process by which malignant cells induce new blood vessel growth.
   c. the spread of cancer cells throughout the body.
   d. a synonym for metastasis.

9. The leading cancer killer for both men and women in the United States is
   a. breast cancer.
   b. lung cancer.
   c. skin cancer.
   d. pancreatic cancer.

10. Testicular cancer tends to strike
    a. men in their 70s.
    b. men between the ages of 20 and 34.
    c. teenage males.
    d. boys under age 10.

critical thinkingquestions

1. What is cancer? How does it spread? What is the difference between a benign and a malignant tumor?
2. What are the differences among carcinomas, sarcomas, lymphomas, and leukemia?
3. What are five controllable risk factors for developing cancer?

references

1. American Cancer Society, *Cancer Facts and Figures 2013* (Atlanta: American Cancer Society, 2013). Available at www.cancer.org
2. Ibid.
3. Ibid; G. A. Colditz et al., "Applying What We Know to Accelerate Cancer Prevention," *Science Translational Medicine* 4, no. 127 (2012): 127rv4, doi: 10.1126 /scitranslmed.3003218.
4. American Cancer Society, *Cancer Facts and Figures 2013*, 2013.
5. Ahmedin Jemal et al., "Annual Report to the Nation on the Status of Cancer, 1975–2009, Featuring the Burden and Trends in Human Papillovirus (HPV)–Associated Cancers and HPV Vaccination Coverage Levels," *Journal of the National Cancer Institute* 105 (2013): 175–201.
6. National Cancer Institute, "Understanding Cancer Series: Angiogenesis," Accessed April 2013, www.cancer.gov
7. National Cancer Institute, "Fact Sheet: Angiogenesis Inhibitors Therapy," Reviewed October 2011, www.cancer.gov
8. American Cancer Society, *Cancer Facts and Figures 2013*, 2013.
9. Ibid.
10. L. C. Brody and B. B. Biesecker, "Breast Cancer Susceptibility Genes BRCA1 and BRCA2," *Medicine* (Baltimore) 77, no. 3 (1998): 208–26.
11. American Cancer Society, "Tobacco-Related Cancers Fact Sheet," Revised January 2013, www.cancer.org

12. American Cancer Society, *Cancer Facts and Figures 2013*, 2013.
13. Colette Coyne Melanoma Awareness Campaign, "Melanoma," Accessed April 2013, www.ccmac.org
14. American Cancer Society, *Cancer Facts and Figures 2013*, 2013.
15. Ibid.
16. M. J. Thun et al., "50-Year Trends in Smoking-Related Mortality in the United States," *New England Journal of Medicine* 368 (2013): 351–64, doi: 10.1056 /NEJMsa1211127.
17. Ibid.
18. J. Samet et al., "Lung Cancer in Never Smokers: Clinical Epidemiology and Environmental Risk Factors," *Clinical Cancer Research* 15, no. 18 (2009): 5626–45; American Cancer Society, "Second Hand Smoke," January 2013, www.cancer.org
19. American Cancer Society, *Cancer Facts and Figures 2013*, 2013.
20. Li-Jun Di et al., "Genome-Wide Profiles of CtBP Link Metabolism with Genome Stability and Epithelial Reprogramming in Breast Cancer," *Nature Communications* 4 (2013): 1449, doi: 10.1038/ncomms2438.
21. American Cancer Society, "American Cancer Society Guidelines for the Early Detection of Cancer," Revised January 2013, www.cancer.org
22. U.S. Preventive Services Task Force, "Screening for Breast Cancer," Reviewed July 2010, www .uspreventiveservicestaskforce.org

23. American Cancer Society, *Cancer Facts and Figures 2013*, 2013.
24. Ibid.
25. National Cancer Institute, "Ovarian Cancer Screening (PDQ)," Modified September 2011, www.cancer.org
26. National Cancer Institute, "Endometrial Cancer," Accessed April 2013, www.cancer.org
27. G. Getz et al., "Integrated Genomic Characterization of Endometrial Carcinoma," *Nature* 497 (2013): 67–73, doi: 10.1038 /nature12113.
28. Centers for Disease Control and Prevention, "Human Papillomavirus (HPV): HPV Vaccines," Updated February 2013, www.cdc.gov
29. Ibid.
30. Ibid.
31. American Cancer Society, "Prostate Cancer Overview: What Are the Key Statistics About Prostate Cancer?" Revised January 2013, www.cancer.org
32. American Cancer Society, *Cancer Facts and Figures 2013*, 2013.
33. National Cancer Institute, "SEER Stat Fact Sheet: Testis," 2013, http://seer.cancer.gov
34. American Cancer Society, *Cancer Facts and Figures 2013*, 2013.
35. N. J. Samadder et al., "Elevated Risk of Colorectal Cancer in Relatives of Patients with Colorectal Cancer: A Population-Based Study in Utah," American College of Gastroenterology, 77th Annual Scientific Meeting, October 2012.

36. Ibid.
37. H. Singh et al., "Risk of Colorectal Cancer After Diagnosis of Endometrial Cancer: A Population-Based Study," *Journal of Clinical Oncology* (2013): doi: 10.1200/JCO.2012.47.6481.
38. Y. Qiu et al., "Urinary Metabonomic Study on Colorectal Cancer," *Journal of Proteome Research* 9, no. 3 (2010): 1627–34; Y. Cheng et al., "Distinct Urinary Metabolic Profile of Human Colorectal Cancer," *Journal of Proteome Research* 11, no. 2 (2012): 1354–63, doi: 10.1021/pr201001a.
39. American Cancer Society, *Cancer Facts and Figures 2013*, 2013.
40. Ibid.
41. Ibid.
42. Ibid.
43. Ibid.
44. G. A. Colditz et al., "Applying What We Know to Accelerate Cancer Prevention," 2012; Y. Zhang et al., "Stromal Progenitor Cells from Endogenous Adipose Tissue Contribute to Pericytes and Adipocytes That Populate Tumor Microenvironment," *Cancer Research* 72, no. 20 (2012): 5198, doi: 10.1158/0008-5472.CAN-12-0294; T. Boyle, "Physical Activity and Colon Cancer: Timing, Intensity, and Sedentary Behavior," *American Journal of Lifestyle Medicine* 6 (2012): 204–15, doi: 10.1177/1559827612436932; T. J. Key, E. A. Spencer, and G. K. Reeves, "Symposium 1: Overnutrition: Consequences and Solutions, Obesity and Cancer Risk," *The Proceedings of the Nutrition Society* 69, no. 1 (2010): 86–90.
45. L. E. McCullough et al., "Fat or Fit: The Joint Effects of Physical Activity, Weight Gain, and Body Size on Breast Cancer Risk," *Cancer* 118, no. 19 (2012): 4860–68, doi: 10.1002/cncr.27433; L. A. Healy et al., "Obesity Increases the Risk of Postmenopausal Breast Cancer and Is Associated with More Advanced Stage at Presentation But No Impact on Survival," *The Breast Journal* 16, no. 1 (2010): 95–7, doi: 10.1111/j.1524-4741.2009.00861.x.
46. T. Morikawa et al., "Prospective Analysis of Body Mass Index, Physical Activity, and Colorectal Cancer Risk Associated with B-Catenin (CTNNB1) Status," *Cancer Research* 73, no. 5 (2013): 1600–10, doi: 10.1158/0008-5472.CANM-12-2276; R. F. Zoeller, Jr., "Lifestyle in the Prevention and Management of Cancer: Physical Activity," *American Journal of Lifestyle Medicine* 3, no. 5 (2009): 353–61, doi: 10.1177/1559827609338680.
47. S. A. Kentfield et al., "Physical Activity and Survival After Prostate Cancer Diagnosis in the Health Professionals Follow-Up Study," *Journal of Clinical Oncology* 29, no. 6 (2011): 726–32; R. F. Zoeller, Jr., "Lifestyle in the Prevention and Management of Cancer," 2009.
48. M. E. Martinez et al., "Dietary Supplements and Cancer Prevention: Balancing Potential Benefits Against Proven Harms," *Journal of the National Cancer Institute* 104, no. 10 (2012): 732, doi: 10.1093/jnci/djs195; B. Julin et al., "Dietary Cadmium Exposure and Risk of Postmenopausal Breast Cancer: A Population-Based Prospective Cohort Study," *Cancer Research* 72, no. 6 (2012): 1459–66, doi: 10.1158/0008-5472.CAN-11-0735.
49. National Cancer Institute, "Fact Sheet: Chemicals in Meat Cooked at High Temperatures and Cancer Risk," Reviewed October 2012, www.cancer.org; M. Stott-Miller et al., "Consumption of Deep-Fried Foods and Risk of Prostate Cancer," *The Prostate* 2013; doi: 10.1002/pros.22643.
50. A. Chocarro-Calvo et al., "Glucose-Induced B-Catenin Acetylation Enhances Wnt Signaling in Cancer," *Molecular Cell* 49, no. 3 (2012): 474–86, doi: 10.1016/j.molcel.2012.11.022.
51. G. G. Meadows, "Diet, Nutrients, Phytochemicals, and Cancer Metastasis Suppressor Genes," *Cancer and Metastasis Reviews*, no. 3–4 (2012): 441–54, doi: 10.1007/s10555-012-9369-5.
52. National Cancer Institute Fact Sheet, "Psychological Stress and Cancer," December 2012, www.cancer.org; K. Ross, "Mapping Pathways from Stress to Cancer Progression," *Journal of the National Cancer Institute* 100, no. 13 (2008): 914–5, 917.
53. National Cancer Institute, "Cancer Genetics Risk Assessment and Counseling (PDQ)," Modified September 2011, www.cancer.org
54. American Cancer Society, "Breast Cancer Overview: What Causes Breast Cancer?" Revised February 2013, www.cancer.org
55. National Institute of Allergy and Infectious Diseases, "Viral Infections: Treating Cancer as an Infectious Disease," Updated March 2009, www.niaid.nih.gov
56. National Cancer Institute, "Fact Sheet: Human Papillomaviruses and Cancer," Reviewed September 2011, www.cancer.org
57. U.S. Environmental Protection Agency, "Radon (Rn): Health Risks: Exposure to Radon Causes Lung Cancer in Non-Smokers and Smokers Alike," Updated February 2011, www.epa.gov
58. R. J. Roscoe et al., "Lung Cancer Mortality Among Nonsmoking Uranium Miners Exposed to Radon Daughters," *JAMA* 262, no. 5 (1989): 629–33.

getfitgraphic references

1. W. Liu et al., "LKB1/STK11 Inactivation Leads to Expansion of a Prometastatic Tumor Subpopulation in Melanoma," *Cancer Cell* 21, no. 6 (2012): 751-64, doi: 10.1016/j.ccr.2012.03.048
2. Aim At Melanoma, "About Melanoma and Other Lesions," 2012, www.aimatmelanoma.org
3. Centers for Disease Control and Prevention, "Indoor Tanning," Reviewed July 2013, www.cdc.gov; M. R. Wehner et al., "Indoor Tanning and Non-Melanoma Skin Cancer: Review and Meta-Analysis," *British Medical Journal* 345 (2012): e5909, doi: 10.1136/bmj.e5909.
4. American Association for Cancer Research, "Some Melanoma Survivors Still Use Tanning Beds, Skip Sunscreen," *AACR in the News,* April 8, 2013, www.aacr.org
5. American Cancer Society, "Skin Cancer Protection and Early Detection, How Do I Protect Myself from UV rays?" Revised January 2013, www.cancer.org

Name: _____   Date: _____

Instructor: _____   Section: _____

Purpose: To assess your personal risk of common cancers.

Directions: Read each question and select the number corresponding to your Yes or No answer. Be honest and accurate in order to get the most complete understanding of your cancer risks.

Section I: Breast Cancer	Yes	No
1. Do you check your breasts at least monthly using breast self-examination (BSE) procedures?	1	2
2. Do you look at your breasts in the mirror regularly, checking for any irregular indentations/lumps, discharge from the nipples, or other noticeable changes?	1	2
3. Has your mother, sister, or daughter been diagnosed with breast cancer?	2	1
4. Have you ever been pregnant?	1	2
5. Have you had a history of lumps or cysts in your breasts or underarm?	2	1
Total Section I (Breast Cancer) Points	_____	
Section II: Skin Cancer	Yes	No
1. Do you spend a lot of time in the sun, either at work or at play?	2	1
2. Do you use sunscreens with an SPF rating of 15 or more when you are in the sun?	1	2
3. Do you use tanning beds or sun booths regularly to maintain a tan?	2	1
4. Do you examine your skin once a month, checking any moles or other irregularities, particularly in hard-to-see areas?	1	2
5. Do you purchase and wear sunglasses that adequately filter out harmful sun rays?	1	2
Total Section II (Skin Cancer) Points	_____	
Section III: Cancers of the Reproductive System—Men	Yes	No
1. Do you examine your penis regularly for unusual bumps or growths?	1	2
2. Do you perform regular testicular self-examination?	1	2
3. Do you have a family history of prostate or testicular cancer?	2	1
4. Do you practice safe sex and wear condoms with every sexual encounter?	1	2
5. Do you avoid exposure to harmful environmental hazards such as mercury, coal tars, benzene, chromate, and vinyl chloride?	1	2
Total Section III (Reproductive Cancer) Points—Men	_____	

Section III: Cancers of the Reproductive System—Women	Yes	No
1. Do you have a regularly scheduled Pap smear?	1	2
2. Have you been infected with the human papillomavirus, Epstein-Barr virus, or other viruses believed to increase cancer risk?	2	1
3. Has your mother, sister, or daughter been diagnosed with breast, cervical, endometrial, or ovarian cancer (particularly at a young age)?	2	1
4. Do you practice safe sex and use condoms with every sexual encounter?	1	2
5. Are you obese, taking estrogen, and/or consuming a diet that is very high in saturated fats?	2	1
Total Section III (Reproductive Cancer) Points—Women	_____	

Section IV: Cancers in General	Yes	No
1. Do you smoke cigarettes on most days of the week?	2	1
2. Do you consume a diet that is rich in fruits and vegetables?	1	2
3. Are you obese and/or do you lead a primarily sedentary lifestyle?	2	1
4. Do you live in an area with high air pollution levels or work in a job where you are exposed to several chemicals on a regular basis?	2	1
5. Are you careful about the amount of animal fat in your diet, substituting olive oil or canola oil for animal fat whenever possible?	1	2
6. Do you limit your overall consumption of alcohol?	1	2
7. Do you eat foods rich in flavonoids and antioxidants?	1	2
8. Are you "body aware" and alert for changes in your body?	1	2
9. Do you have a family history of ulcers or of colorectal, stomach, or other digestive system cancers?	2	1
10. Do you avoid unnecessary exposure to ionizing radiation such as X-rays, radon, and ultraviolet radiation?	1	2
Total Section IV (General Cancer) Points	_____	

REFLECTING ON YOUR SCORES

Take a careful look at each question where you marked a "2" and any areas in which you marked mostly 2s. Did you receive total points of six or higher in Sections I through III? Did you receive 11 or more total points in Section IV? If so, you have at least one identifiable risk, and a higher score indicates a higher risk level.

What general nutritional principles have you learned during this course that apply to your own cancer risks?

_____

Which of your lifestyle habits contribute to your cancer risk, and what is standing in the way of your eliminating them?

_____

Which medical screenings do you have each year? How does this compare to public health recommendations?

_____

LAB 12.2

PLAN FOR CHANGE

PLAN FOR CANCER PREVENTION

MasteringHealth™

Name: _____ Date: _____

Instructor: _____ Section: _____

Purpose: To develop a plan to change risky behaviors and employ healthy behaviors for cancer prevention.

Directions: Complete Sections I and II below, outlining your behavior, goals, and plan for cancer prevention.

SECTION I: BEHAVIOR EVALUATION

After reviewing the chapter and completing Lab 12.1, evaluate your behavior and identify patterns and specific things you are doing that may be risky for cancer.

1. What behaviors could you change today?

_____

_____

2. What behaviors could you change next week or next month?

_____

_____

SECTION II: CANCER PREVENTION GOALS

Create goals for cancer prevention. Be sure to use SMART (specific, measurable, action-oriented, realistic, time-oriented) goal-setting guidelines. Select appropriate target dates and rewards for completing your goals.

Behavior Change Goal #1: _____

Target Date: _____ Reward: _____

Behavior Change Goal #2: _____

Target Date: _____ Reward: _____

Behavior Change Goal #3: _____

Target Date: _____ Reward: _____

13 Avoiding Substance Use, Abuse, and Addiction

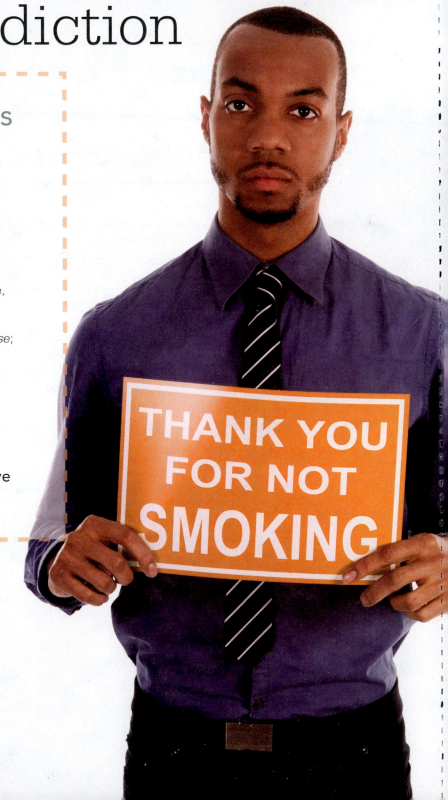

LEARNINGoutcomes

1 Define *addiction* and list four of its symptoms.

2 Describe the short-term and long-term health effects of alcohol use; the characteristics of a "problem drinker"; and strategies for avoiding alcohol abuse.

3 Describe the short-term and long-term health effects of tobacco use and secondhand smoke, and ways to avoid them.

4 Differentiate between *drug use* and *drug abuse*; name some common drugs and their health effects; and discuss ways to avoid their use.

MasteringHealth™

Go online for chapter quizzes, interactive assessments, videos, and more!

casestudy

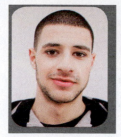

NATHAN

"My name is Nathan. I'm like most people: I experimented with alcohol in high school. But I never smoked or did drugs because I was on sports teams and frankly, I didn't want to get caught and lose my chance at a scholarship. Now that I'm in college, I am constantly exposed to drinking. I've seen some of my friends and fraternity brothers get into huge trouble with it, too. I also have friends who have started smoking and some who grow marijuana in their dorm rooms or go clubbing and do Ecstasy. People make it seem like it's no big deal. So how dangerous are drugs like these? When do people cross the line between having fun and getting in trouble?"

HEAR IT! ONLINE

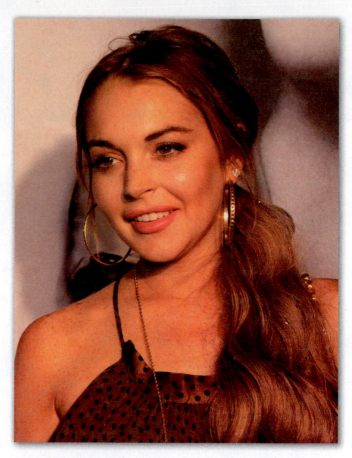

FIGURE **13.1** Actress Lindsay Lohan is one of many celebrities who has earned notoriety for struggling with substance abuse.

These days, it is easy to find high-profile cases of compulsive and destructive behavior. Stories of celebrities and politicians struggling with drug and alcohol addictions are splashed in the headlines and profiled on television news programs (**Figure 13.1**). But millions of "everyday" people throughout the world battle addiction as well. In this chapter, we will focus on the health risks posed by alcohol, tobacco, and other types of drug use. We will cover the short-term and long-term effects of substance use, discuss ways to identify patterns of addiction, and describe treatment options for those struggling with substance abuse.

What Is Addiction?

Addiction is a persistent, compulsive dependence on a behavior or substance, including mood-altering behaviors or activities, despite ongoing negative consequences. Although the mechanism is not well understood, all forms of addiction probably reflect dysfunction of certain biochemical systems in the brain.[1]

LIVE IT! ONLINE
Worksheet 30
Are You
Addicted?

Addictions, whether chemical or behavioral, are characterized by four common symptoms:[2]

- *Compulsion,* or craving for and excessive preoccupation with the behavior (drinking, drug use, gambling, etc.), plus an overwhelming need to perform it
- *Loss of control,* or the inability to reliably predict whether any isolated occurrence of the behavior will be healthy or damaging
- *Negative consequences,* such as physical damage, legal trouble, financial problems, academic failure, or family problems caused by the behavior
- *Denial,* or the inability to perceive that the behavior is self-destructive

Addictive substances or behaviors initially provide a sense of pleasure or stability that the addict cannot achieve in other ways. To be addictive, a substance or behavior must have the potential to produce a positive mood change. Chemicals are responsible for the most profound addictions; they produce dramatic mood changes and cause

addiction Persistent, compulsive dependence on a behavior or substance, despite ongoing negative consequences

cellular changes to which the body adapts so well that it eventually requires the chemical to function normally. *Withdrawal* is the variety of symptoms that occur after use of some addictive drugs is reduced or stopped. Other behaviors, such as gambling, spending money, working, and sex, create somewhat milder changes at the cellular level, along with elevating mood—which explains why these behaviors can also be addictive.

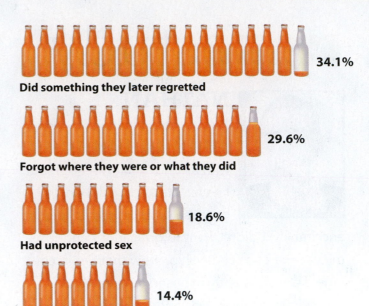

SEE IT! ONLINE
Woman's Shopping Addiction Revealed

What Are the Health Risks of Alcohol Use and Abuse?

Alcohol is the most widely used (and abused) recreational drug in our society. An estimated 51.5 percent of Americans consume alcoholic beverages regularly. Of them, about 7 percent are heavy drinkers, defined as those who habitually consume more than five drinks in one sitting.[3] Nearly half of Americans, however, are light drinkers or nondrinkers: About 13.6 percent drink fewer than a dozen drinks per year. About 35 percent don't drink at all. Globally, 40.6 percent of the adult population drinks, 45.8 percent have always abstained, and 13.6 percent are former drinkers.[4]

Alcohol on Campus

Alcohol is also the most popular drug on college campuses, where approximately 62 percent of students report having consumed alcoholic beverages in the last 30 days.[5] Students have more freedom and more social pressures and opportunities to drink than do other young people. A higher percentage of full-time college students drink more heavily than do same-aged peers who aren't in school.[6] Alcohol use among college students has many negative consequences (**Figure 13.2**).

About 44 percent of all college students engage in **heavy episodic (binge) drinking**; this usually involves drinking five or more drinks in a row (men) or four or more in a row (women) in about two hours.[7] Many students engage in **pregaming** (also called preloading or front-loading), and the incidence escalates rapidly upon college entrance.[8]

Did something they later regretted — 34.1%

Forgot where they were or what they did — 29.6%

Had unprotected sex — 18.6%

Physically injured self — 14.4%

Got in trouble with the police — 3.0%

Physically injured another person — 1.9%

FIGURE **13.2** A significant number of students experienced negative consequences as a result of their alcohol consumption over the past year.

Source: Data from American College Health Association, *American College Health Association—National College Health Assessment II: Reference Group Executive Summary Fall 2012* (Hanover, MD: American College Health Association, 2013).

Pregaming is a form of binge drinking: Students gather to drink heavily before going to a bar, nightclub, or sporting event where the drinks might be expensive or drinking might be prohibited. This and the other forms of binge drinking account for 90 percent of the alcohol young people consume.[9] Binge drinking is dangerous for many reasons: Alcohol-related injuries and death are the number-one cause of preventable death among undergraduate college students in the United States today, and 85 percent of all alcohol-impaired driving episodes involved people who binge drink.[10] Nationally, binge drinking kills over 40,000 people each year in the United States and costs over $167 billion annually in medical costs, legal costs, lost wages, and other economic impacts.[11] Even in young drinkers, binge drinking can damage the liver[12] and blood vessels (leading to heart disease later in life),[13] and it can induce long-lasting deficits in learning, memory, planning, and reasoning.[14]

heavy episodic (binge) drinking Drinking for the express purpose of becoming intoxicated; five drinks or more at one sitting for men; four drinks or more at one sitting for women

pregaming A form of binge drinking during which people gather to drink heavily before going to a bar, nightclub, or sporting event

Alcohol Profoundly Affects Your Body

Alcoholic beverages contain **ethyl alcohol** or **ethanol**. Unlike the molecules found in most foods and drugs, ethanol molecules are sufficiently small and fat soluble to be absorbed throughout the entire gastrointestinal system. A negligible amount of alcohol is absorbed through the lining of the mouth. Approximately 20 percent of ingested alcohol diffuses through the stomach lining into the bloodstream, and nearly 80 percent passes through the lining of the upper third of the small intestine.

Several factors influence how quickly your body absorbs alcohol, including the alcohol concentration in your drink, the amount of alcohol you consume, the amount of food in your stomach, your metabolism, your weight and body mass index, and your mood. The higher the concentration of alcohol in your drink, the more rapidly it will be absorbed in your digestive tract. For example, your body would absorb the alcohol in a one-ounce shot of tequila more rapidly than the alcohol in one ounce of beer because the beer is less concentrated. Carbonated alcoholic beverages, such as champagne and mixed drinks made with soda, are absorbed more rapidly than noncarbonated drinks because the carbonation raises the gas pressure in the stomach and this drives alcohol molecules through the stomach wall more quickly. If your stomach is full of food, alcoholic beverages empty more slowly into the small intestine, slowing absorption. Mixing alcohol with sugar-free diet drinks speeds absorption and increases blood alcohol content compared to using a sugary mixer.[15] Mood affects absorption as well; powerful moods, such as stress and tension, are likely to cause the stomach to dump its contents into the small intestine, speeding absorption.

Blood alcohol concentration (BAC) is the ratio of alcohol to total blood volume. A drinker's BAC depends on weight and body fat, the water content in body tissues, the concentration of alcohol in the beverage consumed, the rate of consumption, and the volume of alcohol consumed. **Figure 13.3** shows approximate BACs based on body weight and number of drinks consumed. The liver can metabolize (break down) about one ounce of alcohol per hour. If you drink more than that, the excess alcohol remains in your bloodstream, increasing your BAC.[16]

The **proof** of an alcoholic drink represents the percentage of alcohol in the beverage—the drink's strength. Alcohol percentage is half of the given proof. For example, 80-proof whiskey is 40 percent alcohol by volume. Lower-proof drinks will produce fewer effects than the same amount of higher-proof drinks. Most beers are between 2 and 5 percent alcohol, and most wines are about 12 percent alcohol (see **Figure 13.4** on page 422).

Short-Term Effects of Alcohol Use

Alcohol has many intertwined short-term effects on the body that start within minutes or hours of taking a drink. **Figure 13.5** on page 423 summarizes both the short- and long-term effects of alcohol on the body.

Nervous System Effects In the central nervous system, alcohol depresses the functioning of nerve and

> **ethanol (ethyl alcohol)** An addictive drug produced during fermentation and found in many beverages
>
> **blood alcohol concentration (BAC)** The ratio of alcohol to blood volume; used as a measure of intoxication
>
> **proof** A measure of the percentage of alcohol in a beverage

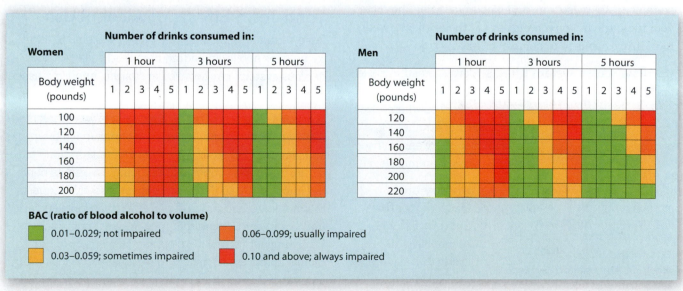

FIGURE **13.3** These charts show the approximate blood alcohol concentration (BAC) for women and men, based on body weight and number of drinks consumed.

Alcoholic beverage	Percentage of alcohol by volume	Amount of alcohol per serving
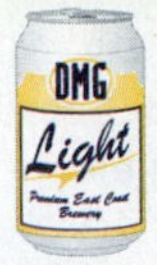 Light beer (12-oz. can)	2.4–4.8%	0.29–0.58 oz.
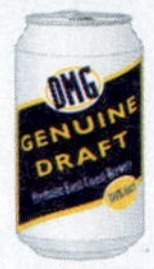 Regular beer (12-oz. can)	3.2–5.0%	0.38–0.60 oz.
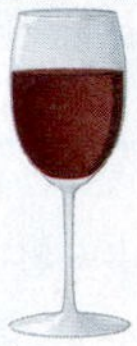 Wine (4-oz. glass)	12%	0.48 oz.
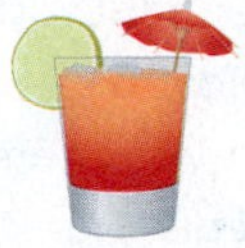 Cocktail (mixed drinks)	40–50%	1 oz.

FIGURE **13.4** This chart shows the approximate amount of alcohol typically contained in four common alcoholic beverages.

brain tissue. It slows your reaction time and impairs your judgment and motor coordination. This is why it is so dangerous to drink and drive. Alcohol also decreases vital functions controlled by the brain including your respiratory rate, pulse rate, and blood pressure. The more you drink, the more pronounced are these effects. Very high BACs can lead to coma and death.

Cardiovascular System Effects Slowed breathing, decreased pulse rate, and lowered blood pressure are all short-term cardiovascular effects. Binge drinkers put themselves at short-term risk for irregular heartbeat or even total loss of heart rhythm, which can disrupt blood flow and damage the heart muscle.

hangover A physiological reaction to excessive drinking, including symptoms such as headache, upset stomach, anxiety, depression, diarrhea, and thirst

blackout Amnesia for the people and events encountered while drinking, especially bingeing

Urinary and Gastrointestinal System Effects Alcohol is a diuretic that causes increased urinary output. The resulting imbalance in body

fluids can cause sluggish activity in your brain and nervous system and the fierce headache and sensory overload that typically accompany a hangover. Alcohol also irritates and inflames the gastrointestinal system. If consumed in large quantities or ingested on an empty stomach, it may cause indigestion, heartburn, and nausea.

Sexual Impairment Drinking alcohol can lower your sexual inhibitions. This can result in poor choices such as having sex with someone you might not choose if you were sober and exposing yourself to greater risk for a sexually transmitted infection. In a large national college student survey, about 19 percent of students had unprotected sex within the past year as a result of drinking, and about 2 percent experienced sex without their consent.[17] Drinking alcohol can also lead to less satisfying sex. Because alcohol is a diuretic and depresses nerve function, it decreases vaginal lubrication in women and can lead to erectile dysfunction in men.

Hangovers and Blackouts Drinkers often experience a **hangover** the morning after a night of heavy consumption. The symptoms of a hangover include headache, muscle aches, upset stomach, anxiety, depression, diarrhea, and thirst. It usually takes 12 hours to recover from a hangover. Bed rest, solid food, fluid intake, and aspirin may help, but the best strategy is to avoid one by abstaining from excessive alcohol use.[18] Hangover is an indicator of neural tissue damage, and it is sometimes paired with memory blackouts or amnesia for the people and events encountered while drinking, especially bingeing.[19] About half of all college students have experienced at least one **blackout**, and this often-frightening effect appears to reflect damage to the brain's hippocampus, a structure central to memory and learning.[20]

Long-Term Effects of Alcohol Use

Long-term use of alcohol can cause problems in addition to the ones above, including chronic diseases of the nervous system, cardiovascular system, and liver, as well as some cancers.

Nervous System Effects Even people who drink moderately may, over time, experience shrinkage in brain size and weight.[21] For example, even moderate drinking can shrink the hippocampus and bingeing can cut its nerve cell numbers by 40 percent.[22] Recent research suggests that humans continue to experience brain development until about age 25, and that teen drinking can significantly impact normal development, especially in the brain's frontal areas, including regions crucial for controlling impulses and thinking through consequences.[23] In addition, research shows that the earlier a teen takes his or her first drink, the more likely they will binge drink in

Short-term effects

- Impaired judgment/reaction time, impaired motor coordination, headache
- Decreased respiratory rate
- Decreased pulse rate and blood pressure; high amounts of alcohol can cause irregular heartbeat
- Irritation of gastrointestinal system, indigestion, heartburn, nausea
- Reduced sexual responsiveness
- Increased urination
- Muscle ache

Long-term effects

- Reduced brain size, damaged brain cells, dependency
- Increased risk of cancers of the mouth and tongue
- High blood pressure, increased heart rate
- Increased risk of breast cancer
- Fatty liver, alcoholic hepatitis, cirrhosis, increased risk of liver cancer
- Increased risk of cancers of the esophagus, stomach, and others
- Chronic inflammation of pancreas, increased risk of pancreatic cancer
- Impaired nutrient absorption
- Increased risk of osteoporosis
- Risk of giving birth to babies with fetal alcohol syndrome

FIGURE 13.5 The short-term and long-term effects of alcohol on the body.

high school or college, the more alcohol-related problems they will experience, and the more likely they will become *alcohol dependent* at some time in their lives compared to those who wait to drink until at least age 21.[24] The average American teen starts between 14 and 15.[25] Other nervous system effects of long-term alcohol use include increased susceptibility to anxiety and disrupted sleep, especially in the second half of the night.[26]

Cardiovascular System Effects The effects of alcohol on the cardiovascular system are complex. Numerous studies have associated light to moderate alcohol consumption with a reduced risk of coronary artery disease. However, a recent British study calculated the *optimal* level of alcohol consumption—the one associated with the lowest rates of Cardiovascular Disease (CVD) and other chronic diseases—and found it to be no more than one-half of a typical drink per day![27] Even moderate alcohol consumption (up to two drinks per day) contributes to high blood pressure and slightly increased heart rate and cardiac output, in part due to the blood vessel damage it can cause and in part due to the blood fats (triglycerides) the body produces after metabolizing alcohol. People who drink regularly have higher systolic blood pressure than people who do not.[28]

Liver Effects Heavy drinking causes the liver to deposit and store fat—a condition known as *fatty liver*. Over time,

fat-filled liver cells can stop functioning. Prolonged heavy drinking can also cause **alcoholic hepatitis**, another alcohol-related liver disease in which the liver becomes inflamed. Alcoholic hepatitis may itself be fatal or it may progress to **cirrhosis**, a condition in which the liver cells are damaged and scarring occurs.[29] Eventually, the liver cells die, damage becomes permanent, and the liver can no longer carry out its functions in the body. Among moderate to heavy drinkers, this damage may begin in the teens and progress rapidly in early adulthood. By middle-age (45 to 65 years old), cirrhosis is the most common cause of death in Americans after heart disease, cancer, accidents, and suicide.[30]

Cancer Alcohol is considered a *carcinogen* (cancer-causing agent). The repeated irritation caused by long-term alcohol use has been linked to cancers of the esophagus, stomach, mouth, tongue, liver, colon, and rectum.[31] There is also substantial evidence that even light drinkers (those who consume one drink per day) have a slightly increased risk for

alcoholic hepatitis A condition resulting from prolonged use of alcohol in which the liver is inflamed

cirrhosis The last stage of liver disease associated with chronic heavy use of alcohol, during which liver cells die and damage becomes permanent

breast cancer. A recent large study attributes 15 percent of breast cancer deaths to drinking alcohol, and about 3.5 percent (or 19,500) of all cancer deaths to drinking. In 48 to 60 percent of these cancer deaths, the drinkers consumed more than three drinks per day, but in about 30 percent, they estimate, the patient drank less than 1.5 drinks per day.[32]

Other Effects Alcohol abuse is a major cause of chronic inflammation of the pancreas, the organ that produces digestive enzymes and insulin. Chronic alcohol abuse inhibits enzyme production, which further inhibits the absorption of nutrients. Drinking alcohol can block the absorption of calcium, which may contribute to a woman's risk of developing *osteoporosis*, a disease characterized by bone thinning due to calcium loss.

Women who are pregnant should avoid alcohol altogether.[33] Alcohol ingested by the mom passes through the placenta, enters the growing baby's bloodstream, and can cause **fetal alcohol syndrome (FAS)**, associated with facial abnormalities and learning disabilities.

Drinking and Driving

In 2010, approximately 31 percent of all traffic fatalities in the United States were alcohol related.[34] Over two-thirds of those killed were driving with BAC levels above 0.08, the legal limit in all states, and one out of three of them were aged 21 to 34.[35] Laboratory and test-track research shows that the vast majority of drivers are impaired even at the legal limit of 0.08 BAC, showing decreased ability in braking, steering, and lane changing.[36]

Alcohol Use Can Lead to Alcoholism

Alcohol use becomes **alcohol abuse** when it interferes with work, school, or social and family relationships—or when it entails any violation of the law, including driving under the influence (DUI).[37] **Alcoholism, or alcohol dependence**, is suspected when personal and health problems related to alcohol use are severe and when stopping alcohol use results in withdrawal symptoms. The four symptoms of alcoholism include craving—a strong urge to drink; loss of control—not being able to stop drinking once started; physical dependence—withdrawal symptoms such as nausea, sweating and shaking after stopping drinking; and the need to drink ever more alcohol to feel drunk due to tolerance—a physiological phenomenon in which the body requires larger and larger doses of a drug or an addictive behavior in order to produce an effect.

Identifying a Problem Drinker Recognizing and admitting the existence of an alcohol problem is often extremely difficult. Alcoholics deny their problem, often making statements such as, "I can stop any time I want to. I just don't want to right now." Their families also tend to deny the problem, making excuses like "He really has been under a lot of stress lately. Besides, he only drinks beer." The fear of being labeled a "problem drinker" often prevents people from seeking help. **Lab 13.1** provides a questionnaire for assessing your risk of alcohol abuse.

DO IT! ONLINE

Recovery from Alcohol Addiction

Many alcoholics and problem drinkers who seek help have experienced a turning point: flunking out of school, getting arrested for drunk driving or other legal troubles, being fired from a job, or having a spouse walk out. He or she has, in many cases, reached a low point and finally recognized that alcohol controls his or her life. The first step on the road to recovery is assuming responsibility for personal actions.

Treatment Programs The problem drinker who is ready for help has several avenues of treatment: psychologists and psychiatrists specializing in the treatment of

---

fetal alcohol syndrome (FAS) A disorder that may affect the fetus when the mother consumes alcohol during pregnancy; among its effects are mental retardation, small head, tremors, and physical abnormalities

alcohol abuse Use of alcohol that interferes with work, school, or personal relationships or that entails violations of the law

alcoholism (alcohol dependence) A condition in which personal and health problems related to alcohol use are severe and stopping alcohol use results in withdrawal symptoms

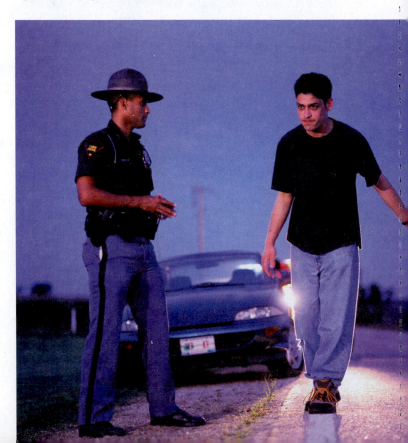

alcoholism, private treatment centers, hospitals specifically designed to treat alcoholics, community mental health facilities, and support groups such as Alcoholics Anonymous.

On some college campuses, the problems associated with alcohol abuse are so great that schools are instituting strong policies against drinking and programs to help students deal with alcohol-related problems: University presidents have formed a leadership group to help curb the problem of alcohol abuse; many fraternities and sororities are maintaining "dry" houses; and student health centers are opening their own treatment programs. For example, the University of Texas sponsors a center where students in recovery can get support services and hang out together. And at 18 schools including Rutgers University, Vanderbilt, Case Western Reserve University, and others, students in recovery can live together in "clean and sober" housing.[38] It can be difficult to recover from an alcohol abuse problem in college, and programs such as these provide the support and comfortable environment recovering students need.

The Family's Role Members of an alcoholic's family sometimes take action before the alcoholic does. They may seek help from an organization or a treatment facility for themselves and their relative. *Intervention*—a planned confrontation with the alcoholic that involves friends, family members, and professional counselors—is an effective method of helping an alcoholic recognize they have a problem.

Learning to Drink Responsibly

The social atmosphere on college campuses encourages drinking in many ways. College students seek peer approval; and drinking is part of many college traditions such as Greek rush and football games. Advertising for the alcoholic beverage industry targets college students. Students believe alcohol will make them feel less stressed, more sociable, and less self-conscious. Many turn 21 while at college and celebrate by getting drunk. In

SEE IT! ONLINE
Sloppy Spring Breaker

- -

 TOOLS FOR **CHANGE**

How to Cut Down on Your Drinking

If you have a severe drinking problem, alcoholism in your family, or other medical problems, you should stop drinking completely. If you need to cut down on your drinking, these steps can help you:

- Write down your reasons for cutting down or stopping.

- Determine a limit for how much you will drink. You may choose to cut down or to not drink at all. If you aren't sure what is healthy for you, talk with your counselor. Write down your drinking goal and post it where you'll see it.

- Keep a diary of your drinking. For three or four weeks, write down every time you have a drink. You may be surprised how much you drink and when. How different is your limit from the amount you drink now?

- Keep little or no alcohol at home. You don't need the temptation.

- Take a break from alcohol. Pick a day or two each week when you will not drink at all. Then try to stop drinking for one week. Think about how you feel physically and emotionally on these days. When you succeed and feel better, you may find it easier to cut down for good.

- Learn to say "no, thank you." You do not have to drink when other people are or take a drink when offered one. Stay away from people who give you a hard time about not drinking.

- Stay active. Use the time and money once spent on drinking to do something fun with your family or friends.

- Get support. Ask your family and friends to help you reach your goal. Talk to your counselor if you are having trouble cutting down.

- Avoid people, places, or events that tempt you to drink. Plan ahead of time what you will do to avoid drinking when you do feel tempted.

- Don't give up! Most people don't cut down or give up drinking all at once. If you don't reach your goal the first time, try again.

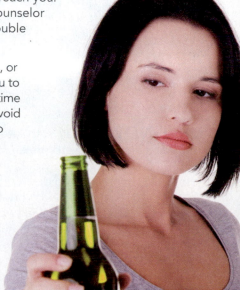

addition, campus communities often have a large number of bars and liquor stores with relatively low prices.

How can you drink responsibly in an atmosphere with so many pressures to drink? Here are some tips:

- Eat before and while you drink.
- Don't drink before a party or event.
- Avoid drinking if you are angry, anxious, depressed, or taking any medication.
- Pace yourself. Drink one alcoholic drink or less per hour.
- Alternate alcoholic and nonalcoholic drinks.
- Determine ahead of time the number of drinks you will have for the evening.
- Avoid drinking games.
- Don't drink and drive. Volunteer to be the sober driver.
- Avoid parties where you expect heavy drinking.

LIVE IT! ONLINE
Worksheet 32 A Dozen Drinking Dilemmas

casestudy

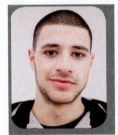

NATHAN

"At some parties, they'll card you to make sure you're over 21, but a lot of the time they don't. I'm underage, but it's easy to get a fake ID. When we go out to parties on weekends, or when we have one here at the fraternity house, I usually have three or four drinks a night. After three drinks, I definitely feel drunk, but I'm pretty moderate compared to other people I know. My friend Chris usually has at least six drinks in a night and I've seen him pass out from it."

THINK! Would you consider Nathan a heavy drinker? What about Chris? Explain. How many times per week do you drink alcohol? Are you a binge drinker?

ACT NOW! Today, calculate what your BAC would have been toward the end of the most recent party you attended. This week, prepare yourself for the next party by writing down three things you can say or do to avoid drinking more than you want to because of social pressure. In two weeks, set a limit for how much you will drink at future parties and stick to it. Remember that switching to nonalcoholic drinks after you've reached your set limit is one good way to cut back.

HEAR IT! ONLINE

If you have trouble doing any of the tips and suspect that you may have a drinking problem, try using the information in the box How to Cut Down on Your Drinking on the previous page.

What Are the Health Risks of Tobacco Use?

Every puff of tobacco smoke causes harm, according to a recent report from the U.S. Surgeon General's office.[39] There is no safe level of tobacco use. Yet, despite the health risks, an estimated 43.8 million people in the United States, or 19 percent of all adults (aged 18 years and older), smoke cigarettes. Cigarette smoking is more common among men (21.6%) than women (16.5%), and is higher among 18 to 44-year-olds (24.2%) than those 45 or older.[40] Smoking causes the typical smoker to lose about 10 years of life expectancy.[41] In addition to the dangers, tobacco use is expensive. The average cost of a pack of cigarettes in the United States is about $8.67, and a pack-a-day smoker can spend more than $3,164 per year on cigarettes. This does not include the costs of higher health care bills and higher insurance premiums for the smoker and those exposed to his or her secondhand smoke. The long-term health consequences are incalculably higher.

LIVE IT! ONLINE
Worksheet 34 Smoke and Snuff Stumpers

Smoking on Campus

Smoking among today's college students appears to be lower than it's been in decades: 13 percent in 2012 compared to 31 percent in 1999.[42] One recent study suggests that over two-thirds of college students are nonsmokers.[43] College-educated people are less likely to smoke than other people, but still more than one in six students do. Why? The largest group, 38 percent, says it helps them control stress. Other less common reasons are social pressure, experimentation, weight control, and addiction. The GetFitGraphic on page 429 explores students' smoking habits (along with alcohol and other drugs).

An important reason that students may be unaware of is advertising. With the number of smokers declining by about 1 million each year, the tobacco industry tries to recruit new smokers by aiming 90 percent of its advertising budget at children and teenagers. The tobacco industry targets young women with pictures of svelte models smoking "slim or light" brands to promote a belief that smoking can help with weight loss. The industry recruits minorities using targeted print ads and neighborhood billboards. It sponsors concerts, races, and other popular events to try to equate social fun with smoking.

Tobacco Products and Tobacco Smoke Contain Many Harmful Substances

The chemical stimulant **nicotine** is the major psychoactive substance in all tobacco products. In its natural form, nicotine is a colorless liquid that turns brown upon exposure to air. When smokers burn tobacco leaves in a cigarette, pipe, or cigar, nicotine is released and inhaled into the lungs. Chewing tobacco releases nicotine into the saliva, and the nicotine is then absorbed through the mucous membranes of the mouth.

Smoking is the most common form of tobacco use and delivers a strong dose of nicotine to the user. Tobacco smoke also contains over 4,000 other chemical compounds, including arsenic, formaldehyde, and ammonia. More than 60 of the chemicals in tobacco smoke are known or suspected to cause cancer. Particulate matter from smoke condenses in the lungs to form a thick, brownish sludge called *tar*, which contains at least 69 known cancer-causing chemicals.[44] Also among the many chemicals in tobacco smoke are various gases and vapors that may have significant effects on the heart and circulatory system. Even exposure to the secondhand smoke from just one cigarette per day accelerates the progression of atherosclerosis,[45] suggesting that even low doses of tobacco smoke exposure could negatively impact heart function.

Of the toxic gases in cigarette smoke, the most dangerous is **carbon monoxide**. The concentration of carbon monoxide is 800 times higher than the level considered safe by the U.S. Environmental Protection Agency (EPA). In the human body, carbon monoxide reduces the oxygen-carrying capacity of the red blood cells by binding with the receptor sites for oxygen, causing oxygen deprivation in body tissues.

The heat from tobacco smoke is also harmful. Inhaling hot gases exposes sensitive mucous membranes to irritating chemicals that weaken tissues and contribute to cancers of the mouth, larynx, and throat.

Main Types of Tobacco Use

Tobacco comes in several forms. Cigarettes, cigars, pipes, bidis, and hookahs are used for burning and inhaling tobacco. Smokeless tobacco is sniffed or placed in the mouth.

Cigarettes Filtered cigarettes designed to reduce levels of gases such as hydrogen cyanide and hydrocarbons may actually deliver *more* hazardous carbon monoxide to the user than nonfiltered brands. Even the use of low-tar and low-nicotine products is self-defeating: Users wind up exposing themselves to the same harmful substances they would with regular-strength cigarettes. Clove cigarettes contain about 40 percent ground cloves (a spice), about 60 percent tobacco, and higher levels of tar, nicotine, and carbon monoxide than regular cigarettes.

Cigars Cigars are no safer than cigarettes.[46] Cigar smoke contains 23 poisons and 43 carcinogens. Smoking as little as one cigar per day can double the risk of several cancers. Daily cigar smoking also increases the risk of heart and lung diseases.

Bidis These small hand-rolled flavored cigarettes are generally made in India or Southeast Asia. They are far more toxic than cigarettes and contain more nicotine. Research clearly indicates that bidi smokers are at the same, if not higher, risk for coronary heart disease and cancer as smokers of regular cigarettes.[47]

Hookahs A *hookah* is a pipe that draws smoke from burning substances through water. Rates of hookah smoking have increased substantially on college campuses.[48] These smokers often think that water filters out the dangerous elements of tobacco smoke, when in fact, hookahs deliver more nicotine, carbon monoxide, and overall smoke than do cigarettes and cause the

nicotine The primary stimulant chemical in tobacco products

carbon monoxide A gas found in cigarette smoke that binds at oxygen receptor sites in the blood

same lung and vascular diseases.

Smokeless Tobacco

Approximately 5 million U.S. adults use smokeless tobacco. *Chewing tobacco* contains tobacco leaves treated with flavorings; it is placed between the gums and teeth. Another type of smokeless tobacco is *snuff*, a fine ground form of tobacco that can be inhaled, chewed, or placed against the gums.

A major risk of chewing tobacco use is *leukoplakia*, a condition characterized by leathery white or gray patches inside the mouth. Three to 17 percent of diagnosed leukoplakia cases develop into oral cancer. It is estimated that 75 percent of the more than 30,000 cases of oral cancer diagnosed in the United States each year result from either smokeless tobacco or cigarette use.[49]

Short-Term Effects of Tobacco Use

In healthy lungs, millions of tiny hair-like projections called *cilia* line the respiratory passageways and sweep away foreign matter, which is then expelled from the lungs by coughing. Nicotine paralyzes the cilia for up to an hour following the smoking of a single cigarette. This allows tar and other solids in tobacco smoke to accumulate and irritate sensitive tissue.

Nicotine is also a powerful central nervous system stimulant that produces a variety of physiological effects. In the cerebral cortex, it produces an aroused, alert mental state. Nicotine also stimulates the adrenal glands, which increase the production of adrenaline. Nicotine stimulation increases heart and respiratory rates, constricts blood vessels, and, in turn, increases blood pressure because the heart must work harder to pump blood through the narrowed vessels.

Nicotine raises blood sugar levels and decreases the stomach contractions that signal hunger. These factors, along with decreased sensation in the taste buds, reduce appetite. Beginning smokers usually feel some or all of the effects of **nicotine poisoning**—including dizziness, light-headedness, rapid and erratic pulse, clammy skin, nausea, vomiting, and diarrhea—with their first puff. The effects cease as tolerance to the chemical develops. Tolerance develops almost immediately in new users, perhaps after the second or third cigarette. Tolerance to most other drugs, such as alcohol, develops over a period of months or years. Regular smokers often do not feel the "buzz" of smoking. They continue to smoke because stopping is too difficult.

Figure 13.6 summarizes both the short-and long-term health effects of smoking.

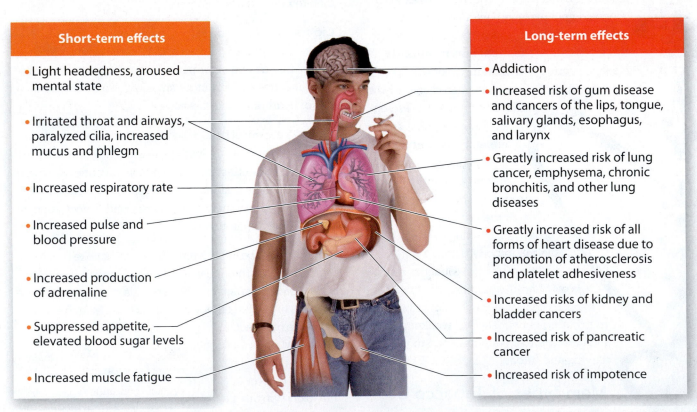

Short-term effects	Long-term effects
• Light headedness, aroused mental state	• Addiction
• Irritated throat and airways, paralyzed cilia, increased mucus and phlegm	• Increased risk of gum disease and cancers of the lips, tongue, salivary glands, esophagus, and larynx
• Increased respiratory rate	• Greatly increased risk of lung cancer, emphysema, chronic bronchitis, and other lung diseases
• Increased pulse and blood pressure	• Greatly increased risk of all forms of heart disease due to promotion of atherosclerosis and platelet adhesiveness
• Increased production of adrenaline	• Increased risks of kidney and bladder cancers
• Suppressed appetite, elevated blood sugar levels	• Increased risk of pancreatic cancer
• Increased muscle fatigue	• Increased risk of impotence

FIGURE **13.6** The short-term and long-term effects of smoking on the body.

DRINKING, SMOKING AND DRUGS IN COLLEGE: NIX THE MIX

THE FACTS

BINGEING & SMOKING

Of the 44% of college students who binge drink, more than half are likely to smoke cigarettes, cannabis, hookas, and/or cigars, as well.[1]

ISN'T OCCASIONALLY SMOKING WHILE DRINKING OK?

NO!

Even occasional smoking raises a college student's likelihood of **developing depression** and of **taking extra risks while driving** or **engaging in sexual behavior**.[2]

44% of students = **17%** + **6.9%** + **9.3%** + **5.5%** + **7.3%**

| Binge Drink | Bingeing Only | Bingeing + Cigarettes | Bingeing + Cigarettes + Cannabis | Bingeing + Cigarettes + Hookahs | Bingeing + Cigarettes + Cannabis + Hookahs + Cigars |

THE FACTS

PRESCRIPTION DRUGS WITH ALCOHOL & CANNABIS

Over 3 in 10 students used someone else's prescription stimulants at some point during their four years in college.[3]

31%

IS MISUSING PRESCRIPTION DRUGS REALLY THAT BIG OF A DEAL?

YES!

Students who misused prescriptions drugs were more likely to skip classes, have lower grade point averages, and experience **problems with alcohol and cannabis use.** Students who abused alcohol and/or cannabis were **more than twice as likely to also misuse prescription "uppers."**

THE FACTS

ALCOHOL & ENERGY DRINKS

During the past month, more than half of all students consumed energy drinks and alcohol in the same drinking session.[4]

WON'T MIXING ALCOHOL AND ENERGY DRINKS CANCEL OUT THE NEGATIVE EFFECTS OF BOTH?

NO!

The likelihood of **being involved in a vehicle crash, being a victim of sexual assault, requiring medical treatment, or riding in a car with a drunk driver** doubled among students who drank alcohol and caffeine compared to students who drank alcohol but no caffeine.

Non-use of Energy Drink + Alcohol **44%**

Energy Drink + Alcohol **56%**

Long-Term Effects of Tobacco Use

With its long list of chronic health effects, cigarette smoking adversely affects the well-being of smokers, as well as the health of everyone nearby. Each day, cigarettes contribute to more than 1,000 deaths from cancer, CVD, and respiratory disorders. In the United States, tobacco use is the single most preventable cause of death. It kills more Americans than alcohol, car accidents, suicide, AIDS, homicide, and illegal drugs combined.[50]

Cancer The American Cancer Society estimates that smoking causes 87 percent of all cases of lung cancer. Fewer than 10 percent of cases occur among nonsmokers.[51] Lung cancer can take 10 to 30 years to develop, and the outlook for its victims is poor. Most lung cancer is not diagnosed until it is fairly widespread in the body; at that point, the five-year survival rate is only 15 percent. By comparison, the five-year survival rate for breast cancer is 88 percent, for colon cancer 74 percent, and for prostate cancer nearly 100 percent.[52]

Tobacco is linked to other cancers as well. The rate of pancreatic cancer is more than twice as high for smokers as nonsmokers. The five-year survival rate for pancreatic cancer is less than 5 percent. Cancers of the lips, tongue, salivary glands, and esophagus are five times more likely to occur among smokers than among nonsmokers. Smokers are also more likely to develop kidney, bladder, and larynx cancers.[53]

Cardiovascular Disease Half of all tobacco-related deaths occur from some form of heart disease.[54] Smokers have a 70 percent higher death rate from heart disease than do nonsmokers and are twice as likely to suffer strokes. In fact, smoking cigarettes poses as great a risk for developing heart disease as do high blood pressure and high cholesterol levels.

Smoking also appears to add the equivalent of 10 years of aging to the arteries.[55] It encourages the buildup of fatty deposits in the heart and major blood vessels (atherosclerosis) and it contributes to *platelet adhesiveness*, the sticking together of red blood cells that is associated with blood clots. Smoking decreases the oxygen supplied to the heart and can weaken tissues. It also contributes to irregular heart rhythms, which can trigger a heart attack. Both carbon monoxide and nicotine in cigarette smoke can precipitate angina attacks (pain spasms in the chest when the heart muscle does not get the blood supply it needs).

Respiratory Diseases Smokers may develop *chronic bronchitis* because their inflamed lungs produce more mucus and constantly try to rid themselves of this mucus and foreign particles. The effort to do so results in "smoker's hack," the persistent cough that most smokers experience. Smokers are also more prone to respiratory ailments such as influenza, pneumonia, and colds.

Emphysema is a chronic disease in which breathing becomes difficult because the alveoli (the tiny air sacs in the lungs) are destroyed, impairing the lungs' ability to obtain oxygen and remove carbon dioxide. There is no known cure for emphysema, and once the damage is done, it is irreversible. Smoking is the major cause of emphysema and smokers are 12 to 15 times more likely to die of emphysema than are nonsmokers. Exposure to secondhand smoke and other environmental exposures also increase risks for this irreversible disease.[56]

Other Effects Other long-term health effects of smoking and tobacco use include chronic cough, sexual dysfunction, increased bone loss, premature aging of the skin, and an increased risk of developing Alzheimer's disease, inflammatory diseases, and gum disease.

Secondhand Smoke

Although only about 20 percent of Americans today smoke, smoking in public places continues to cause an air pollution problem.[57] **Environmental tobacco smoke (ETS)** (commonly called **secondhand smoke**) is divided into two categories: **mainstream smoke** and **sidestream smoke**. Mainstream smoke is emitted from a smoker's mouth. Sidestream smoke is emitted from the burning end of a cigarette. People who breathe smoke from someone else's smoking product are said to be *involuntary* or *passive* smokers.

LIVE IT! ONLINE
Worksheet 31
Passive Smoking

Although involuntary smokers breathe less tobacco than active smokers do, they still face risks from the exposure. About 85 percent of secondhand smoke is sidestream smoke, which contains five times more carbon monoxide and 50 times more ammonia than mainstream smoke (which has already been partially filtered by the lungs of the smoker who exhaled it).[58] A recent study confirms that lung cell damage and lung cancer can result from a nonsmoker's exposure to a cancer-causing agent in the gaseous part of sidestream smoke.[59] The U.S. Surgeon General and the Centers for Disease Control and Prevention estimate that about 100 million Americans breathe in secondhand smoke each year and

---

emphysema A chronic lung disease in which the tiny air sacs in the lungs are destroyed, making breathing difficult

environmental tobacco smoke (ETS) or secondhand smoke Smoke from tobacco products

mainstream smoke Smoke emitted from a smoker's mouth

sidestream smoke Smoke emitted from the burning end of a cigarette

about 50,000 die from it: 3,400 from lung cancer, 46,000 from cardiovascular disease, and 900 newborns from sudden infant death syndrome.[60]

Children, especially those under five, are vulnerable to secondhand smoke and show a greater chance of developing pneumonia, bronchitis, and other infections of the lower respiratory tract as a result of exposure. Additionally, children exposed to secondhand smoke are twice as likely to become smokers during adolescence than children who are not exposed to it.[61] Because of these increased risks, many states have enacted or are considering legislation that prohibits smoking in vehicles when children are present.

Quitting Smoking

About 70 percent of adult smokers want to quit and up to 44 percent make a serious attempt to quit each year, but only 4 to 7 percent succeed.[62] College students who begin smoking regularly want to stop, but only 13 percent are able to.[63]

Smokers must break both the physical addiction to nicotine and the habit of lighting up at certain times of day. A recent study reports that smoking causes the brain to release dopamine, a neurochemical involved in reward and pleasure, and nicotine withdrawal during smoking cessation creates an abnormally large dopamine deficit that magnifies a person's craving for

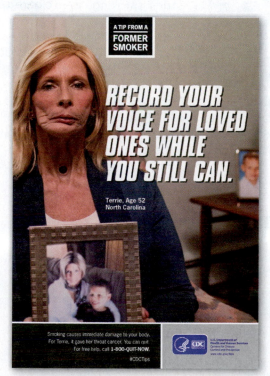

FIGURE 13.7 This ad is part of a campaign designed by the CDC which uses stories of former smokers to motivate people to think about the health risks of smoking and encourage them to quit. The ads appear on TV, on radio, online, and in print.

Source: Centers for Disease Control and Prevention, "Tips from Former Smokers," May 2013, www.cdc.gov

cigarettes.[64] New federally funded ads aim to discourage smoking and encourage quitting (**Figure 13.7**). Local, state, and federal smoke-free laws have the same intent, and studies show that they quickly result in fewer heart attacks and hospitalizations for heart and lung diseases; less smoking at home as well as in public; and significant health care savings to individuals and states.[65]

Breaking Nicotine Addiction Withdrawing from nicotine can cause irritability, restlessness, nausea, vomiting, and intense cravings for tobacco. Several nontobacco products that replace depleted levels of nicotine in the bloodstream, such as nicotine gum, the nicotine patch, prescription nasal sprays, and the nicotine inhaler have helped some people wean themselves off tobacco.

SEE IT! ONLINE
Do Nicotine Patches and Gum Work?

Nonnicotine strategies for breaking addiction include the prescription drugs Zyban and Chantix. Zyban is thought to work on dopamine and norepinephrine receptors in the brain to decrease craving and withdrawal symptoms. Chantix may help smokers quit by providing nicotine-like effects to ease withdrawal symptoms and blocking the effects of nicotine if the patient resumes smoking.[66] A relatively new approach is an antinicotine vaccine now in early testing. The drug stimulates the immune system to generate antibodies that prevent nicotine from entering or acting upon the brain.[67]

How effective are these therapies? A recent study reports that one-third of recent quitters relapse whether using nicotine replacement therapies or going "cold turkey," but that some people do seem to benefit.[68] Those who cannot quit with drug therapies alone may benefit from antismoking behavioral therapy. Some organizations are using text messages, phone apps, and web-based social media to help quitters.[69] Good nutrition can also help; quitters who eat the most fruits and vegetables have a success rate three times higher than those eating the fewest fruits and vegetables.[70] Finally, self-control strategies such as those described in **Lab 13.2** help people resist the temptation to smoke by identifying the specific situations in which they reach for a cigarette.

DO IT! ONLINE

Benefits of Quitting Many tissues damaged by smoking can repair themselves. As soon as smokers stop, the body begins the repair process (see **Figure 13.8** on the following page).[71] Within eight hours "smoker's breath" disappears. Often, the mucus that clogs airways is broken up and eliminated within a month of quitting; 18 to 24-year-olds can see substantially less coughing within two weeks.[72] Many ex-smokers say they have more energy, sleep better, and feel more alert.

Smoking cessation timeline

START HERE

8 hours
- Carbon monoxide level in blood drops to normal.
- Oxygen level in blood increases to normal.

1 to 9 months
- Coughing, sinus congestion, fatigue, shortness of breath decreases.
- Cilia regrow in lungs, which increases ability to handle mucus, clean the lungs, reduce infection.
- Body's overall energy increases.

5 years
- Lung cancer death rate for average former smoker (one pack a day) decreases by almost half.

15 years
- Risk of coronary heart disease is that of a nonsmoker.

20 minutes
- Blood pressure drops to normal.
- Pulse rate drops to normal.
- Body temperature of hands and feet increases to normal.

24 hours
- Chance of heart attack decreases.

2 weeks to 3 months
- Circulation improves.
- Walking becomes easier.
- Lung function increases up to 30%.

1 year
- Excess risk of coronary disease is half that of a smoker.

10 years
- Lung cancer death rate similar to that of nonsmokers.
- Precancerous cells are replaced.
- Risk of cancer of the mouth, throat, esophagus, bladder, kidney, and pancreas decreases.

FIGURE **13.8** The benefits of quitting smoking begin 20 minutes after smoking cessation and continue for years.

What Are the Health Risks of Drug Use and Abuse?

Drug misuse and abuse are huge problems in our society. **Drug misuse** involves using a drug for a purpose for which it was not intended, while **drug abuse** is defined as excessive use of any drug. Each year, such abuse and misuse of drugs contributes to tens of thousands of deaths and costs taxpayers hundreds of billions of dollars in preventable health care costs, extra law enforcement, auto crashes, crime, and lost productivity.[73] Drug use is still on the rise: In the most recent National Survey on Drug Use and Health, 10.1 percent of Americans aged 12 to 17 reported having used illicit drugs during the past month, compared to 9.3 percent reporting past-month use in 2008.[74] For Americans aged 18 to 25, reported use of illicit drugs during the past month rose from 19.7 percent to 21.4 percent in 2011.[75]

Drug Use among College Students

Marijuana is the most commonly used illegal drug on college campuses, and the use of various types of drugs has been on the rise, including club drugs such as Ecstasy, prescription painkillers such as Vicodin and OxyContin,[76] stimulants, tranquilizers, sleeping pills, and Adderall (a stimulant drug for ADHD).[77] Students misuse Vicodin, OxyContin, and Adderall under the mistaken impression that they are a safe way to

drug misuse Use of a drug for a purpose for which it was not intended

drug abuse Excessive use of a drug

casestudy

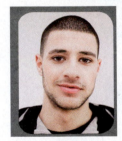

NATHAN

"I went through a phase where I tried smoking clove cigarettes. My friends told me they weren't as bad as regular cigarettes, and I liked the way they tasted. I stopped, though, because the next morning I always woke up coughing and hacking up phlegm and my clothes were starting to smell. My roommate Kevin is still a smoker. He's not allowed to smoke inside the fraternity house, but he does it anyway. He tries to do it when I'm not there, but sometimes when I walk in, I can still see smoke hanging in the air. So my clothes *still* smell!"

THINK! Is Nathan correct that clove cigarettes "aren't as bad" as regular cigarettes? Explain your answer. What hazard is Nathan's roommate exposing him to? What are the dangers involved?

ACT NOW! Today, if you smoke, list three strategies you could employ to limit or eventually stop your tobacco use. This week, notice how often you are around others who smoke, and write down two things you can do to limit your exposure to secondhand smoke. In two weeks, start brainstorming alternative activities or housing situations that eliminate secondhand smoke exposure, then begin to make the necessary changes.

HEAR IT! ONLINE

TABLE **13.1** Annual Prevalence of Use for Various Types of Drugs among Full-Time College Students in One Large National Study	
Drug	% of College Students Reporting Use
Alcohol	79.2
Cigarettes	23.4
Any illicit drug	37.3
Any illicit drug other than marijuana	17.1
Marijuana	34.9
Inhalants	1.5
Hallucinogens	4.5
Cocaine	3.1
Heroin	0.1
Narcotics other than heroin	5.4
Amphetamines, adjusted	11.1
Sedatives (Barbiturates)	2.2
Tranquilizers	3.4
Steroids	0.3

Source: Data from L. D. Johnston et al., *Monitoring the Future, National Survey Results on Drug Use, 1975–2012: Volume 2, College Students and Adults Ages 19–50* (Ann Arbor: Institute for Social Research, The University of Michigan, 2013).

alleviate anxiety or depression, to stay awake for studying, or to increase their stamina for sports.[78] However, abuse of Vicodin and OxyContin increases rates of both depression and suicidal thoughts and Adderall abuse can cause addiction.[79] **Table 13.1** shows annual drug use among full-time college students.

Commonly Used Drugs

In this section, we discuss the health risks of various drugs, including marijuana, so-called club drugs, stimulants, depressants, hallucinogens, inhalants, and steroids.

LIVE IT! ONLINE
Worksheet 35 Test Your Drug I.Q.

Marijuana **Marijuana** is the most popular illicit drug used by college students and the third most popular drug (after alcohol and tobacco) used by students overall. Users usually smoke marijuana in a cigarette, called a *joint*, or in a pipe or bong. The psychoactive substance *tetrahydrocannabinol* (THC)

causes the "high" that marijuana users experience. THC's most noticeable effect is the dilation of the eyes' blood vessels, which produces characteristic bloodshot eyes. Users can also experience coughing, dry mouth and throat, increased thirst and appetite, lowered blood pressure, mild muscular weakness, severe anxiety, panic, paranoia, psychosis, sensory alterations, and slowed reaction time that lead to an impaired ability to drive.[80]

Studies of long-term marijuana users indicate that marijuana causes lung irritation, coughing, and wheezing, but less long-term damage than tobacco smoking.[81] Other risks associated with long-term marijuana use may include diminished oxygen-carrying capacity of the blood, suppression of the immune system, blood pressure changes, and impaired memory function.[82] Pregnant women who smoke marijuana are at higher risk for stillbirth or miscarriage and for delivering low-birth-weight babies with abnormalities of the nervous system. Males who use marijuana are twice as likely to develop certain forms of testicular cancer.[83] Marijuana use appears to increase the addictive qualities of nicotine in those who also smoke tobacco.[84]

Designer or "Club" Drugs **Designer (club) drugs** are produced in chemical laboratories, often in homes, and are sold illegally. They include Ecstasy, GHB, Special K, and Rohypnol. Research has shown that club drugs can produce a range of unwanted side effects, including hallucinations, paranoia, amnesia, and in some cases death. Some club drugs work on the same brain mechanisms as alcohol and using them together can dangerously boost the effects of both substances.

Ecstasy Ecstasy (methylene dioxymethylamphetamine [MDMA]) has had a resurgence of popularity on college campuses. Young people may initially use Ecstasy to improve mood or get energized; it also increases heart rate and blood pressure and may raise body temperature to the point of kidney or cardiovascular failure. Chronic use of this hallucinogen appears to damage the brain's ability to think and to regulate emotion, memory, sleep, and pain. Combined with alcohol, Ecstasy can be extremely dangerous and sometimes fatal.[85]

marijuana Chopped leaves and flowers of a *Cannabis* plant; a psychoactive stimulant

designer (club) drugs Synthetic versions of existing illicit drugs; includes Ecstasy, Rohypnol, GHB, and Special K

Rohypnol and GHB The tranquilizers Rohypnol (the brand name of the prescription drug flunitrazepam) and gamma-hydroxybutyrate (GHB) are a growing problem on college campuses. Sometimes called the "date rape" drug, Rohypnol has been slipped into the drinks of victims in hopes of lowering their inhibitions and facilitating sexual conquest.[86] Like Rohypnol, GHB may be slipped into drinks undetected, resulting in memory loss, unconsciousness, amnesia, and even death for the victim. Other side effects include nausea, vomiting, seizures, hallucinations, coma, and respiratory distress.

Ketamine Ketamine, or "Special K," is used legitimately as an anesthetic in many hospital and veterinary clinics. On the street, liquid Special K is cooked and dried by dealers and ground into powder. Special K is classed as a hallucinogen. The drug inhibits the relay of sensory input, and the brain fills the resulting void with visions, dreams, memories, and intense sensory distortions that can mimic schizophrenia.

Stimulants **Stimulants** generally improve mood and decrease fatigue. Illegal stimulants include cocaine and methamphetamine. Legal stimulants include prescribed Ritalin and Adderall and caffeine.

Cocaine Cocaine is a powerful and addictive stimulant. Snorted cocaine enters the bloodstream through the mucus membranes and binds to receptor sites in the central nervous system, where it produces intense pleasure. This feeling quickly disappears, however, and the desire to regain the initial high makes the user crave more cocaine.

Cocaine is both an anesthetic and a central nervous system stimulant. In tiny doses, it can slow the heart rate. In larger doses, it increases heart rate and blood pressure, decreases appetite, and causes convulsions, muscle twitching, irregular heartbeat, and eventual death. Other effects include temporary relief of depression, decreased fatigue, talkativeness, increased alertness, and heightened self-confidence. As the dose increases, users become irritable and apprehensive, and their behavior may turn paranoid or violent. Regular cocaine use stiffens arteries, increases blood pressure, thickens the heart muscle, and accelerates symptoms of brain aging.[87]

Amphetamines Amphetamines include a large and varied group of synthetic agents that stimulate the central nervous system. Small doses of physician-prescribed amphetamines can improve alertness, lessen fatigue, and elevate mood. With repeated use, however, physical and psychological dependency develops. Amphetamine users may experience insomnia; increases in heart rate, breathing rate, and blood pressure; restlessness; anxiety; appetite suppression; and vision problems.

One type of illegal amphetamine called *methamphetamine* (also known as meth or crystal meth) is an increasingly serious problem. Its use began primarily in the western United States. The problem has spread to all states now, but continues to be highest in California, Nevada, Wyoming, and Montana.[88] Methamphetamine is a potent, long-acting, addictive drug that strongly activates the brain's reward center by producing a sense of euphoria. It can cause brain damage that results in impaired motor skills and cognitive functions, as well as psychosis and increased risk for heart attack and stroke. Researchers are working on a vaccine to prevent meth addiction.[89]

The prescription amphetamines Ritalin and Adderall are used to treat children with attention deficit/hyperactive disorder. Students increasingly misuse these drugs to stay awake for all-night cramming sessions. Many have the false perception that these drugs improve academic performance and carry no risk of addiction.[90]

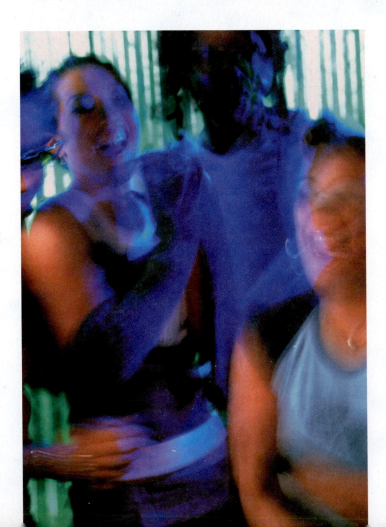

Caffeine While legal, the stimulant caffeine can be abused if consumed to excess. One caffeine pill, such as No-Doz, has about as much caffeine as a cup of caffeinated coffee. An overdose of caffeine can produce confusion, convulsions, breathing problems, sweating, and irregular heartbeat.[91] The caffeine in energy drinks can mask your level of intoxication if you combine them with alcohol, and they double ones risk of alcohol-related driving problems, sexual assaults, and medical emergencies.[92]

LIVE IT! ONLINE
**Worksheet 33
Caffeine
Countdown**

Depressants Depressants include opiates, sedatives and tranquilizers. Among the oldest pain relievers known to humans, **opiates** are derived from the parent drug *opium*, made from the opium poppy seed pod. Illegal opiate drugs (also referred to as *narcotics*) include opium, heroin, black tar heroin, morphine and codeine, and the synthetic opiates Vicodin, Oxycontin, and Percocet that may be prescribed legally as painkillers, but are also frequently abused. All opiates are highly addictive.

SEE IT! ONLINE
**Government
Crackdown on
Painkillers**

Opiates are powerful depressants of the central nervous system. In addition to relieving pain, these drugs lower heart rate, respiration, and blood pressure. Side effects include weakness, dizziness, nausea, vomiting, euphoria, decreased sex drive, visual disturbances, and lack of coordination. Of all opiates, *heroin* has the greatest notoriety as being addictive.

Tranquilizers and sedatives, such as Valium, Ativan, Xanax, and barbiturates, are also nervous system depressants. These drugs may be prescribed legally to reduce anxiety or promote sleep, and they may also be abused. As with the opiates, the depressant effects of tranquilizers and sedatives are increased when taken in conjunction with other depressants, including alcohol. Combining these drugs with alcohol can lead to respiratory failure and death.

Hallucinogens (Psychedelics) **Hallucinogenic** or **psychedelic** drugs include *lysergic acid diethylamide (LSD), mescaline* (derived from the peyote cactus),

psilocybin (one of the active chemicals in mushrooms consumed for their hallucinogenic side effects), and *phencyclidine (PCP)*. The primary pharmacological effect of these drugs is to alter feelings, perceptions, and thoughts. All of them are illegal and carry severe penalties for manufacture, possession, transportation, or sale.

Ketamine and Ecstasy (both discussed above) are technically classed as hallucinogens, as is the most commonly abused over-the-counter drug, *dextromethorphan* (DXM), an ingredient in cough and cold medicines.[93] Often referred to as "robo-tripping," "skittling," or "dexing," the misuse of DXM can cause effects similar to PCP and ketamine, including impaired motor functioning, numbness, nausea and increased heart rate and blood pressure. It can also lead to brain damage and death.[94]

Inhalants **Inhalants** are legal products such as rubber cement and model glue that can be purchased in many stores but are dangerous when misused for mind-altering effects. They contain vapor-producing chemicals that, when sniffed, can cause dizziness, lack of coordination, hallucinations, and euphoria. Their effects usually last for fewer than 15 minutes and users often overlap several "hits." This can create an overdose of fumes that can, in turn, cause unconsciousness. If the user's oxygen intake is reduced during the inhaling process, death can result within five minutes.[95]

Anabolic Steroids **Anabolic steroids** are artificial forms of the male hormone testosterone that promote muscle growth and strength but also cause depression, hostility, and aggression and acne, stunted height, and increased risk of heart disease and cancer.[96] (See Chapter 4 for more details on the health consequences of anabolic steroid use.)

opiates A class of drugs derived from the parent drug opium, characterized by the ability to relieve pain, induce drowsiness, and cause euphoria

hallucinogenic (psychedelic) Refers to substances capable of creating auditory or visual distortions and heightened states

inhalants Products that are sniffed or inhaled in order to produce a high

anabolic steroids Artificial forms of the hormone testosterone that promote muscle growth and strength

relapse Resumption of behavior that one is attempting to cease

Overcoming Drug Abuse

All drug users start out making voluntary, controllable decisions to try drugs just a few times for the experience. However, they often don't realize how quickly a habit can form—until their drug use has already gotten out of control. Once people become addicted, the chance of quitting on their own is very low. Nearly all addicted persons need specialized medical and psychological treatment to recover. However, of the 21.6 million Americans who needed treatment for addiction to alcohol or illicit drugs in 2011, only 2.4 million received it.[97]

Drug programs are designed to help people safely withdraw from chemical dependency, to improve their day-to-day functioning, to avoid future **relapse**, to understand why they became addicted, to return to abstinence after relapses, and ultimately to achieve long-term abstinence and successful functioning in society. Drug treatment usually includes medications (such as the methadone used to block addiction to heroin or morphine) and behavioral therapy involving individuals, groups, or

LIVE IT! ONLINE
Worksheet 36
What Is
Substance Abuse
Worksheet 37
Substance
Use Log

casestudy

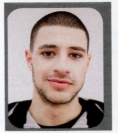

NATHAN

"One thing that's really hard about college is the pressure to drink and do drugs. Most of the parties center around them, and it seems like half the people I know—and most of my fraternity brothers—are into this stuff. Sometimes I feel like a geek because I don't want to get drunk every weekend or do drugs. What's really helped me has been joining an intramural soccer team and volunteering to help with the campus film festival. I like these activities, I've made some great friends, and the focus is on having fun and relaxing through activities instead of substances."

THINK! Do most students on your campus seem to use substances to have fun?

ACT! Name several activities on your campus you could do to have fun or relax that don't involve using drugs or alcohol.

HEAR IT! ONLINE

▶▶ TOOLS FOR CHANGE

If Someone Offers You Drugs

It is likely that you will be invited to use drugs at some point in your life. Here are some questions to consider before you find yourself presented with the opportunity to use illegal drugs or feel pressure to do so:

- Why am I considering trying drugs?
- Am I using this drug to cope? Am I depressed?
- What could taking drugs cost me? Could this cost me my job or career?
- What are the long-term consequences of using this drug?
- What will this cost me in terms of my friendships and family? How would my close family and friends respond if they knew I was using drugs?

Even when you make the decision not to use drugs, it can be difficult to say no gracefully. Some good ways to turn down an offer:

- "Thanks, but I've got a big test (game, meeting) tomorrow morning."
- "I've already got a great buzz right now. I really don't need anything more."
- "I don't like how (insert drug name here) makes me feel."
- "I'm driving tonight."
- "I want to go for a run in the morning."
- "No thanks."

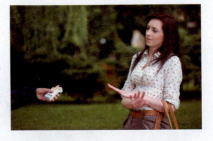

families and led by drug counselors, psychologists, or psychiatrists. Community-based 12-step programs such as Narcotics Anonymous also include a spiritual component.

Because prolonged drug use can ultimately lead to tolerance and dependence, it is vitally important to educate people about drug experimentation and use. Past antidrug strategies have featured total prohibition (as in the alcohol prohibition during the 1920s) and "scare tactics," but both approaches have proven ineffective. Researchers in the field of drug education agree that students should learn the difference between drug use and abuse, how to handle social situations where drugs are present, and how to recognize signs of drug dependence in themselves and their friends. Completing **Labs 13.1** to **13.3** can help you assess your use of alcohol, tobacco, and drugs and determine your potential risk of abuse. Reading the box If Someone Offers You Drugs on the previous page can prepare you in advance to handle social pressure.

DO IT! ONLINE

CHAPTER IN REVIEW

MasteringHealth™

Build your knowledge—and wellness!—in the Study Area of MasteringHealth with a variety of study tools.

SEE IT! ONLINE

videos

Woman's Shopping Addiction Revealed

Sloppy Spring Breaker

Do Nicotine Patches and Gum Work?

Government Crackdown on Painkillers

HEAR IT! ONLINE

audio tools

Audio case study

MP3 chapter review

REVIEW IT! ONLINE

chapter review

Chapter reading quizzes

Glossary flashcards

LIVE IT! ONLINE

programs & behavior change

Take Charge of Your Health! Worksheets:

Worksheet 30 Are You Addicted?

Worksheet 31 Passive Smoking

Worksheet 32 A Dozen Drinking Dilemmas

Worksheet 33 Caffeine Countdown

Worksheet 34 Smoke and Snuff Stumpers

Worksheet 35 Test Your Drug I.Q.

Worksheet 36 What Is Substance Abuse?

Worksheet 37 Substance Use Log

Behavior Change Log Book and Wellness Journal

DO IT! ONLINE

labs

Lab 13.1 Assess Your Alcohol Use and Risk of Abuse

Lab 13.2 Identify Smoking Behaviors and Create a Plan to Quit

Lab 13.3 Learn to Recognize Drug Use and Potential Abuse

review questions

1. Which of the following characterizes addiction?
   a. Compulsion
   b. Ability to control the addictive behavior
   c. Positive consequences
   d. Acceptance and admittance of a problem

2. Consuming five or more drinks in a row (for a male) or four or more drinks in a row (for a female) is called
   a. gorging.
   b. preloading.
   c. periodic drinking.
   d. binge drinking.

3. Blood alcohol concentration (BAC) is
   a. the "proof" value of an alcoholic beverage.
   b. the percentage of alcohol in a beverage.
   c. the level of alcohol in the blood before becoming drunk.
   d. the ratio of alcohol to total blood volume.

4. That last stage of liver disease, which involves the formation of scar tissue, is called
   a. alcoholic hepatitis.
   b. leukoplakia.
   c. fatty liver.
   d. cirrhosis.

5. Smoke emitted from a smoker's mouth is called
   a. mainstream smoke.
   b. sidestream smoke.
   c. active smoke.
   d. chronic smoke.

6. About 85 percent of secondhand smoke is
   a. mainstream smoke.
   b. sidestream smoke.
   c. harmless.
   d. partially filtered by smokers' lungs.

7. The main reason college students cite for smoking is to
   a. stay awake.
   b. control stress.
   c. look cool.
   d. improve academic performance.

8. What is the major psychoactive ingredient in tobacco products?
   a. Carbon monoxide
   b. Tar
   c. Formaldehyde
   d. Nicotine

9. Ecstasy, GHB, and Rohypnol are examples of
   a. inhalants.
   b. "club" drugs.
   c. marijuana.
   d. prescription drugs.

10. Heroin is a type of
   a. stimulant.
   b. opiate.
   c. "club" drug.
   d. steroid.

critical thinkingquestions

1. Why is quitting an addictive behavior so difficult?
2. How would you design alcohol and smoking prevention strategies targeted at college students?
3. Discuss how addiction affects family and friends. What role do they play in helping the addict get help and maintain recovery, whether from alcohol or other drugs?

references

1. R. Goldberg, *Drugs Across the Spectrum*, 7th ed. (Belmont, CA: Thomson/Brooks-Cole, 2014).
2. C. Nakken, *The Addictive Personality: Understanding the Addictive Process and Compulsive Behavior*, 2nd ed. (Center City, MN: Hazelden, 2000); American Society of Addiction Medicine, "Definition of Addiction," Adopted by the ASAM Board of Directors, April 19, 2011, www.asam.org; R. Goldberg, *Drugs Across the Spectrum*, 2014.
3. J. S. Schiller, J. L. Lucas, and J. A. Peregoy, "Summary Health Statistics for U.S. Adults: National Health Interview Survey, 2011," *National Center for Health Statistics, Vital Health Stat* 10, no. 256 (2012).
4. M. J. Friedrich, "Global Alcohol Use," *Journal of the American Medical Association* 309, no. 15 (2013): 1578, doi: 10.1001/jama.2013.3352.
5. American College Health Association, *American College Health Association—National College Health Assessment II: Reference Group Executive Summary Fall 2012* (Hanover, MD: American College Health Association, 2013).

6. Substance Abuse and Mental Health Services Administration (SAMHSA), *Results from the 2010 National Survey on Drug Use and Health: Volume I, Summary of National Findings*, NSDUH Series H-38A, HHS Publication No. SMA 10-4856 (Rockville, MD: Office of Applied Studies, 2011).
7. National Institute on Alcohol Abuse and Alcoholism (NIAAA), "College Drinking," Accessed May 2013, www.niaaa.nih.gov
8. A. L. Haas, S. K. Smith, and K. Kagan, "Getting 'Game': Pregaming Changes During the First Weeks of College," *Journal of American College Health* 61, no. 2 (2013): 95–105, doi: 10.1080/07448481.2012.753892.
9. Centers for Disease Control and Prevention, "Vital Signs: Binge Drinking Prevalence, Frequency, and Intensity among Adults—United States 2010," *Journal of the American Medical Association* 307, no. 9 (2012): 908–10.
10. Ibid.
11. Ibid.
12. S. D. Shukla et al., "Binge Ethanol and Liver: New Molecular Developments," *Alcoholism: Clinical & Experimental Research* 37, no. 4 (2013): 550–7, doi: 10.1111/acer.12011.

13. M. Goslawski et al., "Binge Drinking Impairs Vascular Function in Young Adults," *Journal of American Cardiology* (2013), doi:10.1016/j.jacc.2013.03.049.
14. D. F. Hermens et al., "Pathways to Alcohol-Induced Brain Impairment in Young People: A Review," *Cortex* 49, no. 1 (2013): 3–17, doi: 10.1016/j.cortex.2012.05.021; J. Hopson, "Bad Mix for the Teen Brain," *Scientific American Mind*, July/August 2013, pp. 32–5.
15. C. Marczinski and A. Stamates, "Artificial Sweeteners Versus Regular Mixers Increase Breath Alcohol Concentrations in Male and Female Social Drinkers," *Alcoholism: Clinical and Experimental Research* 37, no. 4 (2013): 696–702, doi: 10.1111/acer.12039.
16. Princeton University Health Services, "Alcohol: Effects of Alcohol on Your Body," Updated December 2013, www.princeton.edu
17. American College Health Association, *American College Health Association—National College Health Assessment II: Reference Group Executive Summary Fall 2012*, 2013.
18. R. Swift and D. Davidson, "Alcohol Hangover: Mechanisms and Mediators," *Alcohol Health and Research World* 22, no. 1, (1998): 54–60.

19. Hopson, "Bad Mix for the Teen Brain," 2013.

20. A. M. White, "Understanding Adolescent Brain Development and Its Implications for the Clinician," *Adolescent Medicine: State of the Art Review* 20, no. 10 (2009): 73–90, viii–ix.

21. J. Ding et al., "Alcohol Intake and Cerebral Abnormalities on Magnetic Resonance Imaging in a Community-Based Population of Middle-Aged Adults," *Stroke* 35, no. 1 (2004): 16–21.

22. M. L. Anderson et al., "Moderate Drinking? Alcohol Consumption Signifcantly Decreases Neurogensis in the Adult Hippocampus," *Neuroscience* 224, (2012): 202–9, doi: 10.1016/j.neuroscience.2012.08.018.

23. D. F. Hermens et al., "Pathways to Alcohol-Induced Brain Impairment in Young People: A Review," 2013; Hopson, "Bad Mix for the Teen Brain," 2013.

24. M. E. Morean et al., "Age of First Use and Delay to First Intoxication in Relation to Trajectories of Heavy Drinking and Alcohol-Related Problems During Emerging Adulthood," *Alcoholism: Clinical and Experimental Research* 36, no. 11 (2012), doi: 10.1111/j.1530-0277.2012.01812.x.

25. Ibid.

26. A. Holmes et al., "Chronic Alcohol Remodels Prefrontal Neurons and Disrupts NM-DAR-Mediated Fear Extinction Encoding," *Nature Neuroscience* 15 (2012): 1359–61, doi:10.1038/nn.3204; I. O. Ebrahim et al., "Alcohol and Sleep I: Effects on Normal Sleep," *Alcoholism: Clinical and Experimental Research* 37, no. 4 (2013): 539–49, doi: 10.1111/acer.12006.

27. M. Nichols et al., "What Is the Optimal Level of Population Alcohol Consumption for Chronic Disease Prevention in England? Modeling the Impact of Changes in Average Consumption Levels," *British Medical Journal Open* 2, no. 3 (2012): e000957, doi: 10.1136/bmjopen-2012-00957.

28. L. Chen et al., "Alcohol Intake and Blood Pressure: A Systematic Review Implementing a Mendelian Randomization Approach," *PLoS Medicine* 5, no. 3 (2008): e52.

29. American Medical Association, "Cirrhosis," *Journal of the American Medical Association* 307, no. 8 (2012): 874, doi: 10.1001/jama.2012.82.

30. National Center for Health Statistics, "FastStats: Leading Causes of Death," Updated January 2013, www.cdc.gov

31. R. Voelker, "Even Low, Regular Alcohol Use Increases the Risk of Dying of Cancer," *Journal of the American Medical Association* 309, no. 10 (2013): 970.

32. Ibid.

33. National Organization on Fetal Alcohol Syndrome, "FASD: What Everyone Should Know," July 31, 2012, www.nofas.org

34. National Center for Injury Prevention and Control, "Impaired Driving: Get the Facts," Updated April 2013, www.cdc.gov

35. Ibid.

36. Insurance Institute for Highway Safety, "Fatality Facts 2011: Alcohol," Accessed May 2013, www.iihs.org

37. Medline Plus, "Alcoholism and Alcohol Abuse," Updated March 2011, www.nlm.nih.gov

38. Association of Recovery Schools, "College Members," Accessed May 2013, www.recoveryschools.org

39. Office of the Surgeon General, "A Report of the Surgeon General: How Tobacco Smoke Causes Disease—The Biology and Behavioral Basis for Smoking-Attributable Disease Fact Sheet," December 2010, www.surgeongeneral.gov

40. Centers for Disease Control and Prevention (CDC), "Vital Signs: Current Cigarette Smoking among Adults Aged ≥18 Years—United States, 2005–2010," *Morbidity and Mortality Weekly Report* 60, no. 35 (2011): 1135–40; American Cancer Society, "Cigarette Smoking," Revised January 2013, www.cancer.org

41. J. Prabhat et al., "21st Century Hazards of Smoking and Benefits of Cessation in the United States," *New England Journal of Medicine* 368, (2013): 341–50, doi: 10.1056/NEJMsa1211128.

42. L. D. Johnston et al., *Monitoring the Future National Survey Results on Drug Use, 1975–2012: Volume 2, College Students and Adults Ages 19–50* (Ann Arbor: Institute for Social Research, The University of Michigan, 2013).

43. K. M. Caldeira et al., "Cigarette Smoking among College Students: Longitudinal Trajectories and Health Outcomes," *Nicotine and Tobacco Research* 14, no 7 (July 2012): 777–85.

44. Office of the Surgeon General, "A Report of the Surgeon General: How Tobacco Smoke Causes Disease," 2010.

45. Ibid.

46. American Cancer Society (ACS), "Cigars: Still Tobacco, Still Dangerous to Your Health," Revised January 2013, www.cancer.org

47. ACS, "What about More Exotic Forms of Smoking Tobacco, Such as Clove Cigarettes, Bidis, and Hookahs?" Revised January 2013, www.cancer.org

48. R. L. Fielder, K. B. Carey, and M. P. Carey, "Predictors of Initiation of Hookah Tobacco Smoking: A One-Year Prospective Study of First-Year College Women," *Psychology of Addictive Behaviors* 26, no. 4 (2012): 963–8, doi:10.1037/a0028344; L. N. Brockman, "Hookah's New Popularity among U.S. College Students: A Pilot Study of the Characteristics of Hookah Smokers and their Facebook Displays," *British Medical Journal Open* 2, no. 6 (2012), doi: 10.1136/bmjopen-2012-001709; P. Jacob et al., "Comparison of Nictotine and Carcinogen Exposure with Water Pipe and Cigarette Smoking," *Cancer Epidemiology Biomarkers & Prevention* 22, no. 5 (2013): 765–72, doi: 10.1158/1055-9965.EPI-12-1422.

49. PubMedHealth, "Leukoplakia," Reviewed July 2011, www.ncbi.nlm.nih.gov

50. ACS, "Cigarette Smoking," 2013.

51. Ibid.

52. Ibid.

53. Ibid.

54. CDC, "Smoking and Tobacco Use: Tobacco-Related Mortality," Updated March 2011, www.cdc.gov

55. American Heart Association (AHA), "Heart Disease and Stroke Statistics 2011 Update: A Report from the American Heart Association," *Circulation* 123, no. 4 (2011): e18–209.

56. CDC, "Smoking and Tobacco Use: Health Effects of Cigarette Smoking," Updated January 2012, www.cdc.gov

57. CDC, "Smoking and Tobacco Use: Secondhand Smoke (SHS) Facts," Updated December 2012, www.cdc.gov

58. Office on Smoking and Health, *The Health Consequences of Involuntary Exposure to Tobacco Smoke: A Report of the Surgeon General—Executive Summary* (Washington, DC: U.S. Department of Health and Human Services, 2006).

59. T. P. Huynh et al., "Na,K-ATPase Is a Target of Cigarette Smoke and Reduced Expression Predicts Poor Patient Outcome of Smokers with Lung Cancer," *American Journal of Physiology: Lung Cellular and Molecular Physiology* 302, no. 11 (2012): L1150–8, doi: 10.1152/ajplung.00384.2010.

60. CDC, "Smoking and Tobacco Use: Health Effects of Secondhand Smoke," 2012; W. Max et al., "Deaths from Secondhand Smoke Exposure in the United States: Economic Implications," *American Journal of Public Health* 102, no. 11 (2012): 2173–80, doi: 10.2105/AJPH.2012.300805.

61. O. Shafey et al., "Chapter 9: Secondhand Smoking," *The Tobacco Atlas*, 3rd ed. (Atlanta: American Cancer Society, 2009).

62. M. C. Fiore et al., *Treating Tobacco Use and Dependence: 2008 Update*, Clinical Practice Guideline (Rockville, MD: U.S. Department of Health and Human Services, 2008).

63. National Center on Addiction and Substance Abuse at Columbia University (CASA), *Wasting the Best and the Brightest: Substance Abuse at America's Colleges and Universities* (New York: CASA, 2007).

64. L. Zhang et al., "Withdrawal from Chronic Nicotine Exposure Alters Dopamine Signaling Dynamics in the Nucleus Accumbens," *Biological Psychiatry* 71, no. 3 (2012): 184–91, doi: 10.1016/j.biopysch.2011.07.024.

65. R. D. Hurt, "Myocardial Infarction and Sudden Cardiac Death in Olmstead County, Minnesota, Before and After Smoke-Free Workplace Laws," *Archive of Internal Medicine* 172, no. 21 (2012), doi: 10.1001/2013.jamainternmed.269; C. E. Tan and S. A. Glantz, "Association between Smoke-Free Legislation and Hospitalizations for Cardiac, Cerebrovascular, and Respiratory Diseases: A Meta-Analysis," *Circulation* 126, no. 18 (2012): 2177–83, doi: 10.1161/CirculationAHA.112.121301; U. Mons et al., "Impact of National Smoke-Free Legislation on Home Smoking Bans: Findings from the International Tobacco Control Policy Evaluation Project Europe Surveys," *Tobacco Control* (2012), doi: 10.1136/tobaccocontrol-2011-050131; J. Lightwood and S. Glantz, "The Effect of the California Tobacco Control Program on Smoking Prevalence, Cigarette Consumption, and Healthcare Costs," *PLoS One* 8, no. 2 (2013): e47145, doi: 10.1371/journal.pone.0047145.

66. Fiore et al., *Treating Tobacco Use and Dependence*, 2008.

67. M. J. Hicks et al., "AAV-Directed Persistent Expression of a Gene Encoding Anti-Nicotine Antibody for Smoking Cessation," *Science Translational Medicine* 4, no. 140 (2012): 140ra87, doi: 10.1126/scitranslmed.3003611.

68. H. R. Alpert et al., "A Prospective Cohort Study Challenging the Effectiveness of Population-Based Medical Intervention for Smoking Cessation," *Tobacco Control* (2012), doi: 10.1136/tobaccocontrol-2011-050129.

69. B. C. Bock et al., "User Preferences for a Text Message-Based Smoking Cessation Intervention," *Health Education & Behavior* 40, no 2 (2013): 152–9, doi: 10.1177/1090198112463020; American Medical Association, "Texting Teens to Quit," *Journal of the American Medical Association* 307, no. 4 (2012): 351, doi:10.1001/jama.2012.4.

70. J. P. Haibach, G. G. Homish, and G. A. Giovino, "A Longitudinal Evaluation of Fruit and Vegetable Consumption and Cigarette Smoking," *Nicotine & Tobacco Research* 15, no. 2 (2013): 355–63, doi: 10.1093/ntr/nts130.

71. American Lung Association, "Benefits of Quitting," Accessed May 2013, www.lungusa.org

72. K. S. Calabro and A. V. Prokhorov, "Respiratory Symptoms After Smoking Cessation among College Students," *Pediatric Allergy, Immunology, and Pulmonology* 24, no. 4 (2011): 215–19, doi: 10.1089/ped.2011.0097.

73. Substance Abuse and Mental Health Services Administration, *Results from the 2011 National Survey on Drug Use and Health: Summary of National Findings*, NSDUH Series H-44, HHS Publication No. (SMA) 12-4713 (Rockville, MD: Substance Abuse and Mental Health Services Administration, 2012).

74. Ibid.

75. Ibid.

76. K. J. Zullig and A. L. Divin, "The Association between Non-Medical Prescription Drug Use, Depressive Symptoms, and Suicidality among College Students," *Addictive Behaviors* 37, no. 8 (2012): 890–9, doi: 10.1016/j.addbeh.2012.02.008.

77. C. L. Hanson et al., "Tweaking and Tweeting: Exploring Twitter for Nonmedical Use of a Psychostimulant Drug (Adderall) among College Students," *Journal of Medical Internet Research* 15, no. 4 (2013): e62, doi: 10.2196/jmir2503.

78. CDC, "CDC Statement Regarding the Misuse of Prescription Drugs," *CDC Online Newsroom*, June 3, 2010, www.cdc.gov

79. K. J. Zullig and A. L. Divin, "The Association between Non-Medical Prescription Drug Use, Depressive Symptoms, and Suicidality among College Students," 2012.

80. National Institute on Drug Abuse (NIDA), "NIDA InfoFacts: Drugged Driving," Revised December 2010, www.drugabuse.gov

81. M. J. Pletcher et al., "Association between Marijuana Exposure and Pulmonary Function over 20 Years," *Journal of the American Medical Association* 307, no. 2 (2012): 173–81, doi: 10.1001/jama.2011.1961

82. NIDA, *Research Report: Marijuana Abuse*, NIH Publication no. 10-3859, Revised September 2010, www.drugabuse.gov

83. J. Charles et al., "Population-Based Case-Control Study of Recreational Drug Use and Testis Cancer Risk Confirms an Association between Marijuana Use and Nonseminoma Risk," *Cancer* 118, no. 21 (2012): 5374–83, doi: 10.1002/cncr.27554.

84. B. M. Kuehn, "Cannabis and Cigarettes," *Journal of the American Medical Association* 309, no. 16 (2013): 1674, doi:10.1001/jama.2013.3888.

85. NIDA, "NIDA InfoFacts: MDMA (Ecstasy)," Revised March 2010, www.drugabuse.gov

86. NIDA, "NIDA InfoFacts: Club Drugs (GHB, Ketamine, and Rohypnol)," Revised July 2010, www.drugabuse.gov

87. AHA, "Recreational Cocaine Use Linked to Conditions That Cause Heart Attack," November 5, 2012, http://newsroom.heart.org; K. D. Ersche et al., "Cocaine Dependence: A Fast-Track for Brain Aging?" *Molecular Psychiatry* 18, no. 2 (2013): 134–5, doi: 10.1038/mp.2012.31.

88. CDC, "Methamphetamine Use and Risk for HIV/AIDS," Modified May 2007, www.cdc.gov

89. M. L. Miller et al., "A Methamphetamine Vaccine Attenuates Methamphetamine-Induced Disruptions in Thermoregulation and Activity in Rats," *Biological Psychiatry* 73, no. 8 (2012): 721–8, doi: 10.1016/j.biophysh.2012.09.010.

90. D. L. Rabiner et al., "Motives and Perceived Consequences of Nonmedical ADHD Medication Use by College Students: Are Students Treating Themselves for Attention Problems?" *Journal of Attention Disorders* 13, no. 3 (2009): 259–70, doi: 10.1177/1087054708320399.

91. Medline Plus, "Caffeine Overdose," Updated January 2010, www.nlm.nih.gov

92. J. Howland and D. J. Rohsenow, "Risks of Energy Drinks Mixed with Alcohol," *Journal of the American Medical Association* 309, no. 9 (2013): 245–6, doi:10.1001/jama.2012.187978.

93. NIDA, "InfoFacts: Prescription and Over-the-Counter Medications," Revised July 2009, www.nida.nih.gov

94. NIDA, "Facts on Dextromethorphan (DXM)," August 2011, http://teens.drugabuse.gov

95. NIDA, "InfoFacts: Inhalants," Revised March 2010, www.drugabuse.gov

96. NIDA for Teens, "Anabolic Steroids," Accessed October 2011, http://teens.drugabuse.gov

97. Substance Abuse and Mental Health Services Administration, *Results from the 2011 National Survey on Drug Use and Health: Summary of National Findings*, 2012.

getfitgraphic references

1. B. A. Primack et al., "Tobacco, Marijuana, and Alcohol Use in University Students: A Cluster Analysis," *Journal of American College Health* 60, no. 5 (2012): 374-86, doi: 10.1080/07448481.2012.663840.

2. E. Sutfin et al., "Tobacco Use by College Students: A Comparison of Daily and Nondaily Smokers," *American Journal of Health Behavior* 36, no. 2 (2012): 218 -29, doi: 10.5993/AJHB.36.2.7; A. C. Halperin et al., "Cigarette Smoking and Associated Health Risks Among Students at Five Universities," *Nicotine Tobacco Research* 12, no. 2 (2010): 96 -104, doi: 10.1093/ntr/ntp182.

3. L. M. Garnier-Dykstra et al., "Nonmedical Use of Prescription Stimulants During College: Four-Year Trends in Exposure Opportunity, Use, Motives, and Sources," *Journal of American College Health* 60, no. 3 (2012): 226-34, doi: 10.1080/07448481.2011.589876; A. M. Arria et al., "Dispelling the Myth Of "Smart Drugs": Cannabis and Alcohol Use Problems Predict Nonmedical Use of Prescription Stimulants for Studying," *Addictive Behaviors* 38, no. 3 (2013): 1643-50, doi: 10.1016/j.addbeh.2012.10.002.

4. J. Howland and D. J. Rohsenow, "Risks of Energy Drinks Mixed with Alcohol," *Journal of the American Medical Association* 309, no. 3 (2013): 245-46, doi:10.1001/jama.2012.187978.

Name: _____   Date: _____

Instructor: _____   Section: _____

Purpose: To assess your patterns of alcohol use and your risk for alcohol abuse, and to explore the possibilities for positive behavior changes.

Directions: Complete Sections I and II below.

SECTION I: EVALUATING YOUR DRINKING PATTERNS AND ABUSE RISK

Select the answer that reflects the best choice for you and add up the points:

	0 Points	1 Point	2 Points	3 Points	4 Points
1. How often do you have a drink containing alcohol?	Never (skip to #9–10)	Monthly or less	2–4 times a month	2–3 times a week	4 or more times a week
2. How many alcoholic drinks do you have on a typical day when you are drinking?	1 or 2	3 or 4	5 or 6	7 to 9	10 or more
3. How often do you have six drinks or more on one occasion?	Never	Less than monthly	Monthly	Weekly	Daily or almost daily
4. How often during the last year have you been unable to stop drinking once you started?	Never	Less than monthly	Monthly	Weekly	Daily or almost daily
5. How often during the last year have you failed to do what was normally expected of you because of drinking?	Never	Less than monthly	Monthly	Weekly	Daily or almost daily
6. How often during the last year have you needed a drink in the morning to get yourself going after a heavy drinking session?	Never	Less than monthly	Monthly	Weekly	Daily or almost daily
7. How often during the last year have you had a feeling of guilt or remorse after drinking?	Never	Less than monthly	Monthly	Weekly	Daily or almost daily
8. How often during the last year have you been unable to remember what happened the night before because of your drinking?	Never	Less than monthly	Monthly	Weekly	Daily or almost daily
9. Have you or has someone else been injured as a result of your drinking?	No		Yes, but not in the last year		Yes, during the last year
10. Has a relative, friend, doctor, or other health worker been concerned about your drinking or suggested you cut down?	No		Yes, but not in the last year		Yes, during the last year
Total for Section I = _____					

Analyzing Your Answers

Scores below 6: Congratulations! You are in control of your drinking behaviors and do a good job of consuming alcohol responsibly and in moderation.

Scores between 6 and 8: Your alcohol consumption is possibly risky. Try taking steps to change your drinking behavior. It might be hard when you are surrounded by friends who participate in the same risky actions, but try to make some positive changes for your health and safety.

Scores above 8: Your drinking patterns are putting you at high risk for illness, unsafe sexual situations, or alcohol-related injuries and may be affecting your academic performance. Look back at how you answered each question and identify some changes you can make to reduce your risk.

Source: "The Alcohol Use Disorders Identification Test: Interview Version" from AUDIT Manual, box 4, p. 17, World Health Organization, Division of Mental Health and Prevention of Substance Abuse. Copyright © 2001 by World Health Organization. Reprinted with permission.

SECTION II: REFLECTION

If you were surprised when evaluating your alcohol consumption behaviors or were not sure how to answer some of the questions, you may want to take steps to change your behavior.

1. Which of your drinking behaviors and patterns are most worrisome to you?

_____

_____

2. Select one drinking behavior that you can change right away and describe it below. What is one drinking behavior that may take more time to change?

_____

_____

3. What are some reasons why you would like to stop or cut down on your drinking?

_____

_____

4. Write a specific short-term goal for your drinking behaviors using the SMART goal-setting guidelines. Set a target date and reward for meeting your goal.

_____

_____

5. Chart your progress in a behavior log or journal. At the end of a week, month, or school session, consider how successful you were in following your plan. What helped you be successful? What made change more difficult? What will you do differently next week?

_____

_____

6. Revise your plan as needed: Are your goals attainable? Are the target dates realistic and the rewards satisfying?

_____

_____

Name: _____   Date: _____

Instructor: _____   Section: _____

Purpose: To identify smoking behavior patterns and to develop a plan to quit smoking.

Directions: Complete Sections I to III, outlining your current and past behaviors, and a plan for smoking cessation.

SECTION I: BEHAVIOR EVALUATION—WHY DO YOU SMOKE?

Identifying why you smoke can help you develop a plan to quit.

Reason #1: Smoking Gives Me More Energy.	Often	Sometimes	Never
I smoke to keep from slowing down.	☐	☐	☐
I reach for a cigarette when I need a lift.	☐	☐	☐
When I'm tired, smoking perks me up.	☐	☐	☐
Reason #2: I Like to Touch and Handle Cigarettes.	**Often**	**Sometimes**	**Never**
I feel more comfortable with a cigarette in my hand.	☐	☐	☐
I enjoy getting a cigarette out of the pack and lighting up.	☐	☐	☐
I like to watch the smoke when I exhale.	☐	☐	☐
Reason #3: Smoking Is a Pleasure.	**Often**	**Sometimes**	**Never**
Smoking is pleasant and enjoyable.	☐	☐	☐
Smoking makes good times better.	☐	☐	☐
I want a cigarette most when I am comfortable and relaxed.	☐	☐	☐
Reason #4: Smoking Helps Me Relax When I'm Tense or Upset.	**Often**	**Sometimes**	**Never**
I light up a cigarette when something makes me angry.	☐	☐	☐
Smoking relaxes me in a stressful situation.	☐	☐	☐
When I'm depressed, I reach for a cigarette to feel better.	☐	☐	☐
Reason #5: I Crave Cigarettes; I'm Addicted to Smoking.	**Often**	**Sometimes**	**Never**
If I run out of cigarettes, it's almost unbearable until I get more.	☐	☐	☐
I am very aware of not smoking if I have no cigarette in my hand.	☐	☐	☐
If I haven't smoked in a while, I get a gnawing hunger for a cigarette.	☐	☐	☐
Reason #6: Smoking Is a Habit.	**Often**	**Sometimes**	**Never**
I smoke cigarettes automatically without even being aware of it.	☐	☐	☐
I light up without realizing I have a cigarette burning in the ashtray.	☐	☐	☐
I find a cigarette in my mouth I don't remember putting there.	☐	☐	☐

Source: Adapted from "Why Do You Smoke?" by U.S. Department of Health and Human Services (NIH Pub. No. 93–1822), 1990.

SECTION II: MOTIVATION AND PAST BEHAVIORS

1. Why do you want to quit smoking?_____

_____

2. Have you tried to quit smoking in the past? What worked and what did not?

_____

_____

SECTION III: SMOKING CESSATION PLAN AND REFLECTION

Answer the following questions to create a plan for quitting smoking.

1. Quit smoking date: _____

2. What family members and friends will you tell about your goal? How can they support you?

_____

_____

3. What health care provider, counseling program, or support groups are available to you?

_____

_____

4. What times in your daily routine do you smoke? What activities can you do instead at those times?

_____

_____

5. What medications have you considered using to help you quit smoking? Make a plan for getting and using the right medications appropriately.

_____

_____

6. What barriers, obstacles, or difficult situations might hinder your smoking cessation goal? Write out specific strategies that you will use with each barrier, obstacle, or difficult situation that may arise.

_____

_____

Name: _____ Date: _____

Instructor: _____ Section: _____

Purpose: To learn the skills necessary to recognize drug use and potential abuse or addiction.

Directions: Review the information and complete Sections I to II.

SECTION I: SELF-ASSESSMENT

How do you know whether you are chemically dependent? Take the following assessment. The more "yes" checks you make, the more likely it is that you have a problem.

Are You Abusing Drugs?	Yes	No
1. In the past month, did you have a hard time paying attention in classes, work, or at home after using drugs?	☐	☐
2. Have you ever felt you should cut down on your drug use?	☐	☐
3. Have you had blackouts or flashbacks as a result of your drug use?	☐	☐
4. Have people annoyed (irritated, angered, etc.) you by criticizing your drug use?	☐	☐
5. Have you ever been arrested or in trouble with the law because of your drug use?	☐	☐
6. Have you lost friends because of your drug use?	☐	☐
7. Have you ever felt bad or guilty about your drug use?	☐	☐
8. Have you ever thought you might have a drug problem?	☐	☐

SECTION II: REFLECTION

1. Investigate specific resources on your college campus (counselor's office, student health service, AA or NA meetings, etc.) that assist students with drug and alcohol use issues. How could you approach one or more of these resource groups for yourself or a friend? What would you say?

_____

_____

2. If you are experiencing social, legal, or academic problems due to drug use but are reluctant to seek help, what personal issues are standing in your way? (These would be good initial topics to discuss with a counselor, professor, physician, or someone you trust.)

_____

_____

14 Reducing Your Risk of Sexually Transmitted Infections

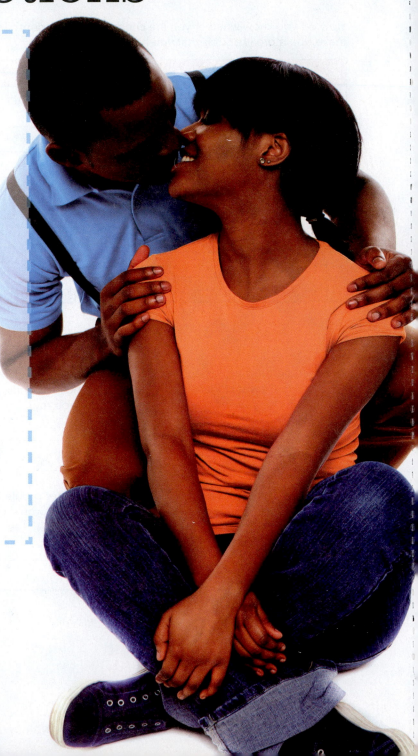

LEARNINGoutcomes

1 Discuss how sexually transmitted infections (STIs) spread.

2 Name several of the major bacteria-caused STIs, as well as their symptoms, risk factors, and typical treatments.

3 List several of the major viral-based STIs, as well as their symptoms, risk factors, and typical treatments. Describe the transmission of the human immunodeficiency virus (HIV), as well as the infection, treatment, and prevention of AIDS.

4 Itemize and discuss other major types of STIs caused by fungi, protozoans, and other agents.

5 Identify strategies to protect yourself from STIs.

MasteringHealth™

Go online for chapter quizzes, interactive assessments, videos, and more!

casestudy

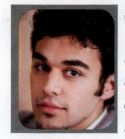

JASON

"Hi, I'm Jason. I have slept with only one person in my life—my girlfriend, Sara. We use condoms most of the time, but I'll admit that once in a while, we drink a few too many at a party and get careless. We've known each other since freshman year in high school, though, so we trust each other completely. I don't consider myself at risk for getting a sexually transmitted infection. Am I wrong not to worry?"

HEAR IT! ONLINE

FIGURE **14.1** People between ages 15 and 24 contract nearly half of all sexually transmitted infections. Protecting oneself begins with learning about risky behaviors.

E ach year, about 20 million Americans contract a **sexually transmitted infection (STI)**, an infection (usually caused by viruses or bacteria) spread through intimate contact.[1] About 10 million of these new STIs occur in young people between 15 and 24.[2] Some STIs, such as chlamydia, are relatively mild and treatable and some, such as genital herpes, are relatively mild but incurable. Others, including HIV/AIDS, are incurable and often fatal. The most recent statistics suggest that more than 110 million Americans are currently living with an STI. Of these, 65 million have an incurable STI—the majority having the herpes virus.[3]

Although Americans between ages 15 and 24 represent only 25 percent of the nation's sexually active population, they contract STIs at twice the rate of those over 25 (**Figure 14.1**).[4] Among college students, about 15 percent report an STI diagnosis within the past year—and many STIs go undiagnosed.[5] Teenagers and young adults are more likely to have three or more sexual partners, to have sex partners who have or had an STI, and to engage in **unprotected sex**, that is, sexual intercourse without a condom or other method of protection.[6]

In this chapter, we cover the major types of STIs, discuss behaviors that put you at risk, and present strategies for protecting yourself from these potentially harmful infections. You can assess your attitudes and beliefs about them in

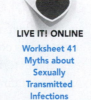

LIVE IT! ONLINE

Worksheet 41 Myths about Sexually Transmitted Infections

Lab 14.1. To check your knowledge about STIs right now, take the quiz in the box What Do You Know about STIs?

DO IT! ONLINE

Early symptoms of an STI are often mild and unrecognizable. Some STIs have no symptoms in one or both sexes. For other STIs, men and women share certain symptoms, but based on anatomy, have some unique indicators of STI (**Figure 14.2**, see page 449). It's important to get checked out if you have any of these symptoms. Left untreated, some STIs can have tragic consequences: sterility, blindness, central nervous system destruction, disfigurement, and even death.

How Do STIs Spread?

STIs are generally spread through some form of intimate sexual contact. Sexual intercourse is the most common mode of transmission, regardless of whether it's oral-to-genital contact, hand-to-genital contact, or anal intercourse. Less likely modes of transmission include mouth-to-mouth contact or contact with fluids from body sores that may be spread by the hands. Although each type of STI involves a specific disease-producing agent or *pathogen* with its own mode of infection, all STI pathogens prefer dark, warm, moist places, especially

sexually transmitted infection (STI) An infection spread through intimate contact with another person's skin or body fluids

unprotected sex Sexual intercourse (vaginal, oral, or anal) without a condom or other method of protection

Q&A What Do You Know about STIs?

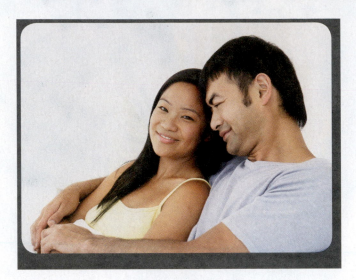

Here are several common beliefs about STIs. Consider each one and then answer: Is it Fact or Fallacy?

1. **Some STIs can be passed on by skin-to-skin contact in the genital area.** ☐ Fact ☐ Fallacy

2. **Herpes can be transmitted only when a person has visible sores on his or her genitals.** ☐ Fact ☐ Fallacy

3. **Oral sex is safe sex.** ☐ Fact ☐ Fallacy

4. **Condoms reduce your risk of both pregnancy and STIs.** ☐ Fact ☐ Fallacy

5. **As long as you don't have anal intercourse, you can't get HIV.** ☐ Fact ☐ Fallacy

6. **All sexually active females should have a regular Pap smear.** ☐ Fact ☐ Fallacy

7. **Once genital warts have been removed, there is no risk of passing on the virus.** ☐ Fact ☐ Fallacy

8. **You can get several STIs at one time.** ☐ Fact ☐ Fallacy

9. **You can get an STI more than once.** ☐ Fact ☐ Fallacy

Now read the answers and see if you were right!

1. **Fact.** Some viruses, including herpes simplex virus and HPV are present on the skin around the genital area.

2. **Fallacy.** Herpes is most easily passed on when the sores and blisters are present, but the virus is also found on the skin around the genital area.

3. **Fallacy.** Oral sex is not safe sex. Herpes, genital warts, and chlamydia can all be passed on through oral sex. Condoms should be used on the penis, and dental dams over the female genitals during oral sex.

4. **Fact.** Condoms significantly reduce the risk of pregnancy when used correctly. Only abstinence provides complete protection against pregnancy and STIs.

5. **Fallacy.** HIV is present in blood, semen, and vaginal fluid. Any activity that allows the transfer of these fluids is risky. Anal intercourse is a high-risk activity, but other sexual activity is also a risk.

6. **Fact.** All sexually active women should have regular Pap smears.

7. **Fallacy.** Genital warts can be removed, but the virus that caused the warts will always be present in the body and can be passed on to a sexual partner.

8. **Fact.** It is possible to have many STIs at one time. In fact, having one STI may make it more likely that a person will acquire more STIs. For example, the open sore from herpes creates a place for HIV to be transmitted.

9. **Fact.** A person can be reinfected many times with the same STI. This is especially true if a person does not get treated for the STI and thus reinfects his or her partner with the same STI.

Source: Adapted from Family Planning Victoria, "Play Safe," Updated 2005, www.fpv.org.au. © Family Planning Victoria; also adapted from "STD Quiz," modified March 2009, from Jefferson County Public Health, Colorado, www.jeffco.us. Used with permission.

---

the mucous membranes lining the reproductive organs. Most of these disease agents are susceptible to light and excess heat, cold, and dryness, and many die quickly on exposure to air. Important elements of prevention are learning to use latex condoms as directed and knowing the STI status of any potential sexual partner through current testing.

What Are the Major Types of Bacterial STIs?

Avoiding sexually transmitted diseases begins with knowing the common types of STIs and how to identify their characteristic symptoms. Let's start by discussing three common STIs—chlamydia, gonorrhea, and

Men only
- A drip or drainage from penis

Men and Women
- Sore bumps or blisters near sex organs or mouth
- Burning or pain when urinating
- Swelling or redness in throat
- Fever, chills, aches
- Swelling of lymph nodes near genitals or swelling of genitals
- Feeling the need to urinate frequently

Women only
- Vaginal discharge or odor from the vagina
- Pain in the lower pelvis or deep in the vagina during sex
- Burning or itching around the vagina
- Bleeding from the vagina at times other than the regular menstrual periods

FIGURE 14.2 Men and women share certain STI symptoms but have separate ones, as well. Many are mild and easy to overlook.

syphilis—that are caused by simple, single-celled, microscopic bacteria.

Chlamydia

Chlamydia is the most common bacterial STI in the United States (**Figure 14.3**) and reported cases are on the rise, due, in part, to more vigorous screening

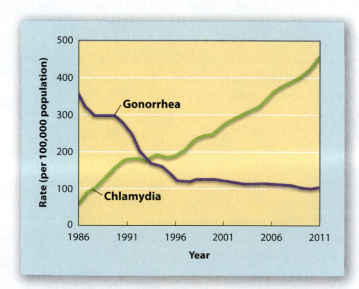

FIGURE 14.3 Chlamydia and gonorrhea are the most common bacterial STIs. Chlamydia rates have been rising for more than 20 years, while gonorrhea rates declined and then stabilized.

Source: Data from the Centers for Disease Control and Prevention, *2011 Sexually Transmitted Disease Surveillance Report* (Atlanta, GA: Department of Health and Human Services, 2012), www.cdc.gov

campaigns. The bacterium *Chlamydia trachomatis* infects an estimated 2.86 million people in the United States each year, mostly women.[7] Chlamydia often presents no symptoms and most cases continue to go unreported; thus, people can transmit chlamydia to sexual partners without realizing they have it.[8]

Symptoms and Complications Most people infected with chlamydia display no symptoms. In women who do experience symptoms, early signs (which usually appear within one to three weeks after infection) include abnormal vaginal discharge or a burning sensation while urinating. Later symptoms may include abdominal pain, lower back pain, and bleeding between periods. In men, early symptoms include painful urination and a watery, pus-like discharge from the penis.

In women, an untreated chlamydia infection can spread to the uterus or fallopian tubes, causing **pelvic inflammatory disease (PID)**. PID can permanently damage reproductive organs and cause infertility. A pregnant woman infected with chlamydia has a high risk for miscarriage and stillbirth. She can also pass the bacteria to her newborn. Long-term complications for men are uncommon, though in rare cases can result in sterility.[9]

Treatment Chlamydia is treatable with antibiotics if detected early. Pregnant women and sexually active women 25 or younger—especially those with new or multiple sex partners—should request chlamydia screening at least once per year as part of their regular gynecological exam. The same is true for men who have sex with men, people with HIV infection, and anyone who has receptive anal sex.[10]

Gonorrhea

Gonorrhea is the second most common bacterial STI in the United States (see Figure 14.3). Cases peaked in the

chlamydia The most common bacterial STI in the United States, caused by the bacterium *Chlamydia trachomatis*

pelvic inflammatory disease (PID) An infection of the female reproductive tract that can result from an untreated sexually transmitted infection

gonorrhea The second most common bacterial STI in the United States, caused by the bacterium *Neisseria gonorrhoeae*

mid 1970s and stabilized at the current high levels. The Centers for Disease Control and Prevention (CDC) estimates that 820,000 persons in the United States contract new gonorrheal infections each year—70 percent of them in 15 to 24-year-olds. However, physicians and clinics report fewer than half of these infections to the CDC.[11]

Symptoms and Complications Men usually notice a white, milky discharge from the penis accompanied by painful, burning urination two to nine days after intimate contact with an infected partner. As a result, men are more likely to seek medical attention and receive an early diagnosis (**Figure 14.4**). Only about 20 percent of males with gonorrhea show no symptoms.

Gonorrhea symptoms in women are often mild, absent, or so nonspecific they are mistaken for a bladder or vaginal infection. Initial signs and symptoms in women may include a painful or burning sensation when urinating, increased vaginal discharge, or vaginal bleeding between periods. About 20 percent of infected women experience a yellowish or bloody discharge or a burning sensation during urination.[12] Most women experience no noticeable symptoms aside from an occasional low-grade fever. A woman could thus be unaware she is carrying the disease and risk infecting sexual partners.

The bacterium *Neisseria gonorrhoeae* primarily infects the linings of the urethra, genital tract, pharynx, and rectum, but it may spread to the eyes or other body regions via the hands or body fluids, typically during vaginal, oral, or anal sex. Undetected, untreated gonorrhea can spread to a man's reproductive and urinary organs where it can cause sterility and in some cases induce a painful curvature of the penis during erection. In a woman, untreated gonorrhea can spread to the reproductive organs, causing PID and potential infertility. In rare cases, gonorrhea bacteria can enter the bloodstream and infect the joints, heart valves, or brain. As with chlamydia, gonorrhea can pass from a woman to her newborn and infect its eyes.

Treatment Health experts recommend that people at risk for gonorrhea—for example, sexual partners of people with gonorrhea, sex workers, and people with multiple sex partners—be screened yearly for the disease. Doctors usually prescribe antibiotics for gonorrhea, but the *Neisseria gonorrhoeae* is notorious for developing drug resistance to one type

syphilis A sexually transmitted disease caused by the bacterium *Treponema pallidum*

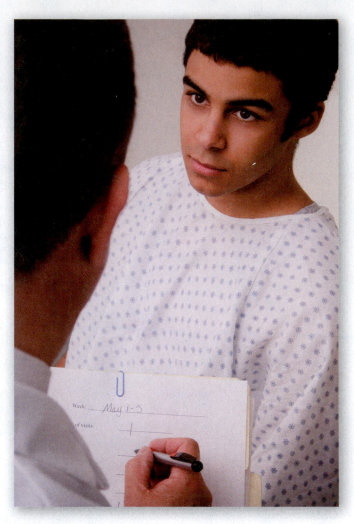

FIGURE **14.4** Bacterial STIs such as chlamydia, gonorrhea, and syphilis can be treated with antibiotics if they are diagnosed early enough, but people with early stage STIs may have no obvious symptoms. However, 80 percent of men with gonorrhea have a burning sensation when urinating and a noticeable discharge from the penis.

of antibiotic after another.[13] The specter of untreatable gonorrhea is all the more reason to use latex condoms and choose partners with care.

Syphilis

Syphilis is caused by the bacterium *Treponema pallidum*. It is generally transmitted via direct contact with a syphilis sore on a partner's sexual organs during intercourse. However, it can also be transmitted via a break in the skin or through deep kissing in which partners exchange body fluids. CDC estimates that about 55,000 people contract new cases of syphilis each year.[14] Most cases (72 percent) are among men who have sex with men. New cases are on the rise (**Figure 14.5**, see the following page),[15] especially among men and women in their teens and 20s, and among young homosexual and bisexual men. African and Hispanic men in these groups experience the highest rates of infection.[16]

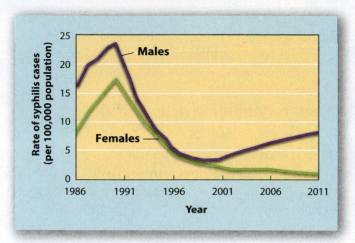

FIGURE **14.5** Cases of syphilis, while less common than either gonorrhea or chlamydia in the United States, have remained steady in recent years.

Source: Data from the Centers for Disease Control and Prevention, *2011 Sexually Transmitted Disease Surveillance Report* (Atlanta, GA: Department of Health and Human Services, 2012), www.cdc.gov

Symptoms and Complications Untreated, syphilis generally progresses through several distinct stages. At the first stage, *primary syphilis*, a **chancre** (pronounced "SHANK-er") may develop. This is a sore most frequently located at the site of initial infection.[17] It usually appears three to four weeks after infection, and although it is painless, the chancre oozes infectious bacteria. Men tend to develop a chancre on the penis or scrotum, but it can also appear in the mouth, throat, or other site of initial infection. In women, the site of infection is often internal, on the vaginal wall or on the cervix, and may go unnoticed. In both men and women, the chancre disappears within three to six weeks, whether or not it is detected and treated.

Symptoms of the second stage, *secondary syphilis*, usually appear one month to a year after the chancre disappears. These include a skin rash and lesions or sores on the mucous membranes of the mouth, throat, or genitals; enlarged lymph nodes; and occasionally hair loss. The sufferer may develop a slight fever or headache. Because symptoms vary so much and appear so much later than the initial sexual contact that caused them, people rarely think to connect them. The underlying infection thus often goes undetected even at the secondary stage.

In the third stage, the *T. pallidum* begins to invade body organs and can cause lesions called "gummas." This stage is called *latent syphilis*. People rarely transmit latent syphilis to others except during pregnancy, when the mother can pass the infection to the fetus, potentially causing death or severe birth defects. If latent syphilis remains unrecognized and untreated for years,

casestudy

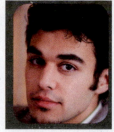

JASON

"After sitting through a lecture about STIs, I started thinking about Sara and me. The summer after high school, we broke up for a while. She went away to Spain, and I spent the summer hanging out at the beach. We got back together when college started, but we never talked much about that summer. Like I said, I completely trust Sara. I think she would tell me if anything had happened in Spain. And she's completely healthy. If she had an infection, I'd know it."

THINK! Can Jason be sure that he and Sara are both free of STIs? If you are sexually active, do you really know everything about your sexual partner(s)? Are you certain?

ACT! Find out the STI status of partners before becoming exposed. Identify all of your own risk behaviors for STIs and come up with a plan to correct them.

HEAR IT! ONLINE

it becomes *late-stage syphilis*. Signs of late-stage syphilis include heart and central nervous system damage, blindness, deafness, paralysis, premature senility, and ultimately dementia.

Treatment If diagnosed early, syphilis can be cured with antibiotics. However, misdiagnosis and lack of access to health care can be obstacles to the successful treatment of syphilis.

What Are the Major Types of Viral STIs?

In the next section, we discuss STIs caused by viruses, including herpes, human papillomavirus (HPV), hepatitis B, and the human immunodeficiency virus (HIV).

Herpes

An estimated 16.2 percent of the American population (or about one out of every six people between ages 14 and 49) is infected with a genital *herpes simplex virus*.[18] There are two types of herpes simplex virus: *herpes*

chancre An open sore most frequently located at the site of an initial syphilis infection

simplex virus 1 (HSV-1) and *herpes simplex virus 2 (HSV-2)*. Women are more likely to have genital HSV-2 (one in five women ages 14 to 49 compared to one in nine men), but men are more likely to transmit the virus to their partners.[19] Racial disparities are also striking in the incidence of herpes: African Americans are three times more likely than Caucasians to contract genital **herpes**.[20] Although HSV-1 is generally associated with "cold sores" around the mouth area and HSV-2 is generally associated with genital herpes sores, both HSV-1 and HSV-2 can infect and cause sores on any area of the body. A person with a cold sore caused by HSV-1, for example, can transmit that virus to a partner's genitals during oral sex.

Symptoms and Complications After the herpes virus has been transmitted but before blisters or sores appear, a tingling or burning sensation and redness at the site of infection may occur. This *prodromal* stage lasts only a day or two and is followed by a second phase in which one or more blisters form, each filled with a clear fluid containing the virus. These crust over, dry up, and disappear within a few days. Whether treated with drugs or not, once a herpes virus becomes established, it remains in the body for life. It typically becomes *dormant*, lurking in nerve roots near the site of infection, until emotional or physical stress triggers the blistering cycle to begin all over again.

Herpes sores can shed highly infectious virus particles even before any blisters show. A person may contract genital herpes through oral or sexual contact with another person who has no awareness of being infected or who shows no outward signs of infection. A pregnant woman can pass genital herpes on to her baby as the baby moves through the birth canal. Genital herpes may also increase the chances of developing cervical cancer.

herpes A condition characterized by sores or eruptions on the skin, caused by *herpes simplex virus 1* (HSV-1) or *herpes simplex virus 2* (HSV-2)

genital warts Small, fleshy growths on the cervix, vagina, vulva, penis, scrotum, or anus; also called *venereal wart* or *condyloma*

human papillomaviruses (HPV) A group of viruses, some of which are linked to cervical cancer, and some of which cause *genital warts*

Treatment There is no cure for herpes. During the prodromal period, taking prescription medications such as acyclovir and over-the-counter medications can lessen the severity of the outbreak. Other drugs, such as famciclovir (FAMVIR), may reduce viral shedding

between outbreaks, lessening the chance that a herpes sufferer will infect a partner. Medical researchers are working to develop herpes vaccines and have had some recent success with preventing HSV-1 in women.[21]

Human Papillomavirus (HPV) and Genital Warts

Genital warts are caused by a small group of viruses known as **human papillomaviruses (HPV)**. An estimated 79 million Americans are infected with HPV, about 14 million more become infected each year, and about 1 percent of sexually active Americans have genital warts.[22] HPV infection occurs during sexual contact, when virus particles penetrate the skin and mucous membranes of the genitals or anus. After six to eight weeks, a person may notice itchy bumps on the cervix, vagina, vulva, penis, scrotum, or anus. However, only some forms of the HPV virus cause "warts"; most people with HPV have no symptoms and have no idea they are infected.

Symptoms and Complications Most HPV infections cause no symptoms at all. Others can cause two types of genital warts, either full-blown warts that are noticeable as tiny bumps or growths, or flat warts that are not usually visible to the naked eye. Either can develop inside the reproductive tract, where they are difficult to see or feel.

The greatest threat from genital warts lies in the apparent correlation between certain HPV strains and cancer. No one is sure how, but HPV infection can lead to cervical cancer; within five years of initial infection, 30 percent of HPV cases in women will lead to precancerous changes in cervical cells. Pap smears and newer kinds of screening can detect these altered cells. Although details are just emerging, oral sex with a partner who carries the HPV virus may also pose a risk for oral HPV infection and cancer of the mouth or throat.[23]

Treatment A vaccine against a common strain of HPV is highly effective at preventing cervical cancer. The vaccine, which is administered via a series of three shots, is recommended for females ages 9 to 26 (**Figure 14.6**, see the following page).[24] Researchers are trying to reduce this dose to two shots to make prevention easier and more affordable.[25] The U.S. Centers for Disease Control and Prevention have approved the current vaccine for use in boys and men to help prevent genital warts as well as viral transmission to females.[26]

Many genital warts eventually disappear on their own, although the virus remains in the body. Physicians can usually treat small genital warts with topical drugs

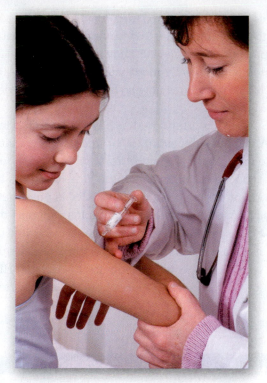

FIGURE **14.6** A vaccine against several common strains of HPV can help prevent cervical cancer.

and can remove large ones by surgical excision or *cryosurgery* (freezing the tissue with liquid nitrogen).

Hepatitis B

Hepatitis B virus (HBV) is one of seven forms of the hepatitis virus that can inflame and damage the liver. Of the 40,000 new cases of hepatitis B in the United States each year most are transmitted via sexual contact.[27] Hepatitis B is also transmitted by the sharing of infected drug needles or from an infected mother to her infant.

Symptoms and Complications Many people infected with hepatitis B have no symptoms.[28] Others may experience jaundice, fatigue, abdominal pain, loss of appetite, nausea, vomiting, and joint pain. Over time, hepatitis B can lead to cirrhosis or liver cancer.

Treatment There is no cure for hepatitis B infection. A preventive vaccine given in three shots over six months is now available; this can protect people from new infections but cannot treat existing ones.[29]

HIV and AIDS

Since 1981, more than 65 million people worldwide have become infected with the **human immunodeficiency virus (HIV)**, the virus that causes **AIDS,** or **acquired immunodeficiency syndrome**.[30] Today, more than 34 million people around the world are living with HIV

or AIDS, and it is a significant global health threat.[31] In 2011 alone, 1.7 million people died of AIDS. Most cases and deaths occur in sub-Saharan Africa. In the United States, about 1.1 million people are currently infected with HIV, and 18.1 percent of them are unaware of their infection.[32] More than 619,400 Americans have died of AIDS since the disease was first identified, with about 18,000 dying each year.[33]

HIV Transmission and Progression

HIV typically enters a person's body when the semen, vaginal secretions, or blood of an infected individual gain entry through a break in the recipient's body surface. Breaks in the mucous membranes of the genital organs and anus—as can occur during sexual intercourse, particularly anal intercourse—provide the easiest route of entry. The virus can also be transmitted through contaminated needles. Some people became infected with HIV through blood transfusions before 1985, when blood donation programs began testing all donated blood products for the virus. An infected mother can pass the virus through the placenta to her unborn baby, and rarely, through breast milk. Antiretroviral drug treatment can prevent this transmission in most cases.

During *primary infection*, HIV multiplication is rapid and the virus invades the bloodstream, destroying immune cells called *CD4 cells*. In response to this invasion, the body produces antibodies. Within one to three months of infection, mild symptoms of illness occur, including night sweats, fatigue, weight loss, skin rashes, mouth ulcers, persistent cold sores, fevers, and fungal infections.

After the primary stage, HIV-infected individuals typically enter an *asymptomatic stage* during which they may look and feel healthy and experience no symptoms of illness. This stage may last for several years. Infected individuals may not know they have the virus and may unknowingly transmit HIV to others.[34]

LIVE IT! ONLINE
**Worksheet 42
Should You Have
the HIV Test?**

hepatitis B virus (HBV) One of seven forms of the hepatitis virus, which infects the liver; hepatitis B is the most common sexually transmitted form

human immunodeficiency virus (HIV) The virus that causes AIDS, transmissible through direct sexual contact or exchange of saliva, semen, vaginal fluid, blood, or other bodily fluids

acquired immunodeficiency syndrome (AIDS) A disease of the immune system caused by human immunodeficiency virus (HIV); characterized by extremely low CD4 counts or susceptibility to opportunistic infections or illnesses

Without treatment, nearly all HIV-positive individuals will progress to full-blown AIDS. HIV-infected individuals are considered to have AIDS when their CD4 levels fall below 200 per cubic millimeter of blood or when they experience illnesses that are considered markers for AIDS, such as the blood cancer *Kaposi's sarcoma* or recurrent opportunistic infections.

With treatment, the asymptomatic phase of HIV can be extended, allowing the person to survive several years with the infection "in check." Throughout all phases, the HIV virus remains transmissible. However, the virus is not highly contagious. Studies of people living in households with an AIDS patient have shown no documented cases of HIV infection due to casual contact. In addition, HIV does not appear to be transmissible by mosquitoes or other insects because the virus cannot replicate inside the insect's body and the bite injects saliva but not blood.[35]

High-Risk Behaviors The following behaviors put you at high risk of contracting HIV:

- *Unprotected sexual intercourse.* The exchange of HIV-infected body fluids (such as blood, semen, or vaginal secretions) during vaginal or anal intercourse is the greatest risk factor. In rare instances, the virus has been found in saliva, but most health officials state that saliva poses a less significant risk than other shared body fluids.

- *Injecting drugs or sharing needles.* An estimated 15 to 25 percent of AIDS cases in the United States result from sharing or using HIV-contaminated needles and syringes.[36] Anyone who shares needles, whether to use illegal drugs or in tattooing and piercing, is at risk.

Although AIDS strikes some minority populations disproportionately, it is not a disease limited to homosexuals or minority groups. People who engage in high-risk behaviors increase their chances of contracting the disease. People who do not engage in these behaviors have minimal risk. **Figure 14.7** illustrates the sources of HIV infection for men and women in the United States.

Drugs and Treatments There is no cure for HIV or AIDS, but drugs can slow the progression from HIV to AIDS and prolong the lives of most HIV patients. The current approach, called antiretroviral treatment (ART), combines several specific types of drugs, especially *protease inhibitors* and *reverse transcriptase inhibitors*. Although no combination has proven to be effective for all patients, annual deaths from AIDS have dropped by two-thirds in the United States based on both treatment and prevention.[37] A recent study reported that in HIV-infected patients with good results on continual ART, the chance of dying is now no higher than in the general population.[38]

Several important studies have shown that taking ART *before* exposure to HIV reduces acquisition of the virus by 73 percent.[39] For infected individuals, ART reduces transmission of the virus to others by 96 percent. Although expensive, ART is potentially life-saving for high-risk groups such as such as men who have sex with men.[40] Experimental vaginal gels and creams that kill microbes and viruses also appear to reduce a woman's chance of acquiring HIV by about 40 percent.[41] Researchers are also working

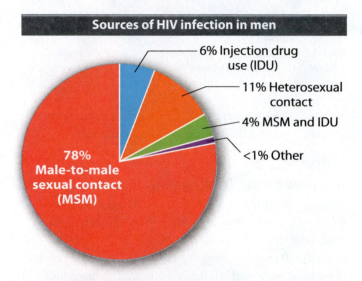

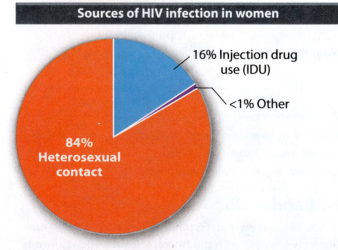

FIGURE **14.7** Sources of HIV infection in men and women with an AIDS diagnosis in the United States.

Source: Data from the Centers for Disease Control and Prevention, *HIV/AIDS Surveillance Report* 17, no. 4 (2012): Table 1, www.cdc.gov

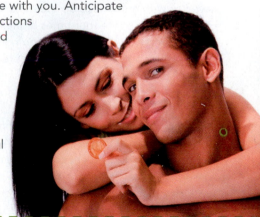

TOOLS FOR CHANGE

Safe Is Sexy

In a world with serious and potentially deadly sexually transmitted infections (STIs), caution is important. Consider this list of protections, always use common sense, and remember this simple phrase: When in doubt, don't!

- Avoid casual sexual partners. Ideally, sex should be limited to long-term, mutually monogamous relationships in which both partners have recently tested negative for HIV and other STIs.

- Avoid unprotected sexual activity that involves the exchange of blood, semen, or vaginal secretions with people at risk for infection. Ask intimate questions about your partner's sexual past, and postpone sexual involvement until you know, through testing, that he or she is not infected.

- If you are not in a lifelong monogamous relationship, practice safer sex by using latex condoms. Always use them properly and remember, condoms can fail. New germicidal products for vaginal insertion are a second line of defense against certain STIs including HIV and hepatitis B and C.

- Never share any instruments through which the exchange of blood could occur, including needles, razors, tattoo instruments, and body-piercing instruments.

- Avoid injury to body tissue during sexual activity.

- Always use a condom or a dental dam during oral sex to prevent the entry of saliva, semen, blood, or vaginal secretions through breaks in mucous membranes.

- Drink responsibly and avoid drug use. Drugs, alcohol, or combinations of the two (e.g., high levels of caffeine plus alcohol or marijuana and alcohol) can cloud your judgment and impair your ability to make responsible decisions about potential sex partners and activities.

- Wash your hands before and after sexual encounters. Urinate after sexual relations and, if possible, wash your genitals.

- Total abstinence is the only absolute means of preventing the sexual transmission of HIV and other STIs. If you are in doubt about a partner's sexual history or infection status, use other means of intimacy such as closed-mouth kissing, hugging, or massages until test results can assure safety.

- Don't risk infecting others: If you are worried about your own status, get tested for STIs.

- Remember that you have a responsibility to your partner to disclose your own status and find out your partner's history and status. Be direct, honest, and determined in talking about sex before you become involved. A person who will not communicate openly and honestly with you may very well fail to take responsibility for his or her actions, as well.

- Decide what you will do if your partner does not agree with you. Anticipate potential objections or excuses, and prepare your responses accordingly. The practice you gain from Lab 14.2 can be very helpful with this.

hard to create a vaccine against the HIV virus, but most of the vaccines tested so far have been largely ineffective.[42]

For now, the only sure way to prevent HIV infection is to avoid the high-risk behaviors described on page 454 and also in the box Safe Is Sexy above. If you are concerned about your risk or the risk of a close friend, arrange a confidential meeting with a health educator or other health professional at your college health center, local public health department, or community STI clinic.

What Are the Other Major Types of STIs?

In addition to bacterial and viral infections, a variety of other parasites and pathogens cause STIs. The box Who Gets STIs? (page 456) goes into more detail about the frequency of all STIs in various populations.

pubic lice Tiny blood-sucking insects that infest human pubic hair; also called "crabs"

DIVeRSiTY
Who Gets STIs?

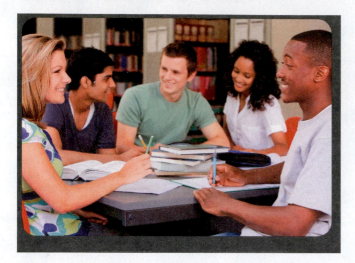

People of both sexes and of all ages, races, and socioeconomic groups contract STIs. Some populations, however, experience higher rates of certain STIs than others.

- **HIV/AIDS.** Three-quarters of the more than 1 million Americans living with HIV or AIDS are male. Men who have sex with men make up the majority of all new HIV infections (a rate four times higher than among females) and about half of all ongoing infections.[1] Individuals who contract HIV through heterosexual contact account for 25 percent of new cases and 28 percent of ongoing infections. Women account for 27 percent of new infections and 25 percent of ongoing ones. Injection drug users make up 8 percent of new infections, 19 percent of ongoing ones. African Americans make up about 12 to 14 percent of the U.S. population but comprise 44 percent of the HIV/AIDS cases.[2] Caucasian Americans account for 31 percent of the cases, Hispanics 21 percent, and all other groups just 2 percent. The incidence of HIV infection among black women is 20 times higher than among white women and nearly 5 times higher than among Hispanic women.[3]

- **Chlamydia.** Women are diagnosed with chlamydia two-and-a-half times more often than men. African American women have rates eight times higher than Caucasian American women; African American men have rates almost 12 times higher than white men.[4] Female Hispanics, Native Americans, and Alaskan natives have rates from three to four times higher than whites.

- **Gonorrhea.** Men and women are diagnosed with gonorrhea about equally, but African Americans accounted for 71 percent of all cases in 2010 and had rates nearly 19 times higher than among Caucasians. Hispanics, Native Americans, and Alaskan natives have rates two to four times higher than Caucasians, while Asian Americans and Pacific Islanders have half as many cases of gonorrhea.[5]

- **Syphilis.** Men are three to ten times more likely than women to be diagnosed with primary or secondary syphilis, depending on race. Rates have been highest in African American and Hispanic males compared to other groups, but have risen rapidly among African American teenaged girls in recent years.[6]

- **Hepatitis B virus.** In the United States, Asian Americans and Pacific Islanders are more likely than other ethnic groups to contract HBV.[7]

Understanding STI Disparities

Public health researchers have identified many factors in an attempt to understand the racial disparities in HIV infection and other STIs.[8] They include poverty, discrimination, and lack of insurance leading to lower quality health care; younger age at the time sexual activity begins; use of illicit drugs; greater numbers of sexual partners; living in communities where STIs are common; higher rates of incarceration leading to a greatly increased risk of STI exposure; and lower rates of circumcision.[9]

Sources:
1. Centers for Disease Control and Prevention, "Estimated HIV Incidence in the United States, 2007 to 2010," *HIV Surveillance Report: Supplemental Report* 17, no. 4 (2012), www.cdc.gov
2. Centers for Disease Control and Prevention, "HIV among African Americans," Updated May 2013, www.cdc.gov
3. Centers for Disease Control and Prevention, "New HIV Infections in the United States," December 2012, www.cdc.gov
4. Centers for Disease Control and Prevention, *2011 Sexually Transmitted Disease Surveillance Report* (Atlanta, GA: Department of Health and Human Services, 2012), www.cdc.gov
5. Ibid.
6. Ibid.
7. Ibid.
8. Ibid; J. Kraut-Becher et al., "Examining Racial Disparities in HIV: Lessons from Sexually Transmitted Infections Research," *Journal of Acquired Immune Deficiency Syndromes* 47, Suppl 1 (2008): S20–7, doi: 10.1097/QAI.0b013e3181605b95.
9. Centers for Disease Control and Prevention, *2011 Sexually Transmitted Disease Surveillance Report*, 2012; A. Tobian et al., "Male Circumcision for the Prevention of HSV-2 and HPV Infections and Syphilis," *New England Journal of Medicine* 360, no. 13 (2009): 1298–309, doi: 10.1056/NEJMoa0802556.

casestudy

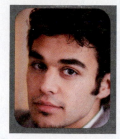

JASON

"The other night, Sara came over and we had a long, awkward conversation. It turns out that there *was* someone else while she was on vacation that summer. She says they slept together only once, and she felt awful about it, but after all, we were broken up. This was more than two years ago, and she says she's only been with me since then. I insisted that we both go to the student health center and get tested for STIs. She thinks I'm crazy—she feels perfectly healthy and says I am being paranoid. But she did agree to go."

THINK! Name three STIs that often show no symptoms in either men or women.

ACT NOW! Today, if you are sexually active, start protecting yourself by learning about the STI screening available on campus. This week, get screened and make sure your partners have been, too. In two weeks, consider if there are changes in your sexual relationships you can make to reduce your potential exposure to STIs, and begin making the changes.

HEAR IT! ONLINE

Pubic Lice

Often called "crabs," **pubic lice** are tiny blood-sucking insects that can be transmitted from partner to partner during sexual contact. Treatment includes using a special soap to kill lice on the body, and washing clothing, furniture, and linens that may harbor lice. Avoid pubic lice by staying away from sexual partners with pubic itching or obvious insect bites and sores in the pubic hair region. Avoid sharing bed sheets, towels, and other linens and clothing. When trying on bathing suits in a store, wear underwear.[43]

Trichomoniasis

Trichomoniasis, or "trich," is caused by a parasitic protozoan that is itself infected by a virus.[44] Symptoms include a foamy, yellowish, unpleasant-smelling discharge accompanied by a burning sensation, itching, and painful urination. There is some evidence that "trich" in males can be associated with later development of prostate cancer.[45] Trichomoniasis is usually transmitted by direct sexual contact, and

can be prevented by using condoms. Trichomoniasis is often treated in both sexual partners with oral metronidazole to avoid the "ping-pong" effect of repeated cross-infection.

trichomoniasis An infection of the genitals caused by a protozoan; also called "trich"

candidiasis A fungal infection often transmitted sexually; also called "yeast infection"

urinary tract infections (UTI) Infections of the urethra or bladder caused by microorganisms; can be sexually transmitted or autoinoculated

Candidiasis

Candidiasis, or a "yeast infection" can occur when the normal chemical balance of the vagina is disturbed, leading to an overgrowth of the fungus *Candida*. Symptoms can include itching, burning and a clumpy white discharge. Over-the-counter creams and suppositories are usually effective in killing the fungi and restoring the normal balance.

Urinary Tract Infections

Some infections of the urethra or bladder can be sexually transmitted when organisms from one partner's genital area or rectum move across and travel up another's urinary tract. Women are more likely than men to contract **urinary tract infections (UTIs)**. Bathing and handwashing with soap and water before sexual intimacy can help prevent some UTIs. Treatment depends on the organism transmitted. It's important to seek treatment for recurrent UTIs.[46]

How Can I Decrease My Risk of STIs?

Twenty million Americans contract an STI each year. To avoid becoming one of them, learn about STIs and how to prevent them, choose a partner wisely, avoid mixing sex with drinking and drugs, and be prepared before challenging situations arise.

Learn about STIs

Reading this chapter is a good step toward educating yourself about STIs. Recognizing the signs and symptoms of STIs can help you identify an infection early on— and prevent transmission to a partner. Evaluate your own beliefs and attitudes toward sexual health by completing Lab 14.1 and viewing the GetFitGraphic on page 459. Part of getting fit and staying well is being aware of your sexual wellness. Consider being screened for STIs, especially if you have any of the risk factors discussed in this chapter. If you choose to be sexually active, know your risk and protect yourself (**Figure 14.8**, see page 458).

Q&A How Reliable Are Condoms?

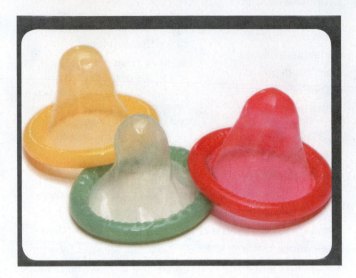

Used consistently and correctly,

condoms provide protection from AIDS and other STIs, as well as prevent pregnancies. But how reliable are they?

Consistent use of latex condoms helps protect against STIs that involve mainly skin-to-skin contact with sores or ulcers (or infected skin that appears normal), including herpes, genital warts (HPV), and skin-to-skin transmission of syphilis. Some skin contact is still possible above and near the condom, however, and these diseases can cause infection in areas not covered by condoms, so the CDC does not consider condoms completely effective in preventing such STIs.[1]

Condoms are better at preventing STIs such as HIV, gonorrhea, chlamydia, and trichomoniasis, which are typically transmitted via semen, vaginal fluid, or other body fluids. The CDC considers condoms "highly effective" at preventing fluid contact, since careful, consistent use can block virtually all fluid exchange. Nevertheless, the CDC

warns that no protective method is 100 percent effective against STIs.[2] In addition, statistics suggest that the best available degrees of protection require a consistency of use that many people can't manage. Explanations for inconsistent condom use include thinking that pregnancy or an STI wasn't a risk at the time, running out of condoms, disliking them, forgetting to use them, getting coerced into unprotected sex by one's partner, not expecting to have sex on that occasion, drinking too much, or being overtaken by passion.

Health experts offer the following warnings about condoms:

- Lambskin and other "real-skin" condoms are not effective in protecting against STIs, as they have pores that can allow the passage of virus-sized particles.
- Storage of latex condoms in warm places (such as wallets and glove compartments) can lead to deterioration and breakage.
- Condoms lubricated with spermicides give no extra protection against STIs, and some studies suggest that nonoxynol-9 spermicides may facilitate the passage of virus particles through microscopic holes in the latex created during manufacture.
- Oil-based lubricants (petroleum jelly, mineral oil, or lotions containing oils) make condoms quickly lose up to 90 percent of their strength and easily tear.
- The time to practice proper condom use is before you get into a sexually charged situation.

The bottom line: Condoms aren't perfect but they can help protect you from a serious—even deadly—STI.

Sources:
1. Centers for Disease Control and Prevention, "Male Latex Condoms and Sexually Transmitted Diseases: Condom Fact Sheet in Brief," Updated March 2013, www.cdc.gov
2. Ibid.

High-risk behaviors	Moderate-risk behaviors	Low-risk behaviors	No-risk behaviors
Unprotected vaginal, anal, and oral sex—any activity that involves direct contact with bodily fluids, such as ejaculate, vaginal secretions, or blood—are high-risk behaviors.	Vaginal, anal, or oral sex with a latex or polyurethane condom and a water-based lubricant used properly and consistently can greatly reduce the risk of STI transmission. Dental dams used during oral sex can also greatly reduce the risk of STI transmission.	Mutual masturbation, if there are no cuts on the hand, penis, or vagina, is very low risk. Rubbing, kissing, and massaging carry low risk, but herpes can be spread by skin-to-skin contact from an infected partner.	Abstinence, phone sex, talking, and fantasy are all no-risk behaviors.

FIGURE **14.8** Sexual behaviors fall on a continuum from high risk to no risk, depending on the level of direct contact with blood, semen, or vaginal secretions.

TESTING FOR **STIs**

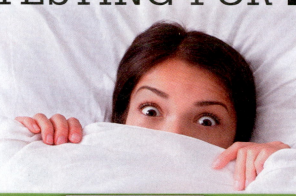

Have you been tested for HIV, chlamydia/gonorrhea, and genital herpes or vaccinated for HPV?

	YES	NO
HIV		
Chlamydia/Gonorrhea		
Genital herpes		
HPV vaccine		

Now see how your answer compares to national college student averages:

College Students Tested[1]	
HIV	33.4%
Chlamydia/Gonorrhea	43.5%
Genital herpes	12.2%
HPV vaccine	45% females

If you haven't been tested for STIs in college, why not?

Check **YES** if this reason sounds like you.

	YES
I don't see myself at risk.	
I've been tested already and I don't need to do it again.	
I'm embarrassed to get tested.	
I don't know how to get tested.	
There are other reasons I haven't been tested.	

Now see how your answers compare to other college students:

College Students Who Say This[2]	
I don't see myself at risk.	68.8%
I've been tested already and I don't need to do it again.	9.3%
I'm embarrassed to get tested.	2.1%
I don't know how to get tested.	2.1%
There are other reasons I haven't been tested.	17.7%

Is unavailability of testing, high costs, or embarrassment holding you back from being tested?

If so, some **STI** and **HIV tests** may be available to you free of charge under the **Affordable Care Act**. Check with your campus health center or insurance provider for availability.

You can test yourself for HIV in the privacy of your home: Oral test kits and home blood test kits for HIV are available over-the-counter; average costs range from **$10** to **$50**. The oral test kit results appear on the test swab. With the home blood kit, you mail a blood sample to a lab for results over the phone.

REMEMBER! Always let your sexual partners know if you test positive for STIs or HIV, and discuss your test results with your health care provider.

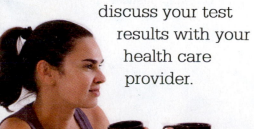

Choose Your Partner Wisely

Choose someone who is willing to engage in low-risk behaviors and is willing to wait for more intimate contact until both partners have been tested for STIs. Keep in mind that a partner with other recent sexual partners or multiple sexual partners represents a high risk. The same is true for a sexually unfaithful partner or a partner with blisters, sores, vaginal or penile discharge, or any other physical signs of an STI, regardless of how recently they may have been tested.[47]

Stay Sober for Sex

Drinking alcohol (and mixing alcohol with the caffeine in energy drinks[48]) is a major factor in high-risk sex. When males are drinking heavily, they are less likely to use a condom, females are less likely to insist on it, and both show poorer judgment in choosing sexual partners and adhering to safe sex practices. As a result, both sexes are more likely to contract STIs, and women are more likely to experience date rape and/or have unintended pregnancies.[49]

Be Prepared

It can be difficult to make good decisions "in the heat of the moment." Complete **Lab 14.3** to develop a plan for preventing STIs. Before you encounter a potentially risky situation, follow these steps:

DO IT! ONLINE

- Make decisions about what you will say and do if, for example, you and your partner want to have sex, but neither of you has a condom.

- Rehearse with a friend what you will say and do before such a situation arises (see **Lab 14.2**).

DO IT! ONLINE

- If your decision involves using condoms or other barriers, learn how to use them properly. Practice using the products by following the instructions on the package *prior* to engaging in sexual activity. Have the supplies when and where you need them. If you have questions, get help from a physician or counselor at the student health service or a community STI clinic. For more information about condom effectiveness, see the box How Reliable Are Condoms? on the page 458.

CHAPTER IN REVIEW

Mastering Health™

Build your knowledge—and wellness!—in the Study Area of MasteringHealth with a variety of study tools.

HEAR IT! ONLINE

audio tools
Audio case study
MP3 chapter review

chapter review
Chapter reading quizzes
Glossary flashcards

REVIEW IT! ONLINE

LIVE IT! ONLINE

programs & behavior change
Take Charge of Your Health! Worksheets:
   Worksheet 41 Myths about Sexually Transmitted Infections
   Worksheet 42 Should You Have the HIV Test?
Behavior Change Log Book and Wellness Journal

labs
Lab 14.1 Assessing Your Attitudes and Beliefs about STIs

Lab 14.2 Effectively Communicating Sexual Information, Boundaries, and Preferences

Lab 14.3 Preventing Sexually Transmitted Infections

DO IT! ONLINE

review questions

1. Each year, the number of Americans who contract an STI is about
   a. 200,000.
   b. 2,000,000.
   c. 20,000,000.
   d. 200,000,000.

2. The number of people aged 15 to 24 who contract an STI is about
   a. 10,000.
   b. 50,000.
   c. 1,000,000.
   d. 10,000,000.

3. Which of the following is a recommended strategy for preventing STIs?
   a. Intermittent abstinence
   b. Occasional condom use
   c. Mutual monogamy with a medically cleared partner
   d. A partner's assurance of infection-free status

4. Chlamydia is a threat to wellness because
   a. it is the most common viral STI.
   b. a small percentage of the afflicted have no symptoms.
   c. there are currently no effective drug treatments.
   d. chlamydia infection can lead to pelvic inflammatory disease.

5. Gonorrhea is a threat to wellness because
   a. about 80 percent of males with gonorrhea show no symptoms.
   b. about 20 percent of females with gonorrhea show no symptoms.

   c. it is the most common STI caused by a protozoan.
   d. untreated gonorrhea can cause scarring and potential sterility in either sex.

6. In what stage of syphilis does a chancre develop?
   a. Primary syphilis
   b. Secondary syphilis
   c. Latent syphilis
   d. Late-stage syphilis

7. Which of these can lead to liver cancer?
   a. Hepatitis B
   b. Syphilis
   c. Chlamydia
   d. HIV antibodies

8. Which of these is a low-risk activity for HIV infection?
   a. Unprotected vaginal intercourse
   b. Unprotected anal intercourse
   c. Sharing needles with another person
   d. Living in the same household as an AIDS patient

9. Chlamydia, gonorrhea, and syphilis are caused by
   a. viruses.
   b. bacteria.
   c. protozoans.
   d. yeast.

10. Herpes, genital warts, hepatitis B, and HIV are all STIs caused by
    a. viruses.
    b. bacteria.
    c. protozoans.
    d. yeast.

critical thinking questions

1. Is chlamydia a more serious health concern for men or for women? Explain your answer.
2. Compare the symptoms of three major bacterial STIs and the long-term problems they can cause.

3. Does a person who has HIV automatically have AIDS? Explain your answer.

references

1. Centers for Disease Control and Prevention (CDC), *Sexually Transmitted Disease Surveillance Report 2011* (Atlanta, GA: U.S. Department of Health and Human Services, 2012.), www.cdc.gov
2. CDC, "Factsheet: Incidence, Prevalence, and Cost of Sexually Transmitted Infections in the United States," February 2013, www.cdc.gov
3. Guttmacher Institute, "In Brief: Fact Sheet—Facts on Sexually Transmitted Infections in the United States," June 2009, www.guttmacher.org
4. CDC, "Factsheet: Incidence, Prevalence, and Cost of Sexually Transmitted Infections in the United States," 2013.
5. American College Health Association, *American College Health Association-National College Health Assessment II: Reference Group Executive Summary Fall 2012* (Hanover, MD: American College Health Association, 2013), www.acha.com
6. E. Wildsmith et al., "Sexually Transmitted Diseases among Young Adults: Prevalence, Perceived Risk, and Risk-Taking Behaviors," *Child Trends Research Brief* #2010-10 (May 2010).
7. CDC, "Chlamydia—CDC Fact Sheet," Updated February 2013, www.cdc.gov
8. Ibid.
9. Ibid.
10. Ibid.
11. CDC, "Gonorrhea—CDC Fact Sheet," Updated February 2013, www.cdc.gov
12. Ibid.
13. G. A. Bolan et al., "The Emerging Threat of Untreatable Gonococcal Infections," *New*

England Journal of Medicine 366, no. 6 (2012): 485–7, doi: 10.1056/NEJMp1112456.

14. CDC, "Syphilis—CDC Fact Sheet," Updated March 2013, www.cdc.gov

15. CDC, *Sexually Transmitted Diseases Surveillance*, 2012.

16. J. R. Su et al., "Primary and Secondary Syphilis among Black and Hispanic Men Who Have Sex with Men: Case Report Data from 27 States," *Annals of Internal Medicine* 155, no. 3 (2011): 145–51.

17. National Institute of Allergy and Infectious Diseases (NIAID), "Syphilis: Symptoms," Updated December 2010, www.niaid.nih.gov

18. CDC, "Genital Herpes—CDC Fact Sheet," Updated February 2013, www.cdc.gov

19. Ibid.

20. CDC, "CDC Analysis of National Herpes Prevalence," Updated April 2010, www.cdc.gov

21. R. B. Belshe et al., "Efficacy Results of a Trial of a Herpes Simplex Vaccine," *New England Journal of Medicine* 366 (2012): 34–43, doi: 10.1056/NEJMoa1103151.

22. CDC, "Genital HPV Infection—CDC Fact Sheet," Updated March 2013, www.cdc.gov

23. M. L. Gillison, "Oral Sex and Risk for Oral HPV Infection and Oropharyngeal Cancer," AAAS 2011 Annual Meeting, Presentation 2872, February 2011, http://aaas.confex.com/aaas/2011/webprogram/Paper2872.html; AAAS symposium, "Oral Sex Is Sex and Can Lead to Cancer," AAAS 2011 Annual Meeting, February 2011.

24. CDC, "Genital HPV Infection—CDC Fact Sheet," 2013.

25. J. Kahn and D. Bernstein, "HPV Vaccination: Too Soon for 2 Doses?" *Journal of the American Medical Association* 309, no. 17 (2013): 1832–4, doi:10.1001/jama.2013.4147.

26. CDC, "FDA Licensure of Quadrivalent Human Papillomavirus Vaccine (HPV4, Gardasil) for Use in Males and Guidance from the Advisory Committee on Immunization Practices (ACIP)," *Morbidity and Mortality Weekly Report* 59, no. 20 (2010): 630–2.

27. CDC, "Hepatitis B: General Information," Publication 21-1073, June 2010, www.cdc.gov

28. CDC, "Hepatitis B FAQs for the Public," Updated June 2009, www.cdc.gov

29. CDC, "Hepatitis B," 2010.

30. UNAIDS, "Global Summary of the AIDS Epidemic, 2012," 2012, www.unaids.org

31. Ibid.

32. CDC, "HIV in the United States at a Glance," July 2012, www.cdc.gov

33. Ibid.

34. Medline Plus, "Acute HIV Infection," Updated March 2013, www.nlm.nih.gov

35. CDC, "HIV Transmission," Updated March 2010, www.cdc.gov

36. CDC, "Cases of HIV Infection and AIDS in the United States and Dependent Areas, 2005," *HIV/AIDS Surveillance Report* 17, Table 17 (updated June 2010).

37. A. S. Fauci and G. K. Folkers, "Toward an AIDS-Free Generation," *Journal of the American Medical Association* 308, no. 5 (2012): 343–4, doi: 10.1001/jama.2012.8142.

38. A. Rodger et al., "Mortality in Well Controlled HIV in the Continuous Antiretroviral Therapy Arms of the SMART and ESPRTIT Trials Compared to the General Population," *AIDS* 27 (2013): 973–9, doi: 10.1097/QAD.0b013e32835cae9c.

39. J. Mermin and K. Fenton, "The Future of HIV Prevention in the United States," *Journal of the American Medical Association* 308, no. 4 (2012): 347–8, doi:10.1001/jama.2012.8693.

40. Ibid.

41. Q. A. Karim et al., "Effectiveness and Safety of Tenofovir Gel, an Antiretroviral Microbicide, for the Prevention of HIV Infection in Women," *Science* 329, no. 5996 (2010): 1168–74, doi: 10.1126/science.1193748.

42. Y. Fukazawa et al., "Lymph Node T Cell Responses Predict the Efficacy of Live Attenuated SIV Vaccines," *Nature Medicine* 18, no. 11 (2012): 1673–81, doi: 10.1038/nm.2934.

43. Medline Plus, "Pubic Lice," Updated April 2013, www.nlm.nih.gov

44. R. N. Fichorova et al., "Endobiont Viruses Sensed by the Human Host—Beyond Conventional Antiparasitic Therapy," *PloS One* 7, no. 11 (2012): e48418, doi: 10.1371/journal.pone.0048418.

45. S. Sutcliffe et al., "Trichomonosis, a Common Curable STI, and Prostate Carcinogenesis—a Proposed Molecular Mechanism," *PLoS Pathogens* 8, no. 8

(2012): e1002801, doi: 10.1371/journal.ppat.1002801.

46. J. M. Torpy, L. A. Schwartz, and R. M. Golub, "Urinary Tract Infection," *Journal of the American Medical Association* 307, no. 17 (2012): 1877, doi:10.1001/jama.2012.3885.

47. T. D. Conley et al., "Unfaithful Individuals Are Less Likely to Practice Safer Sex Than Openly Nonmonogamous Individuals," *The Journal of Sexual Medicine* 9, no. 6 (2012): 1559–65, doi: 10.1111/j.1743-6109.2012.02712.x.

48. K. Miller, "Alcohol Mixed with Energy Drink Use and Sexual Risk-Taking: Casual, Intoxicated, and Unprotected Sex," *Journal of Caffeine Research* (2012), doi: 10.1089/caf.2012.0015.

49. J. Griffin, "Alcohol Use and High-Risk Sexual Behavior among Collegiate Women: A Review of Research on Alcohol Myopia Theory," *Journal of American College Health* 58, no. 6 (2010): 523–32, doi: 10.1080/07448481003621718.

getfitgraphic references

1. E. W. Moore, "Human Immunodeficiency Virus and Chlamydia/Gonorrhea Testing Among Heterosexual College Students: Who Is Getting Tested and Why Do Some Not?," *Journal of American College Health* 61, no. 4 (2013): 196-202, doi: 10.1080/07448481.2013.789880; L. Gilbert, B. A. Levandowski, C. M. Roberts, "Characteristics Associated with Genital Herpes Testing Among Young Adults: Assessing Factors From Two National Data Sets," *Journal of American College Health* 59, no. 3 (2012): 143-50, doi: 10.1080/07448481.2010.497522; L. Lindley et al., "Receipt of the Human Papillomavirus Vaccine Among Female College Students in the United States, 2009," *Journal of American College Health* 61, no. 1 (2013): 18-27, doi: 10.1080/07448481.2012.750607.

2. E. W. Moore, "Human Immunodeficiency Virus and Chlamydia/Gonorrhea Testing Among Heterosexual College Students: Who Is Getting Tested and Why Do Some Not?," 2013.

LAB
14.1

ASSESS YOURSELF
ASSESSING YOUR
ATTITUDES AND
BELIEFS ABOUT STIs

MasteringHealth™

Name: _____ **Date:** _____

Instructor: _____ **Section:** _____

Purpose: To assess whether your attitudes and beliefs may lead you to behaviors that increase your risk of STIs.

Directions: Complete the questionnaire below, indicating whether you believe the statement to be TRUE or FALSE. Score your responses and analyze your score after completing the questionnaire.

STI Attitude and Belief Scale	True	False
1. You can usually tell whether someone is infected with an STI, especially HIV.	☐	☐
2. Chances are that if you haven't caught an STI by now, you probably have a natural immunity and won't get infected in the future.	☐	☐
3. A person who is successfully treated for an STI needn't worry about getting it again.	☐	☐
4. As long as you keep yourself fit and healthy, you needn't worry about STIs.	☐	☐
5. The best way for sexually active people to protect against STIs is to practice safer sex.	☐	☐
6. The only way to catch an STI is to have sex with someone who has one.	☐	☐
7. Talking about STIs with a partner is so embarrassing that it's better not to raise the subject and instead hope the other person will.	☐	☐
8. STIs are mostly a problem for people who have numerous sex partners.	☐	☐
9. You don't need to worry about contracting an STI so long as you wash yourself thoroughly with soap and hot water immediately after sex.	☐	☐
10. You don't need to worry about AIDS if no one you know has ever come down with it.	☐	☐
11. When it comes to STIs, it's all in the cards—either you're lucky or you're not.	☐	☐
12. The time to start worrying about STIs is when you come down with one.	☐	☐
13. As long as you avoid risky sexual practices such as anal intercourse, you're safe from STIs.	☐	☐
14. The time to talk about safer sex is before any sexual contact occurs.	☐	☐
15. A person needn't be concerned about an STI if the symptoms clear up in a few weeks without treatment.	☐	☐

SCORING

All questions are FALSE except numbers 5 and 14, which are TRUE. Give yourself one point for each right answer.

Total correct: _____

A higher correct score indicates a lower risk of contracting an STI. A lower correct score indicates an increased risk. A score of 13 or more means that your attitudes may lower your risk level. However, even one wrong response on this scale can increase your risk of an STI.

LAB 14.2

EFFECTIVELY COMMUNICATING SEXUAL INFORMATION, BOUNDARIES, AND PREFERENCES

MasteringHealth™

Name: _____ Date: _____

Instructor: _____ Section: _____

Purpose: To learn and practice the skills necessary to communicate effectively to a potential sexual partner.

Background: To protect yourself from STIs such as HIV and to honor your own needs and wishes, you must be able to communicate clearly and directly with any potential sexual partner. If you are uncomfortable with anything a partner is proposing, you must be able to say "No," firmly and without hesitation. You must also be able to state what you want and need, whether it is more time to get to know someone, more proof of noninfectious status, a desire for less intimacy at the present, or a different way of being held or touched. *Before* placing yourself in a situation that could escalate beyond your level of safety or comfort, you should practice communicating.

Directions: Choose a trusted, nonsexual friend with whom you can communicate fully and freely. Imagine it is 10 P.M. and you are in a parked car with a potential sexual partner. He or she moves closer to you and puts an arm around your shoulder. In your own words, practice verbalizing the following:

- I don't want intimate contact right now.
- I'm worried about STIs.
- I want to make sure neither of us has an STI before getting intimate, even kissing.
- No matter what, no condom, no sexual activity.
- Hugs are OK, but I don't want to go any further.
- I need to know someone pretty well before getting intimate with them.
- My sexual preference is _____.
- I'm OK with _____ but not _____.
- I like my partner to _____.

Reflection: Were you able to role-play comfortably with your practice partner? How do you think you would you do in a real life situation?

_____

_____

_____

If you had trouble with the role-play, try practicing again or choosing a different friend with whom to practice. When you feel comfortable, try the same exercise with someone who represents a more realistic challenge; for example, if you are heterosexual, try the exercise with someone of the opposite sex but not a potential sexual partner. When you are on a date, try some of your dependable responses (i.e., ones that you can remember and use comfortably even when feeling nervous or stressed). Reassess your ability to answer, and if you need it, return to practicing with a friend.

LAB 14.3

PREVENTING SEXUALLY TRANSMITTED INFECTIONS

MasteringHealth™

Name: _____ **Date:** _____

Instructor: _____ **Section:** _____

Materials: None

Purpose: Develop a plan to prevent getting a sexually transmitted infection.

Directions: Answer the questions below.

1. Do you consider yourself knowledgeable about sexually transmitted infections? Why or why not?

_____

_____

2. Think about three to five behaviors that you can minimize or eliminate in order to reduce your risk of an STI. Write those behaviors here:

_____

_____

_____

3. Think about three to five behaviors that you can add to your lifestyle in order to reduce your risk of an STI. Write those behaviors here:

_____

_____

_____

4. Identify three small action steps that you can take immediately to reduce your risk of an STI:

1. _____

2. _____

3. _____

5. What barriers or obstacles might hinder your STI prevention plan? Indicate your top three obstacles below:

1. _____

2. _____

3. _____

6. Write out three strategies for overcoming your top three obstacles.

1. _____

2. _____

3. _____

7. List resources you will use to get more information or to help you reduce your risk of an STI:

Friend/partner/relative: _____

School-based resource: _____

Community-based resource: _____

Other: _____

Appendix

Answers to End-of-Chapter Questions

Chapter 1
1.b; 2.b; 3.d; 4.a; 5.a; 6.b; 7.b; 8.d; 9.a; 10.d

Chapter 2
1.b; 2.c; 3.d; 4.a; 5.b; 6.d; 7.d; 8.b; 9.d; 10.a

Chapter 3
1.c; 2.a; 3.a; 4.d; 5.c; 6.b; 7.c; 8.a; 9.d; 10.c

Chapter 4
1.d; 2.c; 3.a; 4.d; 5.a; 6.b; 7.c; 8.b; 9.a; 10.c

Chapter 5
1.a; 2.c; 3.b; 4.d; 5.d; 6.b; 7.c; 8.b; 9.c; 10.a

Chapter 6
1.c; 2.d; 3.c; 4.b; 5.b; 6.b; 7.a; 8.c; 9.a; 10.a

Chapter 7
1.d; 2.d; 3.d; 4.c; 5.d; 6.d; 7.d; 8.a; 9.c; 10.d

Chapter 8
1.d; 2.d; 3.b; 4.b; 5.c; 6.a; 7.a; 8.b; 9.a; 10.d

Chapter 9
1.c; 2.b; 3.a; 4.d; 5.d; 6.a; 7.b; 8.d; 9.a; 10.d

Chapter 10
1.d; 2.d; 3.c; 4.a; 5.c; 6.b; 7.d; 8.a; 9.a; 10.b

Chapter 11
1.d; 2.d; 3.d; 4.a; 5.c; 6.d; 7.b; 8.a; 9.d; 10.d

Chapter 12
1.d; 2.c; 3.b; 4.b; 5.a; 6.c; 7.a; 8.b; 9.b; 10.b

Chapter 13
1.a; 2.d; 3.d; 4.d; 5.a; 6.b; 7.b; 8.d; 9.b; 10.b

Chapter 14
1.c; 2.d; 3.c; 4.d; 5.d; 6.a; 7.a; 8.d; 9.b; 10.a

Chapter 15
1.a; 2.d; 3.b; 4.b; 5.c; 6.d; 7.c; 8.c; 9.d; 10.a

Photo Credits

Chapter 1 Chapter Opener: Maridav/Shutterstock; p. 2: Jupiter Images; 1.1: PhotoAlto/Ale Ventura/Jupiter Images; 1.2a: Glow Images, 1.2b: PASIEKA/Science Photo Library/Alamy; 1.2c: Ariel Skelley/Blend Images/Alamy; 1.2d: Alamy; 1.2e: Tetra Images/Alamy; 1.2f: Blend Images/Alamy; 1.3: Alamy; p. 4: Ocean/Corbis; 1.4: Catherine Yeulet/istockphoto; p. 7 (top): holbox/Shutterstock; p. 7 (bottom): arek_malang/Shutterstock; p. 8: Michaeljung/Fotolia; 1.7: Goodshoot/Jupiter Images; p. 10: Masterfile Corporation; p. 12: Wave Royalty Free, Inc./Alamy; p. 14: Radius Images/Alamy; p. 16: manley099/E+/Getty Images; p. 17: Edyta Pawlowska/Shutterstock.

Chapter 2 Chapter Opener: StepStock/Shutterstock; p. 30: Ryan McVay/Photodisc/Getty Images; 2.1 (top): Ken Gillespie Photography/Alamy; 2.1 (middle): Doug Menuez/Photodisc/Getty Images; 2.1 (bottom): Stockbyte/Getty Images; p. 32: Denkou Images Gmbh/AGE Fotostock; p. 35: lculig/Shutterstock; 2.4 (left): Dan Dalton/Digital Vision/Getty Images; 2.4 (center): MIXA/Getty Images; 2.4 (right): Daniel Grill/Alamy; p. 39: FogStock/Thinkstock; p. 41: Lisafx/Dreamstime; p. 42: Bob Daemmrich/Alamy; p. 43: Paul Burns/Blend Images/Jupiter Images; p. 44: Koki Iino/Mixa/Alamy; p. 47 (top): Creativa/Shutterstock; p. 47 (center): Nemlaza/Shutterstock; p. 47 (bottom left): Andrey_Popov/Shutterstock; p. 47 (bottom right): Art4all/Shuttersock and Photastic/Shutterstock; p. 48. Jochen Tack/Alamy; p. 61: Kletr/Shutterstock.

Chapter 3 Chapter Opener: Kenneth Man/Shutterstock; p. 65: JupiterImages/Thinkstock; 3.1: rubberball/Getty Images; 3.2: Radius Images/Jupiter Images; p. 70: Image Source/Alamy; 3.5: Andres Rodriguez/Alamy; 3.6a: Elena Dorfman/Pearson Education/Pearson Science; 3.6b: Elena Dorfman/Pearson Education/Pearson Science; 3.7: Stockbyte/Thinkstock; p. 75: Index Stock Imagery/PhotoLibrary; 3.8a: takayuki/Shutterstock; 3.8b: Lucky Business/Shutterstock; 3.8c: Maridav/Fotolia; 3.8d: La India Piaroa/Shutterstock; 3.8e: Pete Saloutos/Getty Images; p. 79 (top): Rangizzz/Shutterstock; p. 79 (bottom left): serhio/Shutterstock; p. 79 (top right): Africa Studio/Shutterstock; p.79 (bottom right): Leremy/Shutterstock; 3.10: Jack Hollingsworth/Digital Vision/Thinkstock; p. 84: Arman Zhenikeyev/iStockphoto.com; p. 85: Purestock/Alamy; p. 87: Alamy; p. 94. Elena Dorfman/Pearson Education/Pearson Science; p. 102: Flashon Studio/Shutterstock; p. 106: Ljupco Smokovski/Shutterstock; p. 109: Focon/Shutterstock.

Chapter 4 Chapter Opener: Lucky Business/Shutterstock; p. 113: Comstock/Thinkstock; 4.4: Masterfile; p. 119 (top): Leremy/Shutterstock; p. 119 (bottom left): Andresr/Shutterstock; p. 119 (bottom right): Nikiforov Alexander/Shutterstock; 4.5 (left): USDA/ARS/Agricultural Research Service; 4.5 (right): USDA/ARS/Agricultural Research Service; p. 124 (left): Elena Dorfman/Pearson Education/Pearson Science; p. 124 (right): Elena Dorfman/Pearson Education/Pearson Science; p. 126: Masterfile Corporation; p. 133 (left): RubberBall/SuperStock; p. 133 (right): Horst Petzold/Shutterstock; p. 135: Yuri Arcurs/Shutterstock; p.136a: Elena Dorfman/Pearson Education/Pearson Science; p. 136b: Elena Dorfman/Pearson Education/Pearson Science; p. 136c: Elena Dorfman/Pearson Education/Pearson Science; p. 137 (top): Elena Dorfman/Pearson Education/Pearson Science; p. 137 (second): Elena Dorfman/Pearson Education/Pearson Science; p. 137 (third): Rolland Renaud/Pearson Education/Pearson Science; p. 137 (bottom): Elena Dorfman/Pearson Education/Pearson Science; p. 138 (top): Rolland Renaud/Pearson Education/Pearson Science; p. 138 (second): Jac Mat/Pearson Education/Pearson Science; p. 138 (third): Rolland Renaud/Pearson Education/Pearson Science; p. 138 (bottom): Elena Dorfman/Pearson Education/Pearson Science; p. 139 (top): Rolland Renaud/Pearson Education/Pearson Science; p. 139 (second): Elena Dorfman/Pearson Education/Pearson Science; p. 139 (third): Elena Dorfman/Pearson Education/Pearson Science; p. 139 (bottom): Elena Dorfman/Pearson Education/Pearson Science; p. 140 (top): Jac Mat/Pearson Education/Pearson Science; p. 140 (second): Jac Mat/Pearson Education/Pearson Science; p. 140 (third): Elena Dorfman/Pearson Education/Pearson Science; p. 140 (fourth): Rolland Renaud/Pearson Education/Pearson Science; p. 140 (bottom): Elena Dorfman/

Pearson Education/Pearson Science; p. 141 (top): Elena Dorfman/Pearson Education/Pearson Science; p. 141 (second): Creative Digital Visions/Pearson Education/Pearson Science; p. 141 (third): Elena Dorfman/Pearson Education/Pearson Science; p. 141 (bottom): Elena Dorfman/Pearson Education/Pearson Science; p. 142 (top): Elena Dorfman/Pearson Education/Pearson Science; p. 142 (middle): Jac Mat/Pearson Education/Pearson Science; p. 142 (bottom): Elena Dorfman/Pearson Education/Pearson Science; p. 143 (top): Elena Dorfman/Pearson Education/Pearson Science; p. 143 (second): Elena Dorfman/Pearson Education/Pearson Science; p. 143 (third): Elena Dorfman/Pearson Education/Pearson Science; p. 143 (fourth): Elena Dorfman/Pearson Education/Pearson Science; p. 143 (bottom): Elena Dorfman/Pearson Education/Pearson Science; p. 144 (top): Elena Dorfman/Pearson Education/Pearson Science; p. 144 (second): Elena Dorfman/Pearson Education/Pearson Science; p. 144 (third): Elena Dorfman/Pearson Education/Pearson Science; p. 144 (bottom): Elena Dorfman/Pearson Education/Pearson Science; p. 145 (top): Rolland Renaud/Pearson Education/Pearson Science; p. 145 (second): Elena Dorfman/Pearson Education/Pearson Science; p. 145 (third): Elena Dorfman/Pearson Education/Pearson Science; p. 145 (bottom left): Elena Dorfman/Pearson Education/Pearson Science; p. 145 (bottom right): Elena Dorfman/Pearson Education/Pearson Science; p. 146 (top): Elena Dorfman/Pearson Education/Pearson Science; p. 146 (second): Elena Dorfman/Pearson Education/Pearson Science; p. 146 (third): Elena Dorfman/Pearson Education/Pearson Science; p. 146 (bottom left): Creative Digital Visions/Pearson Education/Pearson Science; p. 146 (bottom right): Elena Dorfman/Pearson Education/Pearson Science; p. 147 (top): Elena Dorfman/Pearson Education/Pearson Science; p. 147 (second): Elena Dorfman/Pearson Education/Pearson Science; p. 147 (third): Jac Mat/Pearson Education/Pearson Science; p. 147 (fourth): Elena Dorfman/Pearson Education/Pearson Science; p. 147 (bottom): Elena Dorfman/Pearson Education/Pearson Science; p. 148 (top): Elena Dorfman/Pearson Education/Pearson Science; p. 148 (middle): Elena Dorfman/Pearson Education/Pearson Science; p. 148 (bottom): Elena Dorfman/Pearson Education/Pearson Science; p. 149 (top): Elena Dorfman/Pearson Education/Pearson Science; p. 149 (middle): Elena Dorfman/Pearson Education/Pearson Science; p. 149 (bottom): Elena Dorfman/Pearson Education/Pearson Science; p. 156 (top): Rolland Renaud/Pearson Education/Pearson Science; p. 156 (bottom): Elena Dorfman/Pearson Education/Pearson Science; p. 157: Elena Dorfman/Pearson Education/Pearson Science; p. 164: Warren Goldswain/Shutterstock.

Chapter 5 Chapter Opener: Monika Wisniewska/Shutterstock; p. 169: Plush Studios/Photodisc/Getty Images; p. 171: Dominique Douieb/PhotoAlto/Alamy; p. 172: Tetra Images/Getty Images; 5.2: Elena Dorfman/Pearson Education/Pearson Science; p. 176: Stuart Jenner/Shutterstock; p. 178 (left): Lunamarina/Fotolia; p. 178 (second): Ekaterina Garyuk/Fotolia; p. 178 (third): bradcalkins/Fotolia; p. 178 (right): Hugh Threlfall/Alamy; p. 179: PhotoLibrary/Index Stock Imagery; p. 180: Elena Dorfman/Pearson Education/Pearson Science; p. 183 (top left): sbko/Shutterstock; p. 183 (top right): Neirfy/Shutterstock; p. 183 (bottom left): Flashon Studio/Shutterstock; p. 183 (bottom right): Ljupco Smokovski/Shutterstock; p. 186 (top left): Elena Dorfman/Pearson Education/Pearson Science; p. 186 (top right): Elena Dorfman/Pearson Education/Pearson Science; p. 186 (middle): Jac Mat/PearsonEducation/Pearson Science; p. 186 (bottom): Elena Dorfman/Pearson Education/Pearson Science; p. 187 (top): Elena Dorfman/Pearson Education/Pearson Science; p. 187 (middle): Elena Dorfman/Pearson Education/Pearson Science; p. 187 (bottom left): Elena Dorfman/Pearson Education/Pearson Science; p. 187 (bottom right): Elena Dorfman/Pearson Education/Pearson Science; p. 188 (top): Elena Dorfman/Pearson Education/Pearson Science; p. 188 (middle): Elena Dorfman/Pearson Education/Pearson Science; p. 188 (bottom): Elena Dorfman/Pearson Education/Pearson Science; p. 189 (top left): Elena Dorfman/Pearson Education/Pearson Science; p. 189 (top right): Rolland Renaud/Pearson Education/Pearson Science; p. 189 (middle left): Elena Dorfman/Pearson Education/Pearson Science; p. 189 (middle right): Elena Dorfman/Pearson Education/Pearson Science; p. 189 (bottom): Elena Dorfman/Pearson Education/Pearson Science;

Index